W0106443

CARS 2002

Computer Assisted Radiology and Surgery

Springer-Verlag Berlin Heidelberg GmbH

CARS 2002

Computer Assisted Radiology and Surgery

Proceedings of the 16th International Congress and Exhibition
Paris, June 26–29, 2002

Edited by
H. U. Lemke, M. W. Vannier, K. Inamura, A. G. Farman, K. Doi, and
J. H. C. Reiber

Springer

Professor Heinz U. Lemke, PhD
Technical University Berlin
Computer Graphics and
Computer Assisted Medicine
Secr. FR 3-3
Franklinstrasse 28–29
10587 Berlin, Germany

Professor Kiyonari Inamura, PhD
Osaka University
Faculty of Medicine
School of Allied Health Sciences
Department of Radiological
Technology & Medical Engineering
1-7 Yamadaoka, Suita City
Osaka, 565-0871, Japan

Professor Kunio Doi, PhD
University of Chicago Hospitals
Department of Radiology
Kurt Rossmann Laboratories
5841 S. Maryland Avenue, Mailcode 2026
Chicago, IL 60637, U.S.A.

Professor Michael W. Vannier, MD
The University of Iowa
College of Medicine
Department of Radiology
200 Hawkins Drive
Room 3956 JPP
Iowa City, IA 552242-1077, U.S.A.

Professor Allan G. Farman, PhD, DSc
University of Louisville
School of Dentistry
Department of Diagnosis and
General Dentistry
501 South Preston, Room 222E
Louisville, KY 40292, U.S.A.

Professor Johan H. C. Reiber, PhD
Leiden University Medical Center
Division of Image Processing
Department of Radiology
P. O. Box 9600
Albinusdreef 2
2300 RC Leiden, The Netherlands

This volume of the CARS proceedings is published simultaneously in print and on the web. The web edition contains colour images.

ISBN 978-3-642-62844-3   ISBN 978-3-642-56168-9 (eBook)
DOI 10.1007/978-3-642-56168-9

Library of Congress Cataloging-in-Publication Data

This work is subject to copyright. All rights are reserved, whether the whole or part of the material is concerned, specifically the rights of translation, reprinting, reuse of illustrations, recitation, broadcasting, reproduction on microfilm or in any other way, and storage in data banks. Duplication of this publication or parts thereof is permitted only under the provisions of the German Copyright Law of September 9, 1965, in its current version, and permissions for use must always be obtained from Springer-Verlag or CARS. Violations are liable for prosecution under the German Copyright Law.

http://www.springer.de
http://www.cars-int.de

© Springer-Verlag Berlin Heidelberg 2002 and CARS
Originally published by Springer-Verlag Berlin Heidelberg New York in 2002
Softcover reprint of the hardcover 1st edition 2002

The use of general descriptive names, registered names, trademarks, etc. in this publication does not imply, even in the absence of a specific statement, that such names are exempt from the relevant protective laws and regulations and therefore free for general use.

SPIN 10755372   31/3130 – 5 4 3 2 1 0 –

Honorary President

Kiyonari Inamura, PhD, Osaka University, Faculty of Medicine, Osaka (J)

Congress Organizing Committee

Ulrich Bick, MD
University of Chicago Hospitals (USA)

Kees de Wilde
Philips Medical Systems, Best (NL)

Kunio Doi, PhD
University of Chicago Hospitals (USA)

Allan G. Farman, PhD, DSc
University of Louisville (USA)

Guy Frija, MD
Société Francaise de Radiologie Médicale, Paris (F)

Toyomi Fujino, MD, PhD, FACS
International Med. Information Center, Tokyo (J)

Gary M. Glazer, MD
Stanford Univ. School of Med., Palo Alto, CA (USA)

Kiyonari Inamura, PhD
Osaka University (J)

Takahiro Kozuka, MD
Kaizuka Municipal Hospital, Osaka (J)

J. Thomas Lambrecht, MD, DMD, PhD
University of Basle (CH)

Heinz U. Lemke, PhD
Technical University Berlin (D)

Roberto Passariello, MD
University "La Sapienza", Rome (I)

Pierre Rabischong, MD, PhD
Centre Propara, Montpellier (F)

Johan H.C. Reiber, PhD
Leiden University Medical Center (NL)

Hans G. Ringertz, MD, PhD
Karolinska Hospital, Stockholm (S)

Ramin Shahidi, PhD
Stanford University Medical Center (USA)

Nicola H. Strickland, MD
Hammersmith Hospital, London (UK)

Kintomo Takakura, MD, PhD
Tokyo Women's Medical University (J)

Michael W. Vannier, MD
The University of Iowa (USA)

Industrial Advisory Board

Chairman: Kees de Wilde, Philips Medical Systems, Best (NL)

Heinz-Christoph Blied
Siemens AG, MED, Erlangen (D)

Karel H.P. Cromzigt
IEARC, Den Hague (NL)

Gerhard Kacmaczyk
Image Devices GmbH, Taunusstein (D)

Annelies Kin
Agfa Europe NV, Mechelen (B)

Kenneth A. Marks, MBA
DOME Imag. Syst., Inc., Tiburon, (USA)

Willem Overlaet, PhD
Toshiba Medical Sys., Zoetermeer (NL)

Jürgen Reyinger
GE Medical Systems, Dornstadt (D)

Saeid Mitchell Seyedin
CBYON, Palo Alto, CA (USA)

Kurt R. Smith, DSc
Medtronics, Broomfield, CO (USA)

Chris Varian
Eastman Kodak Company, Hemel (UK)

Stefan Vilsmeier
BrainLAB GmbH, Heimstetten (D)

Program Committee

Andreas Adam, MB, RCP, FRCR
Guy's Hospital, London (UK)

Paul R. Algra, MD, PhD
Medisch Centrum Alkmaar (NL)

David J. Allison, MD
Hammersmith Hospital, London (UK)

Mostafa Analoui, PhD
Indiana University, Indianapolis, IN (USA)

Yutaka Ando, MD
Keio University, Tokyo (J)

Licinio Angelini, MD, FACS
Università "La Sapienza", Rome (I)

Takehide Asano, MD, PhD
Chiba University School of Medicine (J)

Hanna Bachtiar Iskandar, DDS
University of Indonesia, Jakarta (RI)

Frits H. Barneveld Binkhuysen, MD, PhD
Hospital Eemland, Amersfoort (NL)

Elizabeth Beckmann, BSc
Lanmark, Beaconsfield (UK)

Leonard Berliner, MD
Swissray Int., Staten Island, NY (USA)

Silvio Diego Bianchi, MD
Università degli Studi di Torino (I)

Josip S. Bill, MD, DDS
Julius-Maximillians-University, Würzburg (D)

Uldis Bite, MD
Mayo Clinic, Rochester, MN (USA)

Michel Bléry, MD
Hôpital de Bicêtre, Le Kremlin-Bicêtre (F)

Siegfried Bocionek, PhD
Siemens Health Services GmbH, Erlangen (D)

Hugo G. Bogren, MD, PhD
UC Davis Med. Center, Sacramento, CA (USA)

Nicolaas Bom, PhD
Erasmus Universiteit Rotterdam (NL)

Hans G. Bosch, MSc
Leiden University Medical Center (NL)

Carlos A. Bruguera, MD
Inst. de Ensenanza Audiovis., Buenos Aires (RA)

Jean Noel Bruneton, MD
Centre Antoine-Lacassagne, Nice (F)

Richard D. Bucholz, MD, FACS
Saint Louis University (USA)

Gerhard Buess, MD
Nova Med Klinik, München (D)

Jean-Marie Caillé, MD
Groupe Hospitalier Pellegrin, Bordeaux (F)

Davide Caramella, MD
University of Pisa (I)

Ernest V. Carcia, PhD
Emory Univ.., Atlanta, GA (USA)

Robert Cavézian, MD
Cabinet de Radiologie, Paris (F)

Curtis Sau-Kuang Chen, DDS, MSD, PhD
National Taiwan University, Taipei (CHN)

S. James Chen, PhD
University of Colorado, Denver, CO (USA)

Kiyoyuki Chinzei, PhD
Mechanical Engineering Lab. AIST, Ibaraki (J)

John C. Chiu, MD
California Spine Inst., Thousand Oaks (USA)

Hiroaki Chiyokura, PhD
Keio University, Kanagawa (J)

Gary E. Christensen, PhD
University of Iowa (USA)

Philippe Cinquin, MD, PhD
CHU Grenoble, La Tronche (F)

Michel Claudon, MD
Hôpitaux de Brabois, Vandoeuvre (F)

Claus D. Claussen, MD
Eberhard-Karls-Univ. Tübingen (D)

Kevin Cleary, PhD
Georgetown Univ., Washington, DC (USA)

Alan C.F. Colchester, MD, PhD
University of Kent, Canterbury (UK)

Bernard L. Crowe, BA, MPH
Health Inf. Soc. of Australia, Canberra (AUS)

Jack T. Cusma, PhD
Mayo Clinic, Rochester, MN (USA)

Paolo Dario, PhD
Scuola Superiore S. Anna, Pisa (I)

Albert de Roos, MD
Leiden University Medical Center (NL)

Carlo del Favero, MD
Ospedale "Valduce", Como (I)

Anthony M. DiGioia III, MD
Shadyside Hospital, Pittsburgh, PA (USA)

Jouke Dijkstra, PhD
Leiden University Medical Center (NL)

Takeyoshi Dohi, PhD
The University of Tokyo (J)

Huilong Duan, PhD
Zhejiang University Hangzhou (RC)

André J. Duerinckx, MD, PhD
VA North Texas HC System, Dallas, TX (USA)

Masahiro Endo, PhD
National Inst. of Radiological Scie., Chiba (J)

Rolf Ewers, MD, DMD
Allg. Krankenhaus der Stadt Wien (A)

Aly A. Farag, PhD
University of Louisville (USA)

Taeko T. Farman, PhD, DMD, RT
University of Louisville (USA)

Allan G. Farman, PhD, DSc
University of Louisville (USA)

Eckhard Fleck, MD
Deutsches Herzzentrum Berlin (D)

Kevin T. Foley, MD
Image-Guided Surg. Res. Ctr.,Memphis, (USA)

Erik Fosse, MD, PhD
University of Oslo (N)

Bernard Fraysse, MD
Hôpital Purpan, Toulouse (F)

Hiroshi Fujita, PhD
Gifu University (J)

Günther Gell, PhD
Universität Graz - Landeskrankenhaus (A)

Bernard Gibaud
Université de Rennes I (F)

Maryellen L. Giger, PhD
The University of Chicago (USA)

Stephen Golding, FRCR
University of Oxford, Headington (UK)

Dietrich H.W. Grönemeyer, MD
Universität Witten-Herdecke (D)

Chiaki Hamanishi, MD
Kinki University School of Medicine, Osaka (J)

Daijo Hashimoto, MD, PhD
Tokyo Metropolitan Police Hospital (J)

Makoto Hashizume, MD, PhD, FACS
Kyushu University, Fukuoka (J)

Stefan Haßfeld, MD, MDS
Ruprecht-Karls-Universität, Heidelberg (D)

David Hatcher
Univ. of California, San Francisco, CA (USA)

David J. Hawkes, PhD
Guy's, Hospital, London (UK)

J.H.C. Hendriks, MD
University Hospital Nijmegen (NL)

Atsuko Heshiki, MD
Saitama Medical School (J)

Kenneth R. Hoffmann, PhD
University at Buffalo (USA)

Karl-Heinz Höhne, PhD
Universität Hamburg (D)

Steven C. Horii, MD
Univ. of Pennsylvania, Philadelphia, PA (USA)

Alexander Horsch, PhD
University of Munich (D)

Walter Hruby, MD
Sozialmedizinisches Zentrum Ost, Wien (A)

H.K. Huang, DSc, FRCR (Hon.)
Univ. of South. California, Los Angeles, CA (USA)

Junpei Ikezoe, MD
Ehime University (J)

Herwig Imhof, MD
Allgemeines Krankenhaus der Stadt Wien (A)

Hiroshi Iseki, MD, PhD
Tokyo Women's Medical College (J)

Takeo Ishigaki, MD, PhD
Nagoya University (J)

Akira Ito, PhD
Japanese Foundation for Cancer Res., Tokyo (J)

Ian T. Jackson, MD
Inst. f.Craniofacial a.R.Surg., Southfield (USA)

C. Carl Jaffe, MD
Yale Univ. School of Med., New Haven (USA)

Pierre Jannin, PhD
Université de Rennes I (F)

Werner Jaschke, MD
Univ-Klinik für Radiodiagnostik, Innsbruck (A)

Jack Jellins, PhD
Intern. Breast Ultrasound Sch., Sydney (AUS)

Peter Jensch, PhD
OFFIS e.V., Oldenburg (D)

Ferenc A. Jolesz, MD
Harvard Medical School, Boston, MA (USA)

Leo Joskowicz, PhD
The Hebrew University of Jerusalem (IL)

Willi A. Kalender, PhD
Friedrich-Alexander-Universität, Erlangen (D)

Shigenobu Kanda, DDS, PhD
Kyushu University, Fukuoka (J)

Kazuhiro Katada, MD
Fujita Health University, Aichi (J)

Amami Kato, MD, PhD
Osaka University Medical School (J)

Erwin Keeve, PhD
CAESAR, Bonn (D)

Ron Kikinis, MD
Harvard Medical School, Boston, MA (USA)

Reinhard Klette, PhD
University of Auckland (NZ)

Klaus Jochen Klose, MD
Universitäts-Klinikum, Marburg (D)

Goran Knezevic, DDS, PhD
University of Zagreb (HR)

Hidefumi Kobatake, PhD
Tokyo Univ. of Agriculture & Technology (J)

Masahiro Kobayashi, MD
Keio University, Tokyo (J)

Gerhard Koning, MSc
Leiden University Medical Center (NL)

Martti Kormano, MD, PhD
Turku University Central Hospital (FIN)

Uwe G. Kühnapfel, PhD
Forschungszentrum Karlsruhe GmbH (D)

Chikazumi Kuroda, MD
Osaka Medical Center for Cancer (J)

Axel Küttner, MD
Klinik. der Eberhard-Karls-Univ. Tübingen (D)

Frode Laerum, MD, PhD, MHA
University of Oslo (N)

J. Thomas Lambrecht, MD, DMD, PhD
University of Basle (CH)

Alexandra Lansky, MD
Cardiov.r Research Found., New York (USA)

Tore A. Larheim, PhD, DDS
University of Oslo (N)

Stéphane Lavallée, PhD
PRAXIM, La Tronche (F)

Swamy Laxminarayan, PhD
New Jersey Inst.of Techn., Newark, NJ (USA)

Lilian L.Y. Leong, MBBS
Queen Mary Hospital, Hong Kong (RC)

Yves Ligier, PhD
CareON S.A., Grand Saconnex (CH)

Jae Hoon Lim, MD
Sung Kyun Kwan University, Seoul (ROK)

Martin J. Lipton, MD
The University of Chicago Hospitals (USA)

Yu-Qing Liu, MD
FuWai Hosp. & Cardiovascular Inst., Beijing (RC)

Tim C. Lueth, PhD
Campus Virchow-Klinikum, Berlin (D)

Xiu-chen Ma, PhD
Peking Univ. Sch.of Stomatology, Beijing (RC)

Riley H. Lunn, DDS
Chattanooga, TN (USA)

Heber MacMahon, MD
The University of Chicago (USA)

Sumio Makino, PhD
Yokohama-City (J)

Borut Marincek, MD
Universitätsspital Zürich (CH)

Steffen Märkle, PhD
Technical University Berlin (D)

Tom H. Marwick, MD
University of Queensland, Brisbane (AUS)

Herbert K. Matthies, PhD
Hannover Medical School (D)

Hans-Peter Meinzer, PhD
Deutsches Krebsforschungsz., Heidelberg (D)

Andreas Melzer, MD
Mühlheimer Radiologie Inst., Mülheim (D)

Reto A. Meuli, MD
CHUV, Lausanne (CH)

Kazuo Miyasaka, MD
Hokkaido University, Sapporo (J)

Kensaku Mori, PhD
Nagoya University (J)

Seong K. Mun, PhD
Georgetown University, Washington, DC (USA)

Eike Nagel, MD
Deutsches Herzzentrum Berlin (D)

K.S. Nagesh
R.V. Dental College, Bangalore (IND)

Hironobu Nakamura, MD, PhD
Osaka University Medical School (J)

Wolfgang Niederlang, PhD
Krankenhaus Dresden-Friedrichstadt (D)

Robert M. Nishikawa, PhD
The University of Chicago (USA)

Hiromu Nishitani, MD, PhD
The University of Tokushima (J)

Lutz-P. Nolte, PhD
Maurice E. Müller Institute , Bern (CH)

Fridtjof Nüsslin, PhD
Eberhard-Karls-Universität, Tübingen (D)

Takahiro Ochi
Osaka University (J)

Nagaaki Ohyama, PhD
Tokyo Institute of Technology, Yokohama (J)

Silas Olsson, MSc
Telia Research AB, Farsta (S)

Dietrich Onnasch, PhD
University of Kiel (D)

Stelios Orphanoudakis, PhD
Institute of Computer Science, Heraklion (GR)

Michel Osteaux, MD, PhD
Vrije Universiteit Brussels (B)

Helmut Oswald, PhD
T-Systems HCS AG, Bern (CH)

Hiroshi Oyama, MD
Kyoto University Hospital (J)

Paolo Pavone, MD
Università "La Sapienza", Rome (I)

Heinz-Otto Peitgen, PhD
University of Bremen (D)

Prem Pillay, MD
Asian Brain Spine Nerve Ctr., Singapore (SGP)

Gabriel E. Pislaru
Charlotte, NC (USA)

E. James Potchen, MD
Michigan State Univ., East Lansing, MI (USA)

Henri Primo
Siemens Medical Syst., Inc., Iselin, NJ (USA)

Osman M. Ratib, MD, PhD
Univ. of California, Los Angeles, CA (USA)

Hans F. Reinhardt, MD
Bethesda Spital, Basle (CH)

Maximilian Reiser, MD
Klinikum Großhadern, München (D)

Stephen J. Riederer, PhD
Mayo Clinic, Rochester, MN (USA)

Otto Rienhoff, MD
Georg-August-Universität, Göttingen (D)

Rainer K. Rienmüller, MD
Universitätskliniken Graz (A)

Richard A. Robb, PhD
Mayo Foundation, Rochester, MN (USA)

Ichiro Sakuma, PhD
The University of Tokyo (J)

Georges Salamon, MD
NW Univ. Med. School, Chicago, IL (USA)

Richard M. Satava, MD
Yale University, New Haven, CT (USA)

Ronald B. Schilling, PhD
PGI Corporation, Los Altos Hills, CA (USA)

Peter M. Schlag, MD, PhD
Robert-Rössle-Klinik, Berlin (D)

Wolfgang Schlegel, PhD
Deutsches Krebsforschungsz., Heidelberg (D)

Rainer M.M. Seibel, MD
Univ. Witten/Herdecke, Mülheim/Ruhr (D)

Wolfhard Semmler, MD
Deutsches Krebsforschungsz., Heidelberg (D)

Jean Sequeira, PhD
Laboratoire d'Informatique de Marseille (F)

Iekado Shibata, MD, PhD
Toho University, Tokyo (J)

Faina Shtern, MD
Harvard Medical School, Boston, MA (USA)

Robert Sigal, MD, PhD
Institut Gustave-Roussy, Villejuif (F)

Peter Sloot, PhD
University of Amsterdam (NL)

Milan Sonka, PhD
University of Iowa (USA)

Edward V. Staab, MD
National Cancer Inst., Rockville, MD (USA)

Gero Strauss, MD
University of Leipzig (D)

Nobuhiko Sugano, MD
Osaka University Med. School (J)

Predrag Sukovic, MS
University of Michigan, Ann Arbor, MI (USA)

Naoki Suzuki, MD, PhD
Jikei University School of Medicine, Tokyo (J)

Takashi Takahashi, PhD
Kyoto University Hospital (J)

Hiroshi Takeda, MD, PhD
Osaka University Medical School (J)

Shin-ichi Tamura, PhD
Osaka University Medical School (J)

Russell H. Taylor, PhD
Johns Hopkins Univ., Baltimore, MD (USA)

Bart M. ter Haar Romeny, PhD
University Hospital Utrecht (NL)

Andrew E. Todd-Pokropek, PhD
University College of London (UK)

Thomas Tolxdorff, PhD
Freie Universität Berlin (D)

Jun-Ichiro Toriwaki, PhD
Nagoya University (J)

Hikmet Umar, DMD, MSIS, DIC, PhD
Temple University, Philadelphia, PA (USA)

Vlastimil Valek, MD, PhD
University Hospital Brno (CZ)

Rob J. van der Geest, MSc
Leiden University Medical Center (NL)

Ernst E. van der Wall
Leiden University Medical Center (NL)

Rob van Geuns
Philips Medical Systems, Best (NL)

Paul P.F.G.M. van Waes, MD, PhD
University Hospital Utrecht (NL)

Jos Vander Sloten, PhD
Katholieke Universiteit Leuven, Heverlee (B)

Robert H. Vandre, DDS, MS
US Army, Maryland, MD (USA)

Max A. Viergever, PhD
Utrecht University (NL)

Clemens von Birgelen, MD
Universitätsklinikum Essen (D)

Robert F. Wagner, PhD
Food and Drug Admin., Rockville, MD (USA)

Andreas Wahle, PhD
University of Iowa (USA)

Mamoru Wakoh, DDS, PhD
Tokyo Dental College, Chiba (J)

Thomas Wendler, PhD
Philips Research Laboratories, Hamburg (D)

Karl-Jürgen Wolf, MD
Univ.-Klinikum Benjamin Franklin, Berlin (D)

Richard Wootton, PhD, DSc
The Univ. of Queensland, St. Lucia (AUS)

Hirouki Yoshida, PhD
The University of Chicago (USA)

Frans W. Zonneveld, PhD
University Hospital Utrecht (NL)

Past Honorary Presidents

CAR '89	**Heinz Oeser, MD** Berlin (D)
CAR '91	**Auguste Wackenheim, MD** Strasbourg (F)
CAR '93	**J. Oscar M.C. Craig, MD** London (UK)
CAR '95	**Alexander R. Margulis, MD** San Francisco (USA)
CAR '97	**Takahiro Kozuka, MD** Osaka (J)
CAR '98	**Herbert Kaufmann, MD** Berlin (D)
CARS '99	**Raffaella de Dominicis, MD** Florence (I)
CARS 2000	**Pierre Rabischong, MD, PhD** Montpellier (F)
CARS 2001	**Toyomi Fujino, MD, PhD** Tokyo (J)

CARS 2002 in cooperation with

AAOMR	American Academy of Oral and Maxillofacial Radiology
BAR	Bulgarian Association of Radiology
BIR	The British Institute of Radiology
CRS	Czech Radiological Society
CURAC	Deutsche Gesellschaft für Computer- und Roboterassistierte Chirurgie e.V.
DGBMT	Deutsche Gesellschaft für Biomedizinische Technik e.V.
DRG	Deutsche Röntgengesellschaft
ESCR	European Society of Cardiac Radiology
ESEM	European Society for Engineering and Medicine
EuroPACS	European Association for Promotion of Information Exchange on PACS Research
GI	Gesellschaft für Informatik
GMDS	Deutsche Gesellschaft für Medizinische Informatik, Biometrie und Epidemiologie e.V.
Hungarian Society for Computer Assisted Radiology	
IADMFR	The International Association of Dento-Maxillo-Facial Radiology
IEARC	International Exhibitors Association on Radiological Congresses
IEEE	The Institute of Electrical and Electronics Engineers
JCR	Japanese College of Radiology
JRS	Japan Radiological Society
JSOMR	Japanese Society for Oral and Maxillofacial Radiology
NVvR	Nederlandse Vereniging voor Radiologie
ÖRG	Österreichische Röntgengesellschaft
ÖWGTM	Österreichische Wissenschaftliche Gesellschaft für Telemedizin
Polish Section of the Polish-German Radiological Society	
PMSR	Polish Medical Society of Radiology
RCR	The Royal College of Radiologists
EFSUMB	European Federation for Ultrasound in Medicine and Biology
SFR	Société Française de Radiologie Médicale
SGR-SSR	Schweizerische Gesellschaft für Radiologie
SICTECA	Società Italiana di Chirurgia Tecnologica e Computer-Assistita
SIRM	Società Italiana di Radiologia Medica
Chinese Society for Computer Assisted Radiology	
SPIE	The International Society for Optical Engineering
SRS	Slovak Radiological Society
TU	Technische Universität Berlin
WABT	World Academy of Biomedical Technologies

ISCAS - International Society for Computer Aided Surgery

Administrative Council

President:
Kintomo Takakura, MD, PhD
Tokyo Women's Medical University, Tokyo (J)

Past President:
Michael W. Vannier, MD
The University of Iowa (USA)

Vice Presidents:
J. Thomas Lambrecht, MD, DMD, PhD
University of Basle (CH)

Jeffrey L. Marsh, MD
St. Louis Children's Hospital (USA)

General Secretary:
Heinz U. Lemke, PhD
Technical University Berlin (D)

Adjoint Secretary:
Takeyoshi Dohi, PhD
The University of Tokyo (J)

Treasurer :
Toyomi Fujino, MD, PhD
International Med. Information Center, Tokyo (J)

Adjoint Treasurer :
Rolf Ewers, MD, DMD
Allg. Krankenhaus der Stadt Wien (A)

Board Members

Richard D. Bucholz, MD, FACS
Saint Louis University (USA)

Alan C.F. Colchester, MD, PhD
University of Kent, Canterbury (UK)

Daijo Hashimoto, MD, PhD
Tokyo Metropolitan Police Hospital (J)

Richard A. Robb, PhD
Mayo Foundation, Rochester, MN (USA)

Russell H. Taylor, PhD
Johns Hopkins University, Baltimore, MD (USA)

Jun-Ichiro Toriwaki, PhD
Nagoya University (J)

Honorary Board Member:
Pierre Rabischong, MD, PhD
Centre Propara, Montpellier (F)

Preface

Most, if not all, human knowledge is artificially divided into areas or fields by scientific culture and/or social convention. Professional disciplines are therefore man-made frameworks based on shared models, concepts and definitions. This is the ontological basis for communication and action for professionals in medical physics, radiology, surgery or computer science. In general, new knowledge is being squeezed into these existing boundaries or frames of fields of knowledge. Increasingly, however, this fitting process faces difficulties, particularly in rapidly evolving knowledge areas, such as information technology induced activities - to which CAR (Computer Assisted Radiology) and CAS (Computer Assisted Surgery) belong. Rather than allowing a simple fit into the traditional fields of mathematics, physics, engineering, informatics, medicine or management sciences, these new areas occupy knowledge subsets of two or more of these traditional disciplines. They may therefore be termed interdisciplinary. An example of such evolving interdisciplines is given in Figure 1.

Figure 1 shows the distribution of research and development activities in a number of new interdisciplinary fields or themes as demonstrated by the topics covered by the paper and poster abstract submissions to CARS 2002.

These CARS themes contribute towards the extension and/or fading of the boundaries of traditional disciplines, in particular Medical Physics, Informatics, and Medicine.

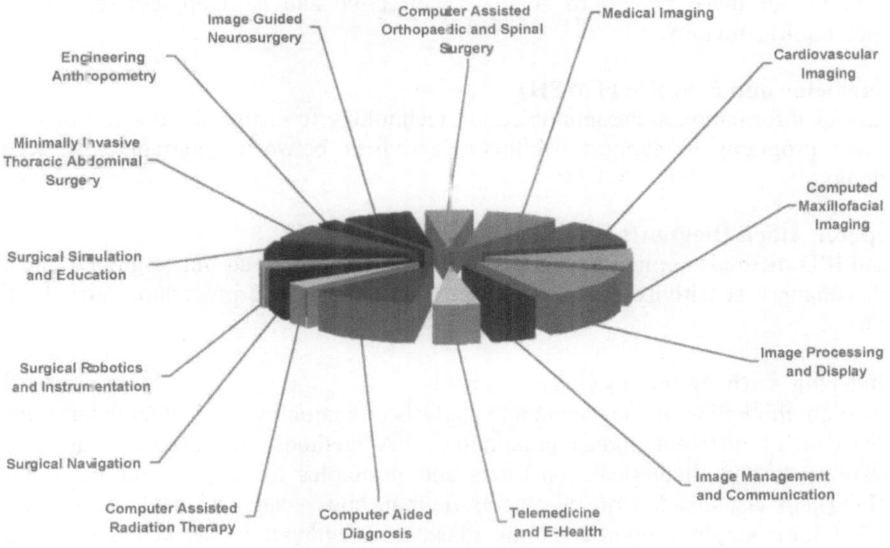

Fig. 1 Interdisciplinary themes of paper and poster abstract submissions for CARS 2002

The following brief definitions of the most important interdisciplines may serve as a guideline regarding the structure on which the CARS 2002 program has been compiled:

Medical Imaging (MI)
The science and engineering needed for the sourcing, acquisition, and processing of signals from the human body to generate multi-dimensional digital images.

Cardiovascular Imaging (CVI)
MI applied to the special requirements of the cardiovascular system and extended with IPD methods to allow quantitatively and qualitatively enhanced medical diagnosis.

Computed Maxillofacial Imaging (CMI)
MI applied to the special requirements of maxillofacial structures and extended with IPD methods to allow quantitatively and qualitatively enhanced medical diagnosis in this area.

Image Processing and Display (IPD)
Processing of elements/objects of images, e.g. pixels, voxels, regions and contours to enhance the quality, understanding, and representation of images. Image processing steps may include enhancement, restoration, registration, segmentation, analysis, interpretation, and multi-modality image fusion. Display steps may include various visualisation algorithms to represent data interrelationships or to enhance reality.

Image Management and Communication/PACS
Systems for storage, transmission, manipulation and display of digital images and the management of these images to enable an effective and hardcopyless (e.g. filmless) healthcare infrastructure.

Telemedicine and E-health (TMEH)
The use of information and communication technology to enable the transfer of medical data and programs to support healthcare activities between geographically separate locations.

Computer Aided Diagnosis (CAD)
MI and IPD methods applied to specific body parts to enable an image-guided diagnosis which enhances sensitivity and/or specificity of a diagnostic procedure carried out by humans.

Engineering Anthropometry (EA)
Acquisition, modelling, management and analysis of anatomic/physical landmarks and 3D surface data of different human populations. EA methods are based on data models, software tools and theoretical constructs and principles to support, for example, the searching and visualisation of 3D objects (human body scans). In healthcare, EA tools may also, for example, support anatomic atlas-based segmentation as well as the design of endoprosthetic devices and implants.

Surgical Navigation (SN)
IT-based systems to assist surgical procedures by guiding instruments within a surgical target volume to an operated volume with maximum accuracy and safety.

Surgical Robotics and Instrumentation (SRI)
IT and MEMS-based systems which use SN or SS to passively assist surgical activities semi-automatically or fully automatically.

Surgical Simulation (SS) and Education
IPD methods and simulation software applied to an surgical target volume to optimize surgical activities for the purpose of training and preoperative planning.

Image Guided Neurosurgery (IGNS)
The use of one or more methods derived from SN, SS or SRI, with a strong bias towards using images, to achieve minimally invasive interventions directed towards surgical target structures including the brain or spinal cord.

Computer Assisted Orthopaedic and Spinal Surgery (CAOS)
The use of one or more methods derived from SN, SS or SRI to achieve minimally invasive interventions directed towards surgical target volume including orthopaedic structures, such as the spinal vertebrae, hip, knee, ankle, or long bones. In a wider definition it may also include rapid prototyping and the design and manufacturing of endoprosthetic devices and implants.

Minimally Invasive Thoracic Abdominal Surgery (MITAS)
The use of one or more methods derived from SN, SS or SRI to achieve minimally invasive interventions directed towards surgical target volume within the thorax (excluding the cardiovascular structures) and the abdomen.

Computer Assisted Radiation Therapy (CART)
Modelling of radiation target structures with IPD methods and the application of radiation dose planning programs to optimize target volume (tumor) radiation treatment.

The subset of knowledge from the traditional fields of mathematics, physics, engineering, informatics, medicine, and management science required to advance the CARS interdisciplines given above is also subject of change. A proper understanding of this may illuminate which traditional profession comes closest to pursuing the respective activities within the CARS themes.

Results derived from CARS methods and applications provide valuable data, information, knowledge and even wisdom, and are changing medicine and associated professions. The impact this will have on current educational curricula as well as on changing the professional profiles of medical physicists, radiologists, surgeons, and computer scientists is substantial and requires further examination. As yet, few teaching institutions have responded to this challenge and are ready to offer appropriate educational courses and training. CARS 2002 and future CARS congresses are aimed at showing the direction into which a significant part of medicine will evolve in research, development and practice.

Heinz U. Lemke
Paris, June 2002

Acknowledgements

Once upon a time, back in the 1960s, when I first had to program a computer it was done in an assembler language. The good thing about this was that this language or interface to the computer, had a finite set of instructions and a finite set of combining these. The bad things were the lack of computational power of the workstation and the user interface to the assembler. On execution, however, the computer did more or less what one wanted it to do. Now, in 2002, times have changed. The good thing now is, that some twelve levels of hardware and software sophistication separate the assembler from the modern "easy to use" graphical user interfaces. Super computational power takes care of everything. The bad thing is, that the computer does not always do what one wants it to do.

Anyone who does not believe this, I should like to invite to do the electronic editing of the next CARS proceedings. The non-believers probably belong to the approx. 5% of authors who submitted their papers according to the author instruction for electronic submission for the CARS proceedings. These authors focused not only on providing excellent content but also on the structure and visual appearance of their papers. The other 95% obviously preferred to focus on content only and have worked, as I like to do, that is, leaving styling and layout of the paper to others.

The move into the electronic age was necessary in order to improve the quality and ensure the timely appearance of the CARS proceedings as a hardbound copy and also on the web. It has meant, however, a considerable amount of extra workload for Franziska Schweikert and her team, in particular Dagmar Harrison, in addition to the "usual" organizational and management work. During a two week period before and at the deadline of paper submission (i.e. 15th March, 2002) approx. 170 papers and 110 posters were received at the CARS Conference Office and electronically prepared and edited. The four weeks in March meant double-shift work for Franziska Schweikert and this is my written promise that next for year's CARS, we will engage additional assistance.

I also should like to acknowledge and thank for the continuing help received from the personnel of my department at the Technical University of Berlin, in particular from Helga Kallan, Steffen Märkle, Kai Köchy and René Tschirley. This is carried out in an environment marked by an increasing number of students in courses and for supervision, against a background of further cuts in teaching staff positions.

We are all delighted to have Prof. Kiyonari Inamura as the Honorary President of CARS 2002. I have known Kiyo Inamura for more than 10 years and had the pleasure to work closely together with him on a number of projects and many congress events. His contributions to research and development in many fields relating to CARS are documented in numerous publications. In particular, I treasure him for his engagement in advancing interdisciplinary and international cooperation. Through his remarkable selflessness, he is a great benefit not only for Japan but also for the rest of the world.

Heinz U. Lemke
Paris, June 2002

Prelude

CARS, Quo Vadis?

It is generally known that CARS involves a very wide spectrum of topics based on medicine, physics, computer science and even sociology. Since the first CAR Conference in 1985 up to the 16th CARS in 2002, there have been more than 60 topics. The terminology of these topics mainly came from the title of the sessions. However, I found that these topics could be grouped into 6 main categories, A to F, as shown below:

A. Modalities and their related topics
   1 MRI, 2. CT, 3. Nuclear medicine, 4. Ultrasound, 5. Digital radiography involving a flat panel detector, 6. Angiography involving DSA, 7. Mathematical modeling for reconstruction etc., Multi-modality imaging and Medical imaging

B. Application of modalities
   8. Radiation therapy and minimal invasive therapy, 9. Computer assisted radiology, Radiology diagnosis and Cardiology, Pediatric radiology, Neurology, IVR, Dosimetry in diagnosis and Computer assisted stereotaxy

C. Image processing, communication, display, interaction and related systems
   10. PACS, RIS, HIS, Electronic med. record, Workflow, Standards such as DICOM, IHE (Integrating Healthcare Enterprise), 11. Telemedicine, 12. Image processing & display, Human-computer interaction and Virtual reality, 13. Workstation and Voice recognition applic., 14. Computer vision, 15. Computer graphics

D. Surgery, orthopaedics, maxillofacial and other related invasive topics
   16. Surgery, Anthropometry, Surgical simulator, Surgical navigation, Neurosurgery, Spinal surgery, Thoracic and abdominal surgery, Standards in information-guided therapy, Surgical robotics, Optical diagnosis & in-situ tissue analysis, Ergonomics & motion analysis, Curved and steerable instr. and Endoluminal, 17. Orthopaedics, 18. Maxillofacial and Implantology, 19. Virtual endoscopy, 20. Cardio-vascular, Coronary and Medical innovation and technology

E. 21. Computer Aided Diagnosis

F. Surrounding and supporting infrastructure
   22. Healthcare infrastructure, Interface between medicine and computer sciences, 23. Technology assessment and/or social implications, 24. Education, Knowledge based systems, Expert systems, Learning systems and Training systems, 25. Planning in the radiology department, 26. Strategic thinking, Decision making and Biointelligence

The chronological change in the number of presentations is shown in Table 1. The bracketed number indicates a double counted number. Example: (5) means that 5 presentations are double counted somewhere else in the same year. 16. Surgery in 2001 has 161 presentations and 72, the latter are broken down into I -VI. Also 16. Surgery in 2002 has 46 presentations and 56, the latter are composed of VII - XII. The features of CARS compared with those of other international conferences would be as follows:

1. Interdisciplinarity
   SPIE, SCAR, ICR and ECR cannot complete or bridge areas as CARS does in the categories shown in D and F in Table 1. Even RSNA is not as comprehensive as CARS.
2. Flexibility and elasticity
   CARS is sufficiently flexible to accept hot topics, new ideas, new concepts and different point of views. As shown in Table 1, sessions have been organized according to problem-oriented thinking. Session names have been revised rather frequently each year compared with other international conferences, because participants in CARS want different but the most appropriate solutions to chronologically changing problems. For example, the topics of "Computer vision" and "Computer graphics" which emerged in 1985 were revised to "Workstation" from 1991 and to "Image processing and display" from 1995, as shown in topics numbers 14, 15, 13 and 12 in Table 1.
3. Extension, penetration, but never fading out
   Depth and originality are respected, but they have often been driven by extension and penetration into other areas such as "medical innovation and technology".

I would like to point out the significance and importance of joint conferences. It was ten years ago, during his stay at Osaka Univ. as a visiting professor in 1992, that Prof. Heinz U. Lemke encouraged me to consider the extension of CAR topics, even outside conventional radiology. His idea was realized in 1995 when CAR collaborated with EuroPACS, ISPRAD, Telerad., The 2nd Congress of the Int. Society for Computer Aided Surgery-ISCAS 95, Computed Maxillofacial Imaging-CMI, and Image Guided Therapy.

In 1997, CAR, in collaboration with the 1st Annual Conference of the International Society for Computer Aided Surgery, was held in Berlin. However, the first CAR outside Europe was in Japan in 1998, and that was the beginning of a new era for CARS which had collaborated with more than 3 international formal annual conferences. Nowadays, for example in 2001, 6 international conferences joined with CARS and most enjoy exchanging common intellectual property. Efficacy, effectiveness and efficiency of knowledge communication as well as "aufheben" of new concepts and/or new ideas are the obvious advantages of joint international conferences. Especially young scientists, who accumulate a wealth of knowledge, will be stimulated intensively each June during 4 days in the last week.

I am sure that, in future, CARS will increasingly contribute to the education and training of young scientists, even though the development of new technologies and highly advanced medicine itself are the targets of CARS. In the field of radiology, the RSNA has its own education system with an educational fund, awards and credits etc, however, they have no consistent training. The disciplines and interdisciplines in CARS must be gradually focus and order to establish a training methodology to acquire and disseminate joint intellectual property among young scientists.

Kiyonari Inamura, PhD, Osaka University, Japan
Honorary President, CARS 2002

Table 1. Chronological change in the number of presentations for each topic in CAR and CARS

Cat	Topics Year→	'85	''87	'89	'91	'93	'95	'96	'97	'98	'99	'00	'01	'02
A	1. MRI	12	14	12	14	6	10	16	13	10	9	16	21(5)	19
	2. CT	4	6	8	20	4	5	4	8	21	17	4	8	(19)
	3. Nuclear Medicine	9	6		2	4		5	1	8	2			
	4. UltraSound		5	4	8	2		6	4	4	4	2	34(13)	
	5. Digital Radiography	16	9	14	20	12	8	12	12	16	11	13	5	
	6. Angiography	5	6	5	6	11		5	8	1	12			
	7. Modeling	3	4		5									
B	8. Radiation Therapy	9	7	6	10	9	6	8	12	16	7	11	9	8
	9. Radiology & Diagnosis	10	12	19	17	17						1		
C	10. PACS, RIS, HIS, EMR	10	16	30	38	44	33	33	54	41	51	36	45	17
	11. Telemedicine	1			9	11	22	35	22	14	9	12	11	8
	12. Image Processing & Display	4	5	3	7	7	36	31	28	33	26	51	48	45
	13. Workstation				15	11	9	7	8	2	10	2	1	1
	14. Computer Vision	12	18	14	21	11								
	15. Computer Graphics	14	13	7		7			3			1		
D	16. Surgery	3	1	3	8	8	30	60	82	65	76	78	161 72(I-VI)	46 56(VII-XII)
	17. Orthopedics	4	10	8	6			19	7	15	31	16	16	10
	18. Maxillofacial						28	36		40	35	39	27	27
	19. Virtual Endoscopy							4		9	13	9	2	
	20. Cardiovascular			7	3								36	40
E	21. CAD	1					9	11	11	17	17	45	32	47
F	22. Healthcare Infrastructure								9				5	
	23. Technology Assessment		6	7	7	9		3	4	4		(7)		
	24. Education					2	10	7	15	7	7	12	15(4)	4
	25 .Planning in Radiology Dept.						17			5	7			
	26. Strategic Thinking									1	1	2	9	
Total		117	138	147	216	175	223	302	298	333	346	350	535	328

I Optical diagn.&in-situ tissue anal. 6 II Erg..&motion anal., curv. steer. instr. 10 III MedCapital 12 IV SMITIMAGE 13 V SMITEndol. 19 VI SMIT Poster 12 VII Anthropometry 9 VIII Surgical Simulator 11 IX Surgical Navigation 7 X Neurosurgery 13 XI Spine Surgery 6 XII Thoracic Abdominal Surgery 10

Contents

6th Annual Conference of the International Society for Computer Aided Surgery - ISCAS

Surgical Simulation

Image Guided Neurosurgery

Robotics and Telesurgery

Surgical Robotics and Instrumentation

Minimally Invasive Spine Surgery

Computer Assisted Orthopaedic Surgery

16th International Congress and Exhibition on Computer Assisted Radiology - CAR

Medical Imaging

Computer Assisted Radiation Therapy

Towards a World Engineering Anthropometry Resource

Telemedicine

Special Session on Electronic Health Record

4th International Workshop on Computer-Aided Diagnosis - CAD

Special Session on Breast CAD

Special Session on 3D CAD

2002 International Symposium on Cardiovascular Imaging - CVI

Invasive Coronary Imaging

Invasive Coronary and Vascular Imaging

Left and Right Ventricular Function

8th Computed Maxillofacial Imaging Congress - CMI

Image-Guidance in Implantology

Image-Guided Cranio-Maxillofacial Surgery

6th Annual Conference of the International Society for Computer Aided Surgery - ISCAS

6th Annual Conference of the International Society for Computer Aided Surgery - ISCAS
President: **Kintomo Takakura, MD, PhD (J)**

Surgical Simulation

©CARS/Springer. All rights reserved.

Towards patient specific, anatomy based simulation of facial mimics for surgical nerve rehabilitation

Stefan Zachow, Evgeny Gladilin, Hans-Christian Hege, Peter Deuflhard
Zuse-Institute Berlin (ZIB), Takustr. 7, 14195 Berlin, Germany
E-mail: (zachow, gladilin, hege, deuflhard)@zib.de
URL: http://www.zib.de/visual/projects/cas

Abstract

Nerve rehabilitation in cases of facial paralysis is an important issue in plastic and reconstructive surgery. However, surgeons need to know which muscles of the mimic musculature are most suited for reinnervation to achieve an optimal rehabilitation of a patient's physiognomy. We present results of our work on the simulation of anatomy based, muscle driven facial mimics on basis of an elaborate volumetric facial tissue model and a physics based tissue modelling approach, that could meet the demands for such a surgery planning task.

Keywords: Facial paralysis, muscular modelling, nerve rehabilitation

1. Introduction

In cases of facial paralysis surgeons are often confronted with the problem of the rehabilitation of specific facial nerves, for the reactivation of certain parts of the facial musculature. From the patient's point of view, facial paralysis often leads to a disability of non-verbal interpersonal communication, i.e. changes in facial expression that reveal the innermost feelings. Restoring function and expression to the highest possible degree, is a difficult task for a plastic and reconstructive surgeon. Thus, predicting the influence of certain muscles on different facial expressions for *individual patients* is the envisioned goal of our project. Although the simulation of facial expressions is not a new topic in computer graphics and animation, we found only a few groups doing research in anatomy based muscular modelling for medical applications [1,2]. Most of the work comes from the field of biomechanics or trauma research. The simulation of muscle based facial expressions for *surgical nerve rehabilitation* to our opinion seems to be rather neglected.

2. Material and methods

This work extends our first results on the simulation of patient specific post-operative mimics, that have been presented in [3-5]. The prediction of a patient's post-operative facial appearance after cranio-maxillofacial surgery, under consideration of some basic facial expressions became an appealing issue for plastic and reconstructive surgeons (figure 1a-c). Thus, we decided to build an elaborate anatomy based model of the entire mimic musculature from an MRI data set of a volunteer's head, that will teach us how combinations of different muscles result in certain facial expressions (figure 1d). Our goal

©CARS/Springer. All rights reserved.

is to determine the contributions of different muscles to a set of basic facial expressions, and to provide a modelling approach for a patient specific simulation of facial mimics.

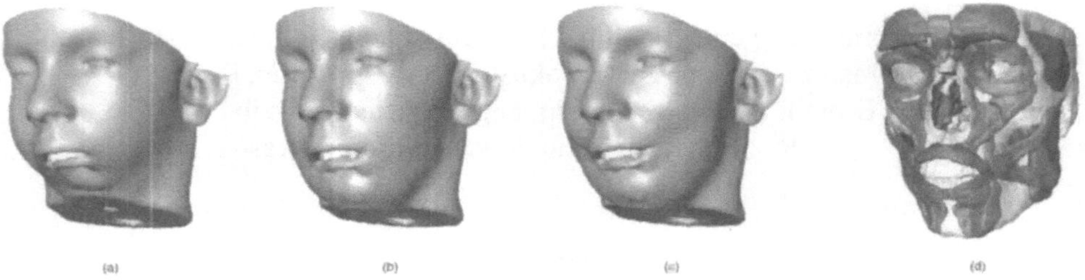

Fig. 1. a–c) simulation of a post-operative facial expression due to the contraction of the zygomaticus major, d) 3D model of the entire mimic musculature

A 3D model of the mimic musculature has been generated from an MRI data set of a volunteer's head. The data have been acquired with a Siemens Magnetom Symphony, 1.5 Tesla MR Scanner, in a T1 weighted spin echo sequence. The exported tomographic slices have a 2mm interslice distance. This dataset has been segmented into a 3D skull model, as well as a 3D model of the facial tissue, with 32 different facial muscles explicitly discriminated. Afterwards, the segmented data set has been supersampled to near cubic voxels, leading to a 512×512×428 data cube. A high resolution surface model as well as an adaptively simplified volumetric tetrahedral grid of the entire facial tissue finally have been generated from the segmented data [6]. Muscle fiber orientations are derived from the muscles' geometry by spline interpolation on medial axis points between origin and insertion area. For sphincter muscles, i.e. the orbicularis oris and the orbicularis oculii, radial fiber directions have been defined manually. The muscle contraction directions, derived from the muscle fibers, are provided as a 3D vector field, that has been assigned to the nodes of the tetrahedral grid. Finally the contraction of each muscle and its impact on the entire facial tissue can be simulated via a finite element approach on the basis of a biomechanical tissue model, as it has been presented by our group for soft tissue prediction in cranio-maxillofacial surgery [7].

3. Results

A template tetrahedral grid with approx. 1.7 million elements as well as appropriate boundary conditions have been generated from an MRI data set. Relevant muscles of the mimic and masticatory musculature have been identified and appropriate vector fields for muscle fiber directions were generated. So far, only three muscles have been contracted along their fiber directions (i.e. zygomaticus major, risorius and orbicularis oris). Furthermore, jaw movements have been simulated. The resulting deformation fields for the entire soft tissue can then be applied to the initial grid, and arbitrary combinations can be assessed by superposition (cf. figure 2). Thus, facial expressions can be simulated and the influence of different muscles to a certain facial expression can be evaluated.

©CARS/Springer. All rights reserved.

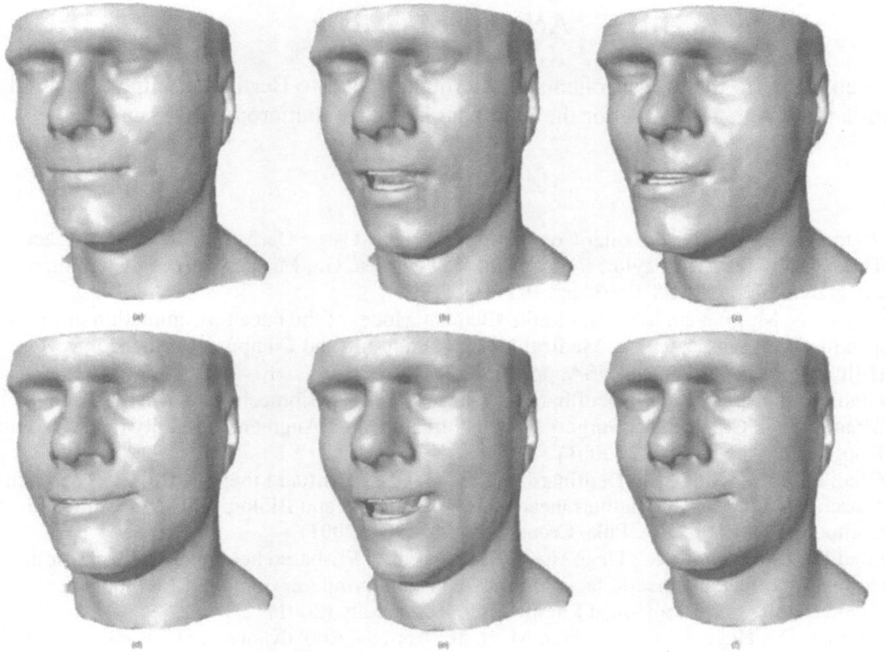

Fig. 2. a) relaxed face as initial situation, b,c) jaw movements, d) contraction of the risorius muscle, e) contraction of the zygomaticus major with open mouth, f) compression of the lips by contraction of the orbicularis oris

4. Conclusions and future work

Our approach of physics and anatomy based simulation of facial expressions seems to be an extraordinary basis for any kind of facial animation. For surgical nerve rehabilitation it is of utmost importance to know the impact of single muscles to the entire facial appearance, since only a few muscles can be reactivated. The correct choice depends on the position and size of individual muscles as well as the thickness of surrounding tissues. A pre-operative simulation of individual muscle contractions as well as combinations out of a few muscles will help a surgeon to find appropriate positions for reinnervation.

We have shown, that the simulation of muscle contractions on basis of an anatomical 3D model leads to realistic facial expressions. The muscle model is supposed to serve as a template for patient specific simulations, where only origin and insertion areas of the muscles have to be identified manually. Thus, a surgeon is even able to plan the procedure of a surgical modification of muscle origin or insertion points. The template model including the deformation fields can then be elastically transformed to meet a patient's anatomical situation. A finite element model of a patient's facial tissue including the warped deformation fields might enable us to simulate patient specific, muscle based mimics in a very simple manner.

©CARS/Springer. All rights reserved.

Acknowledgements

We would like to thank Dr. Johanna Gellermann (Charité Berlin – Campus Buch, Hyperthermia therapy & research) for the kind acquisition of numerous MR scans.

References

1. Waters, K: Synthetic Muscular Contraction on Facial Tissue Derived from Computerized Tomography Data. In Taylor, R ; Lavallée, S. : Burdea, G. ; Mösges, R (eds.) Computer-Integrated Surgery, MIT Press, pp. 191–199 (1996)
2. Chabanas, M. ; Payan, Y.: A 3D Finite Element Model of the Face for Simulation in Plastic and Maxillofacial Surgery. Proc. Medical Image Computing and Computer-Assisted Intervention (MICCAI), Pittsburgh, PA, USA, pp. 1068–1075 (2000)
3. Gladilin, E. ; Zachow, S. ; Deuflhard, P. ; Hege, H.-C.: A Biomechanical Model for Soft Tissue Simulation in Craniofacial Surgery. Medical Imaging and Augmented Reality (MIAR), Hong Kong, China, pp. 137–141 (2001)
4. Gladilin, E. ; Zachow, S. ; Deuflhard, P. ; Hege, H.-C.: Virtual Fibers: A Robust Approach for Muscle Simulation. IX Mediterranean Conf. on Medical and Biological Engineering and Computing (MEDICON), Pula, Croatia, pp. 961–964 (2001)
5. Gladilin, E. ; Zachow, S. ; Hege H.-C. ; Deuflhard P.: FE-based heuristic approach for the estimation of person-specifc facial mimics. 5-th Int. Symp. on Computer Methods in Biomechanics and Biomedical Engineering, Rome, Italy (2001)
6. Stalling, D. ; Hege, H.-C. ; Zöckler, M. et. al.: Amira – An Advanced 3D Visualization and Modeling System, http://www.amiravis.com (2002)
7. Zachow, S. ; Gladilin, E. ; Trepczynski, A. ; Sader, R. : Zeilhofer, H.-F.: 3D Osteotomy planning in cranio-maxillofacial surgery: Experiences and results of surgery planning and volumetric finite-element soft tissue prediction in three clinical cases. In: Lemke, H.U. et al. (eds.): Computer Assisted Radiology and Surgery (CARS), Paris, France (2002)

CARS 2002 – H.U. Lemke, M.W. Vannier; K. Inamura, A.G. Farman, K. Doi & J.H.C. Reiber (Editors)
©CARS/Springer. All rights reserved.

Interactive simulation of the human hand

Leonard Sibille[a], Matthias Teschner[a, b], Sakti Srivastava[c], Jean-Claude Latombe[a]
[a] Robotics Laboratory, Stanford University, USA
[b] National Biocomputation Center, Stanford University, USA
[c] SUMMIT, Stanford University, USA

Abstract

This paper presents techniques for simulating the motion of a human hand on a computer graphics display. This simulation is based on a generic 3D model of the human hand in which the bone structure is described as an articulated linkage. Soft tissue around the bones is represented using mass-spring meshes. A predictor-corrector method, including the treatment of incompressibility and collision constraints, is used to compute soft-tissue deformation while bones are moving. Tendons responsible for the movement of the fingers are not explicitly represented as distinct objects, but their mechanical effect on the bone structure (application of forces) is included in our model. The implemented software simulates a human hand, including bone movement, soft-tissue deformation, and collision handling, at interactive rates on a PC. This software may be used as a tool to teach anatomy or simulate surgical operations.

Keywords: Human hand simulation, articulated system, mass-spring model

1. Introduction

Virtual-reality techniques have increasing applications in medicine. For instance, they can be used to teach anatomy to medical students. Surgeons can also train and develop their skills on virtual models before operating real patients. In this paper, we describe methods that we have integrated into a software system to simulate a generic human hand. We describe the hand skeleton as an articulated linkage. Visco-elastic soft tissue around the bones is represented using damped mass-spring meshes. A predictor-corrector method computes the deformation of the meshes by taking both incompressibility and collision constraints into account. Tendons responsible for the movement of the fingers do not have a separate geometric model, but their mechanical effect is explicitly represented by means of forces and rotational springs at the joints between finger bones. The implemented software simulates a human hand, including bone movement, soft-tissue deformation, and collision handling, at interactive rates on a PC. It may be used as a tool to teach anatomy or simulate surgical operations. Another possible application is in the simulation of digital actors for movies and video games.

The interactive simulation of human hands is studied in [1,6] as part of broader efforts to create digital actors. Video streaming techniques (instead of models) augmented by haptic interaction is proposed in [4] to teach hand anatomy. The representation of skeleton structures by mechanical linkages is investigated in [5,7,8]. The modeling and simulation of visco-elastic human-body tissue is studied in many publications, using either mass-

©CARS/Springer. All rights reserved.

spring meshes, finite-element methods, or a combination of both. See [1]. Techniques for adapting an external skin layer to the motion of underlying structures are presented in [2].

2. Simulation of the Bone Structure

2.1. Anatomy

The human hand consists of 29 bones (Fig.1). In our system, all bones are explicitly represented by geometric models, but only the movement of the phalanxes is simulated. Each finger (except the thumb) consists of three phalanxes: proximal, intermediate, and distal. We consider its four degrees of freedom, which are controlled by five tendons: Extensor EXT, Interosseus Left INL, Interosseus Right INR, Flexor Digitorum Profundis FDP, and Flexor Digitorum Superficialis FDS. EXT, FDP, and FDS create phalanx motions in the flexion-extension plane, while INL and INR are responsible for abduction-adduction movements, accompanied by partial extension. One end of each tendon connects to hand muscles and the other is attached to the bone structure. Some tendons are attached to more than one phalanx (e.g., EXT), whereas others are attached to both the top and bottom sides of a phalanx (e.g., FDP). When a tendon is pulled, another tendon acts in the opposite way, thus ensuring the mechanical stability of the hand. The thumb is made of two phalanxes. Our model only considers the two degrees of freedom in the flexion-extension plane.

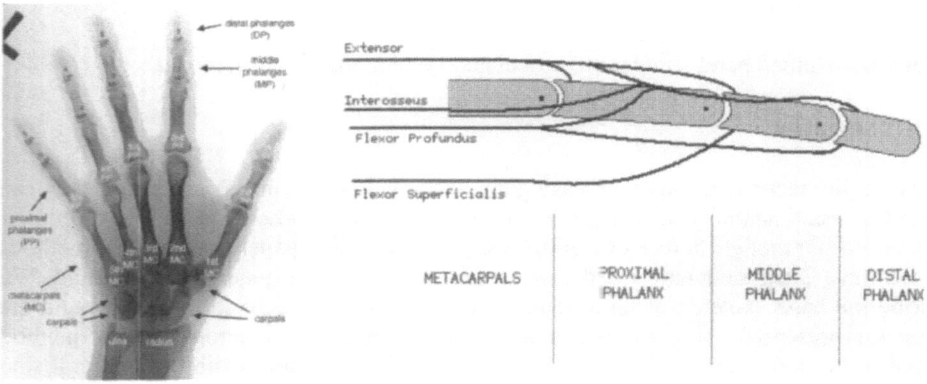

Figure 1: Anatomy of the hand

2.2. Kinematic Model

The surface of each bone is modeled by a mesh of about 200 triangles. The entire geometric model contains approximately 6000 triangles. As mentioned above, we only simulate the motion of the phalanxes. Each finger (except the thumb) is modeled as a serial linkage of three phalanxes with four revolute joints. See Fig.2. Three degrees of freedom are in the flexion-extension plane, and one is in the abduction-adduction plane. In our model, each joint connects a phalanx P to a previous bone B, and allows P to rotate around a point that is fixed relative to B. The thumb is modeled as a linkage of two phalanxes with two degrees of freedom, both in the flexion-extension plane.

©CARS/Springer. All rights reserved.

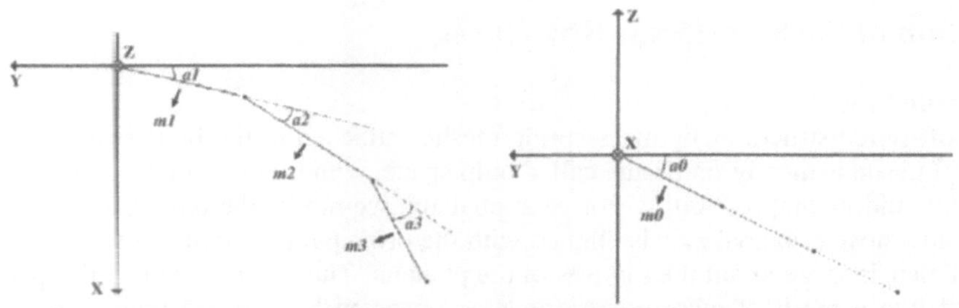

Figure 2 Kinematic model of a finger. Left: Three degrees of freedom in the flexion-extension plane. Right: Single degree of freedom in the abduction-adduction plane.

2.3. Mechanical Model

The motion of the hand results from the application of forces by tendons. We do not explicitly represent the geometry of the tendons, but we model the result of their combined actions on the bone structure. This is done by means of a simple linear transform that maps the set of tendon forces to forces applied at specific points on each phalanx. In turn, these forces create torques m_i, $i = 0$ to 3, applied at the four joints.

The feedback action of the tendons is modeled by rotational springs, each of which is associated to one degree of freedom. Therefore, our finger model contains four rotational springs (only two for the thumb): two at the proximal-metacarpal joint, one at the intermediate-proximal joint, and one at the distal-intermediate joint. Given a set of angular variations a_i, these springs induce reaction torques $-k_i a_i$, where k_i are the spring constants. When the hand is at rest, the torque at each joint is null. When new forces are exerted on the tendons, some joints between phalanxes rotate. Rotational springs then induce reaction torques opposed to this motion. This leads to a new equilibrium of the hand.

Numerical integration techniques are often used to compute angular variations caused by torques. Instead, we opted for a quasi-static approach [1], by assuming that the hand achieves static equilibrium at any one time, hence ignoring inertial effects on the motion. This assumption is valid for a wide range of common hand motions. The equilibrium state of a finger is defined by the angles a_i, $i = 0$ to 3, such that the torques induced by the tendons at the joints are exactly balanced by the reaction torques of the rotational springs. We compute these angles by minimizing the potential energy of the hand. In practice, these angles must also satisfy anatomical boundary conditions [5]. From these limits, we can easily infer the minimum and maximum torques that can be applied at a specific joint.

Assume that the finger is initially (time 0) in equilibrium with a set of applied tendon forces F_1. To generate the motion leading to the equilibrium corresponding to a new set of forces F_2 at time t, we first sample the time interval $[0,t]$ at a fixed step δ. At each successive time sample $t_k = k\delta$ we compute a set of forces F by linearly interpolating between F_1 and F_2. Then, we compute the angles a_i corresponding to the equilibrium when F is applied. Finally, we refresh the graphic display with those new angles. To simulate the motion of the entire hand, we simply perform the same computation for each finger, plus the thumb.

©CARS/Springer. All rights reserved.

3. Simulation of the Soft-Tissue Structures

3.1. Soft-Tissue Model

We model soft-tissue structures by mass-spring meshes attached to the bone structure of the hand. Soft tissue is mostly fat tissue, called pulp space, with two important properties: visco-elasticity and incompressibility. For each phalanx, we model the pulp space at rest by an ellipsoid whose principal axis is aligned with the principal direction of the phalanx, and whose dimensions are about the same as of the phalanx. The volume of the pulp space is discretized into a mesh of mass points (nodes) connected by damped linear springs. Some of these nodes are attached to the bottom side of the phalanx. Similarly, we model the soft tissue of the palm by an incompressible damped mass-spring mesh. We explicitly represent the external surface of each mesh not in contact with a bone as a collection of triangles whose vertices are the surface nodes of the mesh.

3.2. Simulation Process

The bone movements are responsible for the motion and deformation of soft tissues. At each step of the hand simulation, we first compute the new configuration of the bone structure (Section 2). Since each mass-spring mesh *M* is attached to a single phalanx or to the rigid palm, the new positions of the nodes are easily derived from this configuration. But adjacent meshes may have collided. We first detect collisions and "resolve" each of them by shifting penetrating nodes backwards. In turn, such shifts produce spring forces inside meshes and we compute the resulting deformation of these meshes. Overall, the simulation the soft tissue consists of (1) computing the new position/orientation of each mesh (from the current configuration of the bone structure), (2) detecting and resolving collisions, and (3) computing the deformation of the colliding meshes. In (1) the shape of each mesh is the one computed at the previous step of the simulation process.

3.3. Collision Handling

To detect collisions between two meshes, we consider two layers of nodes for each mesh (Fig.3): one layer is simply the mesh surface, while the other layer is obtained by translating each node of the first layer inwards by some small distance *L* along the surface normal. *L* is selected so that all nodes move by no more than *L* during a single simulation step (we assume that *L* is small enough for the second layer to be homeomorphic to the first). Each pair of corresponding triangles from the two layers defines a prism. For any two adjacent meshes that may have collided, we compute all sets of intersecting prisms, and we determine all the nodes of one mesh that may have penetrated the other one. The collision is then "resolved" by projecting these points onto a separation plane computed as the plane passing through the barycenter of the penetrating nodes and perpendicular to the average of the surface normals at these points. The contact between the two colliding meshes is flattened along the separating plane during this last step. This process is illustrated (in two dimensions) in Fig.3. To speed-up collision detection, we pre-compute a hierarchical bounding representation of the prisms, using Axis-Aligned Bounding Boxes (AABB) as described in [3]. Because objects deform, the AABB hierarchies are recomputed at each simulation step.

©CARS/Springer. All rights reserved.

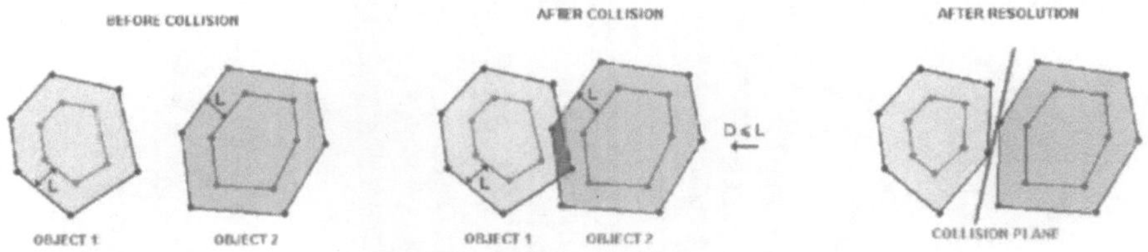

Figure 3. Collision treatment.

3.4. Soft-Tissue Deformation

In a colliding mesh, the relative positions of the penetrating nodes have changed relative to the other nodes. Internal spring forces are induced by these changes, leading the mesh to undergo some global deformation. Various techniques exist to compute the deformation of a mass-spring mesh. Here, we use a predictor-corrector method, in which spring forces in a mesh are predicted and node positions are corrected accordingly. More specifically, all spring forces $\boldsymbol{F}_t$ in a mesh are computed at time t according to the current lengths of the springs and a predicted set of new node positions $\check{\boldsymbol{S}}_{t+dt}$ is derived using explicit Euler integration. From $\check{\boldsymbol{S}}_{t+dt}$ we compute the corresponding set of predicted spring forces. A second Euler step, using these predicted forces applied to the current positions $\boldsymbol{S}_t$ leads to the corrected node positions $\boldsymbol{S}_{t+dt}$.

We also take soft-tissue incompressibility into account. Each pair of original and displaced triangles defines a prism. The sum of the signed volumes of all such prisms is an approximation δV of the volumetric variation of the mesh during the deformation steps. To neutralize this variation, we translate every surface node that is not involved in a collision by the same amount in the direction of the surface normal computed by averaging the normals to the triangles adjacent to this node.

4. Implementation

Our software is written in C++, uses the SGI's OpenInventor library, and runs on a Linux PC with two 1-GHz processors and 1GB of memory. The overall geometric model of the bone structure contains approximately 6000 triangles. For each phalanx, the pulp space is modeled with a mesh of 40 mass points connected by 80 springs. In total, the soft-tissue model of the whole hand (including the palm) contains 700 mass point and 1400 springs.

In addition, our current software creates a "skin surface" wrapped around the bone structure and the soft tissue. This surface is created by extruding vertices of the bone and soft tissue structures by a small amount. Our skin model consists of 2000 triangles.

The time step of the simulation needed to perform all simulation operations – update of bone structure, collision resolution, soft-tissue deformation, adjustment of the skin – is approximately 10 milliseconds. Fig.4 shows two computed configurations of the hand.

©CARS/Springer. All rights reserved.

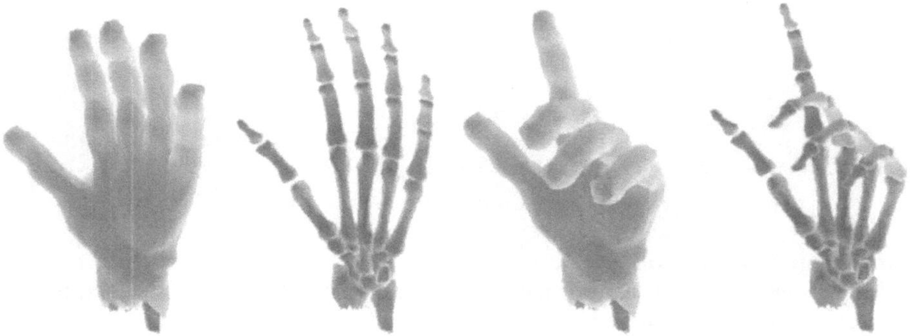

Figure 4. Left: Initial configuration of the hand. Right: Flexion of three fingers.

Our future research will aim at incorporating a better model of the skin, modeling additional degrees of freedom, simulating grasping operations of rigid and flexible objects, taking into account reaction torques exerted by soft tissue on the joints of the bone structure, and generating patient-specific hand models.

Acknowledgements

This research was funded by NSF Grant IIS-9907060. The geometric data of the hand model used in our research was provided by the Stanford-NASA Biocomputation Center.

References

1. J. Brown, S. Sorkin, C. Bruyns, J.C. Latombe, K. Montgomery, M. Stephanides. Real-Time Simulation of Deformable Objects: Tools and Application. *Proc. Computer Animation 2001*, 2001.
2. J. E. Chadwick, D. R. Haumann , R. E. Parent. Layered Construction for Deformable Animated Characters. *Proc. SIGGRAPH '89*, 23(3), pp. 243-252, 1989.
3. J. D. Cohen, M. C. Lin, D. Manocha, M. K. Ponamgi. "I-Collide: An Interactive and Exact Detection System for Large-Scale Environments." *Proc. ACM Interactive 3D Graphics Conf.*, pp. 189-196, 1995
4. D. Gutierrez, A. Shah, and D.A. Harris. Performance of Remote Anatomy and Surgical Training Applications under Varied Network Conditions. *Proc. ED-MEDIA 2002, World Conf. on Educ. Multimedia, Hypermedia and Telecom.*, 2002.
5. R. Mas, D. Thalmann. A Hand Control and Automatic Grasping System for Synthetic Actors. *Proc. Eurographics '94*, 13(3), pp. 167-178, 1994.
6. L. Moccozet, N. M. Thalmann. Multilevel Deformation Model Applied to Hand Simulation for Virtual Actors. *Proc. Int. Conf. on Virtual Syst. and MultiMedia*, 1997.
7. H. Rijpkema, M. Girard. Computer Animation of Knowledge-Based Human Grasping. *Proc. SIGGRAPH '91*, 25(4), pp. 339-348, 1991.
8. Y. Yasumuro, Q. Chen, K. Chihara. 3D Modeling of the Human Hand with Motion Constraints." *Image and Vision Computing*, 17(2), pp. 149-156, 1999.

CARS 2002 – H.U. Lemke, M.W. Vannier; K. Inamura, A.G. Farman, K. Doi & J.H.C. Reiber (Editors)
©CARS/Springer. All rights reserved.

Planning and training of minimally invasive surgery by integrating soft tissue cuts with surgical views reproduction

Megumi Nakao[a], Tomohiro Kuroda[b], Hiroshi Oyama[b], Masaru Komori[c], Tetsuya Matsuda[a], Takashi Takahashi[b]

[a] Graduate School of Informatics, Kyoto University
[b] Department of Medical Informatics, Kyoto University Hospital
[c] Computational Biomedicine, Shiga University of Medical Science

Abstract

This paper gives integrated methods that perform virtual reality based planning and training of minimally invasive surgery. The authors propose an advanced framework of volumetric soft tissue cutting, which consistently combines topological changes into deformable models. Collision detection and physical constraint are provided in simulated surgery space. Time series MRI dataset are applied to a visual and haptic system with a force feedback device. The reconstructed environment enables to identify approachable region, and to discuss optimum strategy. Figures and evaluations assure that the developed methods are effective in preoperative planning as well as in learning surgeries.

Keywords: Soft tissue cutting, planning and training, minimally invasive surgery

1. Introduction

Minimally invasive surgery (MIS) is focused in the medical fields because small incision contributes to patient's beauty and risk reduction. Although MIS benefits patients, surgeons have to learn high procedural skills and have to experience more surgeries. One reason lies in the fact that surgeons insufficiently acquire anatomical and geometrical information from localized surgical view. Another reason is caused by difficulty of proper treatments when unexpected cases like bleeding happen. The result of the latest difficult surgeries such as minimally invasive cardiac surgery (MICS) mostly depends on how to settle surgical environments and local views [1]. However, surgeons are forced to make decisions on surgical strategies empirically or intuitively using conventional 2D images.

For these requirements, an advanced virtual reality based simulation has possibilities of providing a solution to both preoperative planning and training. So far, many studies reported surgery simulators that provide manipulating, suturing, and sculpting of tissues [2-6]. The authors also presented haptic reproduction and interactive visualization of a beating heart [7]. In the next step, this study aims to present advanced surgical planning and training with soft tissue cutting in MICS, which helps us to optimise incision (cutting point and length), surgical path (direction and approach) and surgical environment (view and space). Note that both simulation accuracy and interactive realism are also essential subjects to realize practical simulators.

©CARS/Springer. All rights reserved.

In order to provide realistic surgery simulator described above, this paper proposes to establish an advanced framework that simulates interactive soft tissue incision and dissection. After cutting into muscle and fat of a virtual chest wall, simulated surgical view is reproduced. Both collision detection and force feedback scheme gives geometrical and physical constraint of the localized area. Combination of these methods performs an effective environment for planning and training in MICS. The proposed methods are implemented on a visual and haptic system with measured dataset. Finally, both efficiency and limitation are discussed based on some evaluations.

2. Methods

This chapter describes overall methods that provide basics of a surgical planner in MICS. First of all, details of the proposed cutting framework are given. Secondly, interaction model between virtual instruments and reconstructed surgical environments is presented. To provide interactive surgery simulation, computational structure for large medical dataset is also mentioned.

2.1 A framework for soft tissue cutting

Cutting simulation for a virtual 3D object is performed based on physical and geometrical methods: physical balance and transition of soft tissues and adaptive subdivision of tetrahedral objects.

Physical balance and transition of soft tissues

From the viewpoint of consistent physical approaches, the proposed framework focuses on internal tension: biomechanical characteristics of soft tissues including skins, fats, muscles and organs. Actually, all tension between soft tissues is in equilibrium at ordinary state, and physical balance changes into the next stable state after cutting. In a particle system (Fig. 1 (a)), such initial state that internal tension is acting on tissues is represented by setting initial length of edges shorter than initial distance between two vertices.

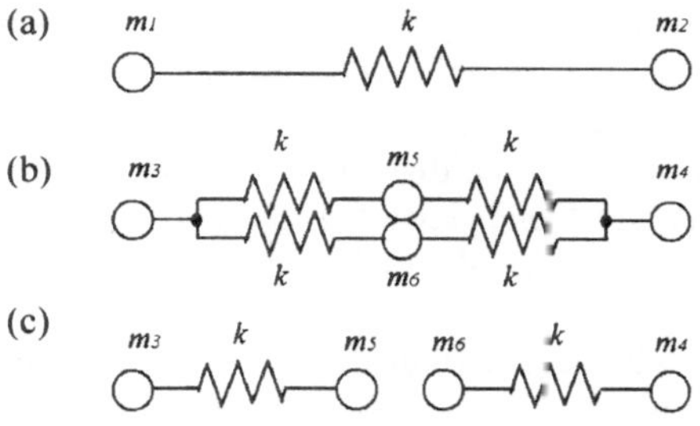

Fig. 1. Remodeling the particle system: (a) initial particle system, creation, (b) distribution of new vertices, (c) physical transition after elimination of the edges

Cutting simulation has to combine physical transition and topological change in order to represent relaxation of the tissues. A pair of new vertices is created at the same coordinates on a certain edge of cut, and the particle system is modified on condition that the system has the same characteristics towards adjacent external vertices (Fig. 1 (b)). Mass of the vertices is distributed to the created vertices. As a result, we can cut into the system by elimination of alternative tensor elements connected to different neighbours

©CARS/Springer. All rights reserved.

(Fig. 1 (c)). If the physical system has the internal tension described above, the vertices physically spread apart to new stable positions. The movement of the vertices produces dynamic movement while cutting tissues.

Adaptive subdivision of tetrahedral objects

In order to visualize volumetric cuts, both new edges and polygons are required on the cut surfaces that spread apart from each other. So far, related works reported that zigzag cut is a key problem in cutting simulation [4]. Radical increase of the elements also becomes a serious drawback to interactive simulation that has to keep update rate stable and small. To solve such problems, the authors propose adaptive tetrahedral subdivision that gives compact and intelligent topological change.

Movement of a virtual scalpel defines a clipping plane *C*, which clips a cut surface *S* from tetrahedral objects *T*. Figure 2 (a) illustrates the relationship between these three elements. Note that incomplete intersection can be occurred at some tetrahedra because *C* is given as a partial plane by cutting manipulation. This incomplete intersection is shown at the rightmost tetrahedron of *T* in Fig. 2 (a). For this situation, the authors define the cut surface *S* by removing incomplete intersection instead of handling complex patterns of whole intersections. Definite solution that removes incomplete intersection is illustrated in Fig. 2 (b), which represents movement of vertices on the clipping plane *C*. For example, the vertex *A* is updated to the vertex *A'* on the boundary *B* of the clipped area *C*. The movement vector of the vertex is given as an average of edge vectors (v_1, v_2) that intersect at *B*. According to this scheme, all adjacent vertices outside of the area *C* are moved and replaced on its boundary *B*.

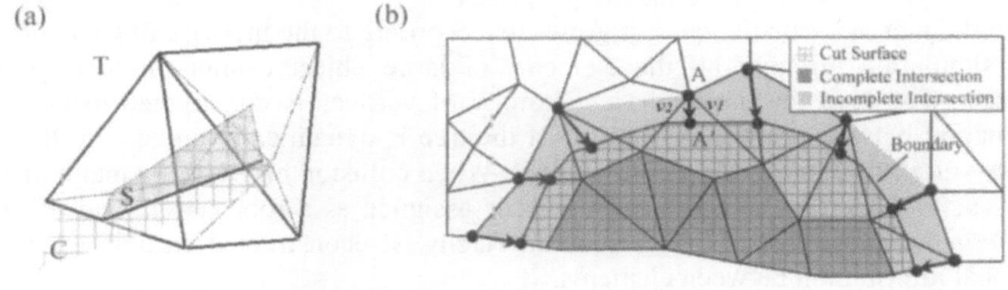

Fig. 2. Definition of cut surface (*C*: clipping plane, *S*: cut surface, *T*: tetrahedral object): (a) Intersection between a clipping plane and tetrahedra, (b) movement of vertices on the clipping plane

Consequently, the cut surface *S* can be simply represented as a combination of the two patterns of intersection in Fig. 3. The generated cut surface *S* displays volumetric cut. The remodeling scheme of particle systems presented above is applied to all edges that are clipped by *C*. Implementation of the methods is simple because complex description of subdivision patterns is not required. Moreover, this approach provides more efficient solution that reduces growth rates of vertices than that proposed in foregoing works [5, 6]. Because degree of freedom of created vertices is still low, some edges are inserted into the object in order to simulate realistic cuts. Minimal tetrahedral subdivision in Fig. 3 gives consistent and effective patterns of edge insertion. This work also concerns accurate shape of cuts. The adaptive scheme optimises tetrahedral mesh quality for calculation and solves best subdivision pattern that is insensitive to 3D topology of the object. Dihedral angle of

©CARS/Springer. All rights reserved.

a tetrahedron is used as the indicator of the mesh quality, and max-min and min-max approach is applied. In other words, the scheme selects the subdivision pattern that maximizes the minimum dihedral angle and minimizes the maximum dihedral angle.

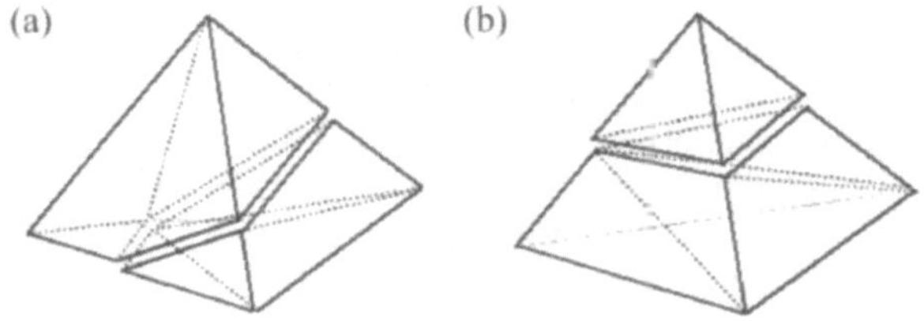

Fig. 3. Tetrahedral subdivision: (a) four-edge intersection, (b) three-edge intersection

2.2 Reproduction of surgical environments

After decision of the cut point and length on the breast wall, the localized view during surgeries is reconstructed. The geometrical and physical constraint in the localized area disturbs movement of a virtual instrument. These facts are simulated visually and haptically using collision detection and force feedback through haptic devices. The body of virtual instruments like a scalpel and a clamp is simply modelled as a cylinder. The interaction between the instrument and the beating heart is described as the 4D extension of the God Object based method [7, 8]. Haptic rendering and force feedback during cutting operations is simulated using the friction and rotation model described in [4, 5].

2.3 Computational structure for large dataset

Due to the fact that calculation cost grows up according to the increase of elements, large-scale simulation utilizing all the elements of large object cannot produce interactive feedback. To solve this problem, a hierarchy of vertices is constructed using adjacent information between vertices. The root of the tree is dynamically updated to the nearest surface vertex from a tip of a virtual scalpel. When collision between the manipulator and the tissue is detected, the contacted vertex is assigned as a root vertex, and its children become adjacent vertices. Note that the hierarchy is reconstructed partially using stored relational information between elements.

The hierarchical structure performs suitable traverse in regional order, and the depth d briefly manages the level of local calculation. Using the depth d as a threshhold of localization, the lower vertcies are fixed and the upper vertices are freed to move. Since actual cutting does not influence on large area, it is reasonable to assume that most of vertices further away from the contacted point do not move. The frozen vertices allow not only controlling calculation cost, but also keeping the physical system stable.

3. Results

Dataset of human body structures with a beating heart was obtained from ECG-gated 3D MRI of a normal volunteer. The whole dataset consist of time series 15 volumetric data (256*256*64 voxels) for one cardiac cycle. After semi-automatic region extraction from surroundings, 3D surfaces of the breast and the heart are extracted, and then each internal region is divided into tetrahedra (Fig. 4 (a)). The tetrahedral objects have 17582 vertices,

©CARS/Springer. All rights reserved.

100807 edges, 19964 polygons and 73279 tetrahedra on average. In this work, a beating heart is represented by sequential animation of the dataset, and the chest wall is fixed. Overall algorithms of the proposed methods are implemented on a standard PC (Dual CPUs: Pentium III 933MHz, Memory: 2GB). The PHANToM (Sensable Technologies Inc.) is applied to the simulation system as force feedback device. As parameters, the elastic coefficient 100N/m, the damper coefficient 0.05Ns/m, the density 0.90g/cm3 and the level of localization 4 are applied.

Figure 4 (b-f) illustrates an example of procedures in planning and training of minimally invasive pericardiotomy. 3D line is directly drawn on the pericardium of the virtual heart as a surgical plan using transparent display (Fig. 4 (b-c)). Then, small incision into the chest wall is given. The next two frames (Fig. 4 (d-e)) show interactive volumetric cutting. After stretching incised chest wall, a part of pericardium and planed line appears (Fig. 4 (f)). Collision detection and response between virtual instruments and the chest wall enable surgeons to check approachable region, and to discuss both optimum approach and more appropriate cutting point and length. Thus, reconstructed surgical environments are effective in preoperative planning as well as in learning surgical views.

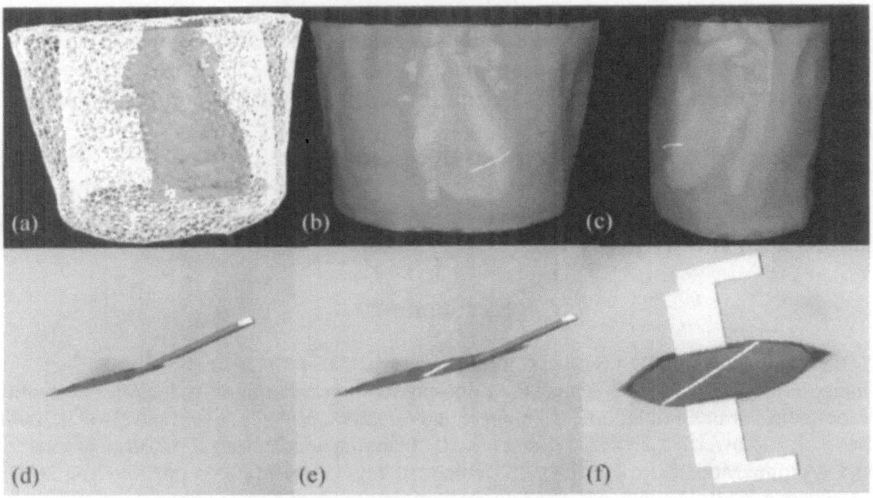

Fig. 4. Preoperative simulation for minimally invasive cardiac surgery: (a) rendered heart and tetrahedral mesh of chest wall, (b-c) input of a plan for pericardiotomy, (d-e) interactive cutting into the chest wall with the virtual scalpel, (f) reconstructed surgical view

Simulation accuracy of the cuts is evaluated by comparing the proposed adaptive cuts with non-adaptive cuts using total area of the created cut surface as a quantitative indicator. The average growth rate of the proposed model becomes 1/3 of that of the other, which means zigzag cuts are reduced. As a result of measurement of calculation time, overall algorithms (i.e. collision detection, deformation, topological change) are calculated within 5 msec. Force feedback architecture is also managed strictly by parallel thread computing and valid complementation using dual CPU system. Consequently, the system achieves real time refresh rate for interactive and realistic simulation.

©CARS/Springer. All rights reserved.

4. Discussion

Figures and evaluations in the previous chapter demonstrate that overall methods enable interactive cutting and improve shape of cuts. However, some problems still lie in absolute accuracy, because physical behaviour was simulated based on the standard mass-spring model. One solution for more reliable simulation is to apply the proposed framework to other advanced particle based models like the tensor mass model [6], which is based on the liner elastic finite element formulation. To provide advanced simulation such as non-linear biomechanical deformation and physiological description of human bodies is an essential subject for realistic surgery simulation. Detailed anatomical models and interaction methods between multiple deformable organs are also necessary.

5. Conclusion

This paper first gives a framework to provide soft tissue cutting for surgery simulation. The proposed methods are simple to implement, and integrate topological change into deformable models based on physically consistent manner. Both collision detection and physical constraints between virtual instruments and tissues simulates localized surgery environment in MICS. Time series MRI dataset acquired from an adult man was applied to a prototype system with a force feedback device. The results assure that the overall framework contributes to preoperative planning and training in MIS. Clinical trial and improvement of overall applicability are future works for practical surgery simulators.

Acknowledgements

This work was supported by the Ministry of Education, Science, Culture of Japan, Grants-in-Aid for JSPS Fellows No.0103889

References

1. R. Omoto et al, Minimally Invasive Cardiac Surgery, ISBN4-7878-1099-5, 1999.
2. Kuhnapfel U., Cakmak H.K., Mass H., "Endoscopic Surgery Training Using Virtual Reality and Deformable Tissue Simulation", Computers and Graphics, Vol.24, No.5, pp.671-682, 2000.
3. Pflesser B., Leuwer R., Tiede U. Hohne, K. H, "Planning and Rehearsal of Surgical Intervention in the Volume Model", Proceedings of Medicine Meets Virtual Reality, pp. 259-264, 2000.
4. C. Basdogan, Chih-Hao Ho, M. A. Srinivasan, "Simulation of Tissue Cutting and Bleeding for Laparoscopic Surgery Using Auxiliary Surfaces", Proceedings of Medicine Meets Virtual Reality 8, pp.38-44, 1999.
5. D. Bielser, M. H. Gross, "Interactive Simulation of Surgical Cuts", Proceedings of Pacific Graphics, pp.116-125, 2000.
6. S. Cotin, D. Herve, N. Ayache, "A Hybrid Elastic Model for Real-Time Cutting, Deformations, and Force Feedback for Surgery Training and System", The Visual Computer (Springer), Vol. 16, pp.437-452, 2000.
7. M. Nakao, M. Komori, H. Oyama, T. Matsuda, T. Takahashi, "Haptic Reproduction and Interactive Visualization of a Beating Heart Based on Cardiac Morphology", Proceedings of Medical Informatics, pp.924-928, 2001.
8. D. Ruspini, K. Kolarov, O. Khatib, "The Haptic Display of Complex Graphical Environments" Proceedings of Computer Graphics (SIGGRAPH), pp. 345-352, 1997.

CARS 2002 – H.U. Lemke, M.W. Vannier; K. Inamura, A.G. Farman, K. Doi & J.H.C. Reiber (Editors)
©CARS/Springer. All rights reserved.

An integrated system for maxillo-facial surgery simulation

M. Maggio Binucci[1], C. Lamberti[1], R. Gori[2], L. Montagna[1], A. Sarti[1]
[1]Dept. of Electronics, Computer Science and Systems
University of Bologna
[2] Cineca, High Performance Computing Center
Interuniversity Consortium, Bologna
clamberti@deis.unibo.it

Abstract

Computer-aided surgery simulation represents a rapidly emerging and increasingly important area of research that combines a number of disciplines for the common purpose of improving health care. Generally, the goal of computer-based surgery simulation is to enable a surgeon to experiment with different surgical procedures in an artificial environment. This study introduces a mathematical modelling and a numerical simulation of maxillo-facial surgery taking into account biomechanical properties of soft tissues. The approach for elastic modeling of human tissue is based on the use of embedded boundary condition techniques. Models obtained with this method allow to simulate the cranio-facial surgery directly on the natural grid of the 3D CT image of the patient avoiding any need of regridding and mesh tuning [1]. The associated matrix is solved using iterative and multi-scale methods. The integration of a distributed data management component has been developed into virtual surgery environment, to make the system distributed and suitable for clinicians involved in. The application of this approach for modeling the elastic deformation of human tissue in response to movement of bones is demonstrated both on the Visible Human Data Set of the National Library of Medicine and on the CT dataset of real patients.

Keywords: Maxillo facial virtual surgery, surgery simulation, bioengineering

1. Introduction

Virtual surgery, a new discipline which recently appeared among the medical sciences, is an excellent example of contribution from medical and computational knowledge to health development and progress. Cranio-facial surgery is a surgical branch regarding study and treatment of any kind of disease (malformations, trauma and tumors) affecting the face. Peculiar to this kind of surgery is that any surgical procedure has not only functional but even aesthetical implication such important for all patients' life. Anatomical and functional complexity of the face and skull, characterized by the presence of the eyes, ear, nose, mouth, facial nerve ad the proximity of very important organs as the brain and the respiratory system, make this area extremely hazardous for any skilled surgeons and a very dangerous field for practitioners. Moreover cadaver anatomical dissection which in the past was the best way to learn surgery, is extremely difficult to be

©CARS/Springer. All rights reserved.

performed in the face. For these scientific and teaching reasons 3D computer simulation of cranio-facial surgery can be extremely useful in clinical practice.
The most important aim of computer-based surgery simulation is to enable a surgeon to experiment with different surgical procedures in an artificial environment, in order to predict the outcome of a cranio-facial intervention before the real surgery.
The first problem in the development of a surgical simulator consists in the modelling of the target organ. The geometry is usually obtained from medical imaging device like CT and MR, while models of continuum biomechanics determine the behaviour of the soft tissues.
Several methods to simulate the elastic nature of the soft tissue have been proposed, but generally they suffer the problem to approximate the anatomical geometry with a computational mesh. The 3D tessellation of the geometric model into finite elements is indeed non trivial for complex anatomical structures like bones and soft tissues in the head.
In this study we propose to simulate cranio-facial surgery directly on the grid of the 3D CT data taking an eulerian approach instead of the classical lagrangian, typical of the previous methods.
This method allows reduction of computational costs without loosing details in anatomical structures.
Our purposes are:

- to realize a physically based computational model allowing the simulation of soft tissue deformation as a consequence of the surgery planning. This module allows simulating and predicting the post-surgical aspect of the patient's face, working directly on the 3D CT data;
- to realize an interactive user interface for surgery planning, improving the 3D data manipulation to provide a more natural way to the surgeons to execute the virtual operation;
- to obtain numerical/visual tools for results visualisation and for comparison between prediction and post-operation CT data for error evaluation;
- to make portable software module suitable both for the integration within a PACS server in a hospital environment or even into the graphics work-station, as a standalone solution;
- to develop data handler modules to keep track of all the data involved in the planning, and perform data compression for speeding up the data exchange in case of a distributed framework;
- to provide transparent access to patients data (input, output, and parameters of the simulation) using a web application, that allows surgeons to easily compare different planning hypotheses and share the results.

2. Methodology

The Surgery Simulation workflow is composed of several steps, performed by different actors (DEIS and CINECA of Bologna), and supported by different modules of integrated Hospital Information Systems (Rizzoli Hospital's Radiology Unit of Bologna and Bufalini Hospital's Maxillo-Facial Workgroup of Cesena).

©CARS/Springer. All rights reserved.

2.1 CT Acquisition

A 3D CT scan is acquired from the patient before the surgery. The acquisition is performed employing a High Speed Spiral CT in helical mode using parameters (slice distance = 3mm / 1.3s, 120 Kw, 160 mA) and modalities specified in a suitable acquisition protocol. Normally data consist of approximately 120 images for patient in the ACR-NEMA DICOM3 format. A low radiation acquisition protocol has been recently introduced.

2.2 Efficient access to patients data

One key component of the user interface is the data front-end, able to help the surgeon to keep track of all the data involved in the surgical simulation. The main task of this component is to provide a consistent interface to the different DBMS or PACS protocol. All the data relative to an intervention planning are handled: input CT scans, all the parameters defining the planning hypotheses (osteotomies) and simulation outputs as shown in Fig. 1.

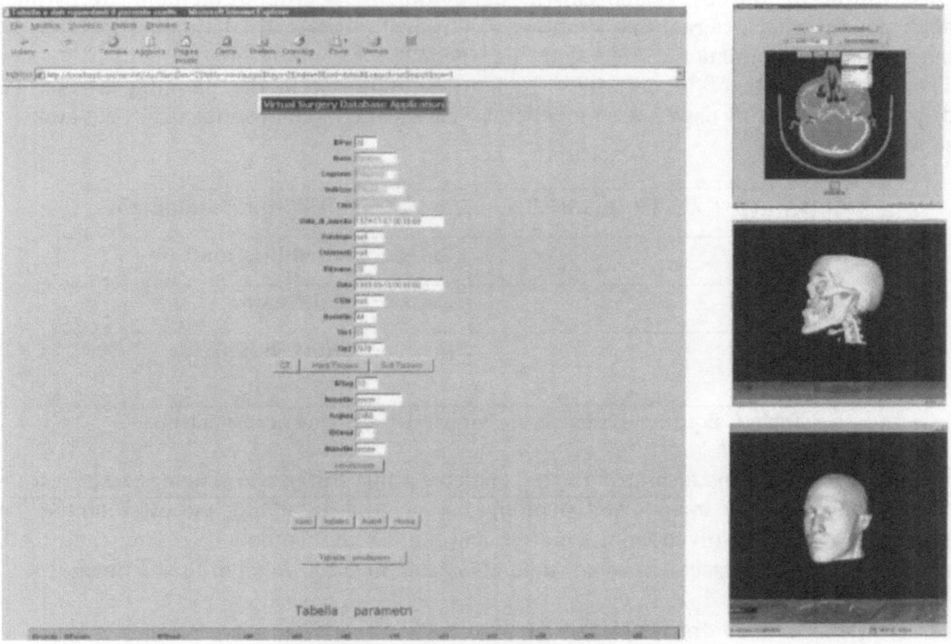

Fig. 1: Interface to the virtual surgery Data Base: all patient's data, as CT scans, reconstructed 3D models, planning hypotheses and simulation outputs, can be managed.

The system has been integrated into the graphical user interface, allowing the user to browse through the patient data and to select input data, that are locally cached, to avoid unnecessary network transmission (all the data are time stamped). All the data are be stored and transferred in compressed form.

Of course security, privacy and more in general private data managing ethical aspects, always relevant in medical applications, are kept in necessary consideration.

©CARS/Springer. All rights reserved.

2.3 Tissue Segmentation, Classification and 3D Reconstruction

By selecting suitable value of CT parameters, soft tissue and bone tissue can be separated. We developed a set of automatic and semi-automatic tools to process 2D real patients' CT slices and obtain 3D volumes necessary for surgery simulation.

2.4 Input visualization and Surgical Planning

A 3D graphical interface allows the user to interact directly with the hard and soft tissues reconstructed models. The code has been written in Tcl/Tk and based on the Vtk library to be cross-platform [2][3]. Using a force feedback 3D virtual reality bistoury (Haptic device) [4] or simply a mouse, osteotomy lines can be traced and anatomical regions can be moved and relocated according to the established surgical procedure. Relocations are quantified in terms of translational and rotational parameters. At the end of the surgical planning a new geometry of bones is hypothesized.

2.5 Numerical Simulation

Description of tissues' visco-elastic behaviour is a crucial element to estimate deformations after external interventions. A physically based simulation kernel computes the soft tissue deformation caused by the new geometry of bones [5][6].
The displacements of hard tissues (bones) are imposed in the planning phase. The displacements of soft tissues are modelled by classical continuous mechanics equations as shown in Table 1.

$\mu\Delta\mathbf{u}(\mathbf{x}) + (\mu+\lambda)\nabla(\nabla\cdot\mathbf{u}(\mathbf{x})) = \mathbf{0}$	for $\mathbf{x} \in$ **soft tissues subdomain**
$\Delta\mathbf{u}(\mathbf{x}) = \mathbf{0}$	for $\mathbf{x} \in$ **embedding material**
$\mathbf{u}(\mathbf{x}) = \mathbf{u}_0(\mathbf{x})$	for $\mathbf{x} \in$ **hard tissues**
$\frac{d\mathbf{u}(\mathbf{x})}{dn} = \mathbf{0}$	for $\mathbf{x} \in$ **volume boundary**

Table 1. Equation system for the virtual surgery numerical simulation.

The equation system is discretized using centered finite difference schemes respect to the natural grid of the CT image itself, avoiding any need of regridding and mesh tuning. The associated matrix is solved using iterative and multi-scale methods [7]. The result of the simulation is the displacement vector field associated to every voxel of the CT image.

2.6 Output Visualization

The original CT image is warped following the physically based displacement field obtained by numerical simulation. The new hypothetical face of the patient can be visualized inside the same graphical interface (see Fig. 2).

3. Data

The application of our approach for modelling the elastic deformation of human tissue in response to movement of bones has been tested both on the Visible Human Data Set of the National Library of Medicine and on the CT datasets of real patients.

©CARS/Springer. All rights reserved.

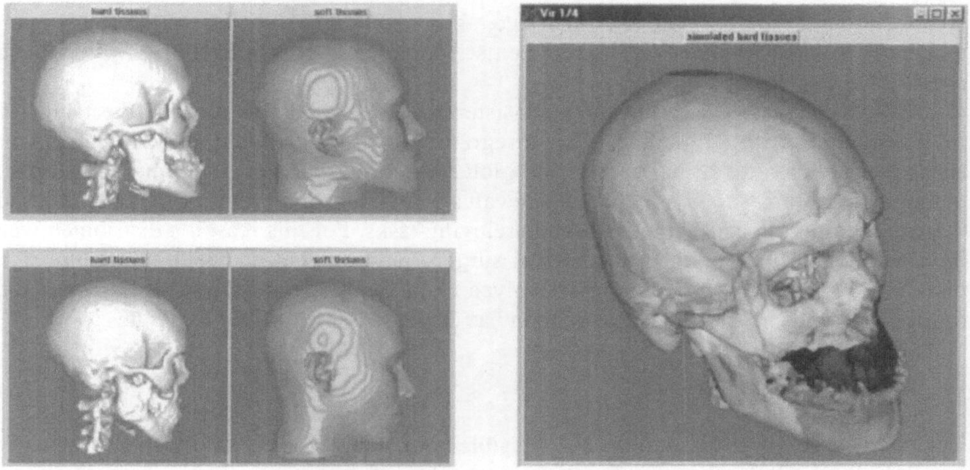

Fig. 2: Example of surgical intervention planning on the skull of a real patient: **Top left**: From CT data, hard tissues and soft tissues 3D models are reconstructed. **Right**: Bones have been selected, cut and relocated. In this phase the operator can experiment different surgical procedure. **Down left**: After planning, numerical simulation provides prediction of patient's face's final aspect by simulating the mechanical behaviour of real soft tissues (remodelling) in response to bone's replacement.

The set of patient involved in our research is for 50% females and 50% males, aged between 10 and 37 with average age of 25.1, affected by cranio-facial deformities.
The surgeons performed several kinds of procedures. For the validation of the application, no extra CT acquisitions have been required, because pre- and post-operative exams were just suitable. The following Table 2 shows a number of validated cases.

Patients	Procedures
9	Le Fort I maxillary advancement
6	Le Fort I high maxillary advancement extended to zigoma Bilateral sagittal split osteotomy Genioplasty (2 cases) Mandibular border osteotomy
3	Bilateral sagittal split osteotomy Genioplasty (1 case)
1	Le Fort III
1	Le Fort III, fronto orbital advancement

Table 2. Surgical procedures.

4. Results

A complete system has been developed, able to be used in a clinical routine to plan maxillo-facial surgical intervention. The proposed structure, through the development of a portable, scalable and progressive computational kernel, embedded in a distributed

©CARS/Springer. All rights reserved.

architecture and in a portable user interface, allows to build a real time surgical planning tool with reasonably low HW requirements. Moreover a cross-platform SW has been used.
The 80% of the studied cases resulted consistent with the validation procedure established in accordance with clinicians. The integration of a distributed data management component allows to further reduce the global time required for the complete surgical planning, enabling surgeons to quickly evaluate different intervention hypotheses, and helping them in the data acquisition and archiving tasks. For this reason a distributed web interface has been developed into virtual surgery environment, to make the application distributed and suitable for clinicians involved in. Actually the mean overall time required for planning and simulating an intervention has decreased down to 10-15 minutes.

5. Conclusions

The 3D CT surgery simulation is a feasible tool, which could allow the surgeon to simulate the real (hard and soft tissues) outcome of cranio-facial surgery procedures, limiting the risk of operation failure. The final goal of this research will be to better understand for each kind of surgery (osteotomies, graft, implants etc.) the true distribution of the soft tissue due to the different modality of their incompressibility and in this way to improve the quality and likelihood of the simulation.
For this reason, a useful and reliable tool capable to be routinely integrated in the daily clinical practice has been realized.

Acknowledgements

The work presented in this paper has been partially supported under the Activity No IST-1999-20226/VISU of the European Take-Up of Essential Information Society Technologies for Medical Application (EUTIST-M).

References

1. A. Sarti, R. Gori, A. Bianchi, C. Marchetti and C. Lamberti, *Information Technologies in Medicine, Vol II*, 183-199, John Wiley & Sons, New York, 2001.
2. W. Schroeder, K. Martin and B. Lorensen, *The Visualization Toolkit. An Object-Oriented Approach To 3D Graphics, 2nd Ed.*, Prentice-Hall, New Jersey, 1999.
3. B. Welch, *Practical programming in Tcl and Tk, 3rd Ed.*, Prentice Hall, New Jersey, 1999.
4. *GHOST® SDK, Programmer's Guide, Version 3.1*, SenSable Technologies Inc.®, 2001.
5. Y.C. Fung, *Biomechanics: Mechanical Properties of Living Tissues, 2nd edition*, Springer Verlag, New York, 1993.
6. F. M. Montevecchi, *Meccanica nei tessuti biologici*, Patron Ed., Bologna, 1997.
7. Y. Saad, *Iterative Methods for Sparse Linear Systems*, PWS Publishing Company, Boston, 1996.

©CARS/Springer. All rights reserved.

Towards functional simulation of soft tissue deformation for preoperative planning and postoperative evaluation

Peter Zerfass[a], ErwinKeeve[a]
[a] Research center caesar
Friedensplatz 16, 53111 Bonn, Germany

Abstract

In this paper we present in depth one of the preprocessing steps of our software system for the simulation of soft tissue behaviour and biomechanical processes. The entire system can be used by surgeons for preoperative planning and prediction of postoperative results. The software creates a pipeline to automatically construct meshed datasets for finite element modelling from presegmented patient data. In further parts of the system resulting deformations of soft tissue from surgical interventions and motion of bones are computed for visual and haptic display.

Keywords: Meshing, finite elements, biomechanic modelling

1. Introduction

Simulation of soft tissue deformations for virtual surgery has many applications in medicine. Preoperative simulation of interventions may be used to decide upon a best course of action while simulation of post operative outcomes can give a good idea of the functional effects of the operation (e.g. in maxillofacial or prosthetic knee surgery). A number of systems for these tasks have been proposed which either utilise mass spring type models [1], finite elements [2] or a combination thereof [3]. For accurate and stable prediction of soft tissue deformations finite element models are favoured although they have a number of drawbacks which special attention must be given to. First, with a large number of elements they become computationally expensive - this is especially important in view of the realtime aspect of virtual surgical simulators. Second, they rely on the quality of the underlying mesh for numerical stability. This leads to the conclusion that the mesh is a critical component in the makeup of the entire system. Most mesh generators operate on parametrized surfaces (e.g. [4],[5],[6]) which can be extracted from patient datasets. However the extraction usually leads to at a loss of detail. Additionally they generally set no hard limit on the number or quality of elements they create. The mesh generators proposed in this paper work directly on the volume data acquired from medical imaging devices, guarantee preset quality criteria and provide a mesh with a limited amount of elements. These three criteria set the best possible basis for accurate, fast and stable simulation of soft tissue deformation via finite element methods.

©CARS/Springer. All rights reserved.

2. Methodology

2.1 Overview of mesh creation

To create a mesh with the mentioned properties from voxel data five steps are performed. Initially, the maximum number of allowable elements and their lower quality criteria are set by the user. Then the data is subsampled to create a blocky representation. In a third step the subsampled data is meshed with hexahedra into an initial brick mesh. Further subdivison follows, depending on whether an all hexahedral or tetrahedral mesh is to be created. Finally, the mesh is grown to fit the contours of the original object while the interior nodes are relaxed to improve mesh quality.

2.2 Subdivision schemes

Depending on whether a tetrahedral or hexahedral mesh is to be created different subdivision schemes are employed. To create a tetrahedral mesh suitable for growth and relaxation each element of the initial brick mesh is subdivided into five tetrahedra (Fig. 1). Alternating neighbouring bricks between the shown split and its mirror image ensures consistency. A subdivision into 6 or even 12 tetrahedra without alternating configurations are also possible, but the quality of these elements is inferior and those subdivisions introduce a large number of extra elements.

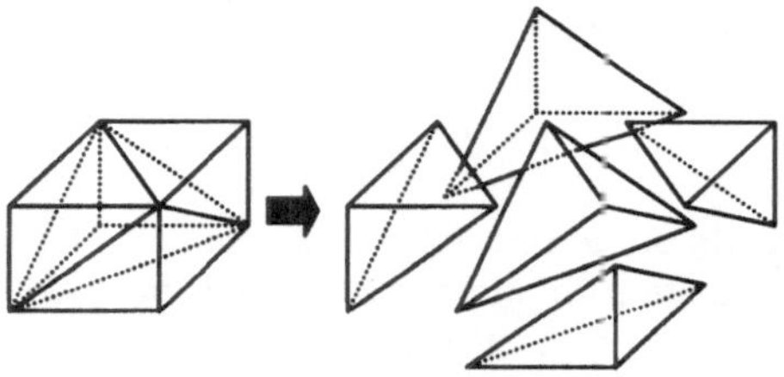

Fig. 1: Splitting of brick into 5 tetrahedra.

For hexahedral meshes the initial brick mesh is not ideal because we learned from creating tetrahedral meshes that any element which has more than one of its faces on the boundary of the initial mesh is in danger of becoming flattened during the growth phase. This would result in numerical instability for the following finite element simulation. Consequently for hexahedra a subdivision scheme is employed which guarantees that each created element has maximally only one such boundary surface. Bricks from the initial net are therefore divided into 8 or 32 elements (Fig. 2) depending on whether the brick has at most one or more than one of its sides on the initial mesh surface.

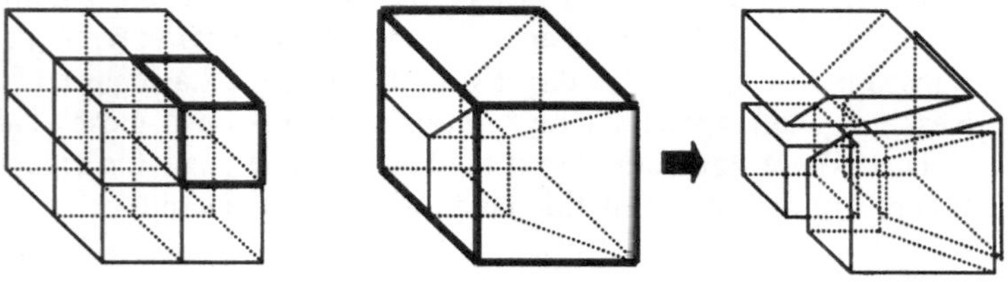

Fig. 2: Left: Subdivision of brick into 8 elements.
Middle and Right: Subdivision into 32 elements splits each subelement (bold) into 4 hexahedra.

©CARS/Springer. All rights reserved.

2.3 Subsampling and initial mesh creation

It is straightforward to create the initial brick mesh based on the voxels already present in the image data i.e. setting one brick per voxel (Fig. 3a). However, this would result in a mesh with an inordinate amount of elements defeating any attempts to achieve realtime performance in the following simulation step. Therefore a subsampling needs to be performed.

Medical image datasets from CT or MRi scanners usually have different spacing in x, y and z directions. In an anisotropic subsampling the subsampling rate of the coordinate axes are consecutively increased. The current axis stepwidth to increase by one is chosen so that the voxels in the output volume will be as cuboid as possible (Fig 3b). A filter is run over the volume using the current stepwidths for the axes which creates an element in the initial brick mesh if all of the voxels in the original volume within a stepwidth in x, y and z directions are part of the object. This ensures that in the growth phase only expansion of mesh will occur. A region growing algorithm extracts the largest connected area from the resulting brick mesh and estimates how many elements the final mesh will contain from the subdivision schemes proposed in 2.1. If the number of projected elements is larger than the maximum desired value then the process is repeated until a suitable coarsening of the volume is found (Fig 3 c)

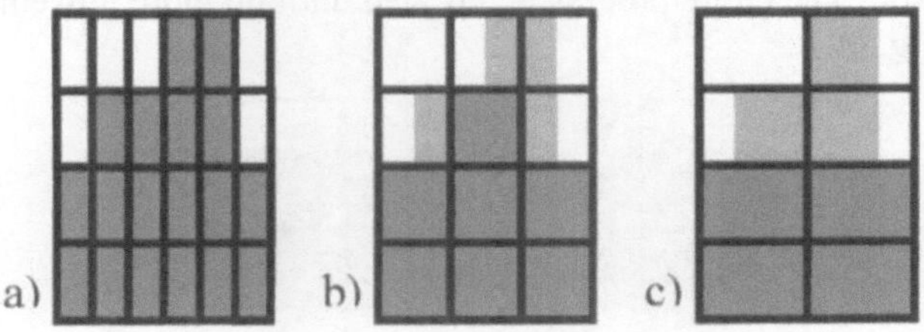

Fig. 3: 2D example of consecutive subsampling steps.
Grey: Object voxels. Dark grey: Areas that will produce a brick in the initial mesh.

2.4 Tetrahedral Mesh Generation

For possible post processing certain elements are tagged before growing the exterior mesh nodes to the image surface because they may be flattened during the process (Fig. 4). These critical elements can be indentified by having 3 border faces and consequently 4 border nodes (peak elements). If their quality drops below the set values they are simply eliminated.

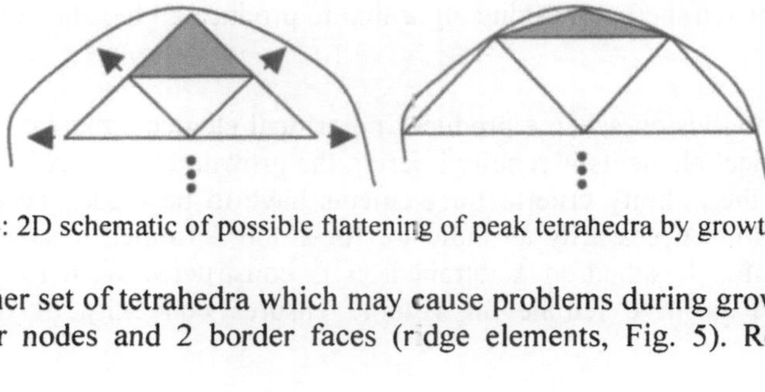

Fig. 4: 2D schematic of possible flattening of peak tetrahedra by growth process.

There is another set of tetrahedra which may cause problems during growth, namely those with 4 border nodes and 2 border faces (ridge elements, Fig. 5). Removing these is

©CARS/Springer. All rights reserved.

impossible because this would again create other peak or ridge tetrahedra which fit the removal criteria and so on until no elements are left. The only way to handle these dangerous elements is by limiting the node movement during the growth phase in a way to keep the tetrahedrons quality measurement within the specified limits.

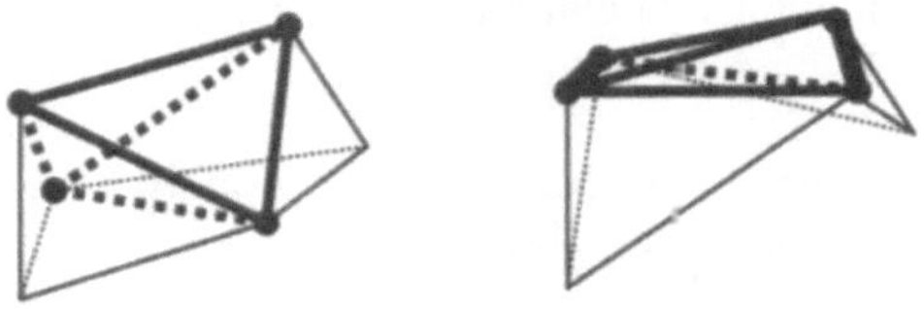

Fig. 5: Possible flattening of ridge tetrahedra by growth process if no limiting criteria are enforced.

Nodes on the surface of the mesh are grown in small steps towards the borders of the original image by moving in direction of the nearest contour voxel. During each step the validity of the elements is ascertained by checking for positive element volume, maximum and minimum angles as well as aspect ratio of the cell (weighted ratio of sum of side lengths to volume). If any of these criteria are violated movement of the relevant node is halted until the next microstep. Peak elements are removed as necessary. After each microstep interior nodes are relaxed to increase element quality with respect to interior angles and aspect ratio. The entire process is repeated until no more movement within the mesh takes place (Fig. 6).

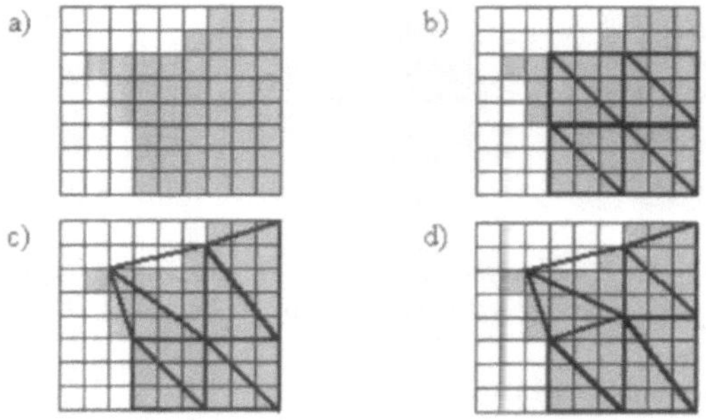

Fig. 6: a) Image data. b) Subsampling and tetrahedralization. c) Gowth of exterior nodes. d) Relaxation of interior nodes

2.5 Hexahedral Mesh Generation

[7] reports that in finite element simulations hexahedra outperform tetrahedra. Therefore the extension of the tetrahedral meshing algorithm to produce all hexahedral meshes is the next logical step.

The hexahedral subdivision scheme produces no critical elements therfore no tagging or elimination of critical elements is required during the growth and relaxation phases. Only small changes to the validity criteria for elements have to be made because a positive element volume is not necessarily an indicator for a non-deformed hexahedron. Instead, for each corner of a hexahedron a tetrahedron is constructed from the neighbouring element nodes. A positive tetrahedral volume ensures convexity of the corner. In

©CARS/Springer. All rights reserved.

conjunction with an adequate corner angle criterion - user defined minimum and maximum angles -. convexity of all 8 corner nodes guarantee a valid element.
Note: there is another possible subdivision which renders elements with only maximally one border surface, but these elements can be flattened irrecoverably. The above described subdivision leaves the mesh with the ability to relax interior nodes to keep the mesh valid even if the surrounding hexahedron is nearly completely flattened (Fig. 7).

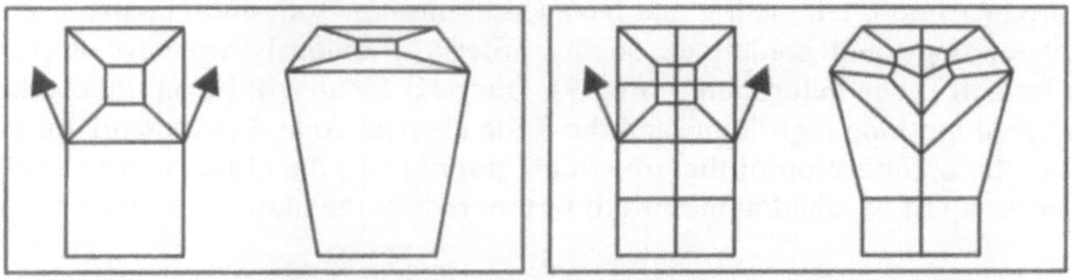

Fig. 7: Left: Alternative subdivision can still lead to individual elements being flattened
Right: Proposed subdivision retains good interior angles and can even relax into adjacent elements.

3. Results

Results from the tetrahedral meshing algorithm are promising for a range of synthetic and real datasets (Fig. 8). Results from the Hexahedral mesher are forthcoming.

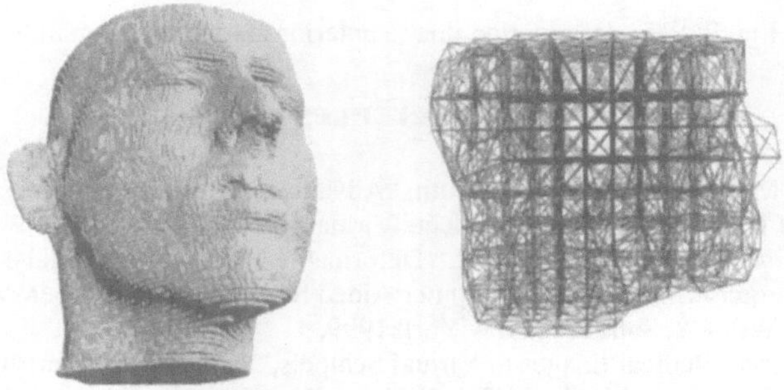

Fig. 8: Patient head meshed with tetrahedral mesher

One of the criteria we optimized the tetrahedral meshes for is the aspect ratio (1). Optimal aspect ratio for a tetrahedron is 1. For example tests on synthetic data (voxelized sphere) with a mesh made up of 276 elements show an average aspect ratio of 3.16 with the worst element having a ratio of 7.6 and 87% of all element ratios below 5. This indicates that while the original shape of the object can be closely approximated no invalid or even severely degenerate elements were created

$$A_Y = \frac{\left(\frac{1}{6} \sum_{i=1}^{6} l_i^2 \right)^{3/2}}{6\sqrt{2} \cdot V_{el}} \tag{1}$$

l_i : Edge lenghts

V_{el} : Volume of an element

©CARS/Springer. All rights reserved.

4 Discussion and future work

To put biomechanic modelling on a sound mathematical basis finite elements are the method of choice. High quality meshes with a relatively low number of elements are an important factor in retaining the ability for realtime virtual surgery simulations and the numerical stability during motion. We therefore have implemented a meshing algorithm which produces both tetrahedral and hexahedral meshes from digital patient images with arbitrary topology and predefined quality criteria. Previously we have implemented a system for soft tissue deformation (Fig. 9). Our next focus will be on the combination of the described meshing algorithms and the finite element code. Future work on the mesher will lie in the optimisation of the growth algorithm to fit the object more closely and the post-processing of hexahedral meshes to further reduce the number of elements produced.

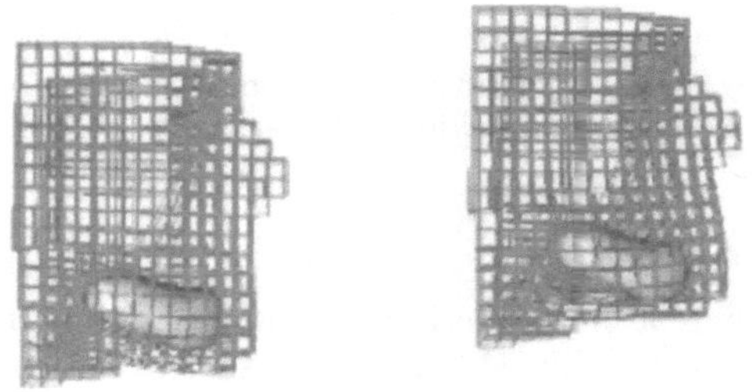

Fig. 9: Skin deformation due to anterior motion of the mandible.

References

1. C. Bruyns; K. Montgomery, S. Wildermuth, "Advanced Astronaut Training/ Simulation System for Rat Dissection," Medicine Meets Virtual Reality 2001
2. E. Keeve, S. Girod, R. Kikinis, B. Girod, "Deformable Modeling of Facial Tissue for Craniofacial Surgery Simulation," Computer Aided Surgery, invited paper, Vol. 3, No. 5, pp. 228-238, John Wiley & Sons Inc., New York,1999.
3. N. Ayache, "From Medical Images to Virtual Scalpels," caesarium, Bonn, 2001
4. T. Tautges, T. Blacker, S. Mitchell, "The Whisker Weaving Algorithm: A Connectivity-Based Method for Constructing All-Hexahedral Finite Element Meshes," International Journal for Numerical Methods in Engineering, Vol 39, pp. 3327-3349, Wiley, New York, 1996
5. X-Y.Li, T. Shang-Hua, A. Ungor, "Biting Spheres in 3D," Proceedings , 8th International Meshing Roundtable, pp. 85-95, October 1999
6. M. Katsuhiro and T. Blacker "Hexahedral Mesh Generation Using Multi-Axis Cooper Algorithm," Proceedings, 9th International Meshing Roundtable, Sandia National Laboratories, pp. 89-97, October 2000
7. S. Benzley, E. Perry, K. Merkley, B. Clark and G. Sjaardema "A Comparison of All-Hexahedral and All-Tetrahedral Finite Element Meshes for Elastic and Elasto-Plastic Analysis," Proceedings, 4th International Meshing Roundtable, Sandia National Laboratories, pp. 179-191, October 1995

CARS 2002 – H.U. Lemke, M.W. Vannier; K. Inamura, A.G. Farman, K. Doi & J.H.C. Reiber (Editors)
©CARS/Springer. All rights reserved.

Force feedback master arms, from telerobotics to robotics surgery training

J.P. Friconneau[1], M. Karouia[2], F. Gosselin[1],
Ph. Gravez[1], N. Bonnet[2], P. Leprince[2]
[1] CEA-LIST, CEN/FAR BP6, F92265 Fontenay-aux-Roses, France
[2] Cardiovascular Surgery Department, Pitié-Salpêtrière Hospital,
47-83, Bd de l'hôpital 75013 Paris, France

Abstract

Good performance of a force feedback input device is achieved when the surgeon would have the feeling in his hands of holding directly the surgical instruments interacting with the patient. This type of needs for high performance force feedback input device are similar to the requirement in telerobotics. In nuclear application, due to hazardous environment, remote operation are necessary. During maintenance phases, the operator should operate his set of tools remotely through a force feedback master/slave system. Advanced technics and technology have been developed sofar and many similarities could be pointed out with the surgical robotics applications. Therefore we aim benefits to apply this telerobotics background to develop surgical robotics systems. The development of a new input device calls first for a precise understanding of the application requirements. A complete bibliographic study as well as specific experiments were therefore undertaken to understand both the operators manipulative abilities (amplitude of movements, forces, bandwidth, …) and the requirements of the tasks to be done (workspace, environment's behaviour, …). A new methodology was then developed to use these information to obtain precise design guidelines for the master arm.

Keywords: Telerobotics, surgery, haptic device.

1. Introduction

Since 10 years, endoscopic surgery has deeply changed surgical practice. Absence of direct viewing and direct access to the workspace associated with reduced dexterity and sensory feedback led surgeons to develop new skills, requiring long experimental trainings on animals and cadavers. Robotics assisted surgery recently introduced in surgical blocks constitutes a new revolution in surgical practice and will also need a new training phase. In fact, surgeons need to become familiar both with robotics systems and the surgical techniques before moving to clinical applications. Moreover, animal and cadaver experiments are more and more difficult because of high costs, regulations and risks of contamination (AIDS, Creutzfeld Jacob). Finally, surgery training requires changes. Today, mentors have direct access to the field of operation. Tomorrow, when considering endoscopic surgery, direct action to assist trainee surgeons becomes hazardous due to lack of space. Training methods must therefore be reconsidered. Virtual Reality Technology, featuring haptic feedback through proper input devices, offers a

©CARS/Springer. All rights reserved.

particularly attractive solution as it will allow to develop surgical simulators allowing surgeons to learn and train with enhanced technics.

2. Master arm design requirement

A large consensus exists on the characteristics a 'good' input device must exhibit [1] [2] [3]. Whether considering virtual reality, telesurgery or heavy arms teleoperation, all authors have the same conclusions. A 'good' master arm must be 'transparent'. The operator must have the feeling that he performs the task directly in the remote environment. He must be free in unencumbered space (which requires a large and singularity free workspace, low inertia and low friction) and he must feel crisp contacts against the obstacles encountered by the slave arm (which requires a sufficient force feedback, a high bandwidth and a large stiffness).

All existing input devices were designed using these qualitative criteria. They exhibit, however, very different performances [4] [5] and are therefore more or less adapted to different applications. It is however essential in the design phase of an input device to know if it will fit a particular task efficiently. Precise requirements must thus be associated with each criterion.

In order to achieve this goal, we developed a method allowing the designer to specify the master arm and its control board (which drives data transmission between the operator and the slave arm, with or without advanced functions like amplifications, reductions or tremor cancellation) level of performance necessary to take advantage of the best operator's and slave arm's capacities within the limits of the desired tasks [6]. This method takes two types of limitations into account :

- Intrinsic limitations due to the operator's capacities : workspace, force range, position and force resolution are closely related with the operator. On one side, the ability of the master arm to generate movements or forces below the level of detection of an operator is useless but all significant information coming from the slave must be felt by the operator. On the other side, all the operator's voluntary movement or force must be measured but the operator's hand tremor computed on the slave side must be in accordance with the precision needed to perform all desired tasks with the slave arm.
- Limitations due to the master-slave system's characteristics : in teleoperation, the master arm must be designed in accordance to the slave arm. Its position resolution must be high enough to restore to the operator slave arm behaviour. Moreover, low friction (required for force resolution), mass and inertia drives comfortable feeling in the master side and efficiency on the slave side. Conversely, master arm electric stiffness must be tuned in a way that the slave limits of stability are always reached before the master ones. Finally, Master direct force and position bandwidths must be high enough to follow the operator's motor dynamics and to transmit all of his orders to the slave arm. Master inverse bandwidths must be higher than the sensitive bandwidth of the operator (considering the limitations introduced by the slave).

This method requires a correct understanding of both the operator's manipulative abilities and tasks to perform. This is necessary to extract precise specifications for the master arm

©CARS/Springer. All rights reserved.

which direct influence the master slave system performances. Main Master arm parameters are the workspace, the position resolution, the maximum force capacity and force resolution, and finally the electric stiffness, apparent mass and bandwidth.

3. Master arm design drivers

Once specified, the new input device must be designed according to these specifications. The design and optimisation of a robot are however quite complex problems as results depend on the parameters taken into account.

The first design driver taken into account is the workspace of the robot. It is defined as the set of configurations the robot can reach. To study this parameter, we scan the Cartesian space and check which positions the robot can effectively reach using its inverse geometric model $q=g(X)$. This model is used to tune the size of the robot until its workspace encompasses the specified workspace.
The second design driver to consider is the force capacity defined as the minimum amount of force applicable in any direction. To study this parameter, we use the notion of force ellipsoid defined as the operational forces produced by 1 N.m motor torques. Calling J_{mot} and G_{mot} the direct and inverse Jacobian matrices from motor to operational space, this ellipsoid can be defined by $F^T.(J_{mot}.J_{mot}^T).F \leq 1$. It allows to compute for each reachable configuration the minimum force the robot can apply in all directions. It is used to tune the reduction ratios until it is equal to the specified amount of force feedback.

The third design driver taken into account is the master arm's electric stiffness. It is defined as the minimum static gain in any direction deduced in the operational space from the maximum stable static gain of the motor's control loops. To study this parameter, we use the apparent stiffness ellipsoid defined as the operational forces produced by a normalised displacement (1m). Calling K_{mot} the motor static gain ($\tau_{mot}=K_{mot}.dq_{mot}$), this ellipsoid can be defined by $F^T.(K.K^T)^{-1}.F \leq 1$, with the apparent stiffness matrix $K=G_{mot}^T.K_{mot}.G_{mot}$. This ellipsoid allows to compute for each reachable configuration the minimum apparent stiffness in all directions. It is used to tune the reduction ratios until this stiffness is higher than specified.

Finally, the fourth design driver taken into account is the apparent mass of the robot. It is defined as the maximum mass experienced in all directions by the operator when moving the end tip of the robot in free space (the motor torques at zero). This parameter requires use of apparent mass ellipsoid defined as the operational forces produced by a normalised acceleration of 1 m/s^2. Calling $A_{mot}(q)$ the kinetic energy matrix of the robot, this ellipsoid can be defined by $F^T.(M.M^T)^{-1}.F \leq 1$, with the apparent mass matrix $M=G_{mot}^T.A_{mot}(q).G_{mot}$ computed under the following simplification assumptions : the centrifugal and Coriolis forces are neglected as the end tip of the robot manipulated by the operator experiences relatively small speeds and the gravity forces are neglected as the master arm will be statically balanced. This ellipsoid allows to compute for each reachable configuration the maximum apparent mass in all directions. It is used to optimise the size of the robot in order to minimise this maximum mass.

CARS 2002 – H.U. Lemke, M.W. Vannier; K. Inamura, A.G. Farman, K. Doi & J.H.C. Reiber (Editors)
©CARS/Springer. All rights reserved.

By means of four criteria, this methodology is based on a designer controlled constrained optimisation scheme that aim to minimise the apparent mass and the compactness. Optimisation parameters are the geometry and size, as well as joints torques and stiffness. The constraints are a given workspace and a minimum amount of force feedback and electric stiffness in every direction along full workspace.

4. Application in telerobotics and virtual reality

This method was first applied to design new master arm for real and simulated nuclear remote handling application. Input data, essential for the design, such as operator's manipulative abilities, were obtained from many data source such as medical science, ergonomics or robotics. Assuming remote handling application conditions, this drive the choice of the grasping interface of the master arm (Force grasping). As the master/slave system force reflective system is coupled, slave characteristics are essential for the master design. We took the assumption of the use of an electric robot such as a Staübli RX90 industrial robot. Using this information and considering a passive bilateral coupling scheme (both arms are reversible and torque controlled), we obtained the following design drivers [6].

	Design Drivers	Final Design	Identified Performances
Useful Workspace	300x300x300mm	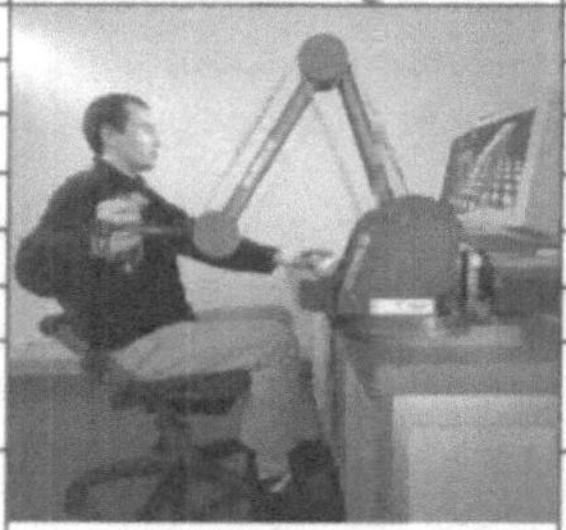	300x300x300 mm
Total Workspace			420x490x920 mm
Position resolution	60µm		
Force capacity	>40N full range		34 to 55 N
Force resolution	0.4N		0.3 to 0.6 N
Apparent mass	<500g full range		
Electric stiffness	>5000N/m full range		2350 to 6000 N/m
Mechanical stiffness			3650 to 7500 N/m
Bandwidth	16Hz		

Table 1 : Virtuose 3D Specifications

Several candidate structures were optimised to reach these specifications. The results obtained were used to design Virtuose 3D (cf. table 1). This master arm features a four bar mechanism serially connected to a rotational axis. This simple and efficient solution allows to obtain 3DOF with motors close to the base thus reducing inertia. Both arm and forearm are 350mm long as higher values increase cumbersomeness without significant mass decrease. It uses also capstan reducers. This technology allows to minimize clearance and friction. It limits however the reduction ratios that can be obtained in a small volume. As optimisation results exhibited such large reduction ratios, we choose to limit the force capacity in order to keep the device compact. Moreover, the structure is decoupled due to the use a centred wrist. This property allows ergonomic one hand operation as no cross-coupling between translations and rotations appears when moving the arm in free or encumbered space. As the first axis of the wrist is permanently maintained horizontal, this allows to reject singularity from the translational workspace.

©CARS/Springer. All rights reserved.

Finally, the arm and forearm are statically balanced using spiral springs. Virtuose 3D is thus less tiring and intrinsically safe.

First tests shows high transparency compared to existing systems. Friction and inertia are small enough to feel unencumbered space as free. Stiffness and force capacity are high enough to feel crisp contacts with the environment. A 6 degrees of freedom upgrade of this arm is now available on the market (V6D RV, www.haption.com).

5. Design of a new input device for telesurgery

Robotic telesurgery systems are basically composed of three main subsystems : the master console, the slave robot holding the endoscope and the surgical instruments and the communication channel conveying positions and efforts bilaterally between master and slave arms, allowing the slave arms to mimick human gesture and instrument/tissues interaction to be sensed through force/displacement feedback.

On the master side of the system, the surgeon is seated in front of a video monitor displaying images from the surgical site. He manipulates two master arms conveying his movements into orders for the slave robots, thus controlling the movements of surgical instruments as well as of the camera. In order to allow fine movements, a precision grasp is used (stylus grasp). Moreover, a support is provided to allow armrest manipulation. Design drivers associated with these constraints are summarized in table 2. They integrate and combine results obtained previously for telerobotics applications [6] and specific surgery constraints [7].

	Translation	Rotation	Design
Useful Workspace	200x200x200mm	160x160x180°	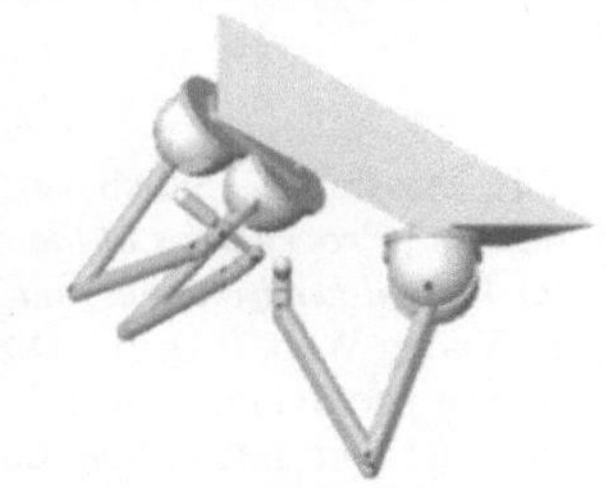
Force capacity	15N	1N.m	
Force resolution	0.15N		
Electric stiffness	2500N/m		

Table 2 : Virtuose 6D Design Drivers

A new input device satisfying these requirements is actually under development. This master arm is based on a parallel structure (cf. table 2) that exhibits particularly good performances while being simple to implement [6].

4. Conclusion

Robotics employed in the industrial field since many years is beginning to be used in the medical field. Existing robotic systems requires however improvements to be adapted to mini-invasive surgical procedures in order to increase the patient benefits. This evolution

©CARS/Springer. All rights reserved.

towards MIS procedures calls for telesurgery systems whose performance depends on the quality of the input device allowing the surgeon to control the system.
This evolution will also introduce a new and different way of surgery practice, which will probably require changes in methods of work and health organisations. In order to train and familiarize the medical staff (surgeons and operating room staff) to these new technologies, surgical simulators with realistic virtual models will be an efficient training tool.

The advances in VR technologies (real time simulation, complex numeric models, haptic interfaces...) will contribute to develop more and more realistic surgical simulators and optimize the training costs. Surgical simulators have a double benefit. Firstly, it will permit to minimize animal and cadaver experiments, and to provide nearly realistic training environment (virtual human anatomy, 3D models, force feedback, life simulation…). Secondly, the simulators will allow to search and develop new surgical techniques via pre-operative preparation. It will also allow to update surgeon skills (training, valuation) via scenarios simulation of special cases and emergency situations in operating room environment (patient, medical staff, nurses, materials…).

Performances of such simulators as well as performances of new telesurgery systems will however depend on input devices performances and adaptation to the tasks performed. We therefore developed new generic methodologies to design performant master arms. These tools were used to design a new input device for telerobotics and virtual reality (now available on the market). Based on the success of these methods, and due to the similarities between telerobotics and telesurgery requirements, we are now using these tools to design a new input device for telesurgery.

References

1. T.H. Massie, J.K. Salisbury, 'The PHANToM haptic interface : a device for probing virtual objects', *Proceedings of the ASME Winter Annual Meeting, Symposium on Haptic Interfaces for Virtual Environment and Teleoperator Systems*, Chicago, November 1994
2. K. Young Woo, B.D. Jin, D.S. Kwon, 'A 6-DOF force reflecting hand controller using the fivebar parallel mechanism', *Proceedings of the 1998 IEEE International Conference on Robotics and Automation*, Louvain, Belgium, pp1597-1602, May 1998
3. R. Baumann, R. Clavel, 'Haptic interface for virtual reality based minimally invasive surgery simulation', *Proceedings of the 1998 IEEE International Conference on Robotics and Automation*, Louvain, Belgium, pp381-386, May 1998
4. D.A. McAffee et P. Fiorini, 'Hand Controller Design Requirements and Performance Issues inTelerobotics', *ICAR 91, Robots in Unstructured Environments*, Pisa, Italy, pp186-192 ,June 1991
5. G. Burdea, P. Coiffet, 'La réalité virtuelle', Hermès Publishing, Paris, 1993
6. F. Gosselin, 'Développement d'outils d'aide à la conception d'organes de commande pour la téléopération à retour d'effort', Ph.D. diss. (in French), University of Poitiers, June 2000
7. L. Toledo, 'Analyse des Actions Elémentaires en chirurgie Endoscopique: Applications au Développement d'un Instrument Basé sur le Concept du Poignet Articulé', DEA diss. (in French), University Paris 5, 1995

CARS 2002 – H.U. Lemke, M.W. Vannier; K. Inamura, A.G. Farman, K. Doi & J.H.C. Reiber (Editors)
©CARS/Springer. All rights reserved.

The generalized implementation of virtual instruments for surgical simulation

Kevin Montgomery[a], Cynthia Bruyns[a,b], Anil Menon[a,b]
[a]National Biocomputation Center, Stanford University,
701A Welch Rd, Suite 1128, Palo Alto, CA 94305
[b]BioVIS Center, NASA Ames Research Center, Moffett Field, CA 94035

Abstract

The proliferation of surgical simulators would be increased if a common framework and set of virtual instruments existed for use by the application developer. We describe such a framework consisting of a powerful abstraction of a user interaction device, which can be attached to any virtual instrument. A functional taxonomy of instruments is also provided.
Keywords: Virtual instruments, surgical simulation.

1. Introduction

The benefits of computer-based surgical simulation have been widely discussed and quantitatively demonstrated by many researchers. The benefits include the ability to broaden surgical training by easily providing different training scenarios, objectively quantify surgical performance, and accelerate the acquisition of baseline surgical skills without risk to real patients.

Two key areas of implementation for these simulators are the interface to user interaction devices (such as haptic and non-haptic tracking devices) and the development of virtual instruments. As in other areas of development, each research group must implement this infrastructure and this time consuming, repetitious, and error-prone coding takes time and resources away from development of the simulation application itself.

Instead, the field would derive great benefit from a general framework for tools and device interface. Functionally, this framework should support mapping from any hardware device to a suite of virtual instruments, to allow any available hardware to control any required surgical instrument.

The purpose of this paper is to describe such a framework that is part of a simulation system which we have been developing called ***Spring***[1]. The system has been used to develop a number of applications[2-7] and been refined and enhanced over time. It is our intent to share these details of implementation and to release the code and corresponding virtual instruments in order to help the field achieve faster development and, hopefully, greater proliferation and adoption within the medical community.

©CARS/Springer. All rights reserved.

2. Methods

The Spring surgical simulator is cross-platform and runs on Unix (Sun Solaris, SGI Irix, and Linux) and Windows (98/NT/2000/XP) platforms. It is written in C++ and uses OpenGL for graphics; GLUT, GLUI, and MUI for user interface; and supports parallel processing. It allows for the easy introduction of patient-specific anatomy and supports many common file formats. It performs soft-tissue modeling[8], limited rigid-body dynamics, and suture modeling[8]. The simulator interfaces to many different interaction devices and provides for multi-user, multi-instrument collaboration over the Internet. Many surgical and non-surgical virtual tools have been created and their interactions with tissue have been implemented. Collision detection is provided through an enhanced[9] bounding-sphere algorithm[10]. In addition, extra features such as voice input/output, real-time texture-mapped video input, stereo and head-mounted display support, and replicated display/rendering facilities are provided.

2.1 Device I/O

One key element in the production of a surgical simulator is the interface to the user. While many devices exist, the appropriate device depends upon the surgical application. However, in order to provide a general simulation framework, a generalized method of device I/O is also needed.

2.2 Abstraction: Sensor Class

A Sensor is an abstraction of a 6D tracking and/or haptic device. It contains a position in 3D space, along with orientation information (rotation matrix). In addition, it contains an array of floating-point activation values to store information from any buttons, handles, or other controllers associated with the device. For interfacing with haptic devices, the Sensor class also contains a 'force' variable, which is the force vector that should be applied upon the device. A Sensor can then be linked to a particular virtual object (typically a virtual instrument such as a scalpel, scissors, etc) and, when that object is updated, it will derive its new position/orientation from the Sensor value and articulate its parts based on the activation values. After collision detection and resolution has taken place, the simulation can then send the appropriate force vector back to the device for haptic rendering. This abstraction is powerful because it insulates the simulation from the particular haptic hardware that the user happens to have and provides a flexible framework for mapping devices to virtual instruments.

2.3 Local Sensors

The Sensor superclass is inherited by subclasses that communicate directly with their individual devices. These include haptic and non-haptic devices such as electromagnetic trackers, inertial trackers, mechanical trackers. Each of these devices can be plugged into the computer using its native method, yet Spring is isolated from dealing with the communications protocol and interfacing issues. In any case, the subclass instantiation implements the communication with the device and fills in the position, orientation, and activation values of the Sensor superclass.

©CARS/Springer. All rights reserved.

2.4 Networked Haptics/Sensors

Because many devices can only be interfaced through methods available only on PC platforms, and due to the desire to have the simulation capable of running on the most appropriate (perhaps non-PC) hardware, the system also provides for a network-based module that communicates with a sensor or haptic server program running on a different (perhaps dedicated) computer over the network. In this way, we can decouple the interfacing restrictions of these devices from the simulation itself[11].

When the network sensor is created, it forms a TCP/IP connection with the hapticserver computer. Then, as the simulation processes, the hapticserver sends the position, orientation, and activation values over the network, which, in turn, updates the Sensor fields in the simulator. Then, as the simulator processes the object (virtual instrument) and any collisions it may be experiencing, it calculates the resulting haptic force and updates a force vector value within the Sensor. Upon the next sensor update, this value is sent to the haptic device where the force is rendered. Note that this streaming forces model is dependent upon the latency of the network and this latency produces an upper bound on the haptic update rate. In a local-area network at 100Mbps, we have noted over 5000 updates per second, but clearly, as one moves to a wide-area network, router, signal propagation and congestion-based delays will quickly begin to impact this update rate. For these reasons, we have also developed other, latency-moderated methods for wide-area, networked haptics[12].

This method of network-based sensor- and hapticservers inherently provides for multi-user and multi-instrument interaction and easily supports collaborative procedures. No matter what the method of device interface may be, the Sensor is assured of having the most recent information possible and this information can be used to define the position, orientation, and articulation of virtual instruments within the simulation.

2.5 Virtual Instruments

Virtual instruments are specified in geometry files in industry-standard formats (SMF, STL, Wavefront, Mesh, Cyberware, Inventor, VRML). Within each file, geometrically disconnected components denote the subparts of an object.

When a particular instrument is selected by the user, its geometry is read in and the subpart information is maintained by the simulation. The virtual instrument is then linked to a particular Sensor that it will later use to articulate and transform itself based upon this information. The location of the attachment point of the sensor to the virtual instrument is given as the *sensor offset* of the tool.

In order to generalize the implementation of these instruments, it is first necessary to classify surgical instruments into functional categories, based upon their methods of operation. These instrument classes are defined below.

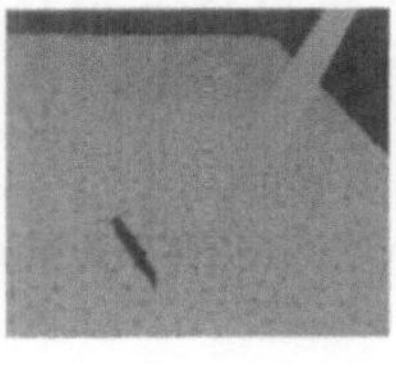

Some instruments are *monolithic* (such as a scalpel, dilator, probe, retractor, etc) and, as the name implies, have a single part and no dependence upon the activation value of their attached Sensor. They

©CARS/Springer. All rights reserved.

merely transform themselves based on the rotation matrix and position value provided by the Sensor.

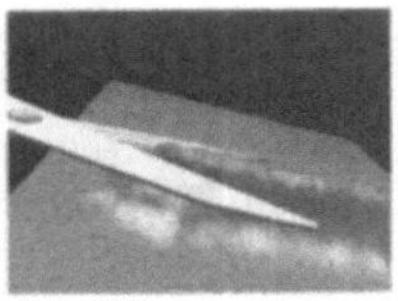

A typical *hinged* tool (forceps, scissors, endoscopic scissors, graspers) may have 3 parts: one part that will rotate with a positive angle based on the activation value, one part that will rotate with a negative angle based on that value, and one part that is not dependent upon the activation value (for the shaft of a grasper or for the hinge itself). A *multihinged* tool (such as a 3-prong grasper) may have multiple articulating subparts dependent upon a single activation value, along with a fixed component. Both of these classifications are implemented with an identical, underlying framework.

For each hinge, we specify the hinge location, axis of rotation, and activation value upon which it depends. We then provide the list of subparts that are dependent upon that hinge (if the subpart id provided is negative, it denotes that it should move with the negative angle of the hinge). Therefore, when the object is transformed, the individual subparts are transformed by the hinge on which they depend first, then are transformed by the overall rotation/position information of the sensor.

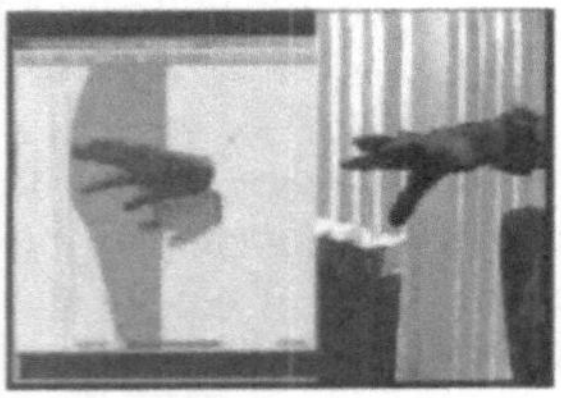

Note that some tools are *dependent-hinged* (for example, a multiaxis endoscopic grasper, or a grasping hand), where the location of one hinge is dependent upon another. In this case, a particular subpart can have multiple hinges upon which it depends and, when updated by the simulation, each particular subpart will be transformed by each hinge, in order, and finally by the overall rotation/position of the Sensor.

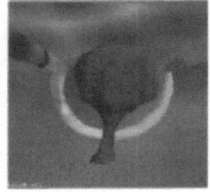

Telescoping instruments, (such as a resectoscope or plunger of a syringe) have one part that slides in relation to another, based upon the activation value of the attached Sensor. In this case, the direction vector and minimum and maximum values along that vector are specified. The activation value is then used to parameterize a translation along this vector of the subpart before it is transformed by the overall rotation/position information.

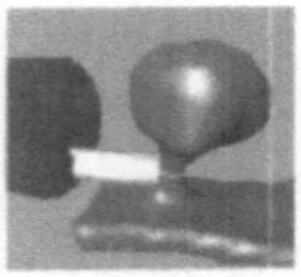

A *lasso* instrument (such as a biopsy snare) has a fixed part, and one that constricts based upon the activation value. In this case, the lasso is modeled as a set of nodes with single edges between them which constrict based upon the activation value specified.

Some tools are *combinations* of these classes (for example, have hinged telescoping parts) and are implemented by mixing and matching the techniques above. Finally, some instruments are *multitools*, which have working channels for the insertion of tools of the kinds stated above.

This facility provides a general framework for the interfacing of a vast array of virtual instruments to their corresponding devices through the abstraction of the *Sensor* class. The

©CARS/Springer. All rights reserved.

details of how these instruments interact with virtual tissue is described in greater detail elsewhere[1-7].

3.0 Results

All major haptic and non-haptic tracking devices have been integrated within the system using this framework. This includes all haptic devices from Sensable Technologies (Phantom) and Immersion Corporation (LapIE, Bimanual LapIE, 3GM), as well as tracking devices from Ascension Technologies (Flock of Birds, pcBird), Polhemus (FasTrak), Immersion (Microscribe, CyberGloves), InterSense (InterTrax), among others. These devices operate at their peak rates with optimized drivers and effectively insulate the main simulator from the many nuances of communication that are required.

In addition, a large number of virtual instruments have been created (currently over 85). These virtual tools are easily linked with the device-based Sensors, articulate effectively with the activation values, and are available within any simulation application.

Monolithic	*Hinged/Multi*	*Dependent Hinged*	*Telescoping*	*Lasso*	*Miscellaneous*
Scalpels/Saws	Forceps	Multiaxis grasper	Syringes	Biopsy snares	*Combo Tools*
Dilators	Scissors	Hands	Resectoscopes		*Multitools*
Probes/Picks	Endo graspers	Virtual robot	Roller ablators		Sutures
Retractors	Endo scissors		Loop cautery		Stents
Needles, Hooks, rasp	Needle holders, Shears, clamps, clip				Pens, Pipettes

Table 1: Implemented virtual instruments, by class

For example, the Immersion LapIE device has an endoscopic handle for user interaction and, as this handle is opened and closed, the linked virtual instrument (e.g., an endoscopic grasper) similarly opens and closes smoothly. A virtual instrument can also easily provide an endoscopic view by rendering graphics from the tip of the instrument.

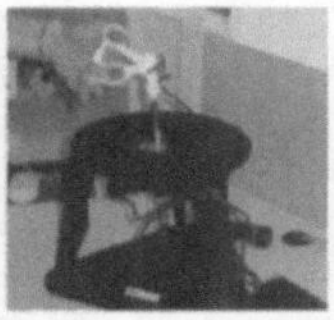

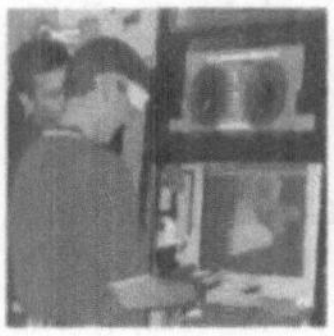

As a further example, the Immersion CyberGlove input devices can be worn by a user and the values of the user's hand joint angles are provided as a set of activation values stored in the Sensor. This is then provided to a virtual instrument (a virtual hand), which similarly uses the activation values to smoothly articulate its joints.

An instrument with spinning parts (such as a drill) can also be easily represented in this framework. In this case, the value used for articulating the part is not an activation value of the attached sensor, but can be based on a timer or counter variable.

4. Conclusion

We have presented a flexible framework for the interfacing of haptic and non-haptic devices and a method for the generalized implementation of virtual instruments. This framework allows for the realistic implementation of a large number of virtual

©CARS/Springer. All rights reserved.

instruments, and has been refined and enhanced while developing a number of applications. It is our intent to not only present this method, but to release the code and the suite of instruments to the wider surgical simulation community in order to facilitate collaboration, speed development, and hopefully contribute to the ultimate adoption of surgical simulators within the medical curriculum.

Acknowledgements

The authors would like to thank Julien Durand, CJ Slyfield and the BioVIS lab (NASA Ames Research Center), Simon Wildermuth (IDR, Zurich), Leroy Heinrichs and Parvati Dev (SUMMIT) and Michael Stephanides and Stephen Schendel (Stanford). This work was supported by grants from NASA (NCC2-1010), NIH (NLM-3506, HD38223), NSF (IIS-9907060), and a generous donation from Sun Microsystems.

References

1. Montgomery, K; Bruyns, C; Brown, J; Sorkin, S; Mazzella, F; Thonier, G; Tellier, A; Lerman, B; Menon, A; "Spring: a General Framework for Collaborative, Real-time Surgical Simulation", Medicine Meets Virtual Reality(MMVR02), Newport Beach, California,Jan 2002.
2. Montgomery, K; Bruyns, C; Wildermuth, S; Hasser, C; Ozenne, S; Bailey, D; Heinrichs, L; "Surgical Simulator for Hysteroscopy: A Case Study of Visualization in Surgical Training", IEEE Visualization 2001, San Diego, California, October 21-26, 2001.
3. Montgomery, K; Heinrichs, L; Bruyns, C; Wildermuth, S; Hasser, C; Ozenne, S; Bailey, D; "Surgical Simulator for Operative Hysteroscopy and Endometrial Ablation", Computer-Aided Radiology and Surgery (CARS 2001), Berlin, Germany, June 27, 2001.
4. Montgomery, K; Stephanides, M; Brown, J; Latombe, JC; Schendel, S; "A Virtual Environment for Training in Microsurgery", SPIE, v3639(1), pp. 398-403, Jan 1999.
5. Brown, J; Montgomery, K; Latombe, JC; Stephanides, M; "A Microsurgery Simulation System", Medical Image Computing and Computer-Assisted Interventions (MICCAI 2001), Utrecht, The Netherlands, October 14-17, 2001.
6. Bruyns, C; Montgomery, K; Wildermuth, S; "A Virtual Environment for Simulated Rat Dissection: A Case Study of Visualization for AstronautTraining", IEEE Visualization 2001, San Diego, California, October 21-26, 2001.
7. Montgomery, K; Stephanides, M; Schendel, S; "Development and application of a virtual environment for reconstructive surgery", Journal of Computer-Aided Surgery, v5(2), ISSN: 1092-9088, 2000, pp:90-97.
8. Brown, J; Sorkin, S; Bruyns, C; Latombe, JC, Montgomery, K; Stephanides, M; "Real-Time Simulation of Deformable Objects: Tools and Application", Computer Animation 2001, Seoul, Korea, November 6-8, 2001.
9. Sorkin, S; "Distance Computation Between Deformable Objects", Honors Thesis, Computer Science Department, Stanford University, June 2000.
10. Quinlan, S, "Efficient Distance Computation Between Nonconvex Objects", Proc. IEEE Int Conf on Robotics and Automation, pp. 3324-3329, 1994.
11. Montgomery, K; Lerman, B; Stephanides, M; Schendel, S; "Haptic Devices in Medical Applications", 2nd International Workshop on Haptic Devices in Medical Applications, Computer Assisted Radiology and Surgery (CARS), July 1, 2000.
12. Mazzella, F; Montgomery, K; Latombe, JC; "The Forcegrid; A Buffer Structure for Haptic Interaction with Virtual Elastic Objects", 2002 IEEE International Conference on Robotics and Automation, Washington DC, May 11-15, 2002.

CARS 2002 – H.U. Lemke, M.W. Vannier; K. Inamura, A.G. Farman, K. Doi & J.H.C. Reiber (Editors)
©CARS/Springer. All rights reserved.

Models of the human heart for simulation of clinical interventions

F.B. Sachse, G. Seemann, M.B. Mohr, L.G. Blümcke, C.D. Werner
Institut für Biomedizinische Technik, Universität Karlsruhe (TH)
76128 Karlsruhe, Germany
E-mail: Frank.Sachse@ibt.uni-karlsruhe.de

Abstract

Detailed models of the human heart are introduced which can serve in conjunction with virtual reality techniques as basis for the simulation of cardiac interventions. The models describe the anatomy, electrical excitation propagation and force development. The anatomical models were constructed with methods of digital image processing basing on photographic images delivered by the Visible Human Project, National Library of Medicine, USA. Appropriate models of electrophysiology and force development are chosen subject to the tissue types. The models are applied to simulate electrical and mechanical processes in the heart.

Keywords: Human heart model, cardiac electrophysiology, cardiac force development, surgical interventions

1. Introduction

The simulation of clinical interventions can be a valuable tool for the development and assessment of therapeutic strategies as well as for educational purposes. Particularly, the computer based simulation of cardiological interventions offers information, which are not directly accessible neither in patients nor in animal models. Computer based simulations allow the examination and optimization of therapeutic strategies as well as their comparison with pharmaceutical interventions.

The physiologic function of the heart necessitates regular, coupled electric and mechanical processes, which are strongly dependent on the variant anatomical structures. In pathophysiologic cases the heart shows irregular processes and the anatomy can be altered. The advances in computing resources as well as the availability of detailed measurement data allow the simulation of the physiology as well as of the pathophysiology of the human heart with increasing realism. Simulations of the whole heart necessitates knowledge concerning the macroscopic distribution of tissue and the orientation of cardiac cells.

In this work highly detailed anatomical models of the human heart are presented in conjunction with efficient models of the electrical excitation propagation and the force development. Appropriate models of electrophysiology are chosen subject to the tissue types. The models are applied to simulate electrical and mechanical processes in the heart. In conjunction with virtual reality techniques the models can serve as basis for the simulation of cardiac interventions.

©CARS/Springer. All rights reserved.

2. Modeling

2.1.1. Anatomical Modeling

The basis of this work form two anatomical heart models, which were constructed with methods of digital image processing basing on photographic images delivered by the Visible Human Project, National Library of Medicine, USA [1,2,3,4]. The images show transversal views of the cadavers of a 38 year old man and a 59 year old woman. Each image consists of 2048 x 1280 pixels with 24 bit color information. The stack of 2D cryosection images was pre-processed to obtain 3D-data sets. The 3D-data set was segmented and classified using different techniques of digital image processing, e.g. interactively deformable contours, thresholding, region growing, and morphological operators.

The anatomical models include the orientation of fibers of the myocardium [3]. The determined fiber orientation can be viewed as the averaged macroscopic orientation of the principal axis of the cardiac muscle cells (myocytes). The orientation of myocardial fibers was interpolated based on sets of restrictions. The sets of restrictions were determined with automatic methods inside and on the surface of myocardial structures. For each structure an individual rule-based method was chosen. The rules were derived from anatomical studies.

Special focus was given to the excitation conduction system, which is of importance for the electrical excitation process through the heart. The excitation conduction system was constructed manually and with rule-based techniques [5]. The system is partly represented in a tree like data structure.

The models and the processing tools are resulting from the MEET Man project (Models for Simulation of Electromagnetic, Elastomechanic and Thermal Behavior of Man), a project of the Institut für Biomedizinische Technik, Universität Karlsruhe (TH), Germany [4]. The purpose of this project is the creation of models for computer-based simulation of the physical behavior of man.

2.1.2. Modeling of Cardiac Electrophysiology and Force Development

The electrical excitation propagation and the force development in the heart are simulated with a so-called cellular automaton consisting of a regular, discrete, infinite network representing the underlying spatial structure, i.e. the volumetric model of cardiac anatomy and the tree like data structure of the excitation conduction system, and a finite automaton working at each node, so-called cell, of the network [5].

The cellular automaton is parameterized by numerical experiments with continuum electrophysiologic and excitation-contraction coupling models [5,6]. Therefore, a large number of numerical simulations was performed varying the cell model and the frequency of an electrical stimulus.

The simulations deliver tissue and stimulus frequency specific courses of the cellular transmembrane voltage, of the excitation velocity and of the force development in the contractile units of the myocytes. The ventricular and atrial cellular electrophysiology is described with recently developed, mathematical models, e.g. derived from measurements in human ventricles and atria, resp.. The force development is reconstructed with mathematical models basing on the simulations of cellular electrophysiology [8].

©CARS/Springer. All rights reserved.

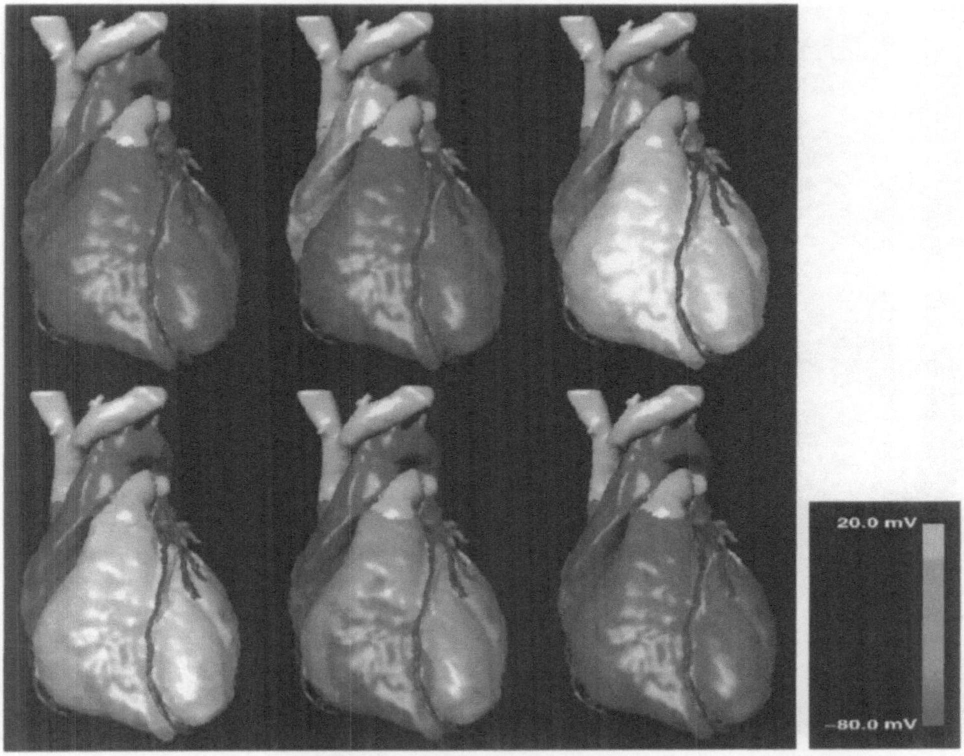

Fig. 1: Electrical excitation of human heart at different time steps. The distribution of transmembrane voltage of myocytes is visualized at surface of Visible Man heart model. The excitation starts at the sinus node, propagates over the atria and via specialized pathways over the ventricles. The palette at right side shows the coding of the transmembrane voltages.

3. Results

Two models of the cardiac anatomy are available. The model of the Visible Man heart is represented in a three dimensional data set consisting of approximately 360,000 cubic voxels with a size of 1 mm x 1 mm x 1 mm. Each voxel was assigned to one out of 16 different tissue classes, e.g. left and right ventricle, left and right atrium, arterial and venous blood, and fat as well as different kinds of vessels. The model of the Visible Female heart is stored in a three dimensional data set, which consists of approximately 80 million cubic voxels. Each voxel has a size of 0.33 mm x 0.33 mm x 0.33 mm and was assigned to one out of 20 different tissue classes. The models can be reduced to fulfill requirements concerning computing and storage demands.
The models are applied for the simulation of the electrical excitation propagation and force development. The result of a simulation with the cellular automaton is the temporal and spatial distribution of the intracellular and extracellular electrophysiologic states, e.g. the transmembrane voltage, for each voxel (see Fig. 1 and 2). Furthermore, the developed force can be calculated (see Fig. 3 and 4). The simulations can be performed both in the whole heart as in specific regions.

©CARS/Springer. All rights reserved.

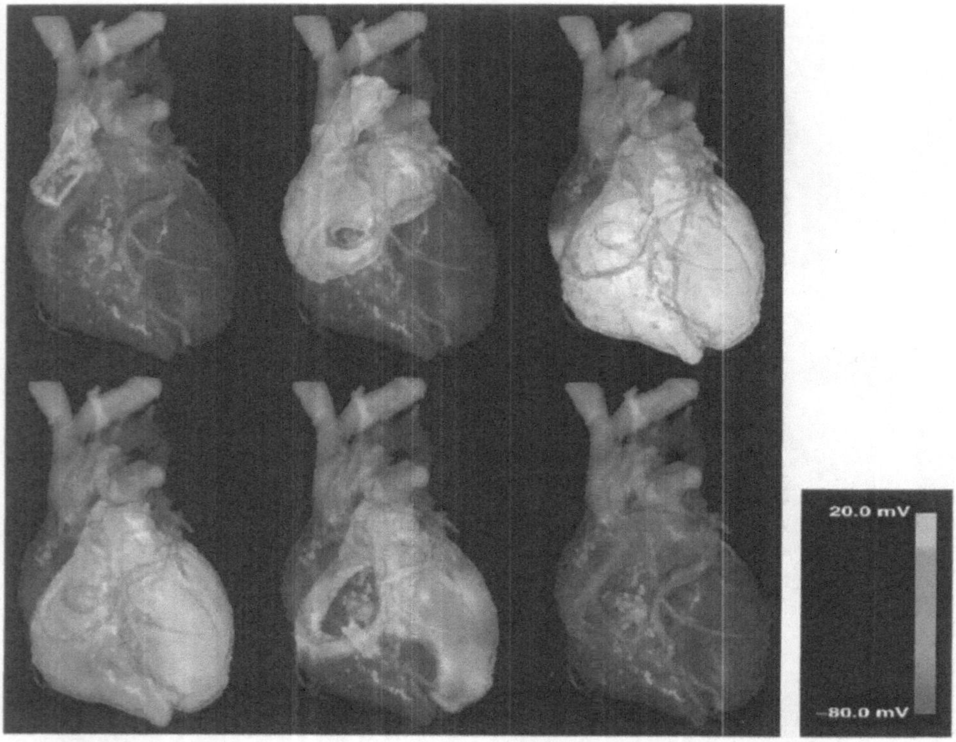

Fig. 2: Electrical excitation of human heart in volume-based representation. The distribution of transmembrane voltage in the heart is visualized at different time steps. The excitation starts at the sinus node, propagates over the atria and via specialized pathways over the ventricles.

4. Discussion and Conclusions

The high spatial resolution of the models and the detailed description of the cardiac anatomy enhances the repertoire of anatomical models of the human heart. Particularly, the incorporation of the myocardial fiber orientation makes the models of interest for applications in the scope of surgical planning and medical education. The model can be applied for the simulation of radio-frequency (RF) ablation for the treatment of atrial and ventricular flutter [5]. The model can provide important information concerning cardiological interventions, surgical corrections and pharmaceutical therapies in conjunction with their influence on the cardiac electrophysiology and mechanical contraction [6,7].

Furthermore, the models can be applied in simulations of elasto- and fluid-mechanics as well as microscopic electrophysiology of the human heart [8,9]. Therefore, a change of the model representation might be necessary, e.g. to surface and irregular volume meshes. Of interest in future works is the adaptation of the models to patient data by inclusion of medical images and multi channel electrocardiograms. Furthermore, the inclusion of elastomechanical models and of electro-mechanical feedback mechanisms can prove to be of advantage for specific applications [8].

©CARS/Springer. All rights reserved.

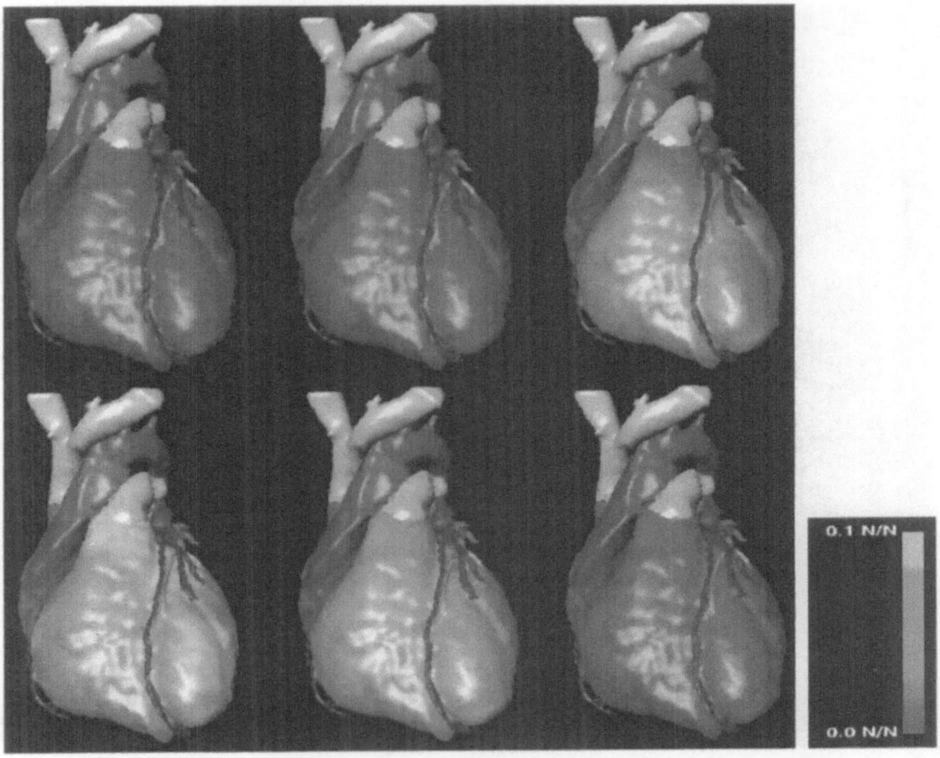

Fig. 3: Force development in human heart at different time steps. The distribution of forces developed in myocytes is visualized at heart surface. The palette at right side shows the coding of the forces. The force is normalized with the maximal developable forces and acts in fiber direction.

Acknowledgements

The Rechenzentrum, Universität Karlsruhe (TH), particularly Mr. R. Mayer, supported our work by providing the necessary visualization and computing resources.

References

1. M.J. Ackerman "Viewpoint: The Visible Human Project", *Journal Biocommunication*, Vol. 18, No. 2, page 14, 1991
2. F.B. Sachse, M. Glas, M. Müller, and K. Meyer-Waarden, "Segmentation and tissue-classification of the Visible Man dataset using the computertomographic scans and the thin-section photos", *Proc. 1st Users Conference of the National Library of Medicine's Visible Human Project*, 1996.
3. F.B. Sachse, C.D. Werner, M.H. Stenroos, R.F. Schulte, P. Zerfass, and O. Dössel, "Modeling the anatomy of the human heart using cryosection images of the Visible Female dataset", *Proc. Third Users Conference of the National Library of Medicine's Visible Human Project*, 2000.
4. MEET-Man Project, IBT, Karlsruhe, http://www-ibt.etec.uni-karlsruhe.de/forschung/meetman
5. C.D. Werner, *Simulation der elektrischen Erregungsausbreitung in anatomischen Herzmodellen mit adaptiven zellulären Automaten*, PhD thesis, Universität Karlsruhe (TH), Institut für Biomedizinische Technik, TANEA, Berlin, 2001.

©CARS/Springer. All rights reserved.

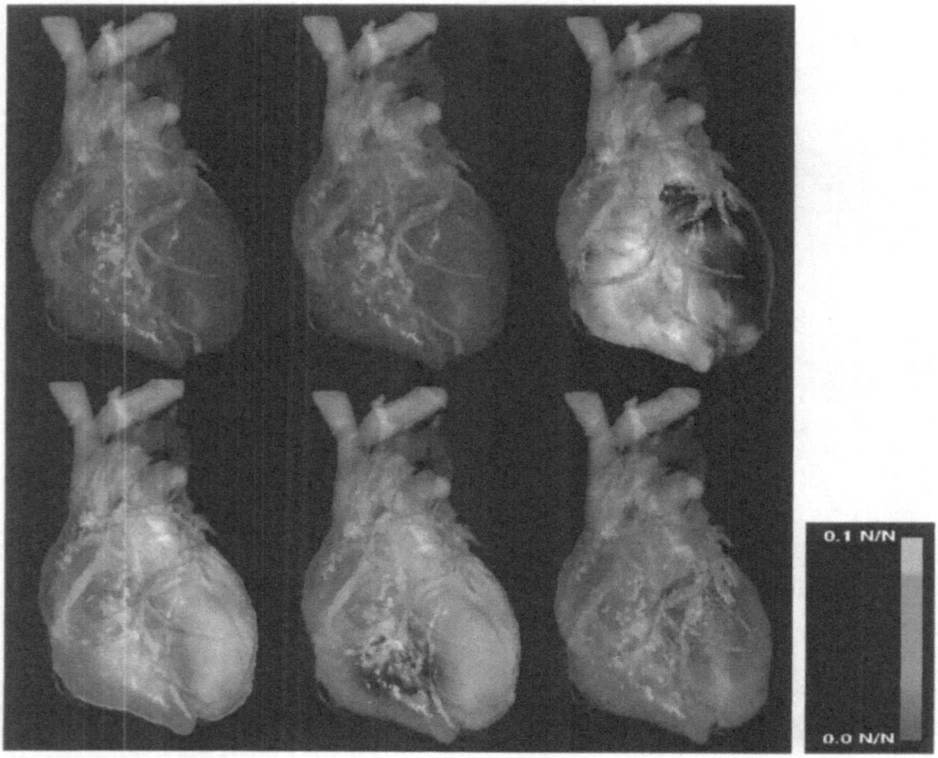

Fig. 4: Force development in human heart in volume-based representation. The distribution of forces developed in myocytes is visualized at different time steps.

6. F.B. Sachse, C.D. Werner, and G. Seemann, "Simulation of cardiac electrophysiology and electrocardiography", *Computer Simulation and Experimental Assessment of Cardiac Electrophysiology*, N. Virag, O. Blanc, and L. Kappenberger, pages 97–104, Futura Publishing, Armonk, New York, 2001.
7. G. Seemann, F.B. Sachse, C.D. Werner, and O. Dössel, " Simulation of surgical interventions: Atrial radio frequency ablation with a haptic interface ", *Proc. CARS 2002*, H.U. Lemke, M.W. Vannier; K. Inamura, A.G. Farman, K. Doi and J.H.C. Reiber, Springer, Berlin, 2002.
8. F. B. Sachse, G. Seemann, C. Riedel, C. D. Werner, and O. Dössel. Modeling of the cardiac mechano-electrical feedback. Int. J. Bioelectromagnetism, 2(2), 2000.
9. F. B. Sachse, G. Seemann, and C. D. Werner. Combining the electrical and mechanical functions of the heart. Int. J. Bioelectromagnetism, 3(2), 2001.

CARS 2002 – H.U. Lemke, M.W. Vannier; K. Inamura, A.G. Farman, K. Doi & J.H.C. Reiber (Editors)
©CARS/Springer. All rights reserved.

Simulation of surgical interventions: atrial radio frequency ablation with a haptic interface

G. Seemann, F.B. Sachse, C.D. Werner, O. Dössel
Institut für Biomedizinische Technik, Universität Karlsruhe (TH)
76128 Karlsruhe, Germany
E-mail: Gunnar.Seemann@ibt.uni-karlsruhe.de

Abstract

A prototype of a real-time simulation environment for atrial radio frequency ablation therapy with a haptic interface is presented. The environment can be used to plan surgical interventions and to educate physicians in using ablation therapy with respect to the cardiac electrophysiology. Therefore, the electrophysiology is simulated with a time efficient cellular automaton on a human heart model. The cellular automaton is also capable of simulating pathologies, like atrial flutter and tachycardia. The electrophysiological properties can be changed interactively by applying virtually ablation therapy with the haptic interface. The electrophysiological states of the heart model and the virtual operation tool are visualized nearly in real-time. An exemplary simulation of the atrial radio frequency ablation is presented in this work.

Keywords: Human heart model, cellular automaton, virtual reality

1. Introduction

Atrial flutter is an electrical intra-atrial re-entrant mechanism frequently including an anatomical obstacle, e.g. the venae cavae, the tricuspid valve ring or previously applied surgical incisions [1]. It leads to a reduced contraction of the atrium and therefore to a reduced filling of the ventricles. Nearly 0.4 percent of the populations of industrial nations suffer from atrial flutter [2]. Atrial flutter is in medium term not a critical cardiac pathology but it leads to an increasing mortality in the long term and reduces the competitiveness of the patient. Frequently, radio frequency (RF) ablation therapy via a catheter is used to terminate atrial flutter [3]. Therefore, radio frequency currents are applied to destroy the excitability of the surrounding cells. A large number of patients are not healed, because the pathways of the pathologic excitation propagation are not terminated completely or the flutter uses other pathways.

Aim of this work is to provide a simulation environment in virtual reality for surgical interventions for the treatment of atrial flutter. Therefore, the cardiac excitation propagation and the effects of the therapy on the electrophysiology are considered. The environment consists of an anatomical heart model, a model for simulating cardiac electrophysiology, a haptic interface to interact with the models, a visualization tool and a graphic workstation to run the tools efficiently in parallel. The electrophysiological model is a rule based adaptive cellular automaton. It allows efficient simulations in large and complex models.

Within the final version of this environment, the catheterization of the virtual patient will be included. Finally, it should be possible to plan and verify surgical interventions on individual patient data sets and educate physicians in using ablation therapy.

©CARS/Springer. All rights reserved.

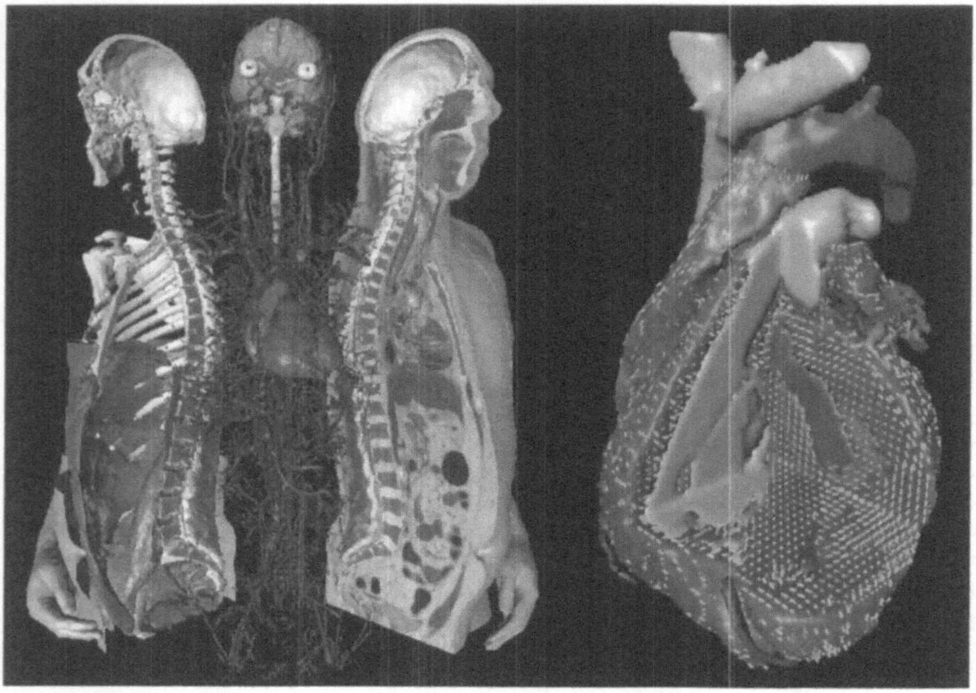

Fig. 1: (left) Detailed anatomical model of the human body (MEET-Man) in an opened view and (right) MEET-Man heart model with a white texture of the muscle fiber orientation in a sliced view.

2. Data

A foundation of this work is the computer based tissue classified anatomical model of the human body (see Fig. 1 left, MEET-Man project [4, 5]). This model is derived from the cryosection images of the Visible Man data set provided by the National Library of Medicine, Bethesda, Maryland [6] using digital image processing. A part of it is the anatomical model of the heart (see Fig. 1 right). It is a cubic voxel based data set with a resolution of 1 mm and consists in the physiologic case of 16 tissue classes for different types of myocytes e.g. sinus node, right atrium, Purkinje fiber and left ventricle. For each voxel the fiber orientation is determined to enable simulations regarding anisotropic properties [7]. A specialized cardiac conduction system is created semi-automatically, because of the low resolution and contrast of the image data. A tree composed of nodes and edges represents it.

3. Methodology

3.1. Cellular Automaton

Rule based cellular automata are used in several disciplines to model the course of natural processes [8, 9]. They are also capable of simulating efficiently the excitation propagation in the whole heart [8, 10]. A cellular automaton can be divided into two components: A regular, discrete, infinite network representing the underlying spatial structure and a finite automaton working at each node of the network.

©CARS/Springer. All rights reserved.

In this work, the network consists of the presented anatomical model of the human heart. The tissue specific excitation velocity and the anisotropy of the myocardium based on a myocyte orientation data set are considered. The finite automaton at each node point represents the physiological state by modeling the course of the transmembrane potential depending on tissue type, stimulation frequency and refractory periods.
The finite automaton is configured from simulations with complex electrophysiological cell models, e.g. Luo-Rudy or Beeler-Reuter, in conjunction with a bidomain model as an excitation propagation approach [11]. A large number of simulations were performed varying the cell model and the stimulus frequency. For atrial and ventricular tissue types electrophysiological models of human cells were used. The simulations deliver tissue specific and stimulus frequency specific courses of the transmembrane voltage (see Fig. 2) as well as excitation velocities.

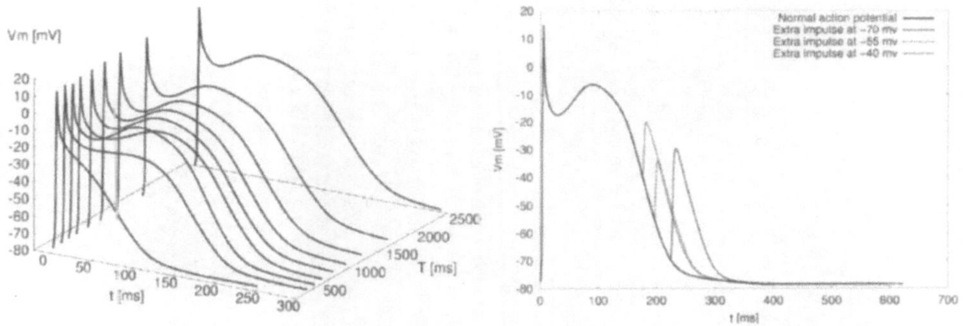

Fig. 2: (left) Dependency of the action potential courses on the heart rate and (right) extra impulses in the refractory period lead to changes in the courses of the action potential.

Atrial flutter can be simulated with a cellular automaton e.g. by applying a spatial and temporal suitably positioned extra stimulus following the physiological sinus node excitation [12]. This modeled electrical stimulus leads to a unidirectional block in the repolarization phase of parts of the atrial myocardium. In this case the excitation propagates in the opposite direction of the block. Afterwards, a spiral wave is rotating around the blocked area and can lead to a re-entry circle e.g. around the vena cava inferior or superior. This re-entry mechanism leads to a stable atrial flutter. In some cases, this rotating wave splits up into several wavelets and leads to atrial fibrillation.
Applied radio frequency currents destroy the pathways of the excitation propagation in these areas of the atrial myocardium. Commonly, lines of myocardium are ablated with endpoints at the orifices of the atrium, e.g. at the vena cava superior and inferior. The location of the lines has to be chosen suitably in such a way that propagation from the sinus node via the atrium to the atrioventricular node is still possible and the atrial flutter is permanently terminated.

3.2. Haptic Interface

Haptic interfaces expand the functionality of ordinary input devices with force feedback output. Force feedback is used in virtual reality to give the impression that one perceives interaction with the model. Therefore, haptic interfaces can be used to simulate surgical interventions. In this work, a PHANToM (SensAble Technology Inc.; Cambridge) [13] is

©CARS/Springer. All rights reserved.

used that provides a six-dimensional input device with force feedback in three dimensions (see Fig. 3). The PHANToM consists of a movable arm with force feedback for positioning. At its end a pin is installed with another three degrees of freedom without force feedback for the orientation. Advantages of the PHANToM are the modest mass of the manipulator, the large working area and the easy handling of the tip.
The force is calculated dynamically depending on the collision of the ablation tip with the surface of the volumetric model, its physical properties and the depth of the intrusion. By pressing the switch at the tip, voxels of the anatomical model can be manipulated. This simulates the application of the radio frequency current and leads to changes of the electrophysiological properties.

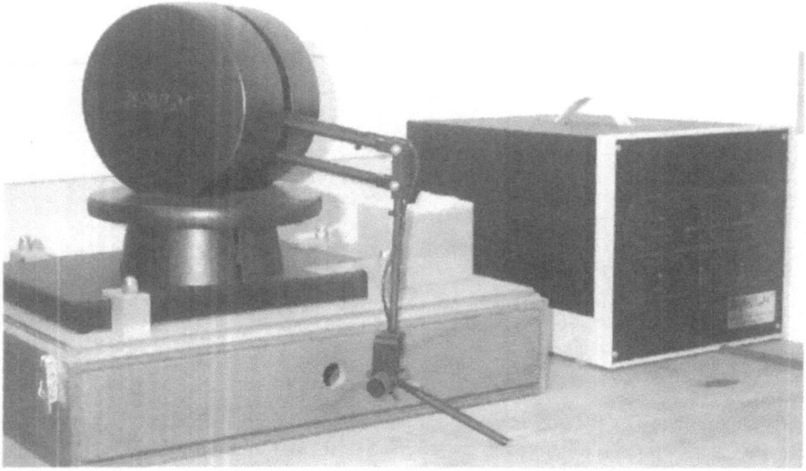

Fig. 3: The haptic interface with its arm and pin. The control unit is shown in the background.

3.3. Visualization

Specific software tools were developed to visualize the anatomical heart model, the changes of the transmembrane voltages of the electrophysiological model that are blended on the heart model and the virtual ablation tip [14]. The visualization software is used considering surface and volume based techniques with a suitable update rate. The visualization software is based on OpenInventor.

3.4. Computational environment

The processes of the simulation environment run in parallel and use inter process communication. This includes shared memory, synchronization of the processes via semaphores and exchanging messages with message queues. These techniques are necessary for complex and parallel simulations in real-time e.g. to prevent dead locks. Furthermore, a workstation with high computational and visualization power is applied. For this work, a SGI Octane with two 400 MHz processors is used in conjunction with a Graphic Board V6.
With this environment it is possible to calculate a heart cycle on an anatomical model with 444.000 voxels and a resolution of 2 mm including haptic interaction in 30 s with an update rate of five pictures per second.

©CARS/Springer. All rights reserved.

4. Results

The described methods were combined to a simulation environment that is controlled by a single, easy to handle graphical user interface. The environment permits the simulation of the RF-ablation of atrial flutter. In an exemplary simulation the atrial flutter is represented by a rotating wave around the vena cava superior. The simulated treatment of the atrial flutter is the ablation therapy with the haptic interface considering the effects of the ablation to the electrophysiology in real-time. Because of the force feedback, the ablation tip can be positioned on the surface of the atrium and a therapy can be applied.
In the exemplary simulation the rotating wave is terminated after execution of two ablation lines set with the haptic interface (see Fig. 4). A first line is set in the dorsal right atrial wall from the vena cava superior to the vena cava inferior. The first line results in a rotating wave around the vena cava inferior and the ablation line, which leads to an increase of the cycle duration of the flutter. A second line is set in the bottom area of the right atrium leading to a termination of the flutter. The ablation still permits the propagation from sinus node to the ventricles via the atrioventricular node, but a reinitiating of flutter with the same stimulus sequence is not possible.

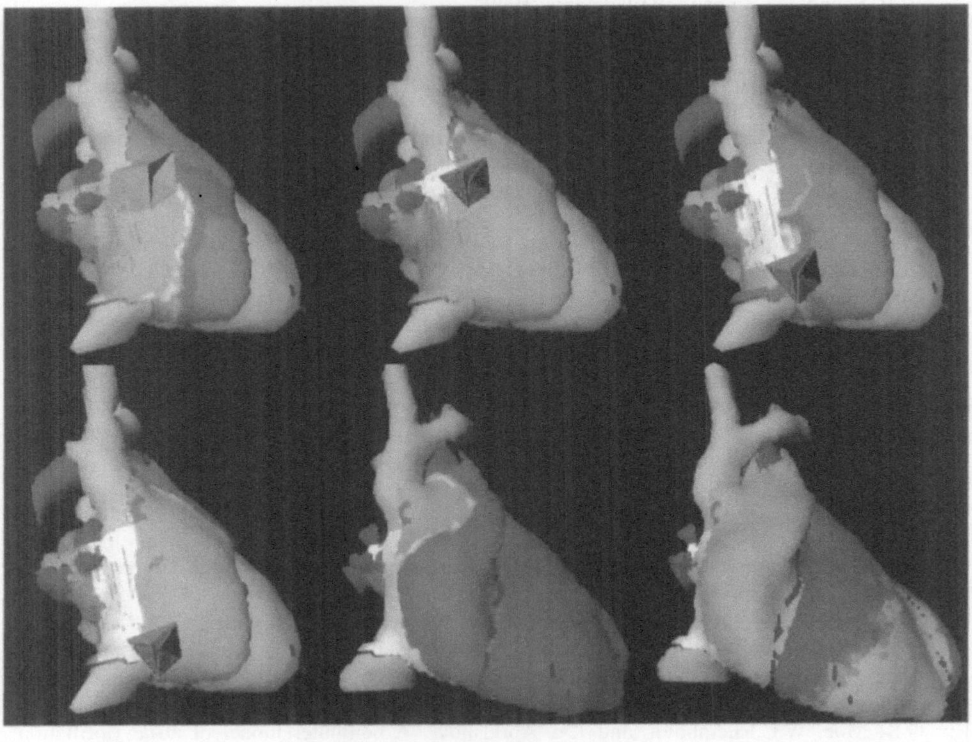

Fig. 4: RF-ablation therapy applied with the simulation environment. The ablation was carried out epicardially for visualization purpose. The projection of the transmembrane potential on the heart surface is color-coded. (upper row) The first ablation line set from vena cava superior to inferior leads to increasing cycle duration of the flutter. (lower row) After application of the second ablation line the electrical excitation propagation is physiologic again.

©CARS/Springer. All rights reserved.

5. Conclusions

The simulation environment is capable of simulating atrial flutter, of executing ablation with the haptic interface and of incorporating electrophysiological effects of the ablation therapy. The environment can facilitate the preceding training of a surgical intervention for the designated physician and can lead to better results of the treatment, because of the additional knowledge of the effects on electrophysiology.

Anatomical models with higher resolution will be used in future. Furthermore, the contraction of the heart will be modeled for a more realistic simulation. After detailed validations of the methods and models, this environment can be used on individual patient data sets for planning, simulating and validating the treatment. This can help to reduce the risks for the patient and to minimize the costs for the health services. Additionally, other interventions like the aneurism surgery will be modeled with this simulation environment.

References

1. A.L. Waldo, "Atrial Flutter: Mechanism, Clinical Features, and Management", *Cardiac Electrophysiology. From Cell to Bedside*, D.P. Zipes and J. Jalife, 3rd Edition, pages 468–476, W.B. Saunders Company, Philadelphia, 1999
2. Framingham Heart Study, NHLBI, http://www.nhlbi.gov/about/framingham
3. M.D. Lesh, "Catheter Ablation of Atrial Flutter and Tachycardia", *Cardiac Electrophysiology. From Cell to Bedside*, D.P. Zipes and J. Jalife, 3rd Edition, pages 1009–1027, W.B. Saunders Company, Philadelphia, 1999
4. F.B. Sachse, M. Glas, M. Müller, and K. Meyer-Waarden, "Segmentation and tissue-classification of the Visible Man dataset using the computertomographic scans and the thin-section photos", *Proc. 1st Users Conference of the National Library of Medicine's Visible Human Project*, 1996.
5. MEET-Man Project, IBT, Karlsruhe, http://www-ibt.etec.uni-karlsruhe.de/forschung/meetman
6. M.J. Ackerman "Viewpoint: The Visible Human Project", *Journal Biocommunication*, Vol. 18, No. 2, page 14, 1991
7. F.B. Sachse, C.D. Werner, M.H. Stenroos, R.F. Schulte, P. Zerfass, and O. Dössel, "Modeling the anatomy of the human heart using cryosection images of the Visible Female dataset", *Proc. Third Users Conference of the National Library of Medicine's Visible Human Project*, 2000.
8. C.D. Werner, *Simulation der elektrischen Erregungsausbreitung in anatomischen Herzmodellen mit adaptiven zellulären Automaten*, PhD thesis, Universität Karlsruhe (TH), Institut für Biomedizinische Technik, TANEA, Berlin, 2001.
9. M. Delorme, *Cellular Automata Machines*, chapter 1, Kluwer, Dordrecht, 1999.
10. F.B. Sachse, C.D. Werner, and G. Seemann, "Simulation of cardiac electrophysiology and electrocardiography", *Computer Simulation and Experimental Assessment of Cardiac Electrophysiology*, N. Virag, O. Blanc, and L. Kappenberger, pages 97–104, Futura Publishing, Armonk, New York, 2001.
11. F.B. Sachse, G. Seemann, C. Riedel, C.D. Werner, and O. Dössel, "Modeling of the cardiac mechano-electrical feedback", CardioModel 2000, Computer models of the heart: Theory and clinical application, *Int. J. Bioelectromagnetism*, Vol. 2, No. 2, 2000, http://www.ee.tut.fi/rgi/ijbem/volume2/number2/
12. G.K. Moe, W.C.Rheinboldt, and J.A. Abildskov, "A computer model of atrial fibrillation", *American Heart Journal*, Vol. 67, pages 200–220, 1964.
13. SensAble Technologies, Inc. Cambridge, http://www.sensable.com
14. F.B. Sachse, C.D. Werner, and O. Dössel, "Techniken zur Visualisierung der elektrischen Aktivität des Herzens", *Bildverarbeitung für die Medizin 1999*, H. Evers, G. Glombitza, T. Lehmann, and H.-P. Meinzer, Springer, Berlin, pages 427–431, 1999.

CARS 2002 – H.U. Lemke, M.W. Vannier; K. Inamura, A.G. Farman, K. Doi & J.H.C. Reiber (Editors)
©CARS/Springer. All rights reserved.

An interaction model between multiple deformable objects for realistic haptic force feedback in surgical simulations

Yoshihiro Kuroda[a], Megumi Nakao[a], Silke Hacker[b]
Tomohiro Kuroda[c], Hiroshi Oyama[c], Masaru Komori[d]
Tetsuya Matsuda[c], Takashi Takahashi[c]
[a] Graduate School of Informatics, Kyoto University, Japan
[b] IMDM University Hospital Hamburg-Eppendorf, Germany
[c] Medical Informatics, Kyoto University Hospital, Japan
[d] Biomedical Science, Shiga University of Medical Science, Japan
e-mail: ykuroda@kuhp.kyoto-u.ac.jp

Abstract

This paper proposes an interaction model between multiple physically-based deformable object. This model achieves both accurate force feedback and visualization of surgical manipulations (like hold, push and move organs) while approaching the tissues of interest. Accurate force feedback improves surgical realism and enables exact simulation for diagnosis and procedural training. Interaction is represented by mutual iterative procedures of forcible displacement, calculation of deformation and reaction force. The proposed model has been applied to a simulation where a manipulating point pushes a deformable object, which is in contact with a neighboring one, and the influence of interaction on haptic force feedback has been examined.

Keywords: Multiple deformable objects, haptic force feedback, surgical simulations

1. Introduction

Interest on medical simulation based on Virtual Reality has been growing in medical and computer scientists in this decade. The mechanics and deformation of soft tissue, which are essential to achieve surgical simulations, have been intensively studied in both biomechanics and computer graphics fields [1,2]. Although several surgical simulators have been developed using those techniques [2,3], most simulators display haptic force feedback with a single object in no contact with neighboring objects. However, in real-life surgery, dynamic relations among neighbouring organs affects force feedback at a surgeon's hand and changes the surgeon's manipulation. Force feedback is key information to identify organs and its status, especially under the limited views in endoscopic surgery. Therefore, to produce accurate force feedback is important in surgical simulations. The representation of the interaction between multiple deformable objects is a big challenge because of two issues: accurate interaction between multiple deformable objects in the discrete world and fast computation. The interaction model described below represents the interaction so that improved accuracy of force feedback enables us to distinguish slight haptic differences in surgical simulations.

©CARS/Springer. All rights reserved.

2. Methodology

2.1 Representation of interaction

Many existing applications deal with the interaction between multiple rigid objects or between a rigid and a deformable object. The interaction model between multiple deformable objects must be represented in order to achieve purposes described above. In the proposed model, interaction is represented by a series of procedures: update of pairs of nearest nodes, collision detection, collision procedures, calculation of deformation and conveyance of reaction with pairs of nearest nodes. Physical properties of both objects are also considered. Following paragraphs describe the procedures and process flow of the proposed interaction model.

- **Pair of nearest nodes** The authors propose a "pair of nearest nodes" to handle collision, action and reaction. A pair of nearest nodes consists of two nodes, each of which belongs to a different object. All pairs are registered in the list. For explanation, {A:a1, B:b1} represents a pair consisting of the node "a1" of object A and the node "b1" of object B.
- **Updating pairs of nearest nodes** Pairs of nearest nodes have to be checked and, if necessary, updated when the nodes are moved.
- **Collision detection** Collisions are detected based on the coordinates of a node and the normal vector on the polygons. Although many algorithms are proposed in the field of computer graphics [4], most of them require large computational cost for accurate collision detection. Fast calculation and high accuracy of detection cannot be achieved together. Accuracy has to be reduced for real-time simulation with haptic force feedback.
- **Collision procedures** When a collision between the nodes in a pair is detected, one node is forcibly displaced to the location of the other node and, if necessary, new pairs are added to the management list.
- **Calculation of deformation** The deformation of the collided object is calculated. The models and the computational methods of objects are described in section 2.3.
- **Conveyance of reaction** The calculated stress is conveyed to the other object as reaction via a pair of nearest nodes. Reaction is conveyed as soon as the required force is calculated, and used in the next calculation. Conveyance of reaction results in equilibrium at each collision.
- **A series of procedures** Figure 1 illustrates a series of procedures in the case of the collision between object A and B. The nodes 'a1' and 'b1' belong to object A and B respectively and the nodes are registered as a pair of nearest nodes before collision. The procedures consist of two main steps. During the first step, the collision between node 'a1' and object B is examined. Fig. 1-1 illustrates the initial state when no collision is detected between two objects. If a collision is detected (see Fig. 1-2), the location of 'b2' is updated to the coordinates of 'a1' (see Fig. 1-3). The deformation of the collided object B is calculated and reaction force is conveyed to 'a1', which is used at the next calculation of the deformation of object A (see Fig. 1-4). During the second step, the collision between node 'b1' and object A is examined. If a collision is detected (see Fig. 1-5), the location of 'a1' is updated to the coordinates of 'b1' (see Fig. 1-6). The deformation of the collided object A is calculated and reaction force is conveyed to 'b1', which is used at the next calculation of the deformation of object B (see Fig. 1-7). This series of procedures is carried out iteratively.

©CARS/Springer. All rights reserved.

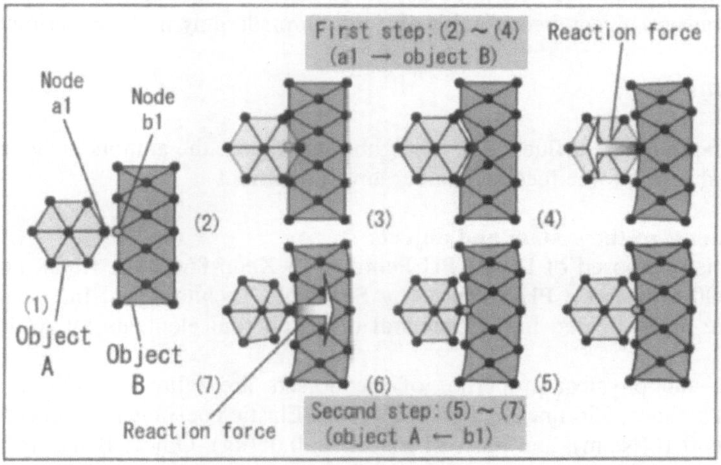

Figure 1: A series of procedures (1-7)

2.2 Addition of pairs

New pairs of nearest nodes have to be added when nodes are collided in order to represent touching surfaces. Neighboring nodes are registered in the management list as pairs of nearest nodes. In Fig. 2-1, a pair of nearest nodes {A:a1, B:b1} is handled before the collision between two objects, A and B. In Fig. 2-2, two pairs of nearest nodes {A:a2, B:b2},{A:a3, B:b3} are added to the list.

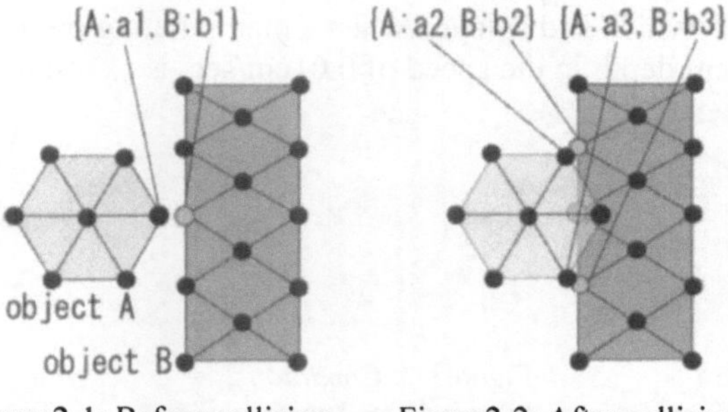

Figure2-1: Before collision Figure2-2: After collision

2.3 Physically-based models and computational methods

The mass spring model is applied to the object directly pushed by a manipulating point and the finite element method is applied to its neighboring object. The mass spring model is calculated by applying Euler' method to Newton's movement equation. Finite element based simulations take large cost in calculation, although the accurate and stable deformation based on continuum mechanics equations is achieved. Some methods for fast calculation must be applied for real-time simulation and then some restrictions follow. Hirota's method [5], which enables us to calculate force instantly after the collision, and Condensation method [6] have been applied to the linear finite element method. Linear

CARS 2002 – H.U. Lemke, M.W. Vannier; K. Inamura, A.G. Farman, K. Doi & J.H.C. Reiber (Editors)
©CARS/Springer. All rights reserved.

model cannot represent realistic large deformations. The mass spring model is applied to the directly pushed object, because this object deforms largely in the experiments.

3. Experiments

In order to examine the influence of a neighboring object, the authors have experimented and measured haptic force feedback under three conditions.

3.1 Components of the system and objects

The system is composed of Dual CPU Pentium III Xeon 866MHz, Main memory 2GB, Windows2000 OS, and a PHANToM (by SensAble Technologies, Inc.) haptic device. Objects have been divided into tetrahedral or hexahedral elements by Amira2.3 (TGS, Inc.).

Components and physical properties of the objects are following. Object A has 112 elements, 112 nodes, 556 lines and 160 polygons. Elastic coefficient is 100(N/m), damper coefficient is 0.10(Ns/m), and mass of a node is 0.05(kg). Object B has 1448 elements, 1,906 nodes, 5165 lines and 540 polygons. Young modulus is 0.0971(MPa) and Poisson ratio is 0.2160(-).

3.2 Three conditions (contacted, free and fixed)

Pushing tests are performed under three conditions. In all conditions, object A is fixed on a certain plain as shown in Fig. 3. *Condition 1* holds two objects, A and B, which are in contact with each other, as shown in Fig. 3-1. *Condition 2* holds a single object, A, and let all nodes on the indicated surface move free as shown in Fig. 3-2. *Condition 3* makes the nodes to be fixed as shown in Fig. 3-3.

Haptic force feedback, which is displayed when a manipulating point pushes a surface of object A towards 0.5cm depth in the speed of 0.01cm/sec, is examined.

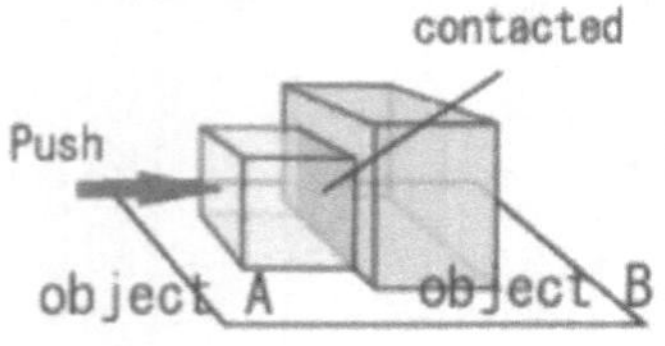

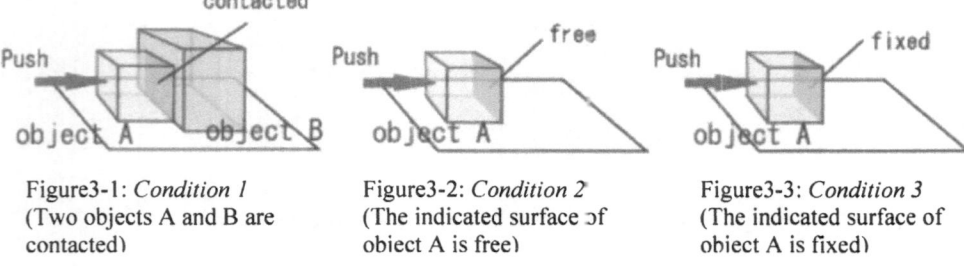

Figure3-1: *Condition 1* (Two objects A and B are contacted)

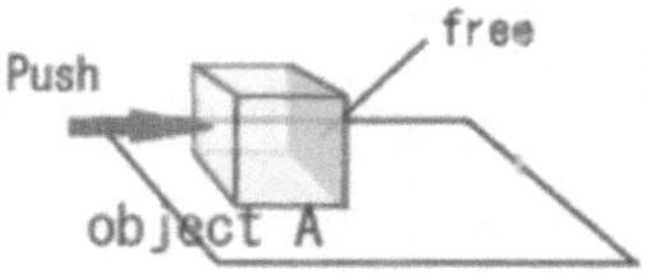

Figure3-2: *Condition 2* (The indicated surface of object A is free)

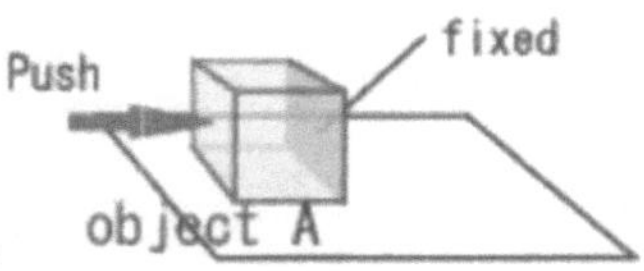

Figure3-3: *Condition 3* (The indicated surface of object A is fixed)

4. Results

Figure 4 shows the results under three conditions. High degree of force is marked under condition 1. The forces under condition 2 and 3 are shown in the low area with some differences, which is easier to see subtle differences in the enlarged graph, Fig. 5. The experimental results show the influence of the neighboring objects on the haptic display.

©CARS/Springer. All rights reserved.

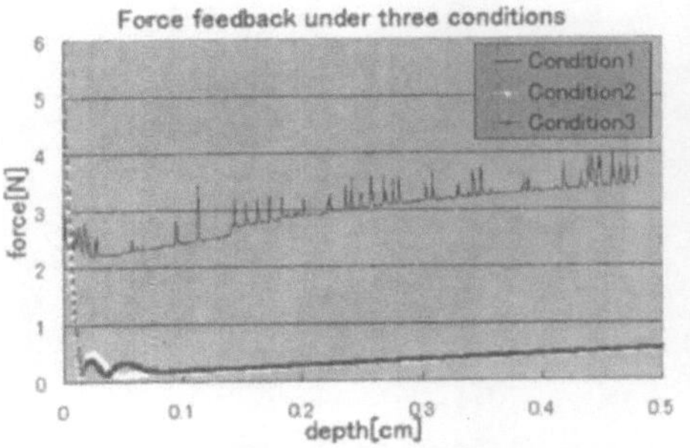

Figure 4: Force under three conditions

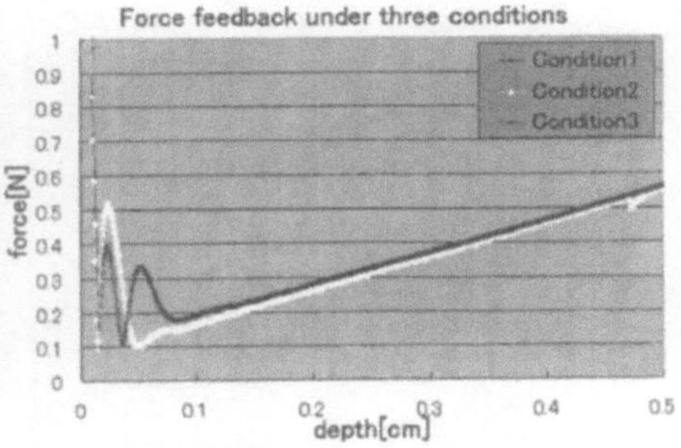

Figure 5: Differences between condition 1 and 2

5. Conclusion

This paper has described an advanced interaction model between multiple deformable objects for accurate haptic force feedback reflecting the influence of neighboring organs. Interaction has been represented by mutual iterative procedures of forcible displacement, calculation of deformation and reaction force. The remarkable feature of the proposed model is that the physical properties of each object are considered for force feedback calculations. The proposed model has been implemented on a standard PC and some experiments have been done. The results show the influence of the interaction between multiple objects on haptic force feedback.
More discussions about the interaction between multiple deformable objects are required in order to achieve advanced surgical simulations. The improved simulation system enables surgeons to regard force feed back into decision consciously or subconsciously.

Acknowledgements

This work was partially supported by the Ministry of Education, Science, Culture of Japan, Grants-in-Aid for JSPS Fellows No.0103889.

References

1. S. F. F. Gibson and B. Mitrich, "A Survey of Deformable Modeling in Computer Graphics", Technical report, http://www.merl.com, TR-97-19, MERL, Nov.1997
2. H. Delingette, "Toward Realistic Soft Tissue Modeling in Medical Simulation", Proceedings of the IEEE, Vol.86, No.3, pp.512-523, Apr.1998
3. C. Basdogan, "Integration of Force Feedback into Virtual Reality Based Training Systems for Simulating Minimally Invasive Procedures", http://eis.jpl.nasa.gov/~basdogan/Tutorials/basdogan.html
4. Y. Kitamura, A. Smith, H. Takemura and F. Kishino, "A Real-Time Algorithm for Accurate Collision Detection for Deformable Polyhedral Objects", PRESENCE, Vol.7, No.1, pp. 36-52, MIT Press, 1998
5. K. Hirota and T. Kaneko, "A Method of Representing Soft Object in Virtual Environment", IPSJ (Information Processing Society of Japan) JOURNAL, Vol.39 No.12, Dec 1998
6. M. Bro-Nielsen, "Finite element modeling in surgery simulation", Journal of the IEEE, 86(3), pp.490-503, 1998

Surgical Navigation

CARS 2002 – H.U. Lemke, M.W. Vannier; K. Inamura, A.G. Farman, K. Doi & J.H.C. Reiber (Editors)
©CARS/Springer. All rights reserved.

Accuracy evaluation of a 3D ultrasound-based neuronavigation system

Thomas Langø, Jon Bang, Frank Lindseth, Toril A Nagelhus Hernes
SINTEF Unimed, 7465 Trondheim, Norway

Abstract

We have investigated the 3D navigation accuracy of an ultrasound-based neuronavigation system for surgical planning and intraoperative image guidance. In addition, we present a detailed description and review of the error sources associated with conventional MRI-based and ultrasound-based surgical neuronavigation. A phantom with 27 precisely defined points was scanned with ultrasound by various translation and tilt movements of the ultrasound probe (180 3D scans), and the 27 image points in each volume were located using an automatic detection algorithm. These locations were compared to the physically measured locations of the same 27 points. The accuracy of the neuronavigation system and the effect of varying acquisition conditions, were found through a thorough statistical analysis of the differences between the two point sets. The accuracy was found to be 1.40 ± 0.45 mm (arithmetic mean) for the system in our laboratory setting. Improper probe calibration is the major contribution to this number. Based on our extensive data set and evaluation, we expect the accuracy found in the laboratory setting to be close to the overall clinical setting in ultrasound-based neuronavigation. Our analysis indicates that the overall clinical accuracy may be as low as 2 mm when using intraoperative imaging to eliminate the brain shift.

Keywords: 3D ultrasound, neuronavigation, accuracy

1. Introduction

In image guided surgery, established imaging techniques like conventional MRI and CT imaging provide high quality 3D data for surgical planning and overview of the patient's anatomy during the operation. However, significant anatomical changes may occur during the operation. Alternative approaches like intraoperative MRI have been developed for detecting and monitoring such changes as surgery proceeds [1, 2]. This is a costly and time-consuming option, which may have considerable impact on the workflow of many standard operation procedures. Intraoperative ultrasound offers real-time capabilities at relatively low cost, and with relatively small impact on established operation routines.

The delicacy, precision, and extent of the work the surgeon can perform based on image information, rely on his/her confidence in the overall clinical accuracy of the system and the anatomical or pathological representation. The overall clinical accuracy in image-guided surgery is the difference between where a surgical tool is located relative to some structure as indicated in the image information presented to the surgeon and where the

©CARS/Springer. All rights reserved.

tool is actually located relative to the same structure in the patient. This accuracy is difficult to assess in a clinical setting, due to the lack of fixed and well-defined landmarks inside the patient that can be reached accurately by a pointer. Common practice is therefore to estimate the system's overall accuracy in a controlled laboratory setting using precisely built phantoms [3, 4]. In order to conclude on the potential clinical accuracy, the differences between the clinical and the laboratory settings must be carefully examined.

We present a thorough analysis on an extensive data set obtained using a commercial system. The method is based on a precisely built and accurately measured wire phantom and an automatic 3D template-matching (by correlation) algorithm [5]. Advantages of an automated procedure are rapid execution so that an extensive evaluation can be performed, and avoidance of subjective influence upon the results. The accuracy and robustness of the automatic algorithm was determined in [5].

First, however, to gain a better understanding of the relation between laboratory and clinical accuracy, we describe and compare the most relevant error sources associated with MRI-based neuronavigation to the error chain associated with ultrasound-based neuronavigation. The overview is based on a combination of available literature and our own experience during 7 years of ultrasound-based image-guidance in neurosurgery.

1.1 Error chains for conventional MRI- and ultrasound-based neuronavigation
The different actions and corresponding sources of error for MRI-based neuronavigation and ultrasound-based neuronavigation are shown in Table 1 and Table 2, respectively.

Action items		Error sources		mm error		
				<1	1-2	>2
1	Glue fiducials to skin					
2	Position patient in MR-scanner	A	Skin/fiducial slide	√	√	√
3	Perform 3D MRI	B	Geometric distortion in MR data	√	√	√
4	Load images and generate volume	C	Quantization in volume reconstruction	√		
5	Position patient on operating table	D	Brain shift due to gravity	√	√	
		E	Skin/fiducial slide due to gravity	√	√	√
6	Mark fiducials in MR images	F	Fiducial identification	√	√	
7	Touch fiducials with pointer	G	Skin/fiducial slide due to pointer pressure	√	√	√
		H	Position system and pointer tip definition	√		
		I	Pointing	√	√	
8	Match images to patient	J	Patient registration/matching algorithm	√	√	
9	Point and reconstruct images with overlaid color cross	K	2D image extraction	√		
		L	Quantization, color cross	√		
		M	Interpretation	√		
		N	Position system and tool tip definition	√		
10	Surgery and brain movements	O	Discrepancy between anatomy and images	√	√	√

Table 1. Error chain associated with conventional MRI-based neuronavigation.

An important advantage of ultrasound-guided navigation is the ability to do repetitive 3D imaging during surgery and thus work with a data set that has recently been updated according to possible changes in the brain anatomy. The error or discrepancy between the images and the anatomy during surgery (error source O') will therefore be small or negligible compared to the case for MRI-based navigation (error source O).

©CARS/Springer. All rights reserved.

Action items		Error sources		mm error		
				<1	1-2	>2
11	Probe calibration	P	Sensor to scan plane transformation	√	√	√
12	Mount position sensor	Q	Sensor attachment repeatability	√		
13	Acquire 3D ultrasound data	R	Position sensor tracking	√		
		S	Synchronization between position data and images	√	(√)	
		T	2D image position discretization	√		
14	Load images and reconstruct volume: 3D scan conversion	U	Sound speed value	√	√	
		V	Resolution (mm/voxel)	√		
		W	Interpolation algorithms	√		
9	Point and reconstruct images with overlaid colored cross	K	2D image extraction	√		
		L	Quantization, colored cross	√		
		M	Interpretation	√	(√)	
		N	Position system and tool tip definition	√		
10	Surgery and brain movements	O'	Brain shift (between repetitive 3D ultrasound acquisitions)	√	(√)	

Table 2. Error chain associated with ultrasound-based neuronavigation.

1.2 Overall accuracy versus overall clinical accuracy

The overall clinical accuracy of a navigation system will be determined by the contribution from all the individual error sources described in Table 1 and Table 2. The net effect will not be the sum of all error sources, but rather a stochastic contribution from all terms. Ultrasound-based navigation does not require patient registration and, thus, this modality is less susceptible to user- and procedure-dependent error sources. Error sources M and O' (Table 2) are affected by the user, while the remaining sources are in control of the system vendor. In MRI-based navigation, the user and procedure affect error sources {A}-{G}, {M} and {O} (Table 1), while the remaining six error sources are in control of the vendor ({H}-{L}, {N}). This indicates that the overall clinical accuracy of an ultrasound-based system may be closer in value to the overall laboratory accuracy than is the case with conventional MRI-based systems.

The purpose of this study was to perform a 3D accuracy evaluation of an ultrasound-based navigation system in the laboratory setting to get an impression of the potential overall clinical accuracy of ultrasound-based neuronavigation. Error sources {P} and {R}-{W} in Table 2 were included in the analysis.

2. Methods

The wire phantom (27 precisely defined wire crosses) was submerged in a water bath and scanned with ultrasound by various translation and tilt movements of the ultrasound probe and different experimental settings (180 3D scans in total). The 27 image points in each volume were located using the automatic detection algorithm and compared to the physically measured locations of the same 27 points. The accuracy of the neuronavigation system and the effect of varying acquisition conditions, were found through a thorough statistical analysis of the differences between the two point sets.

©CARS/Springer. All rights reserved.

The neuronavigation system used in this study (SonoWand®, MISON AS, Trondheim, Norway) differs from conventional neuronavigation systems in that it is integrated with a high-performance digital ultrasound scanner for updating the 3D map during surgery. Further, the system comprises a computer for image processing and navigation and an optical 3D position tracker (Polaris®, Northern Digital, Ontario, Canada). A direct link between the ultrasound scanner and navigation computer provides rapid transfer of 3D ultrasound data. The system can function as a conventional ultrasound scanner, as a conventional neuronavigation system based on MRI or CT-images, or more important, as a combined system where both the features and advantages of preoperative MRI and intraoperative 3D ultrasound are fully utilized. The system thus enables the surgeon to navigate directly by means of intraoperative 3D ultrasound.

Important parameters that have an effect on imaging accuracy in the reconstruction of the freehand 3D ultrasound scans are: probe calibration to determine the position of the image relative to the position sensor attached to the probe; synchronization of position and image data; the speed of sound used in the scan conversion algorithm (to convert raw data into a geometrically correct 3D volume); and the desired output resolution measured in millimeter per voxel. We measured the temperature of the water bath containing the phantom to determine the sound speed, following published data to set a proper value. The effect of probe calibration, synchronization of position and image, and sound speed was investigated in detail.

3. Results

From the total of 4860 points (180 volumes and 27 wire crosses in each volume), we have obtained an overall laboratory accuracy of 1.40 ± 0.45 mm (arithmetic mean) for the navigation system investigated in this study [6] (Fig. 1). Only a minor fraction of this number should be attributed to random noise. First, the variations in coordinate biases and in error vector length seemed to be correlated to camera position and acquisition method. Second, a repeatability test (each scan type was repeated three times) shows that the random contribution is typically one order of magnitude less than the overall variations.

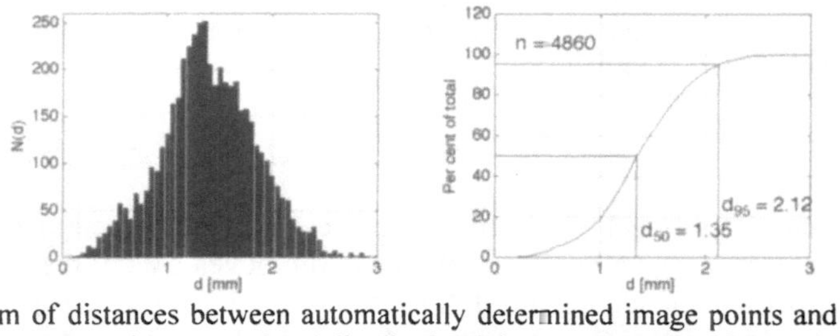

Fig. 1: Histogram of distances between automatically determined image points and the physically measured wire crosses. In the accumulated distribution it is seen that 50% of the values are less than 1.35 mm (median) and 95% of the values are less than 2.12 mm. The mean value is 1.40 mm.

We considered the following systematic error sources: bias in the automatic method, time synchronization in tagging of each 2D ultrasound image with position and orientation, and sound speed and probe calibration transformation used in converting the raw data into a

©CARS/Springer. All rights reserved.

geometrically correct 3D volume. We investigated how each error source individually would affect the results under varying acquisition conditions. Detailed analysis of the data material indicated that inappropriate probe calibration is the main error source in this study. Further investigation of the other error sources and more results can be found in [6].

3.1 Overall clinical accuracy

The most important parameter for the surgeon is the overall clinical accuracy. Although this parameter is difficult to assess, we believe that an estimate can be made, based on our laboratory evaluation and a thorough understanding of the significant additional error sources that occur in the clinical setting. This calculation is summarized in Table 3.

Our starting point is the laboratory accuracy for all tilt scans at the best camera setting (1.3 mm), since this configuration is considered to be most relevant in the clinical situation. Our study does not include calibration and tracking errors of a rigid pointer or surgical tool, which are of the order of 0.6 mm [7]. Furthermore, we have not considered errors associated with the extraction and presentation of a 2D image from the 3D volume; however, such errors should be rather small for a system using good interpolation routines and a high-resolution monitor.

By adding these error numbers, we obtain an estimate of the overall laboratory accuracy. The error sources are assumed to be stochastically independent; hence, their contributions are added on a sum-of-squares basis.

Laboratory accuracy (tilt scans, one camera position)	1.3 mm
+ Calibration and position tracking of rigid surgical tool	0.6 mm
+ Interpolation 2D slice from 3D / tool cross indication	0.1 mm
= Overall laboratory accuracy	**1.4 mm**
+ Sound speed uncertainty	0.5 – 3 mm
+ Brain shift	1 – 10 mm
+ Interpretation of images on monitor	0.5 mm
= Overall clinical accuracy	**1.9 – 10.6 mm**

Table 3. Estimate of overall clinical accuracy based on laboratory experiments and additional error sources in the clinical situation. The numbers are added in a stochastic manner.

For a rigid phantom, the overall laboratory accuracy may be better for an MRI system than for the ultrasound-based system. However, in the clinical setting, the MRI option will also require patient registration, which is unnecessary when using ultrasound.

4. Conclusions

We have developed a novel method for automatic assessment of the accuracy of 3D ultrasound-based navigation systems. The method applies a correlation-based template-matching algorithm that locates well-defined structures in ultrasound volumes. The present implementation is designed for a precisely built wire phantom with 27 wire crosses within a volume of 5^3 cm^3.

©CARS/Springer. All rights reserved.

The application to accuracy evaluation has been demonstrated on an extensive set of ultrasound volumes acquired using a commercial neuronavigation system. Based on this extensive data set and a thorough evaluation, we expect the accuracy found in the laboratory setting to be close to the overall clinical setting in ultrasound-based neuronavigation. This is partly due to the fact that patient registration is unnecessary. In addition, intraoperative ultrasound imaging may eliminate the brain shift problems, which is the potentially largest error source. Our analysis indicate that the overall clinical accuracy may be as low as 2 mm when using intraoperative imaging to eliminate the brain shift.

Acknowledgements

This work was supported by grants from the Research Council of Norway through the Strategic University Program in Medical Technology at the Norwegian University of Science and Technology (NTNU), the Strategic Institute Program at SINTEF Unimed, and the Norwegian Ministry of Health and Social Affairs.

References

1. C. Nimsky, M. D. Ganslandt, H. Kober, M. Buchfelder, and R. Fahlbusch. "Intraoperative magnetic resonance imaging combined with neuronavigation: a new concept", Neurosurgery, vol. 48, pp. 1082 - 1091, 2001.
2. C. R. Wirtz, M. M. Bonsanto, M. Kanuth, V. M. Tronnier, F. K. Albert, A. Staubert, and S. Kunze. "Intraoperative magnetic resonance imaging to update interactive navigation in neurosurgery: Method and preliminary experience", Comp Aided Surg, vol. 2, pp. 172-179, 1997.
3. M. Cartellieri, J. Kremser, and F. Vorbeck. "Comparison of different 3D navigation systems by a clinical "user"", Eur Arch Otorhinolaryngol, vol. 258, pp. 38-41, 2001.
4. N. L. Dorward, O. Alberti, J. D. Palmer, N. D. Kitchen, and D. G. T. Thomas. "Accuracy of true frameless sterotaxy: in vivo measurement and laboratory phantom studies", J Neurosurgery, vol. 90, pp. 160-168, 1999.
5. F. Lindseth, J. Bang, and T. Langø. "A robust and automatic method for assessing the 3D accuracy in ultrasound-based image guidance", Submitted to IEEE Trans Biomed Eng, 2001.
6. F. Lindseth, T. Langø, J. Bang, and T. A. N. Hernes. "Evaluation of the 3D accuracy of an ultrasound-based neuronavigation system", Submitted to Comp Aided Surg, 2001.
7. F. Chassat, and S. Lavallée. "Experimental protocol of accuracy evaluation of 6-D localizers for computer-integrated surgery: Application to four optical localizers", Lecture notes in Computer Science, Medical Image Computing and Computer-Assisted Intervention - MICCAI'98, 1998;1496:277-284.

CARS 2002 – H.U. Lemke, M.W. Vannier; K. Inamura A.G. Farman, K. Doi & J.H.C. Reiber (Editors)
©CARS/Springer. All rights reserved.

Ultra-fast image registration embedded in intraoperative MR imaging

Junichi Tokuda[a], Shigehiro Morikawa[b], Takeyoshi Dohi[c], Nobuhiko Hata[c]
[a] Faculty of Engineering, The University of Tokyo, 7-3-1, Hongo, Bunkyo-ku, Tokyo 113-8656, Japan
[b] Molecular Neuroscience Research Center, Shiga University of Medical Science, Seta-Tsukinowa-cho, Otsu, Shiga 520-2192, Japan
[c] Graduate School of Information Science and Technology, The University of Tokyo, 7-3-1, Hongo, Bunkyo-ku, Tokyo 113-8656, Japan

Abstract

Fast image registration for Magnetic Resonance Imaging (MRI) guided surgery using projection profile matching embedded in MR pulse sequence is proposed. The method can perform two-dimensional image registration by matching projection profiles acquired before and after the motion of the object, and it doesn't need any post-processing of image data. The study involved an experiment performed on a 2.0 Tesla experimental MR scanner and phantom to evaluate the accuracy and feasibility of the method. We scanned moving phantom using customized pulse sequence that acquired echoes for imaging and projection profiles simultaneously, while the laser Charge-Coupled Device (CCD) displacement sensor was tracking the phantom. The standard deviation of the error between projection profile matching and laser CCD sensor is 0.3 [mm], and the mean computing time is 0.024 [ms] per one matching. The method successfully performed on phantom study with enough accuracy and speed.

Keywords: Image registration, projection profile matching

1. Introduction

Intraoperative Magnetic Resonance Imaging (MRI) guided surgery is becoming widely recognized reflecting the trend of minimally invasive therapy. Intraoperative MRI has many advantages of contrast, spatial resolution and radiation safety over any other modalities such as intraoperative ultrasound and Computed Tomography (CT). Before surgery, patients usually undergo some radiological and other diagnoses for pre-operative surgical planning. In order to fuse information of pre-operative multi-modal image diagnoses into intraoperative images, techniques of medical image registration between pre- and intra-operative images have been proposed [1,2]. The important roles of medical image registration are combining images of same subject from different modality or at different times, and compensate for motion of the subject between scans [3]. But previously published methods, including large scale post-processing of pre- and intra-operative images, inherently require a few seconds or minutes to complete registration after an intra-operative image is obtained. Furthermore, post-processing approach cannot compensate for motion of the subject while scanning and constructing images.

©CARS/Springer. All rights reserved.

This paper describes our new registration approach and evaluates its accuracy in phantom study. Our solution for this problem, proposed in this paper, is embedded in MR pulse sequence. The technique is designed to follow large-scale registration to correct small miss-alignment especially caused by the fast motion of body between scans.

2. Method

2.1 Theory

In standard 2-dimensional Fourier encoding method, the signal received by Radio Frequency (RF) coil is given by:

$$S(t) = \int_{-\infty}^{\infty}\int_{-\infty}^{\infty} M(x,y)\exp\{-i(\gamma G_x xt + \gamma G_y yt_y)\}\,dxdy \quad (1)$$

where $M(x,y)$ is the distribution of magnetization, γ is the gyromagnetic ratio, and G_x, G_y is the magnetic field gradient. Considering the case that the RF coil receives echo without phase encoding ($G_y = 0$), the received signal is

$$S(t) = \int_{-\infty}^{\infty}\int_{-\infty}^{\infty} M(x,y)\exp(-i\gamma G_x xt)\,dxdy\,. \quad (2)$$

For notational convenience, we can rewrite this equation as

$$S(k_x) = \int_{-\infty}^{\infty}\int_{-\infty}^{\infty} M(x,y)\exp(-ik_x x)\,dxdy \quad (3)$$

where $k_x = \gamma G_x t$. By applying Fourier Translation to equation (3), we obtain the projection profile along x-axis.

$$\begin{aligned} p(x) &= \frac{1}{2\pi}\int_{-\infty}^{\infty} S(k_x)\,dk_x \\ &= \int_{-\infty}^{\infty} M(x,y)\,dy \end{aligned} \quad (4)$$

Under the condition of rigid body motion, the 2-dimensional translation of the subject causes the 1-dimensional translation of projection profiles along each axis. The shape of projection profile is not deformed by the translation. This means that the displacement of the subject can be quantified by matching projections before and after the motion. Now we are given two projection profiles: $p_0(x)$ and $p_n(x)$. $p_0(x)$ is the baseline projection

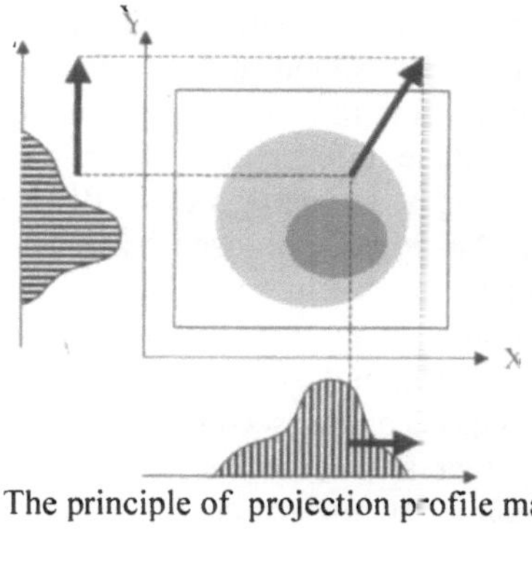

Fig. 1: The principle of projection profile matching.

©CARS/Springer. All rights reserved.

profile along x-axis, and $p_n(x)$ is the nth projection profile along x-axis. Estimating the x-directional translation of the subject between the baseline and n^{th} profile acquisition at Δx, $p_n(x)$ is almost identical to $p_0(x+\Delta x)$ when the parameter Δx is actual value. Thus we can determine the translation parameter Δx by maximizing the similarity measure between $p_n(x)$ and $p_0(x+\Delta x)$. We used cross correlation for this similarity measure. The problem is denoted as follows:

$$\Delta x = \arg\max(C(p_0(x+\Delta x), p_n(x))) \quad (5)$$

where $C(p_0(x+\Delta x), p_n(x))$ is cross correlation between $p_0(x+\Delta x)$ and $p_n(x)$. The method can be applied to the other direction by exchanging the direction of phase encoding and frequency encoding.

Our method requires the assumption that the subject is rigid, but it can be applied to the case that there are moving rigid objects and static objects in one image by segmenting the baseline image. We call this method "segmented projection profile matching". In this method, we segment baseline image into dynamic region and static region before starting profile matching, and calculate the projection profile of dynamic region and static region from this segmented baseline image. The projection profiles of the moving object during scans were calculated by subtracting the baseline profile of the static object from each projection profiles.

2.2 Experiment

We conducted a phantom experiment to evaluate the feasibility and accuracy of the proposed method in a 2.0 Tesla experimental scanner (CSI Omega System, Bruker, Fremont, CA). The specially designed placement stage is installed on the scanner's bore. The movement of the stage was restricted to only frequency-encoded direction for imaging. The moving phantom was fixed on the stage (Fig. 2).
The pulse sequence is modified gradient echo (TR/TE: 40ms/7ms, field of view (FOV) 100mm, matrix 256x128), which is near the sequence of semi-real time imaging used in intraoperative MRI. In this pulse sequence, non-phase-encoded pulse excitation and echo acquisition process was inserted every other echo acquisition for imaging. Total of 64 projection profiles per each axis were obtained during one imaging (approx. 10 seconds). The stage was moved manually up to 30-40 mm while scanning, and the stage was tracked

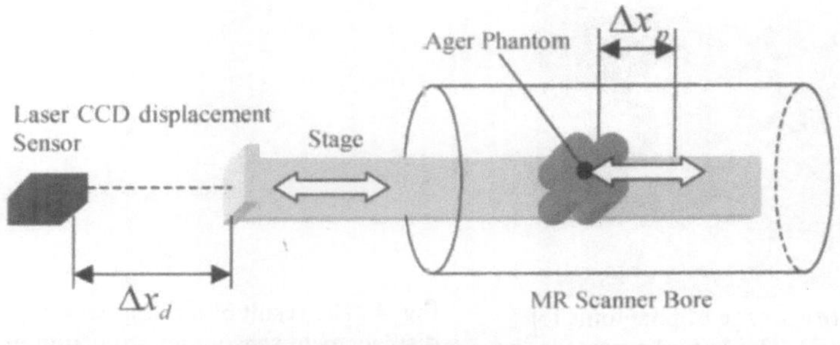

Fig. 2: The configuration of phantom experiment. The stage was tracked by the laser CCD displacement sensor during scans.

©CARS/Springer. All rights reserved.

by Charge-Coupled Device (CCD) laser displacement sensor (LK-500, Keyence, Osaka, Japan) with resolution of 50 μm and sampling cycle of 1024 μs. Both scanning and laser displacement sensor were synchronized by a shared pulse generator.

Two experiments were performed changing the configuration of the phantom.

(A) Non-segmented projection profile matching: The phantom consisted of four cylindrical agar phantoms (20mm in diameter) which were all fixed on the stage and move together. There was no other object in the FOV.

(B) Segmented projection profile matching: The phantom consisted of four cylindrical phantoms fixed on the stage and 6 cylindrical phantoms fixed in the bore of the scanner. The all phantoms are in the FOV, but only the former four phantoms were moved with the stage while the others didn't change their position. Projection profile matching was applied to the profiles of four moving phantoms.

Projection profile matching process is executed retrospectively on a workstation (SunBlade1000, Sun Microsystems, Palo Alto, CA) after all data acquisition had been completed. All matching software is developed with MATLAB (The MathWorks, Natick, MA). In the experiment (B), we segmented the region of moving phantom on the baseline image in order to separate the baseline projection profile into the component of moving phantom and stationary phantom before projection profile matching started.

3. Results and Discussion

18 images (1152 projection profiles for each direction) were acquired for each experiment and 1140 were successfully completed for experiment (A), while 1131 were successfully completed for (B). The standard deviation of the error between the value of the phantom displacement computed from projection data and the value measured by the CCD laser displacement sensor was 0.3 mm for (A), and 0.4 mm for (B). Optimization of each projection profile was completed in 36 ms (CPU time) in average for both configurations. The accuracy of matching is affected by signal-to-noise ratio (SNR). The reason for the result that the accuracy of matching for phantom (A) is better than (B) is that the noise in

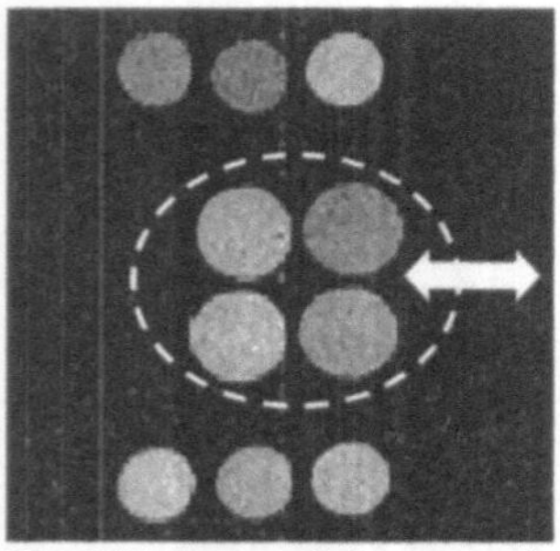

Fig. 3: The MR image of phantoms for experiment (B). The four phantoms in the broken line moved along the axis of the scanner bore. The other phantoms were at the standstill.

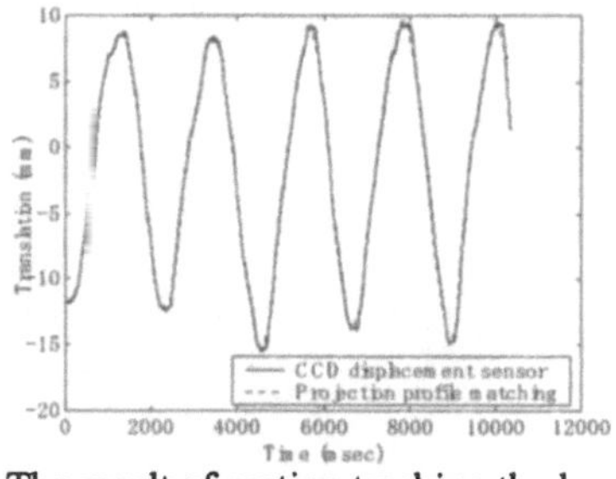

Fig. 4: The result of motion tracking the laser displacement sensor and projection profile matching.

©CARS/Springer. All rights reserved.

baseline projection profile of static phantom was added to the profile of moving phantom. The accuracy is also affected by inhomogeneity of coil sensibility. Since coil sensitivity is highest in the center of the coil, the larger the displacement of phantom becomes, the weaker the signal from phantom is. This is one reason why large displacement caused the failure of matching in experiment (B).

4. Conclusion

We have demonstrated the method for fast image registration embedded in MR pulse sequence. The method successfully performed on phantom study with enough accuracy and speed. This method has capability to apply to 3-dimensional Fast Fourier Transformation (FFT) imaging, and estimate the 3-dimensional motion of the subject.

Acknowledgements

This work was supported in part by Szuken Memorial Foundation and Grant-in-Aid for Scientific Research (B) 13558103 from Japan Society for Promotion of Science (JSPS).

References

1. Gering DT, Nabavi A, Kikinis R, Hata N, O'Donnell LJ, Grimson WEL, Jolesz FA, Black PM, Wells WM, "An integrated visualization system for surgical planning and guidance using image fusion and an open MR", *Journal of Magnetic Resonance Imaging*, Vol. 13, No. 6, pp. 967-975, 2001.
2. Hata N, Nabavi A, Wells WM, Warfield SK, Kikinis R, Black PM, Jolesz FA, "Three-dimensional optical flow method for measurement of volumetric brain deformation from intraoperative MR images", *Journal of Computer Assisted Tomography*, Vol. 24, No. 4, pp.531-538, 2000.
3. Derek LG Hill, Philipp G Batchelor, Mark Holden and David J Hawkes, "Medical image registration", *Physics in Medicine and Biology*, Vol. 46, pp. R1-R45, 2001.

©CARS/Springer. All rights reserved.

A virtual environment for navigating and controlling intraoperative magnetic resonance images

Eigil Samset[a], Anne Talsma[b], Marius Kintel[a]
[a] The Interventional Centre, Rikshospitalet, University of Oslo, Norway
[b] Department of Radiology, University Hospital of Groningen, The Netherlands

Abstract

Intra-operative MRI has recently entered the OR as a new imaging modality. Customised visualisation systems might further facilitate the use of this imaging technology. A visualisation system for use in the interventional MRI was made, providing a virtual environment for navigation in real-time images and for controlling the scanner. The visualisation system has customised features for certain clinical applications. A training- and testing facility was also assembled. The introduction of the visualisation system in the intervention MRI overcame several ambiguities and inconsistencies previously present, and resulted in a more transparent man-machine interface approach. Augmentation of real-time MR images with 3D rendering and customised navigation features opens new possibilities in intra-operative MRI. The described system might also be extended to other intra-operative imaging modalities.

Keywords: Intra-operative MRI, virtual reality, surgical navigation

1. Introduction

Recently interventional MRI has entered the field of image-guided surgery as a new intra-operative image modality [1-2]. Interventional MRI brings the power of three-dimensional imagery and real-time cross-sectional scanning with high soft tissue contrast into the OR. This overcomes the problems involved in using pre-surgically acquired MR image sets for surgical navigation, where the changes of anatomy during the course of surgery are not accounted for.

In spite of its obvious advantages, interventional MR has some shortcomings that have limited its acceptance and utilisation in surgery. Some of the shortcomings of interventional MRI are; long acquisition time, sub-optimal image quality, real-time images are only single slice and a confined working environment. In addition, most interventional MRI systems does not have the powerful navigation and visualisation features as found in most surgical navigation systems - like a neuro-navigation workstation.

The aim of this study was to design a visualisation system, based on intra-operative real-time image acquisition, utilising 3D rendering techniques. Images, instruments and other information with links to physical space were visualised together in a 3D scene. The visualisation system was designed generically, to enable the later integration of other

©CARS/Springer. All rights reserved.

image modalities. The navigation tools and features was a combination of general navigation tools, and features targeting specific clinical applications. The visualisation system was also designed to give the operator control of the scanner and the software from inside the magnet bore. A separate aim was to design a training facility, which would work as an emulator of the MR scanner. This facility would also facilitate development and testing.

2. Materials and Methods

2.1 MRI Scanner

The open MRI scanner, Signa SP/*i* (General Electric Medical Systems, Milwaukee, WI, USA) was used. Probe localisation by optical tracking (Flashpoint 5000, Image Guided Technologies, Boulder, Colorado, USA) is part if the magnet setup. These cameras detect the infrared signal transmitted by LED's mounted on the localisation probe. The coordinate system of the tracking system and the coordinate system of the MR scanner are made identical by calibration.

2.2 Training and testing facility

A MR Mock-Up was made for testing and training purposes. The Mock-Up consists of a large rack, where the distance between the sidewalls is 60cm. Three infrared cameras is mounted in the top of the rack, facing down. Together with a Flashpoint 3000 computer these facilitates optical probe localisation. A plastic skull was placed in the centre of the rack, to act like a phantom, and a monitor was installed. The Flashpoint computer was connected to a PC that emulated the functionality of the MR workstation.

2.3 Software architecture

The software was split in two parts; a server part and a client part, in order to facilitate the development process, ease code maintenance and spread CPU load. The server part retrieves images, tracking information and controls the imaging platform while the client part is performing the visualisation of this data. Two versions of the server part were implemented, one to interact with the interventional MRI system, and one to interact with the MR mockup. The server worked as an abstraction of the imaging hardware, by having identical interfaces regardless of platform. A client application was made to communicate through a network connection with any of the two server versions. This software runs on an SGI O2 (SGI, Mountain View, CA). The server and the client applications communicate through a special designed network protocol. This protocol was made to facilitate real-time two-way communication of requests, images and coordinate information.

In this application a 3D scene was made, where 2D image slices, acquired with 2-7 sec. intervals, were displayed together with the optical trackable localization probe. The camera position could change depending on operator mode. The 3D scene was implemented, using the retain-mode object oriented scenegraph API «Coin3D» (Systems in Motion, Trondheim, Norway) [4].

©CARS/Springer. All rights reserved.

3. Results

3.1 Features

The results are presented in terms of the features implemented. The software, as developed for the open MRI system, has different modes in guidance, visualisation and control of the scanner. The details of each mode are described below.

3.1.1 Standard operation

In this mode the scanner continuously acquires images relative to the position and direction of the localisation probe. The user is able to select from nine different image orientations. Common to all scan orientations is that the images are centered at the projection of the iso-center in the image plane.

Pressing the footswitch could save probe position and direction of a point of interest. As a result a «ghost-pen» was displayed at the saved position. Positions and directions could also be manually entered into the application through a GUI or a file.

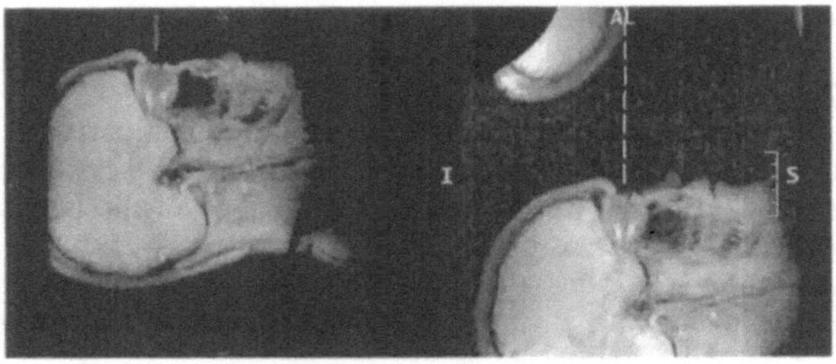

Figure 1 - Comparison of images from conventional realtime display and the implemented visualization system. On the right is a screenshot from the real-time display of the interventional MR scanner. On the left is a screenshot from the implemented visualization system. Different image centers are evident as well as the effect on wrap-around artefacts.

The standard operation mode was tested by simulating presurgical planning on a healthy volunteer (fig. 1). The feature of centering the image plane at the projection of iso-center in the plane gave a more intuitive navigation than the original setup where all images where centered around the probe position. It did not give the feeling of the anatomy moving around, but rather the localization probe. This solution also gave less wrap-around problems since images where not acquired in the periphery of the imaging volume.

©CARS/Springer. All rights reserved.

3.1.2 Find target mode

Returning the localization probe to a saved position was facilitated in this mode. An image plane is acquired at the position of the saved pen. The virtual camera is placed approximately at the position and direction of the user's eyes. This made a simple relationship between the images on the display and the user's view. The virtual pen acted like a laser pointer where a red dot appeared at the point where the trajectory of the virtual pen intersected the image plane. The virtual pen was made to change colour when it was aligned with the saved pen direction and in addition the tip of the pen changes colour when the position of the pen is at the saved position. This is illustrated in figure 2.

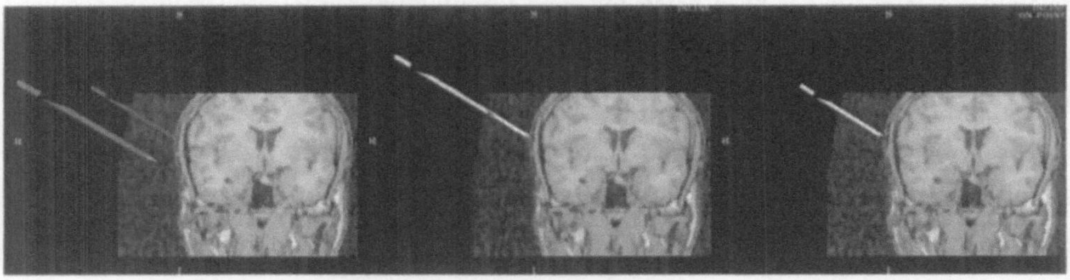

Figure 2 - Illustration of 'find target' mode. The green pen is the saved position. The red pen is first placed in line with the green pen, making both pens white. The red pen is then advanced to be on the saved point, making the tip of the pen blue.

In find target mode a dualplane functionality was also implemented. This functionality made alternate scanning between two different scan orientations possible. The 3D scene would thus show the two last acquired images simultaneously. A typical combination could be in-plane with the probe trajectory and perpendicular to the probe trajectory. The scanplanes would be updated in an alternating fashion. One half of both planes where clipped away to avoid ambiguity, which halves to be clipped could be selected by the user.

3.2 Display

As described above two flat-panel monitors are used for display in the MR. In the mock-up head mounted displays (HMD) were tested in addition to a flat-panel monitor. The software was designed to transmit field-interlaced stereo on the video-output. In combination with the HMD this enabled separate eye-addressing from two cameras in the scene, with stereo separation. The HMD used was i-Glasses (i-O Display Systems, Sacramento, CA, USA) with a resolution of 320x200 per display.

A study was done to evaluate the benefit of stereo vs. mono vision in this application. 7 persons where asked to use the «find target mode» and align the localization probe with 17 pre-planned positions using the HMD. For every hit the HMD were switched between stereo and mono display. All positions were hit twice, once in stereo and once in mono. The time to hit was recorded for every point. A hit was accepted when tip of the handpice was within 3 mm from the save position, and the direction was within 10 degrees from the saved direction.

©CARS/Springer. All rights reserved.

7 test persons conducted 17 hits with mono display and 17 hits with stereo display, giving a total of 119 pairs of time-to-hit records. The mean time-to-hit in mono was 24.9s (STD=36.3s), and in stereo 15.1s (STD=11.3). The paired mean difference was 9.8s (STD=35.7s) in favour of stereo rendering. This difference was statistically significant (p=0.003) with a 95% confidence interval from 3.3s to 16.2s.

4. Discussion

A merge of a navigation system, and an interactive scan guidance system for intra-operative MR image has been presented. The scanning time in intra-operatively acquired MR images is on a scale that makes navigation difficult. The interactive delay makes the total latency very unpractical. Despite this, the ability to navigate with real-time images in contrast to a pre-acquired dataset, is compelling. While the images are not true real-time, the tracking information is. The utilisation of this together with 3D rendering and visualisation of points of interest as virtual objects in the 3D scene narrows the gap between intra-operative MR and neuro-navigation with respect to interaction [4].

Intuitive hand-eye coordination is important in all image-guided surgery applications. Standard radiological view-directions on MR images can often be difficult to navigate from, since the view-direction is patient relative and not user relative. In non-conventional patient positioning it is not always easy to interpret scan orientations. Having the ability to move the camera to the surgeons view-point may thus facilitate both the understanding of scan orientations and correct movement of the tracked probe. The results revealed conceptual differences in how images are translated and rotated with respect to the localization probe. We have presented an implementation where all images are translated to be centered at the projection of the MR scanners iso-center into the image plane. This was only unpractical when using a small field of view, and the periphery of the imaging volume was the focus of attention. It had the benefit of making the image stable while moving the probe in the plane - it is conceptually consistent with the fact that the observer looks at the image from a fixed point relative to the iso-center of the scanner.

The benefit of stereo-scopic views has been discussed in the video-scopic community [6-7]. In the presented applications, the benefit might be clearer, since there are no free hands to move the virtual scope the same way as a laparoscope is moved, although adding head-tracking may give a similar effect. The task of aligning two graphic objects, like the situation is in the find target mode of the presented system, is also well suited for the use of stereoscopic vision. The results showed a large standard deviation for time-to-hit in mono mode. This reflected the observation that some test-persons used long time on some difficult positions. It was also clear that untrained persons had a larger difference between stereo and mono vision that trained persons. It can be concluded that the benefit of stereo is largest for untrained persons and in some locations where the direction ambiguity in mono is predominant.

In conclusion, we have developed a framework for navigation and control in conjunction with an intra-operative image modality. The potential of this framework was exemplified by the features described. The concept of presenting the image- and navigation

©CARS/Springer. All rights reserved.

information in a virtual environment, with a simple relationship with the surgical environment will be an interesting path to explore further.

Acknowledgements

Eigil Samset was supported by a grant from the Norwegian Research Council. We acknowledge the support of Ole Jakob Elle and Lars Aurdal for fruitful discussions and help in this project.

References

1. Alexander, E., III, Moriarty, TM, Kikinis, R., and Jolesz, F. A., "Innovations in Minimalism: Intraoperative MRI." Clinical Neurosurgery , 43, 338-52, 1996
2. Schenck, J. F., Jolesz, F. A., Roemer, P. B., Cline, H. E., Lorensen, W. E., Kikinis, R., Silverman, S. G., Hardy, C. J., Barber, W. D., Laskaris, E. T., Dorri, B., Newman, R. W., Holley, C. E., Collick, B. D., Dietz, D. P., Mack, D. C., Ainslie, M. D., Jaskolski, P. L., Figueira, M. R., vomLehn, J. C., Souza, S. P., Dumoulin, C. L., Darrow, R. D., St.Peters, R. L., Rohling, K. W., Watkins, R. D., Eisner, D. R., Blumenfeld, S. M., and Vosburgh, K. G., "Superconducting Open-Configuration MR Imaging System for Image-Guided Therapy", Interventional Radiology, 195, 805-14, 1995
3. Coin3D. http://www.coin3d.org
4. Gering, D. T., Nabavi, A., Kikinis, R., Hata, N., O'Donnell, L. J., Grimson, W. E., Jolesz, F. A., Black, P. M., and Wells, W. M., III., "An Integrated Visualization System for Surgical Planning and Guidance Using Image Fusion and an Open MR", J.Magn Reson.Imaging 13(6), 967-75, 2001
6. Tendick, F., Bhoyrul, S., and Way, L. W., "Comparison of Laparoscopic Imaging Systems and Conditions Using a Knot- Tying Task", Comput.Aided Surg., 2(1), 24-33, 1997
7. Crosthwaite, G., Chung, T., Dunkley, P., Shimi, S., and Cuschieri, A., "Comparison of Direct Vision and Electronic Two- and Three-Dimensional Display Systems on Surgical Task Efficiency in Endoscopic Surgery", Br.J.Surg., 82(6), 849-51, 1995

©CARS/Springer. All rights reserved.

Collision avoidance in robot assisted surgery

A. Austad[a], O. J. Elle[b], L. Aurdal[b], E. Samset[b], H. Fontenelle[c], E. Fosse[b] and K. E. Malvig[a]
[a]Department of Engineering Cybernetics, Norwegian University of Science and Technology. O.S Bragstads plass 2D, N-7491 Trondheim, Norway
[b]The interventional Centre, National Hospital of Norway
[c]SimSurgery AS

Abstract

The use of surgical robots is growing in order to solve some of the problems encountered in endoscopic surgery. But the use of robots also introduces new problems to the surgical procedure like collision between robotic arms or between instruments. To reduce these problems a prototype of a collision warning system is made. The positions of the robots are measured in real-time and the distances between them are calculated. Before a collision occurs a warning is given. Different types of feedback to the surgeon are tested. The prototype is shown to work properly and give valuable information to the surgeon.

Keywords: Endoscopic surgery, robotics, collision detection

1. Introduction

The dexterity of the human hand is reduced when using endoscopic techniques, where rigid instruments are introduced through small incisions (trocars) allowing in/out, up/down, right/left and rotational (about the length axis of the instrument) movements. Because of this, conventional endoscopic surgery has 4 degrees of freedom (d.o.f) compared to the 6 d.o.f that are necessary for reaching an arbitrary position from all directions. The delicate tactile feedback by the surgeons fingers touching the organs are also partially missed during the minimal invasive procedure, and the procedures typically rely heavily on good visual feedback.

Medical robotic technology can in some cases improve existing procedures or make new procedures possible. Robotic surgery also provides better working ergonomics and possibly reduced healthcare costs. The dexterity, accuracy and the reduction of the tremulous in the human hand makes the robotic arms ideal for precise microsurgical procedures e.g. on the eye, heart or brain. In combination with image-guided procedures, robotic devices are now under implementation in many fields of endoscopic surgery: cardiac surgery, abdominal surgery, orthopaedic surgery, neurosurgery and others.

©CARS/Springer. All rights reserved.

Two robotic systems, the Zeus-system[1] and the DaVinci-system[2] are routinely used in thoracoscopic surgery. While solving some of the problems encountered in endoscopic surgery, the use of robots also introduces new problems to the surgical procedure.

- Extra-thoracic robotic arm collision
  Several researchers have reported on collisions between the robotic arms, and the importance of correct initial arm set-up is stressed [1,2]. We have previously addressed the problem of collision between the robotic arms using the Zeus-system [3]. Even small changes in robotic set-up or patient position can turn the procedure into failure. There are 21 independent variables to be set in the initial robot set-up so it is almost impossible to predict intuitively the effect of changing each variable.

- Intra-thoracic instrument collision
  Using endoscopic robots, the surgeon only has visual feedback from the position of the instruments. Usual, only the tip of the instrument is visible, and collision between the shaft of the instrument and the endoscope can be hard to detect. This might cause danger due to uncontrolled instrument movements if the instrument slip off from the tip of the scope.

- Instruments outside image
  If the instruments are outside the image the surgeon has no feedback from the position of the instruments, and the lack of force feedback makes it impossible to know if the instrument hits human tissue. In order to prevent damage to the patient, manual repositioning of the instrument is often the only solution.

This motivates for development of a "Computer Aided Planning System for Robot Assisted Endoscopic Surgery". This tool will both be used preoperatively to plan the procedure and to train personnel as well as inter-operatively to warn the surgeon about possible collisions before they happen and help him out of the situation.

2. Materials and Methods

A prototype of collision warning system is made in MATLAB. During use of the robots, the position of the end effector (the instrument holder) is measured using the optical navigation system Flashpoint[3] and read into a computer. Calculating the inverse kinematics, the positions of each joint are found, and the minimum distances between the arms are then calculated. If the calculated distance is less than a certain limit, a warning is issued. A graphical model of the robotic system shows if and where a collision is about to occur (Fig 1). The graphical model is updated in real-time and the surgeon can at any time change the angle of view.

---

[1] ComputerMotion, Goleta, California, USA
[2] Intuitive Surgical, Mountain View, California, USA
[3] Image Guided Technologies, Bulder, Colorado, USA

©CARS/Springer. All rights reserved.

When two arms gets closer than a specified distance the arms in conflict change colour from black to yellow. If a collision occurs the colour change to red. The distances between each arm are shown as colour bars (green, yellow or red) with length proportional to the distances. It is optional too show the colour bars only in the main window or as a picture-in-picture in the video image (Fig 3). The distance limits can be pre-set by the surgeon.

When an intra-thoracic instrument collision occurs, the instrument changes colour to red, but the distance is not shown.

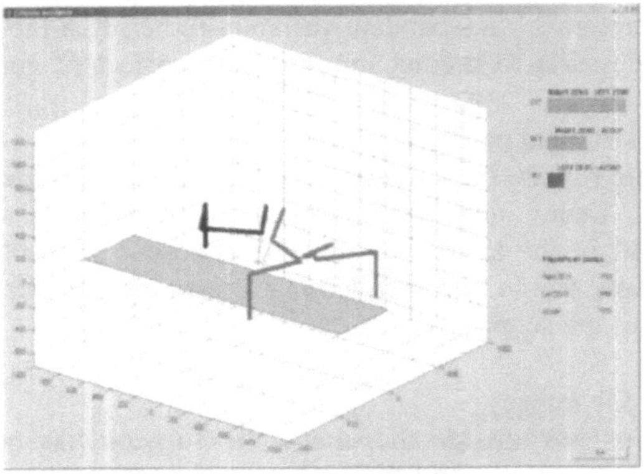

Fig 1: Snapshot of MATLAB program

An experiment in an endoscopic trainer is performed to find what kind of feedback that is considered to be most useful by the surgeon. Fig 2 shows the experimental robotic set-up with the optical probes mounted.

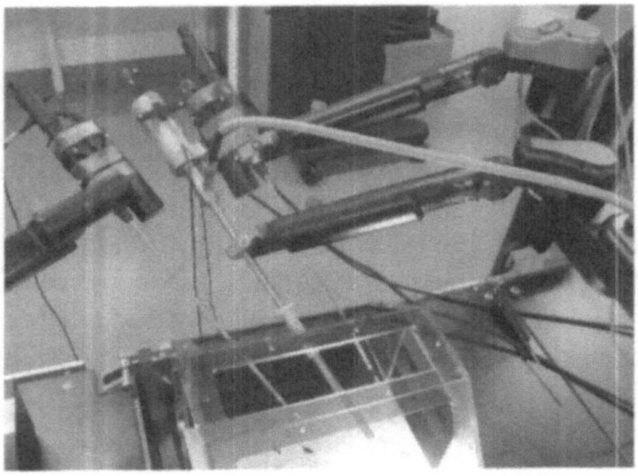

Fig 2: Dry lab robotic set-up. Flashpoint probes are mounted on each instrument

©CARS/Springer. All rights reserved.

3. Results

The collision warning system works properly, but several possible improvements were found:

- During surgery the surgeon has to deal with a number of information sources. Thus it is important to keep all information at a need-to-know level. The picture-in-picture distance information should only be visible when the robotic arms are closer than the given distance limit.
- The instruments are commonly close to the endoscope, and to correctly detect intra-thoracic instrument collision the accuracy of the position measurement has to be high. The Flashpoint probes are mounted direct on the instruments and high accuracy can be achieved. However, accuracy may be a problem if using encoder signals from the robot joints as position measurement, since accurate position of the robots and incision points have to be known to calculate the position of the instruments.
- A common problem in robot assisted endoscopy is to find instruments outside the image. In the graphical model of the robot system, a line extending from the instrument is drawn. This line shows the path of the instrument if moved forward in a straight line, and helps to choose the correct movements to get back into the image. A further improvement will be to automatically have the view in the graphical model to follow the view of the endoscope (similar to the flight-by-wire in aeroplanes).
- The ability to change the angle of view was found very helpful. Looking at the robots from another angle may give more information of their mutual positions.
- The use of the Flashpoint navigation system is ideal for prototype testing since position measurements can be done without access to the hardware of the robotic system. However, using Flashpoint in the OR is not trivial. Thus, for clinical use, encoder signals from the robot joints should be used as position measurements.

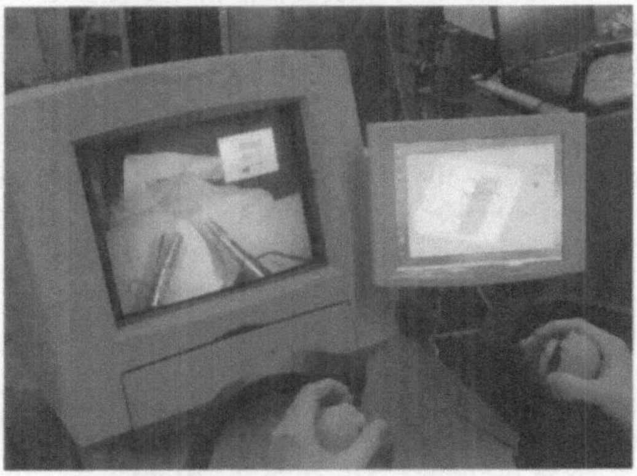

Fig 3: Endoscopic image with calculated distances (picture-in-picture) and graphical model of the ZEUS robotic system (LCD screen)

©CARS/Springer. All rights reserved.

4. Discussion

Limited workspace and possible collision between robotic arms or between the arms and the surrounding environment is a challenge in all multi-arm robotic systems. In medical applications were there should be few restrictions on instrument movements, collision can hardly be completely avoided, unless each arm have redundancy (i.e. more than 6 d.o.f). To minimise the problems, two steps should be taken:

- Proper planing and optimisation of the set-up of the robotic system such that the probability of collision is minimised.
- Before collision happens, the surgeon should get a warning and guidance on how to avoid the collision.

Several groups are working on robotic simulators for training and planning prior to endoscopic surgery [4,5]. This paper focuses on anti collision during surgery. The prototype presented give warnings about collision and some guidance on how to overcome the problem while using the robotic system. The graphical model of the robots shows the position of the surgical instruments, even if they are outside the image. Furthermore the surgeon is able, from his seat at the master console, to look at the robot positions from any angle. The prototype is programmed in MATLAB and Flashpoint is used to measure robot positions. Neither is ideal for a user-friendly tool for clinical use. The next generation tool should implement the improvements suggested and encoder signals form the robot system should be used as position measurements.

Other types of feedback, which is not implemented in our prototype, should also be considered:

- One solution will be to use force feedback in the master console, giving force resistance when the arms gets too close. This is not trivial and has to be implemented in the control software of the robot system. The force feedback can also be used to guide the surgeon trough the problem.
- A warning sound may be given with a single beep at the given distance or with beeps increasing in frequency when the arms get closer (like the proximity alarms in some cars). Another aspect is whether to have one alarm sound or to have different sounds for different kind of collisions, like arm-to-arm or arm-to-environment. If sound signals are used as feedback, care should be taken to keep the feedback at need-to-know level. Sound signals can easily be more irritating than informative.

Numerous surgical teams report on successful surgery using robots. Our experience is that robots is a helpful and often necessary tool in standardised procedures, but deviation from these procedures often cause problems. To solve the problems stated, a tool like the one proposed seems necessary.

©CARS/Springer. All rights reserved.

5. Conclusion

The prototype is shown to work properly and give valuable information to the surgeon. However, further improvements are necessary, and other types of warning feedback to the surgeon should be tested.

References

1. V. Falk, A. Diegler, T. Walther, J. Banusch, J. Brucerius, J. Raumans, R. Autschbach and W.O. Mohr, "Total endoscopic computer enhanced coronary artery bypass grafting", *European Journal of Cardio-thoracic Surgery*, 17:38-45, 2000.
2. D. Loulmet, A. Carpentier, N. d'Attellis, A. Berrebi, C. Cardon, O. Ponzio, B. Aupècle and J.Y.M. Relland, "Endoscopic coronary artery bypass grafting with the aid of robotic assisted instruments", *The Journal of Thoracic and Cardiovascular Surgery*, 118(1):4-10, 1999.
3. A. Austad, O. J. Elle, J. S. Røtnes and K. E. Malvig, "Computer aided planning of trocar placement and robot settings in robot-assisted surgery", In *Proc. of the 15th Int. Congress and Exhibition: CARS 2001 Computer Assisted Radiology and Surgery*, Elsevier Science B.V., Berlin, 2001
4. A.M. Chiu, D. Dey, M. Drangova, W.D. Boyd and T.M. Peters, "3-D Image Guidance for Minimally Invasive Robotic Coronary Artery Bypass", *The Heart Surgery Forum*, 3(3):224-231, 2000.
5. J.S. Røtnes, J. Kaasa, G. Westgaard, E.M Eriksen, P.O. Hvidsten, K. Strøm, V. Sørhus, Y. Halbwachs, O.J. Elle and E. Fosse,"Digital trainer developed for robotic assisted cardiac surgery", *Stud Health Technol Inform,* 81:424-30, 2001

©CARS/Springer. All rights reserved.

Single-step robot guided bone resection and individual reconstruction of the skull

S. Weihe[a], D. Engel[b], M. Wehmöller[c], J. Raczkowsky[b], C. Rasche[a], S. Hassfeld[d], H. Eufinger[a]

[a] Dept. of Oral & Maxillofacial Plastic Surgery, Ruhr-University Bochum, Germany

[b] Inst. of Process Control & Robotics, University of Karlsruhe, Germany

[c] Inst. of Production Systems, Ruhr-University Bochum, Germany

[a] Dept. of Oral & Maxillofacial Surgery, Ruprecht-Karls-University Heidelberg, Germany

Abstract

The TICC (Tomography Image processing CAD-CAM) processing chain allows the supply of existing craniofacial defects with individually prefabricated implants based on helical CT data [1, 2]. In combination with individual templates single-step bone resection and reconstruction is available [3, 4, 5, 6]. New developments in navigation and robotics allowed a robot guided bone resection according to the preoperative planning with the CAD system [7, 8, 9, 10]. This study shows results of resection experiments on ovine cadaver heads.

Keywords: CAS, Resection, robotics

1. Introduction

The TICC-processing chain developed by an interdisciplinary research group at the Ruhr-University Bochum in Germany allows the supply of existing craniofacial defects with individually prefabricated implants based on helical CT data. Until now more than 250 implants made of pure titanium have been inserted successfully with great benefit for the patients (Fig. 1).

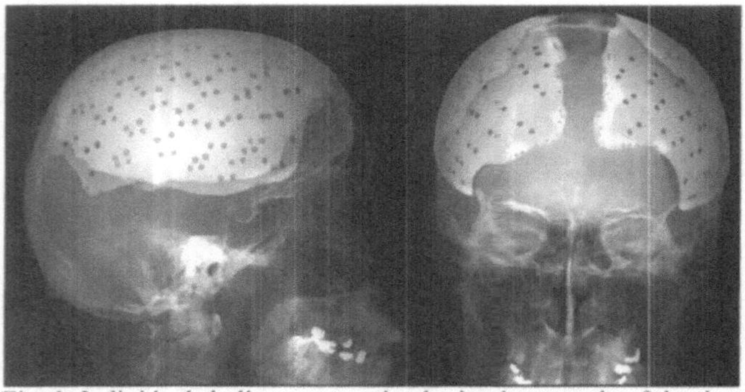

Fig. 1: Individual skull reconstruction by implants made of titanium.

©CARS/Springer. All rights reserved.

Special indications as tumour or osteomyelitis require a single-step bone resection and reconstruction with the preoperatively fabricated implant. So far a resection template was necessary to perform the bone resection corresponding to the prefabricated implant.

New developments in intraoperative navigation and robotics allow a robot guided bone resection of the cranial and facial bone according to the preoperative planning with the CAD system. In consequence a single-step operative approach becomes possible without a resection template (Fig. 2).

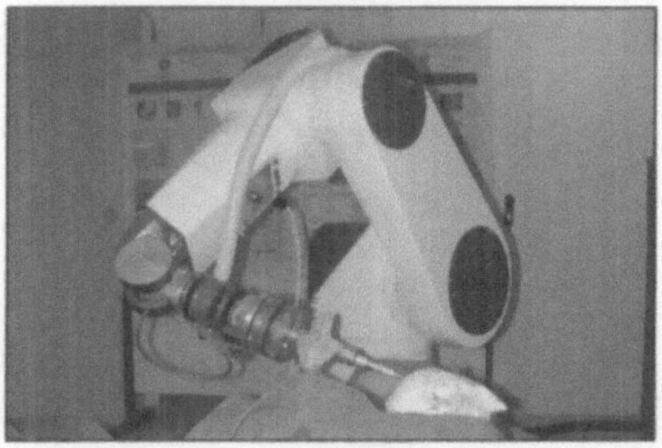

Fig. 2: Robot resection at the Inst. of Process Control & Robotics, University of Karlsruhe, Germany.

2. Materials and Methods

To investigate and evaluate the clinical practicability and the precision of the robot guided bone resection an animal model was evolved: Three ovine cadaver heads were prepared with miniscrews (Medicon, Tuttlingen, Germany) as markers and the data acquisition was carried out with helical CT (Somatom Plus 4, Siemens, Erlangen, Germany). The data were transmitted to the CAD system (STRIM 100 Matra-Datavison, Paris, France) and three complex bony defects were planned in relation to the markers (Fig. 3,4,5).

n°	figure	defect description	extension
#1	3	parietotemporal, right side	6.5 by 4.5 cm
#2	4	parietal, bilateral	5.0 by 4.5 cm
#3	5	orbitotemporal, left side	5.0 by 3.0 cm

Table 1. Defects of the ovine heads.

For the defects #2 and #3 an individual implant and the trajectories for the robot resection were planned with the CAD system. Afterwards the trajectories were transmitted to the control unit of the robot by an ASCI-interface. After referencing the markers with an infrared navigation system and with the manually guided robot's arm the bone resections were performed with the robot system CASPAR (Stäubli RX90CR, Orthomaquet/URS, Schwerin, Germany). During the bone resection of defect #1 the operation table and the holding fixation of the ovine head were not connected to the robot and the infrared navigation system was not integrated in the robot's arm.

©CARS/Springer. All rights reserved.

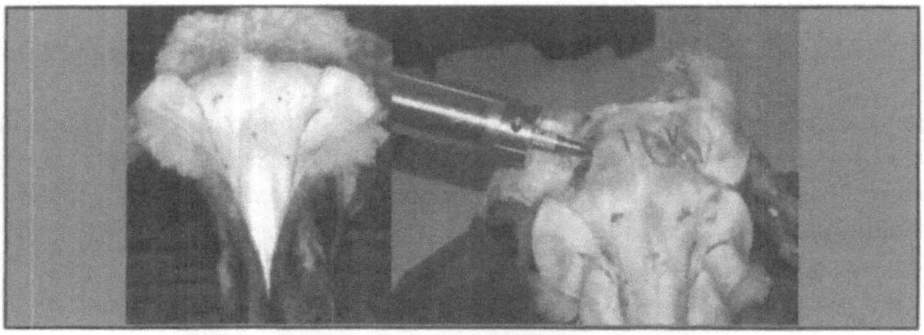

Fig. 3a: Defect #1, *left*: planning, *right*: result.

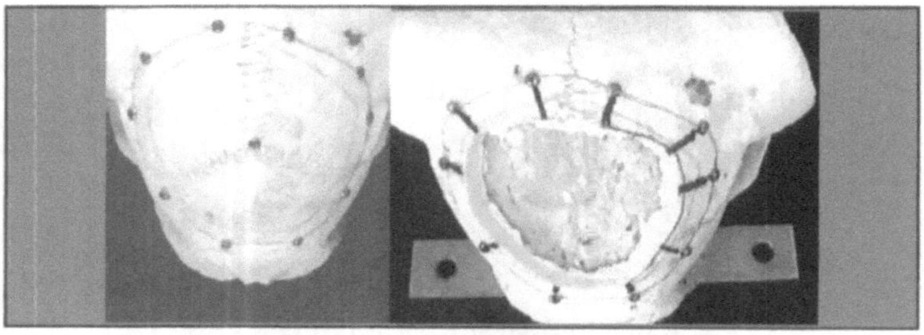

Fig. 3b Defect #2, *left*: planning, *right*: result.

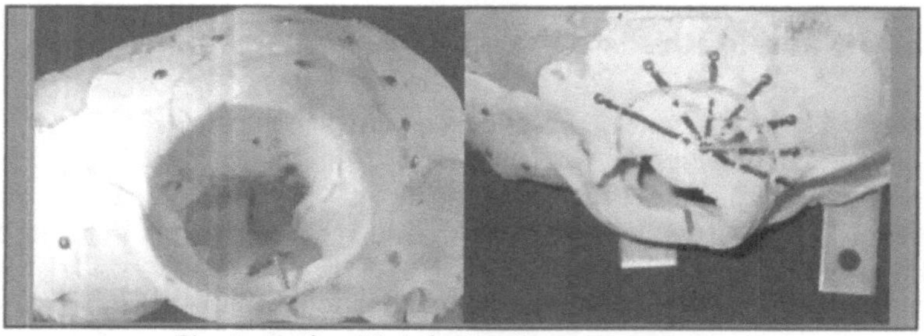

Fig. 3c: Defect #3, *left*: planning, *right*: result.

Defects #2 and #3 were produced by the same robot with the infrared navigation system integrated in the robot's arm. The ovine skulls were fixed in a holder which had a defined position on the operation table connected to the robot during resection. All information (movements, cutting force, cutting speed, cutting depth etc.) were recorded.
For evaluation the resection margins were measured in relation to the markers with a digital sensor, a calliper square and with a ruler by seven persons. The averaged results were compared to the planning data. A preoperatively manufactured implant based on helical CT data was evaluated clinically regarding to the accuracy of the whole procedure.

©CARS/Springer. All rights reserved.

3. Results

During the 18 months between the resection of defect #1 and the resection of defects #2 and #3 a number of modifications and improvements had been developed:
The recorded forces of the resection of defect #1 (x-force of 2 N to 3 N, y-force of -17.5 N to -12.5 N and z-force of –23 N to –22 N) proved to be adequate for milling of bone. All bone cuts were performed with a velocity of the tool of 1 mm/s. The bone was cut up to 8 mm deep, which was partially too deep, so that the meninges were injured. The cutting width was 2 mm corresponding to the tip of the milling cutter.
During this first resection several difficulties had appeared due to the complexity of the chosen trajectories and set up. So the main problem was to determine the optimal configuration of robot and "patient", as the limiting rotation angles of each joint restrict the robot's movements. In this experiment the complete resection had to be carried out in three steps, each time leading to an additional registration error.
During the resections of defects #2 and #3 the accessibility of all positions with the resection tool of the robot could be proved before the resections started, which could therefore be performed in one step.
The cutting depth of resection of defect #2 was too low along the whole resection line caused by incorrect registration of the length of the cutter. After correction of this fault the resection was performed a second time with the right cutting depth, exactly using the first cut. The meninges were not injured and the resected bone could be removed very easily.
The forces of the resection of defect #2 (x-force of -3.1 N to 21.2 N, y-force of -15.2 N to 14.4 N and z-force of -3.3 N to 10.6 N) verified a smooth cutting. The comparison between the planning data and the real dimensions of defect #2 showed deviations of up to 2.42 mm (Fig. 4):

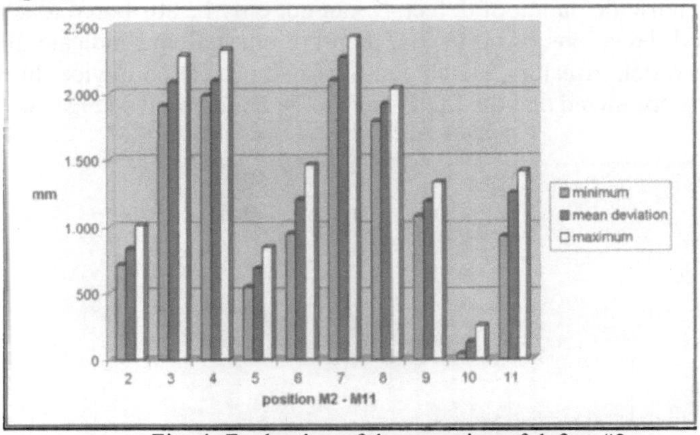

Fig. 4: Evaluation of the resection of defect #2.

The following forces were recorded during the resection of defect #3: x-force of 2.7 N to 15.9 N, y-force of -7.1 N to 3.3 N and z-force of -7.0 N to 7.2 N. The deviations between the planning data and the real dimensions of defect #3 reached up to 1.57 mm (Fig. 5):

©CARS/Springer. All rights reserved.

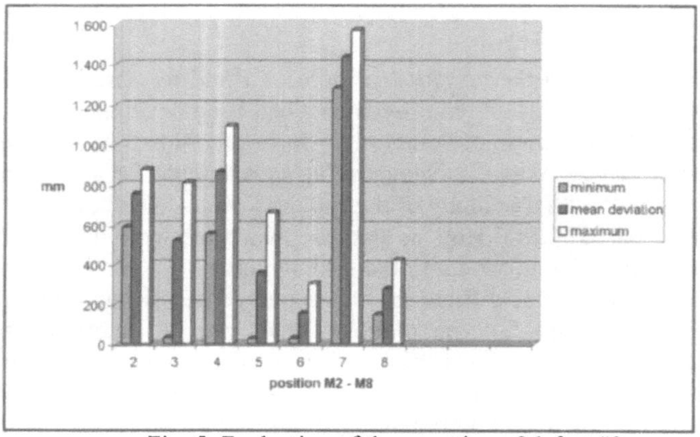

Fig. 5: Evaluation of the resection of defect #3.

4. Discussion

Principally, bone resections in the skull area can be performed by a robot corresponding to a preoperatively manufactured implant based on CT data. The data transfer from CT to the CAD/CAM system and then to the robot control unit was done via an ASCI-interface. So a single data set can be used for the design, the construction, and the production of the implants, as well as for the planning of the resection trajectories.
Even complex defects can be created using the described robotic system. But there are still further developments to be made before using this system in patients:
The described geometric deviation of defect #2 can not only be attributed to a registration error. The measured deviations of up to 2.42 mm are unusual and indicate allowance in the combination of robot, effectors, clutch and overload protection device. In this respect the system has to be optimized and the faults have to be compensated (Fig. 6).

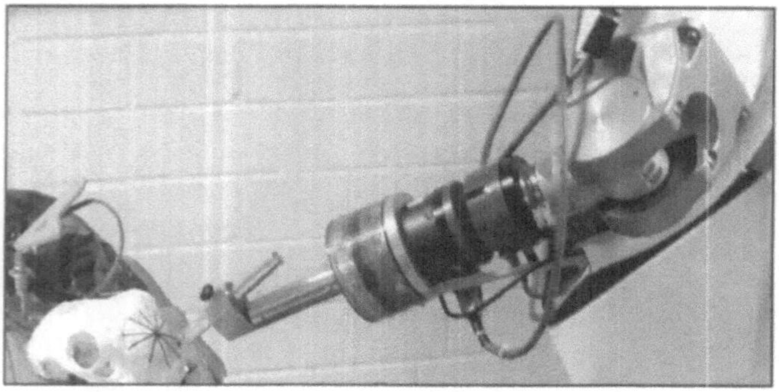

Fig. 6: Clutch and effector of the robot system.

A possibility of visualisation of the whole setup on the CAD system is desirable. The resections should be done virtually before the whole cutting procedure is carried out in reality. Active security concepts have to be put in place, in order to protect patients from

©CARS/Springer. All rights reserved.

system errors as effectively as possible. Additionally the planning of the resection has to take into consideration the possible precision.
As these required improvements are already in the stage of development the first bone resection in the skull area of a patient may take place in the near future.

Acknowledgements

Supported by a grant of the German Research Foundation (DFG - Eu 49/1-2).

References

1. H. Eufinger, M. Wehmöller: Individual prefabricated titanium implants in reconstructive craniofacial surgery - clinical and technical aspects of the first 22 cases. Plast. Reconstr. Surg. 102, 1998, p 300
2. Cranio Construct Bochum: Individual skull reconstruction using titanium. http://www.CranioConstruct.de, 2002
3. H. Eufinger, A.R.M. Wittkampf, M. Wehmöller, F.W. Zonnefeld: Computer assisted cranio-maxillofacial surgery using individual templates and corresponding implants for single-step resection and reconstruction. In: H.U. Lemke, M.W. Vannier, K. Inamura, A.G. Farman (eds.): Computer Assisted Radiology and Surgery, CARS '99, Elsevier, Amsterdam, 1999, p 1024
4. S. Stojadinovic, H. Eufinger, M. Wehmöller, E. Machtens: One-step resection and reconstruction of the mandible using computer aided techniques - experimental and clinical results. Mund Kiefer Gesichtschir. 3 Suppl 1, 1999, p 151
5. K. Radermacher, F. Portheine, M. Anton, A. Zimolong, G. Kaspers, G. Rau, H.W. Staudte: Computer assisted orthopaedic surgery with image based individual templates. Clin. Orthop. 354, 1998, p 28
6. S. Weihe, M. Wehmöller, A. Schramm, N.C. Gellrich, H. Eufinger: Zweizeitiges und einzeitiges Vorgehen bei der Versorgung ausgedehnter Schädeldefekte mit präoperativ individuell vorgefertigten CAD/CAM-Implantaten. 8. Jahrestag der Deutschen Gesellschaft für Schädelbasischirurgie, Leipzig, 2000
7. H. Eufinger, M. Wehmöller: Anwendung und Technik der computerunterstützten Implantatversorgung, Planung und Umsetzung geführter Resektionen. In W. Maßberg, G. Reinhart, M. Wehmöller (eds.): Neue Technologien für die Medizin, WGP 2000, Shaker, Aachen, 2000, p 111
8. S. Weihe, M. Wehmöller, H. Schliephake, S. Hassfeld, A. Tschakaloff, J. Raczkowsky, H. Eufinger: Synthesis of CAD/CAM, robotics, and biomaterial implant fabrication: single-step reconstruction in computer aided frontotemporal bone resection. Int. J. Oral Maxillofac. Surg. 29, 2000, p 384
9. G. Brandt, K. Radermacher, A. Zimolong, G. Rau, P. Merloz, T.V. Klos, J. Robb, H.W. Staudte: CRIGOS: development of a compact robot for image-guided orthopedic surgery. Orthopaede. 29, 2000, p 645
10. S. Hassfeld, J. Mühling: Comparative examination of the accuracy of a mechanical and an optical system in CT and MRT based instrumentation navigation. Int. J. Oral Maxillofac. Surg. 29, 2000, p 400

©CARS/Springer. All rights reserved.

A novel vacuum immobilization device and a novel targeting device for computer assisted interventional procedures

R.J. Bale[a], M. Vogele[a], T. Lang[a], P. Kovacs[a], M. Rieger[a], M. Freund[a], A. Chemelli[a], F. Rachbauer[b], C. Hoser[c], C. Fink[c], B. Dolati[c], R. Rosenberger[c], W. Jaschke[a]

[a] Department of Radiology, Interdisciplinary Stereotactic Interventional Planning Laboratory (SIP Lab), Anichstr. 35, University Clinic Innsbruck
[b] Department of Orthopaedics, Anichstr.35, University Clinic Innsbruck
[c] Department of Traumatology, Anichstr.35, University Clinic Innsbruck

Abstract

Our purpose was the development and evaluation of a patient immobilization device and an aiming device for frameless stereotactic interventional procedures in various body regions. For the CT scan the patient is placed upon a vacuum mattress, wrapped up with special cushions and covered with a plastic sheath. When the vacuum pump is turned on the cushions harden and the patient is sucked against the CT couch resulting in patient immobilization. After the scan the Vertek targeting device is adjusted using the StealthStation navigation system. The aiming device allows for precise alignment of the probe of the navigation system with the preplanned trajectory. The needle is advanced through the aiming device to the target. The novel technique was used for bone-tumor biopsies in 5 patients, vertebral-disc biopsy in two patients and –with a different immobilization technique- retrograde drilling of osteochondral lesions in the talus in 12 patients. Image-fusion revealed a needle displacement within 2-4 mms in all patients. The whole procedure including immobilization, general anaesthesia, adjustment of the targeting device and tissue sampling took about 1-2 hours per patient. Application of navigation systems in combination with the novel devices allows for precise puncturing of different targets in the body.

Keywords: Aiming device, vacuum fixation, frameless stereotaxy

1. Introduction

The most important prerequisites for an accurate puncture are rigid immobilization of the target structure, precise registration and a rigid targeting device [1,2]. Our purpose was the development and evaluation of a whole body immobilization system and a targeting device for computer assisted targeting. We present our novel devices, technique and it's initial clinical applications.

©CARS/Springer. All rights reserved.

2. Methods and Materials

2.1 Immobilization

The BodyFix™ immobilization device (Medical Intelligence, Schwabmünchen, Germany), originally designed to reduce patient motion artefacts during CT/MRI [3] and DSA [4] examinations was modified and adapted to the requirements of computer assisted punctures. It consists of a base plate, a vacuum mattress, a vacuum pump connected to different types of machine-washable cushions which are filled with tiny Styrofoam balls (similar to a vacuum splint) and a plastic foil to cover the region of interest. The patient's part of the body which needs to be immobilised is positioned in a vacuum splint. By evacuating the air the vacuum splint hardens. In addition, the patient is covered with one of the cushions and with the plastic foil. When the vacuum pump is turned on, the air is evacuated from between the covering foil and the vacuum splint. This results in a hardening of the cushion which is sucked against the vacuum splint together with the object to be immobilised, resulting in immobilisation of the patient as long as the vacuum persists. The intensity of fixation can be selected by changing the degree of underpressure built up by the vacuum pump.

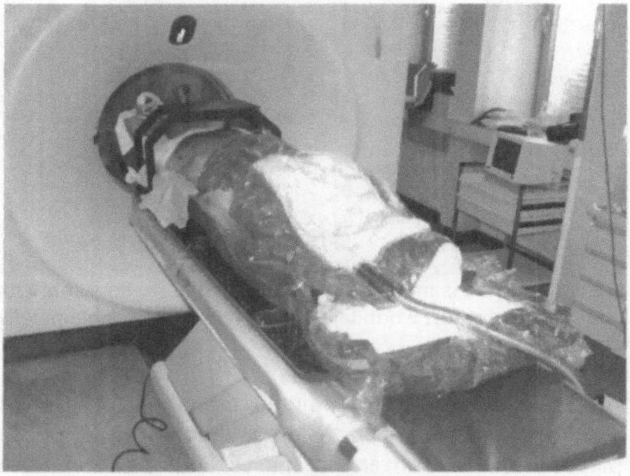

Fig. 1: BodyFix immobilization device - Setup: When the vacuum pump is turned on the air is evacuated from the cushion under the covering sheath . The cushion hardens and is sucked against the CT couch resulting in immobilization of the patient.

2.2 Navigation system

Navigation systems are based on optical localization technology, employing a powerful workstation and an optical position measuring system (OPMS). The OPMS consists of a camera array with two 2D cameras (infrared sensitive charge- coupled device), a variety of hand-held pointer instruments and a dynamic reference frame. The optical sensor array tracks the spatial coordinates of LEDs attached to the instruments. The workstation calculates the coordinates of the sensor and shows the actual position of the instrument in relation to the preoperatively acquired dataset. We used a standard, commercially available stereotactic navigation system, the StealthStation (Medtronic, Memphis, TN, USA). The software and hardware capabilities including the accuracy is comparable to

©CARS/Springer. All rights reserved.

alternate commercially available optical localizing systems, each system having their own characteristics. The system used has implemented a guidance software module allowing development of a surgical plan and interactive execution, respectively.

2.3 Targeting device

For frameless stereotactic targeting we have developed a novel targeting device (Vertek) in collaboration with Medical Intelligence Inc. (Schwabmünchen, Germany) and Sofamor Danek Inc. (Memphis, TN, USA) [5]. The Vertek device consists of an articulating support arm which is mounted to the BodyFix immobilization device via a connector, the aiming device, a guide frame and a reducing tube for the biopsy needle or the pin.

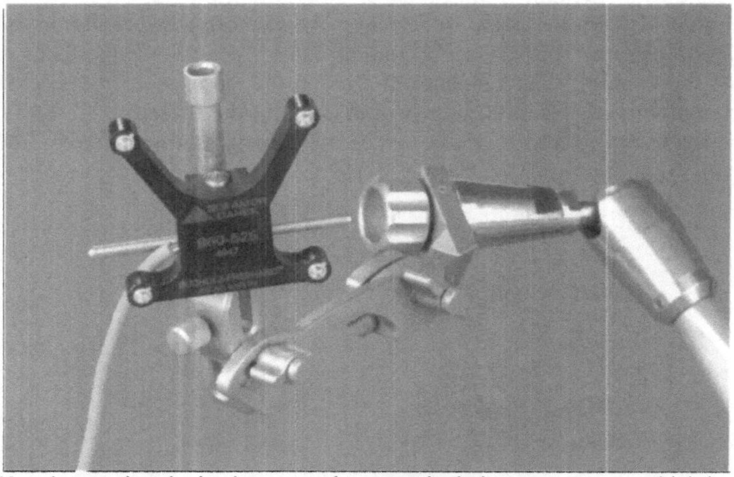

Fig. 2: The Vertek targeting device is mounted to an articulating support arm which is connected to the BodyFix via a universal platform. Two independent pivot joints enable precise alignment of the guide frame with the planned trajectory.

The mechanical arm was designed to overcome the limitations of other „snake-like" arms and remains stable and will not relax or drift into another location, once positioned. The pivots in several places allow for convenient and versatile positioning. All pivots on the arm lock in place with rotation of the locking handle. The guide frame has a LED tracking device to enable the Stealth Station to detect the spatial position of the guide frame. The reducing tube reduces the inner diameter of the guide frame. The aiming device secures a guide frame in place for needle guidance. Two independent pivot joints enable precise alignment of the guide frame (and the biopsy needle) with the planned surgical path.

2.4 Procedure

The patient was immobilized in the BodyFix system. Between six and ten radioopaque markers (Philips Medical Systems, Best, Netherlands) were glued to the BodyFix vacuum matress and to the patient's skin, evenly distributed around the volume of interest.
A Computed Tomography (CT) was obtained with the patient immobilized in the BodyFix. The 3 mm axial CT-scans (increment 3 mm) were performed with the General Electrics HiSpeed CT/i Advantage (GE Medical Systems, Milwaukee, USA) (kV 120,

©CARS/Springer. All rights reserved.

mAs 120). There was a 512*512 -cm matrix, 24-cm field of view, and 0 ° gantry tilt. After CT the patient was anesthetized using oral intubation. In the meantime the CT dataset was transferred to the navigation system located in the CT room via local network.
Three-dimensional reconstructions of the skin, the bone and the radioopaque markers were derived from the original CT – dataset. The pathway was determined on the 3D-navigation system in multiplanar slices, including axial, coronal and sagittal views. In addition, the reformatted planes along the defined path were visualized.
The plastic sheath at the skin entrance point was opened and sterile washing and draping was performed. The sterile dynamic reference frame was mounted to the BodyFix on a a universal platform. After calibration of the probe of the navigation system the sterile image-to patient (fixation device) registration was performed by defining the "virtual" fiducials on the imaged dataset and indicating the respective "real" fiducial markers with the pointer of the navigation system on the BodyFix and on the patient's skin. The system registered the image and BodyFix fiducial positions and derived the root mean square error (RMSE), which is an indicator of registration accuracy. The RMSE was only accepted if it was less than 0.8 mm. If it was higher the registration procedure was repeated. With the pointer of the navigation system the preplanned entrance point on the skin was determined and marked.

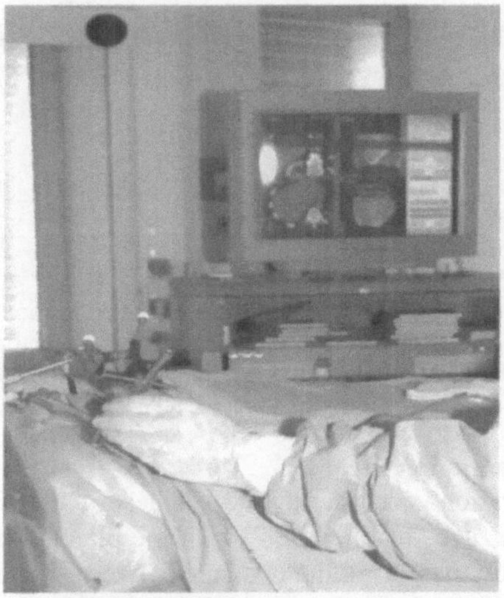

Fig.3: Setup for computer assisted interventional procedure: The Vertek targeting device is adjusted using the navigation system.

The sterile aiming device was connected to the BodyFix via the universal platform. After calibration of the guide frame the arm was positioned such that the guide frame assembly was located above the entry point for the biopsy. The target aim was assessed by using the trajectory views and guidance views of the navigation system software. First the tip of the guide frame was arranged on the line which extends through the predefined entrance position and the target position (i.e. alignment line). The mechanical arm was secured with the locking handle. Second the guide frame was rotated in two axes until the longitudinal axis of the probe was aligned along the preplanned path (i.e. alignment line).

©CARS/Springer. All rights reserved.

These fine adjustments to the aim were performed using two adjustments of the aiming device. When the correct alignment with the trajectory was achieved all adjustments were tightened.

The depth of the biopsy needle insertion was calculated by the navigation system. The guide frame was removed. A stop collar on the biopsy needle was adjusted to the desired depth. The biopsy needle was advanced through the guide frame along the surgical plan to the precalculated target point. After confirming the correct needle position the biopsy was obtained and the needle was retracted.

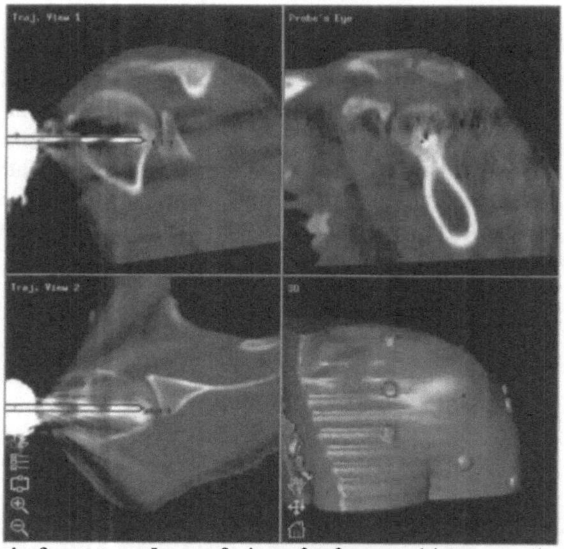

Fig. 4: Quality control of puncture: Image-fusion of reformatted intraoperative scan (with needle in place) with reformatted preoperative scan (with planned trajectory) in a patient with an osteoblastoma of the left humerus for thermocoagulation. Note, that the needle is exactly on the preplanned path.

2.5 Evaluation of localization accuracy

To determine the localization accuracy the 3D – dataset with the biopsy needle in place was superimposed to the 3D – planning CT (with the planned path) and the localization accuracy was evaluated by measuring the distance between the tip of the biopsy needle in the intraoperative scan and the desired target in the plan.

3. Results

The novel technique was used for targeting of bone lesions in 5 patients (2 in the distal tibia, 1 in the humerus, 2 in the femur). In one patient a discography of the disc space between C6/C7 was performed. In another patient with prominent spondylophytes biopsy of the disc space between L5 and S 1 revealed a discitis. In 12 patients retrograde drilling of osteochondral lesions in the talus were performed with a similar technique using the same targeting device but a different immobilization technique (Scotchcast).

©CARS/Springer. All rights reserved.

Image fusion revealed an accuracy of needle placement within 2-4 mms in all 19 patients. In all patients the target point was reached in the first attempt. The whole procedure including immobilization, introduction of general anaesthesia, adjustment of the targeting device and tissue sampling took about 1-2 hours per patient. All patients denied any pain or discomfort related to the immobilization device. A thorough examination of the immobilised extremity after the procedure did not reveal any bruises or swelling directly attributable to the use of the immobilisation device. The device did not interfere with the imaging procedure in any way.

4. Conclusion

Application of navigation systems in combination with rigid immobilization and aiming devices allow for accurate puncturing of different targets in the pelvis, the extremities and the spine at the first attempt. The novel technique offers the possibility to target even very small lesions which are very difficult to localize using conventional puncturing techniques. In contrast to conventional CT-guided punctures angulated approaches can be performed with high precision. However, for precise localization of lesions in organs which are subjects to respiratory movements additional techniques for respiratory triggering have to be developed.

Financial Disclosure / Acknowledgements

Reto Bale, MD and Michael Vogele, MD are co-inventors/developers of the Vertek targeting device and the BodyFix immobilization device and co-shareholders in their financial returns. The authors would like to thank Josef Dummer, Stefan Haselwanter, Helmut Wirtenberger, Martin Knoflach and Christian Müller for their technical assistance.

References

1. Bale RJ, Vogele M, Rieger M, Buchberger W, Lukas P, Jaschke W. A new vacuum device for extremity immobilization. AJR Am J Roentgenol 172(4),1093-4, 1999
2. Bale RJ, Lottersberger C, Prassl A, Vogele M, Czermak B, Dessl A, Sweeney RA, Waldenberger P, Jaschke W. A new vacuum device for extremity immobilisation during digital angiography - initial clinical experiences. European Radiology Pending revision
3. Bale R, Freysinger W, Gunkel AR, Vogele M, Sztankay A, Auer T, Eichberger P, Martin A, Auberger T, Scholtz AW, Jaschke W, Thumfart WF, Lukas PH. Frameless Stereotactic Interstitial Brachytherapy of Head and Neck Tumors – Initial Experience. Radiology 214(2),591-595, 1999
4. Bale RJ, Hoser C, Rosenberger R, Rieger M, Benedetto KP, Fink C. Initial experiences with computer assisted retrograde drilling of osteochondral lesions of the talus – feasibility and accuracy. Radiology 218(1),278-282, 2001
5. Vogele M, Bale RJ. Targeting device (Medtronic, VERTEK™) European Patent 0871407

Surgical Education and Training

CARS 2002 – H.U. Lemke, M.W. Vannier; K. Inamura, A.G. Farman, K. Doi & J.H.C. Reiber (Editors)
©CARS/Springer. All rights reserved.

CathI – catheter instruction system

Ulrike Höfer[a], Thomas Langen[a], Justin Nziki[a], Frank Zeitler, Dr. Jürgen Hesser[a], Ulrich Müller[a], Prof. Dr. Wolfram Voelker[b], Prof. Dr. Reinhard Männer[a]

[a] Institute for Computational Medicine
Universität Mannheim, B6, 23-29, 68131 Mannheim, Germany
hoefer@ti.uni-mannheim.de

[b] Medizinische Universität Würzburg, Josef-Schneider-Str. 2,
97080 Würzburg, Germany

Abstract

Over the last few years the number of minimally invasive cardiological interventions has increased enormously. The equipment has been improved steadily but the education still follows the traditional master-apprentice model. CathI is a new simulation system that allows to train not only the hand-eye co-ordination but also the entire handling with the equipment. The trainee controls everything like in reality with original but insignificantly modified instruments, e.g. guide wire, syringe, control unit for the C-arms, and a foot pedal. According to the real procedure in a catheter laboratory he supervises his activities by using several fluoroscopic screens. The system is based on PC technology (Pentium III, 500 MHz) and generates a frame rate of >12.5 calculated projections/second.

Keywords: Cardiological interventions, simulation, angioplasty

1. Introduction

In the western world most people die because of cardiovascular diseases. Therefore, the number of minimally invasive therapies in this sector has increased enormously over the last few years. Although the cardiological interventions are at low risk, it demands much skill and experience of the cardiologist. In particular, the initial and continued education is considered important. The German Cardiac Society, for example, recommends at least 70 stent implants to stay in good training.

The education follows the traditional master-apprentice model in medicine. An experienced physician supervises the interventions of the learning colleague. This has to be contrasted by the best possible training currently available, since the physician is confronted with typical difficulties and the original setup; and real operation situations. The most severe disadvantage of this model is the accompanied risk for the patients. Hence, it is generally assumed that if a training simulation system can provide the same amount of training experience like real operations, this could solve the current dilemma. Meanwhile, the first systems are available, e.g. in endoscopic surgery [1][2][3]. We assume that in few years, the same will happen in cardiology. Then, training systems will simulate patient and imaging system, and they will allow to harness their near-real setup in the training scenario.

©CARS/Springer. All rights reserved.

Until recently, the only possibility for cardiological surgery training without patients was based on animals or mechanical models. However, except from ethical problems do animals neither have the same cardiovascular morphology like humans nor stenosis. Mechanical models [4] could alleviate these disadvantages, but will require an abundance of complex mechanics to provide a model of the beating heart. Furthermore, in both approaches the trainee receives radiation.

A simulation system without radiation would thus be of a great advantage [5]. But there are rather few systems within the cardiological sector. The ICTS-system [6] and the ICard-system [7] are two examples of training systems that allow the user to navigate with a guide wire in a patient by applying fluoroscopic imaging. The main focus of both systems is the training of the hand-eye co-ordination. The handling of the other instruments within the catheter laboratory is performed by a normal computer mouse and is thus no part of the training program. Only the ICTS-system allows to perform a full angioplasty, which is the aim for our system CathI as well.

2. The catheter instruction system

The aim of the training system CathI (**Cath**eter **I**nstruction System) is to simulate both, the patient and the catheter laboratory.

Figure 1 shows the typical setup of our prototype system. Three computer screens are used as in real catheter laboratories to display the X-ray images of both C-arms and a third for the freeze images. In front, there is the control unit for navigating the C-arms, and a typical setup consisting of a guide wire and a syringe.

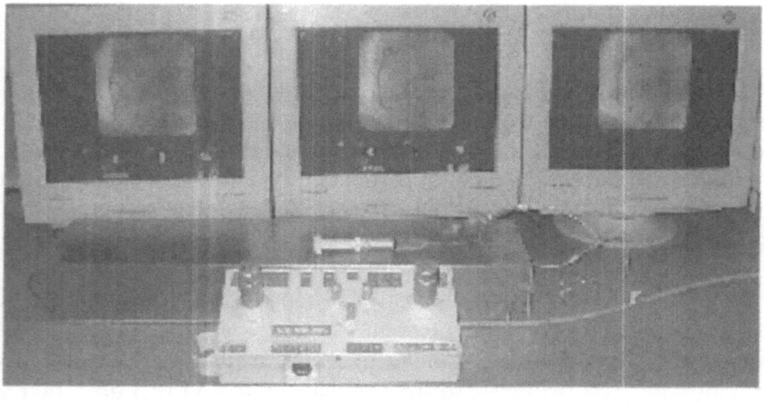

Fig. 1: The prototype design for the CathI simulator for a biplane device

CathI relies on original instruments. Only the X-ray devices and the patient are simulated by computer. The whole system consists of two parts, the input devices and the simulation system. In the following the CathI-system is described in more detail.

©CARS/Springer. All rights reserved.

3. Detailed structure

3.1 Input devices

Besides of the typical control by keyboard and/or joystick the main idea of CathI is to confront the trainee with the typical instruments of a catheter laboratory. The idea is, that the physicians should learn to handle the typical setup. It makes no sense if he learns to move the C-arm by mouse when in practice this interaction is not internalised. The control of the equipment can not be learned during an intervention.

Aside from an original guide wire and a syringe we use an original control unit for the C-arms and a foot pedal for switching on/off the X-ray tube (Fig. 1).

The control units are joysticks that allow the cardiologist to drive the C-arms in different positions. Due to the rotation and angulation angle the fluoroscopy system changes its view. The greatest challenge for a beginner is to position the X-ray optimally with respect to the considered vessel segment. By using the foot pedal he learns to control the X-ray dose. The contrast agent is injected by a syringe. We measure the volumetric flow rate and use this flow to determine the opacity of the vessels. The less contrast agent is injected the lighter are the vessels on the fluoroscopy.

For the therapy, the user must handle with a guide wire inserted into an "artificial patient". This is a tracking system for translational and rotational movements for the guide wire. In contrast to ICard [7] or ICTS [6] our tracking is based on an optical device. The technical solution behind is an optical tracking that measures the movement by changes of optical reflection from a fibre glass rod attached on the guide wire. This is highly advantageous over conventional mechanical tracking systems that have to cope with unrealistic friction and slippage. Since the forces on the guide wire are quite small even slight friction disturb the assumed tactile feedback. Admittedly, it is not possible to unplug the guide wire. But to thread a guide wire into a catheter requires a certain manual prestidigitation and can also be learned without a complex training system.

If the tip of the guide wire hits a hindrance, CathI is able to apply a defined translational force onto the tip. For this purpose the tip contacts a loose plate stick on a slide that can be moved relatively to the guide wire. Due to this construction even hard collisions can be modelled. And like in reality offtake of the guide wire is easily possible. If the friction is applied with clamps the offtake is disproportionately more complex. Finally, friction can be applied by using two rubber blocks pressed on the guide wire. These rubbers simulate the friction agents on the guide wire within e.g. a stenosis.

©CARS/Springer. All rights reserved.

3.2 Simulation system

The second part of the system performs the simulation of the patient and the C-arm devices.

3.2.1 Data acquisition

For the simulation we use a geometric model of a beating heart. The data for these models are obtained from patients during standard interventions. Thus we do not need additional X-ray doses to generate this model and we will be able to upgrade our heart data set. By the use of this procedure we obtain directly a realistic artery topology and the realistic movements of the vessels.

The arteries in the original projections are extracted by a region expansion segmentation approach [8][9]. From this segmentation we obtain a vessel tree. For each artery the skeleton and its local radius are determined. Starting with the information about the two-dimensional structure we reconstruct the three-dimensional geometrical model by biplane reconstruction [10]. By reconstruction of each image pair of one heart cycle we obtain a sequence of 3D-models that is interpreted as a cardiac cycle.

3.2.2 Display

Using this model and the information about the concentration of the contrast agent within the arteries, we generate an X-ray projection according the parameters of the C-arms. The resulting projections are displayed on two respectively three screen, depending on the kind of used device.

The rendering of the arteries is done as follows: A projection matrix composed of internal (like focus, principal point and skew parameter) and external (like translation and rotation) parameters is determined for each X-ray device [11]. The points of the three-dimensional vessel skeleton are projected onto the (virtual) detector. The diameter of the vessel at the point is considered as well. The projected vessel co-ordinates are turned into projected 2D models and then decomposed into triangles that are filled by Gouraud shading. The shading calculation is replaced by assigning opacities to each vertex. This opacity describes the physical attenuation of the vessel, i.e. it considers the thickness and the amount of contrast agent. The latter is calculated by the Hagen-Poiseuille law for the laminar flow of the contrast agent. Finally, this absorption model of the arteries is composited with a pre-calculated X-ray projection of the remaining body of the patient to generate a realistic looking X-ray image. Since the heart moves, the images of each heart cycle are rendered cyclically so that the viewer has the impression of a moving heart.

3.2.3 Guide wire model

The movement of the guide wire is based on the geometric vessel model. It makes physical simplifications like having rigid and circular arteries. The geometric model determines the contact points of the wire/catheter with the wall of the arteries, and it models the bending in between these contact points by direct calculation of the bending of the wire. At the moment we do not consider torsion of the wire/catheter but will include this part soon as well. In addition, we do not yet calculate the force feedback. This part will be finished within the next few months too.

©CARS/Springer. All rights reserved.

4. Results

The current CathI-system runs on a dual Pentium III 500 MHz with three monitors, two for the biplane X-ray device and one for freeze images. The frame rate is guaranteed at least 12.5 frames per second. Thus, we have designed a cost effective, stable system that can be installed in each clinic. In order to understand the functioning of the training simulator we describe a typical training scenario.

At the beginning the physician logs into the system so that user specific training scenarios can be built up. Next a heart model is chosen and the simulation can begin. As in a real catheter laboratory in cardiology one monitor serves for freeze images, others are for projections of the C-arms. The movement of the C-arm is controlled via a joystick on the control unit and X-ray radiation can be switched on by stepping on the foot pedal. Learning to control the C-arm and to use as few radiation as possible is the learning task in this session. In order to see the arteries, the trainee has to inject contrast agent. This has to be co-ordinated with the manipulation of the X-ray system. Hereby, the amount of contrast agent should be minimised as well (just insert as much as necessary to see the vessels). If the user is able to handle these two tasks efficiently, he begins with the navigation of the guide wire. This is again a difficult task that has to be done in parallel with handling the other instruments. The aim is to use as few contrast agent and radiation by having a short an operation time as possible. The results are stored in a personal learning curriculum.
Later scenarios that are currently under development are the simulation of stenosis and complications.

5. Conclusion

CathI was originally developed for catheter interventions in cardiology using guide wires. However, all routines that have been developed for the systems are such flexible that it can be used for any catheter intervention as well. In addition, with this system the handling of C-arm system can be trained without having expensive training centres, simply a PC and the modified instruments are required.

References

1. Ikuta K., Takeichi M., Namiki T.: Virtual Endoscope System with Force Sensation. MICCAI (1998), Cambridge, MA, pp. 293-304
2. McCarthy A.D., Hollands R.J.: A commercially viable virtual reality knee athroscopy training system. Medicine Meets Virtual Reality 6, (1998) San Diego, USA, pp. 302-308
3. Kühnapfel U., Cakmak H.K., Maaß H.: 3D Modeling for Endoscopic Surgery Proc. IEEE Symposium on Simulation, (1999) Delft, NL, pp. 22-32
4. van Walsum T., Zuiderveld K.J., Chin-A-Woeng J.W.C., Eikelboom B.C.,Viergever M.A.: CT-based simulation of fluoroscopy and DAS for endovascular surgery training. Proceedings CVRMed-MRCAS, Lecture Notes in Computer Science, Vol. 1205 (1997), Springer-Verlag, Berlin, pp. 273-282

©CARS/Springer. All rights reserved.

5. Klein L.W.: Computerized Patient Simulation to Train the Next Generation of Interventional Cardiologists: Can Virtual Reality Take the Place of Real Life? Catheterization and Cardiovascular Interventions 51 (2000), pp. 528
6. Dawxon S.L., Cotin S., Meglan D., Shaffer D.W., Ferrell M.A.: Designing a Computer-Based Simulator for Interventional Cariology Training. Catheterization and Cardiovascular Interventions 51 (2000), pp. 522-527
7. Wang Y., Chui C., Lim H., Cai Y.: Real-time Interactive Simulator for Percutaneous Coronary Revascularization Procedures. Journal of Computer Aided Surgery Vol. 3, No 5 (1999), pp. 211-227
8. O'Brien J., Ezquerra N.: Automated Segmentation of Coronary Vessels in Angiographic Image Sequences Utilizing Temporal, Spatial and Structural Constraints. In Proceedings of the Third Conference on Visualization in Biomedical Computing. SPIE, (1994) p. 25
9. Hoffmann K.R., Doi D., Chen S.-H. J., Chan H.-P: Automated Tracking and Computer Reproduction of Vessels in DSA Images. INVESTIGATIVE RADIOLOGY Vol. 25, No.10, (1990) pp. 1069-1075
10. Sarwal A., Dhawan A.P.: Three dimensional reconstruction of coronary arteries from two views. Computer Methods and Programs in Biomedicine Vol. 65 (2001) pp. 25-43
11. Hartley R., Zissermann A.: Multiple View Geometry, Cambridge University Press, (2000)

CARS 2002 – H.U. Lemke, M.W. Vannier; K. Inamura, A.G. Farman, K. Doi & J.H.C. Reiber (Editors)
©CARS/Springer. All rights reserved.

Advanced training environment for gynecologic endoscopy

Wolfgang Müller-Wittig[1], Mario Becker[2], Thomas Elias[1],
Ulrich Bockholt[3], Gerrit Voss[1]
[1] Centre for Advanced Media Technology (CAMTech)
Nanyang Technological University (NTU)
Nanyang Avenue, Singapore, 639798
Tel: +65-6790-6988, Fax: +65-6792-8123
E-mail: mueller@camtech.ntu.edu.sg, URL: http://www.camtech.ntu.edu.sg
[2] Darmstadt Technical University, Darmstadt, Germany
[3] Fraunhofer-Institut für Graphische Datenverarbeitung (Fraunhofer-IGD),
Darmstadt, Germany

Abstract

Rapid development of medical field, expanding knowledge base and new technologies require continuing medical education to achieve life long learning and to keep the surgeons up to date. Consequently, specific training is necessary to guarantee qualification of the surgeons. To overcome the current drawbacks of traditional training systems (on-the-job training, plastic models etc.) for laparoscopy/hysteroscopy an intelligent adaptable training environment has been realized using Virtual Reality (VR), Multimedia (MM) technology, and Intelligent Tutoring Systems (ITS).

Keywords: Surgical training, virtual reality, intelligent tutoring

1. Introduction

This work has been influenced by two paradigm shifts: in medicine there was a transition from open surgery to minimally invasive surgery - surgical interventions are done through small incisions in the body in which a miniature camera and surgical tools are manoeuvred – these complicated techniques require a specific training; and in computer graphics 2-D interaction was replaced by 3-D interaction using Virtual Reality techniques. These innovative technologies open up new possibilities in medicine including anatomical education, preoperative planning, intraoperative support, and surgical training. VR based medical simulation provides a highly realistic surgical environment including anatomical structures and surgical instruments. Especially, a "natural" interaction is guaranteed considering the various human senses. The applicability of VR for rehearsing minimally invasive interventions is proven by a variety of surgical simulators. [1] [2] [3] [4] [5] Billinghurst et al. took the first step towards integration of VR simulation and Intelligent Tutoring Systems for training of ENT surgeons. [6]
The LAHYSTOTRAIN training system is an advanced simulation environment for laparoscopic/hysteroscopic procedures combining virtual reality (VR), multimedia (MM) and intelligent tutoring techniques (ITS). Based on ESHRE (European Society of Human Reproduction and Embryology), the user requirements are specified. Starting with diagnostic procedures and ending with complex therapeutical interventions the whole educational process is covered. In general, due to the various levels in difficulty and

©CARS/Springer. All rights reserved.

complexity the training course can be individually adapted to the level of the trainee addressing all potential „learners“ as students, novices, and experts. The training environment is divided into two scenarios: The basic training system consists of a Web-based training system addressing novice users and focusing on the theory and conceptual aspects of laparoscopy and hysteroscopy. The advanced training system using VR technology addresses more experienced surgeons who want to acquire or improve their skills on minimally invasive techniques. It provides a realistic training environment for rehearsing the various interventions and gives a more intuitive 3-D interaction. The intelligent tutoring architecture detects superficial errors and infers their cause. A tutor proposes different training sessions and exercises according to the user's expertise.

2. Methods

The Advanced Training System (ATS) provides an intuitive training environment for the users of LAHYSTOTRAIN. Moreover, the set up of the training system is similar to the real surgical environment during laparoscopic or hysteroscopic procedures. In general, this environment consists of the patient, the medical instruments - including the endoscope -, video monitor, assistant surgeons, nurses, and the anesthetist. This situation is simulated by the ATS, the VR Simulator - representing the virtual patient, the virtual instruments and the graphics monitor (see Figure 1) and the Intelligent Tutoring System (ITS) - including the assistant surgeons, nurses and the anesthetist.

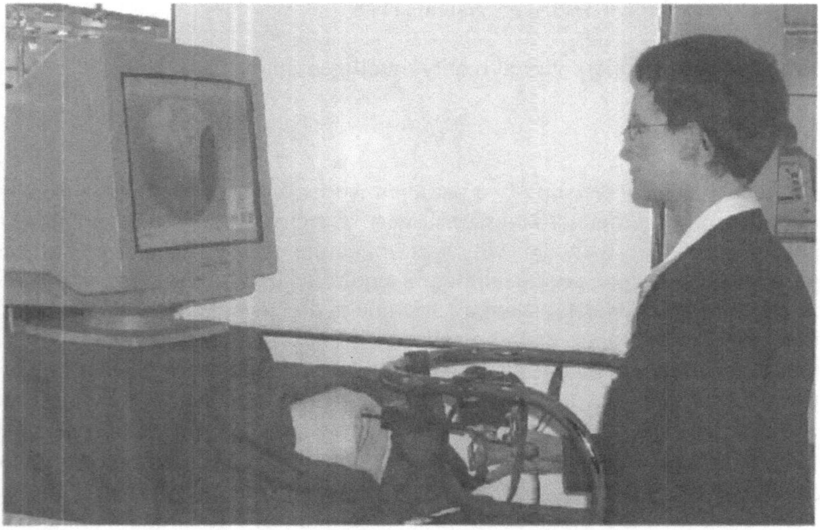

Fig. 1: The hysteroscopy training environment

2.1 Virtual Reality (VR) simulator

The VR Simulator contains virtual anatomical structures and simulates endoscope, surgical instruments, and object behaviour (collision detection, deformation, and cutting). It provides a realistic surgical environment in which training of the various hysteroscopic and laparoscopic interventions is possible. Similar to a real hysteroscopy/laparoscopy, the

©CARS/Springer. All rights reserved.

trainee is able to use surgical instruments interacting with the anatomical region of interest - the virtual situs. The development of the VR simulator is divided into two parts: the generation of the Virtual Environment (VE), and the realization of the 3-D interaction.
Due to analysis of real surgical environment during laparoscopy/hysteroscopy, the Virtual Environment requires a realistic 3-D representation of the abdominal region. Input data for the generation of the virtual situs are CT or MR scans as well as video sequences of laparoscopic/hysteroscopic procedures (see figure 2).

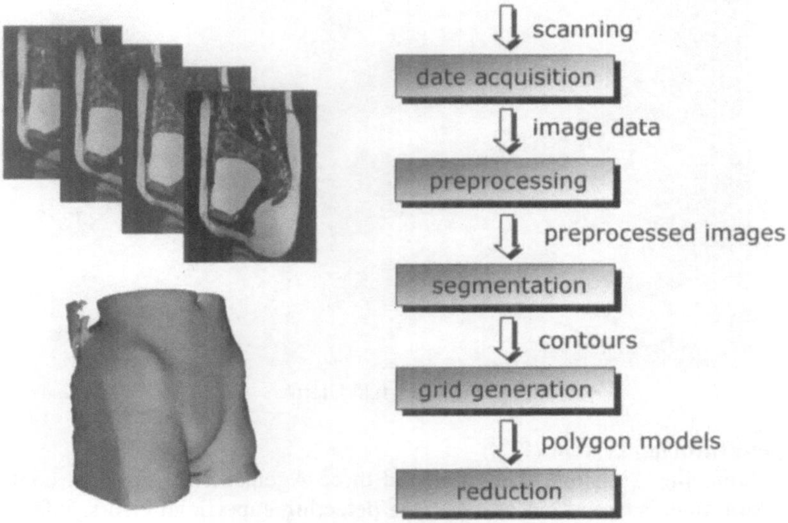

Fig. 2: The 3-D Reconstruction Pipeline

Based on this image data a virtual situs has to be reconstructed suitable for real-time simulation. To provide organ specific textures is indispensable in laparoscopic/ hysteroscopic simulation in order to enhance a realistic appearance and to represent pathological tissue. Input data for the texture generation algorithms are pictures taken from endoscopic video recordings. Finally, these textures are mapped on the virtual anatomical structures (see figure 3).

The simulation model allows a simulation of both rigid instruments and those with moving parts. In addition a virtual endoscope with different optics (e.g., 0°, 12°, 30°) is realised. The hysteroscopic procedure is appropriate for simulation of therapeutic interventions since endoscope and tools are integrated in one single instrument - the resectoscope. Position, orientation and the opening angle of the resectoscope have to be monitored. Providing the simulation origin instruments of KARL STORZ GmbH are integrated into the "Laparoscopic Interface" from Immersion Corporation.)
The trainee handles the instrument and controls the virtual electrodes which are used for the resection of pathologic tissue along the resectoscope´s axis. (see figure 4)

©CARS/Springer. All rights reserved.

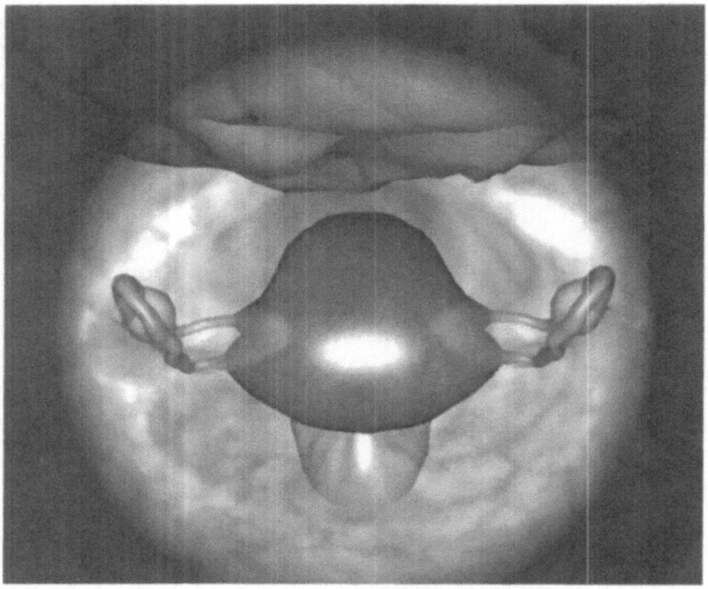

Fig. 3: The Virtual Uterus

2.2 Intelligent tutoring system (ITS)

The ITS includes the Assistant, the Tutor and three Agents. The Assistant controls and supervises the trainee's execution of exercises detecting superficial errors, inferring their cause and providing explanations and remedy suggestions. It provides two types of assistance: reactive and proactive. Proactive assistance consists in the generation of explanations about different aspects of the procedures the surgeons have to carry on. Reactive assistance consists in the generation of explanations whenever the user makes a mistake, or something anomalous is happening at the VR simulator.

The Tutor is in charge of managing the whole training process: rostering and registering student information, acquiring trainee performance data and generating and executing the session according to the user's expertise. The Tutor dynamically modifies this plan adapting it to the trainee's performance during a training session.

Three Agents (Assistant Surgeon, Nurse, and an Anesthetist) will reproduce and emulate the behaviour of some persons of the operating theatre. Surgeons must learn their individual role in the team as well as how to co-ordinate their actions with their team-mates. Intelligent virtual agents, that interact with students through face-to-face collaboration on the virtual world, have already proven in this role [7]. The final subsystem of the LAHYSTOTRAIN architecture is the Student and Instructor Interface which handles all input and output from the advanced training environment:

i) Is the navigation of the endoscope appropriate? What is about the visibility of the therapeutic target in the endoscopic output?
ii) Has the intervention been performed in an appropriate time?
iii) Has all the pathologies been identified correctly?

©CARS/Springer. All rights reserved.

The data for these endoscopic aspects are collected and analyzed by the affiliated Intelligent Tutoring System. The trainee receives an evaluation score of her/his session. Only if she/he has proven her/his skills can she/he pass over to the next level.

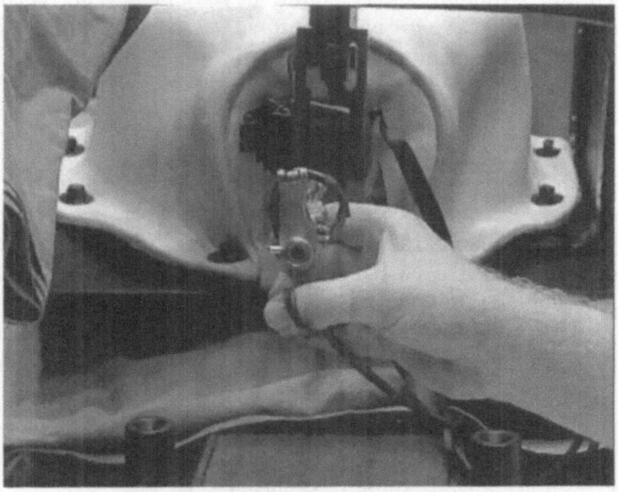

Fig. 4: 3-D interaction with resectoscope

3. Results

The first prototype of LAHYSTOTRAIN includes the treatment of the ovarian cyst. The WWW component provides the learning environment for knowledge acquisition, and the VR simulation system is suitable for skill training. The VR training environment contains virtual anatomical structures and simulates endoscope, surgical instruments and object behavior (collision detection, deformation, cutting). In addition, a force feedback device is integrated into the training system; thus, the trainee is able to feel the give and resistance of the anatomical structures via instruments. The intelligent tutor system guides as the "surgical expert" during the various levels of the training process.

4. Conclusions

This integrative and adaptable training environment provides new opportunities in medical education. Combining intelligent tutor, VR, WWW, and multimedia, this approach demonstrates that the complete educational process can be covered considering the individual training level of the trainee. The LAHYSTOTRAIN system has been validated across European member states in various healthcare environments with existing working methods and practices. Results of the first evaluation showed that the use of medical training simulators has an overall high acceptance. This concept has general applicability to other medical specialties providing standard training situations for objective assessment.

©CARS/Springer. All rights reserved.

The LAHYSTOTRAIN project shows that such surgical simulators are appropriate for practicing surgical techniques without having to advance the learning curve on humans. Considering that several decades were necessary to develop high sophisticated flight simulators, which are available today, rapid developments in recent years and the promising results presented herein give hope that VR based training simulators will be integrated into the medical curriculum in the near future.

Acknowledgements

The European Commission under the Joint Call orchestrated by the Educational Multimedia Taskforce funded this project. We thank Prof. Dr. h.c. Dr.-Ing. José L. Encarnação for providing the environment in which this work was possible. We also thank Dr. Jose Luis Los Arcos (LABEIN, Bilbao), Dr. Peter Oppelt (Universitäts-Frauenklinik Erlangen), Dr. Jan Stähler (Universitäts-Frauenklinik Frankfurt), and all our colleagues and students at our laboratory, especially Berit Klahsen and Albert Schäffer. Without their work we would not have been able to achieve the results presented herein.

References

1. Satava, R.M., "Virtual Reality Surgical Simulator: The First Steps", *Surgical Endoscope*, No.7, Springer-Verlag, New York, 1993, pp. 203-205.
2. Müller, W, and U. Bockholt, "The Virtual Reality Arthroscopy Training Simulator", *Proceedings of Medicine Meets Virtual Reality*, San Diego, 1998, pp. 13-19.
3. Kühnapfel,, U. et al., "3D Modelling for Endoscopic Surgery", IEEE Symposium on Simulation, Delft University, Delft, 1999.
4. Székely, G. et al., "Virtual Reality Based Surgery Simulation for Endoscopic Gynaecology", *Proceedings of Medicine Meets Virtual Reality*, San Francisco, 1999, pp. 351-357.
5. Çakmak, H.K., and U. Kühnapfel, „The Karlsruhe Endoscopic Surgery Trainer for minimally invasive surgery in gynaecology“, 13th Internat. Congress on Computer Assisted Radiology and Surgery (CARS '99), Paris, 1999.
6. Billinghurst, M., J. Savage, P. Oppenheimer, and C. Edmond, "The Expert Surgical Assistant", In Sieburg H., Weghorst S., Morgan K. (editors). Health Care in the Information Age, IOS Press and Ohmsha, Washington DC, 1996, pp. 590-607.
7. Rickel, J., and L.W. Johnson, "Virtual Humans for Team Training in Virtual Reality", 9th World Conference on AI in Education. IOS Press, July 1999.

CARS 2002 – H.U. Lemke, M.W. Vannier; K. Inamura, A.G. Farman, K. Doi & J.H.C. Reiber (Editors)
©CARS/Springer. All rights reserved.

Minimally invasive surgery training by realistic virtual techniques

[a]M. Alcañiz, [b]I. Blanquer, [a]J. García-Collada, [b]V. Hernández, [a]U. Meier, [a,b]C. Monserrat
[a]Medical Image Computing Laboratory (MedICLab),
[b]Departamento de Sistemas Informáticos y Computación (DSIC),
Universidad Politécnica de Valencia.

Abstract

A general simulator for minimally invasive surgery procedures is presented in this paper. Minimally invasive surgical procedures are complex, requiring the surgeons a high training effort. The objective of the simulator is to reduce the casualty due to training. The simulator introduces tools for creating surgical environments and provides interfaces very similar to those used in real interventions. The virtual environments of the simulator comprise actual patient's organs, thus enabling a case-based training, and synthetically generated organs with arbitrary pathologies. The intervention is carried out by means of haptic interfaces with force-feedback. The development of the simulator has been funded by the VRSUR (IST-1999-20783) European Project.

Keywords: Surgery simulation; virtual reality; force feedback

1. Introduction

Training is essential in any specialized task. Training in surgery is even more critical since any mistake can cause patient casualty. Up to now, surgeons train by using cadavers, phantoms, live animals or real patients under the supervision of experts.

The simulator aims at improving the repeatability of the actions. Obviously, training with live animals and human beings do not permit to 'undo' surgical actions or to repeat indefinitely a surgical case until the procedure is correctly learnt. Second objective of the simulator is to train specific pathologies. Live animals are most of the cases sound, and training surgeons start dealing with pathologies when they start training with human beings. The simulator comprises a module for the definition of surgical scenarios, using real medical images, that can present an abnormal anatomy or an interesting pathology. In this case, the trainer surgeon can prepare special cases that will increase the trainees' abilities and skills before they deal with their first real case.

2. Materials and methods

2.1 State of the art

Surgery simulators impose two restrictions to virtual environments: visual realism and physical realism. The first one requires showing organs as similar as in real surgery. The second restriction requires that organs behaviour should be as similar as possible to the physical behaviour of real organs. Dealing with the complexity of these procedures

©CARS/Springer. All rights reserved.

exceeds current computational capacity of standard systems. This implies that surgical simulators have to find a compromise solution between both restrictions.

There are a high number of research groups that have invested important resources in developing surgery simulators. These simulators are focused to training surgeons in a single surgical procedure. Taking into account how the simulators deal with the biomechanical behaviour of organs in a surgery environment, three groups can be set:

- Simulators where organ physical reactions are approximated by simple geometric transformations [1][2].
- Simulators where organ physical behaviour are implemented by using mass-spring models [3][4][5]. These only can simulate deformations of elastic surfaces. The advantage of these models relies on their low computational cost.
- Simulators where organ physical behaviour is modelled by Finite Element Methods (FEM) [6][7][8] or Boundary Element Methods (BEM) [9]. These permit to simulate the deformation of elastic volumes. Their disadvantage is their high computational cost.

In this paper we present the result of developing a new general surgery simulator for training surgeons in minimally invasive procedures (i.e. laparoscopic surgery, arthroscopic surgery, endoscope surgery...). This simulator enables the user to construct environments and to have interaction modes very similar to real surgical intervention. Virtual scenes can be constructed by using either real organs of patients with the pathology or synthetic organs with any type of pathology. The simulator includes two kernels for simulating surface [10] and volumetric [9] rigid, elastic and viscoelastic physical behaviour. Surgery training can be done by using haptic with force feedback devices that provides surgeons with the tactile sense, basic in any surgeon training. The surgery simulator runs on Windows operative system and under PC workstations.

2.2 Modular decomposition of surgery simulator

The simulator comprises two main modules: The image pre-processing module, which comprises the segmentation tool and the scenario generator, and the surgery simulator module, which comprises the simulator workstation and the haptic control system.

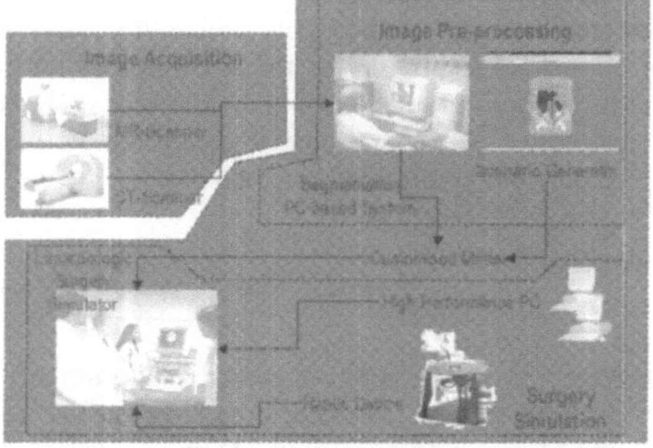

Figure 1: Modular Structure of the Surgery Simulator.

©CARS/Springer. All rights reserved.

Figure 1 show the different modules. Scenarios are generated using synthetic organs or real organs obtained from real images. Real images (coming from CT or MRI) are processed by the segmentation tool which produces VRML models of the organs. These models are read by the scenario generator, which permits to associate textures, dynamic properties and to define the surgical environment. Finally, the scenario is loaded into the surgery simulator which computes the effect of the actions performed by the users, returning the result to the visualisation system and the haptic force-feedback.

2.2.1 The segmentation tool

This tool permits to segment images coming from 3D CT or MRI and compute 3D surface models. On one hand, surface can be obtained from a segmented volumetric image [11], using different approaches, such as Marching Cubes or Snakes [12]. On the other hand, surfaces can be obtained directly by using deformable models and contour interpolation.

Segmentation can be performed either by using Region Growing or Thresholding in 3D. Segmentation and Marching Cubes algorithms have been implemented using High Performance Parallel Computing Techniques to reduce the overhead. Seeds for Region Growing can be obtained automatically by means of a contour identification tool, given that a threshold is provided. Contours can be obtained manually in any case.

The output of this module is a VRML file with the triangular mesh of the surface of each reconstructed organ. This data will be used as input for the scenario generator module.

2.2.2 The scenario generator

This module is used to construct the surgery scene where surgeons want to train in. The process of creating a scenario takes into account several steps: Selection of the organs that comprise the scenario; set-up of the input points for the virtual trocars where the tools and the camera will be introduced; set-up of the dynamic parameters and textures of the organs; and the definition of the relations among the organs.

The scenario generator loads the VRML files with the models of the organs produced in the segmentation tool or from a library of synthetic models, including organs such as liver, ducts, vessels, gall-bladder and peritoneum. Any interesting real organ segmented (e.g. one with an specific pathology) can be added to this library. Physical properties are being associated to each organ from a library of parameters. Two different deformable models are available in the simulator: Mass-spring model and BEM-based model. Textures can be obtained from a set of samples to give more realism to the environment.

Organs inside a real human body present relations among them. The simulator enables the user defining the test case to set-up links among different organs. This permits to divide the organs in different suborgans and associate, to each one, different physical models and behaviour. Moreover, it also permits to create adherences among different organs (for example, it permits to generate adherences between gall bladder and liver surface). This is also used for defining the boundary conditions required for the simulation.

Finally, the scene is complete defining the location of the virtual trocars where the tools will enter in the scene. Up to 9 simultaneous input points (including one for the camera) can be managed.

©CARS/Springer. All rights reserved.

Once the scene in which surgeons want to practice is generated, as well as the tools input points have been established, a virtual surgical environment is defined and can be saved to disk. Then, this file can be read by the Simulator.

2.2.3 The simulator

The simulator module performs the computation of the forces, deformations and reactions as a consequence of the simulation of the surgical procedure. The simulator loads virtual scenes created by the scene generator. In the simulator, organs react to external forces and deformations. These reactions follow the physical properties established in the scene generator. The surgeons interact with the virtual scene through force-feedback haptics.

The haptic devices that are manipulated by the surgeons can be associated with any of the input points established in the scene generator. It is possible to manage all the surgical tools using only one haptic device. The tools that currently can be associated to each input point are: scissors, hook, stapler, pincer and separator. Figure 2 show two screenshots of the simulator during the simulation of a cholecistectomy.

Once s surgeon considers that the virtual intervention is finished, an automatic report on the quality of the intervention is generated. This report includes information such as: temporal cost of the surgical intervention, wrong cuts, cauterizations and number of staples on wrong structures.

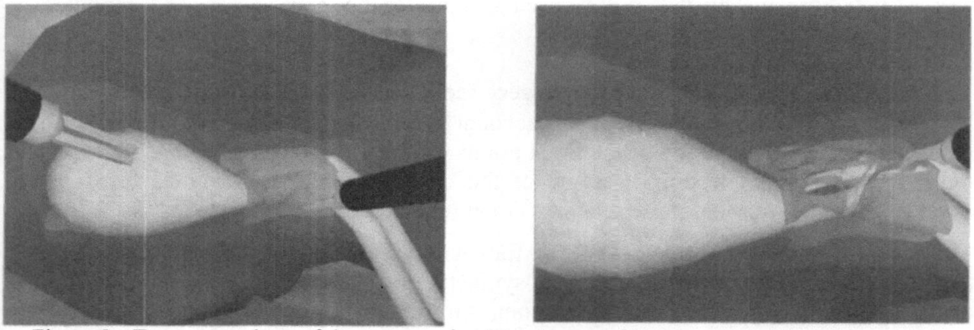

Figure 2.- Two screenshots of the surgery simulator (scene of Laparoscopic Cholecistectomy).

2.3 Hardware structure of the simulator

To provide surgeons with a realistic feeling, the simulator requires fast computing and graphical power. The graphical power is needed for showing a scene believable to surgeons. This high computer graphics power is obtained using an advanced computer graphics board (one that can manipulate textures). With this type of graphic boards, the computer main processor is free of graphic visualization overload. This enables the main processor to calculate exclusively the deformation of the physically based organs. However, high computational power is still required, on one hand, since the visualisation refresh rate should be at least 15 Hz. On the other hand since human tactile sense has a very high resolution, the refresh rate of a haptic with force feedback must be at least of 500 Hz. The computational cost of a single deformation action is also high, since the models comprise a large amount of nodes and a large number of iteration steps are required for the convergence of the process.

©CARS/Springer. All rights reserved.

The system is structured in two parts. The main computer is composed of a multiprocessor PC workstation. This node computes the visual refresh of the simulator and makes all the computations related to the deformation of the organs. This main computer performs at a refresh rate of at least 15 Hz. The haptic control structure is composed of a set of pairs workstation-haptic connected to the main computer. Each computer must assure a correct refresh rate to its respective haptic with force feedback. This implies that computers must send force vectors to each haptic related at a rate above 500 Hz.

However, the main computer calculates the real forces at a frequency of 15 Hz. This implies that the computer associated with each haptic has to estimate the forces between real refreshes. The estimation is used until each computer controlling a haptic receives an exact calculation. For avoiding not desired tool vibrations, the exact calculated force replaces the estimated force smoothly until the calculated force is received.

3. Results

The general surgery simulator developed can be run on a multiprocessor PCs. Tests have been performed for two different hardware configurations:

- Sequential: A mono-processor PC Intel Pentium IV with a clock rate of 1 GHz.
- Parallel: A bi-processor PC Intel Pentium IV with a clock rate of 1 GHz.

Results of the performance for the computation of the deformation of the cholecystectomy scene, comprising 3,180 nodes, are presented in Figure 3. In the parallel environment, the computations are performed 2.32 times faster than in the sequential case.

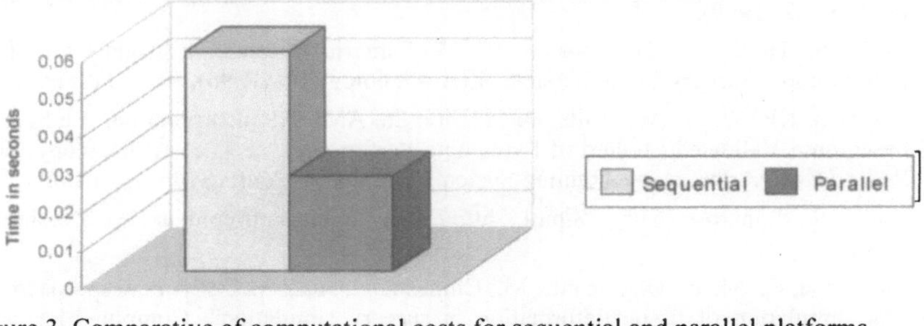

Figure 3. Comparative of computational costs for sequential and parallel platforms.

4. Conclusions

In this paper a virtual surgery simulator has been described. This simulator has several advantages compared with currently available surgery simulators. It permits to construct any scene in which to practice endoscopic, arthroscopic and laparoscopic surgery, as well as dealing with both real organs of patients and synthetic organs (included peritoneum) with any pathology.

The system permits to simulate volumetric physical behaviour as well as surface physical behaviour of the organs that appears in the virtual scene and to control up to 9 simultaneous tools with force-feedback. Finally, it runs on low cost PC workstations.

©CARS/Springer. All rights reserved.

5. Future work

Currently, the simulator prototype is in a first evaluation step. This evaluation is been made by surgeons that have very high experience in laparoscopic surgery from the General Hospital of Valencia (Spain). Once the simulator will be extensively tested, educational advantages of the simulator will be analysed, in comparison to traditional surgical training procedures.

Acknowledgements

This work has been supported by the VRSUR IST-1999-20783 project.

References

1. Reinig, K.D.; Rush, C.G.; Pelster, H.L.; Spitzer, V.M.; Heath, J.A.; "Real-Time Visually and Haptically Accurate Surgical Simulation", Medicine Meets Virtual Reality 4, IOS-Press, 1996.
2. Weghorst, S.; Airola, C.; Oppenheimer, P.; "Formal Evaluation of the Madigan Endoscopic Sinus Surgery Simulator", September R-97-34, Seattle: Univ. of Washington, Human Interface Technology Laboratory, 97.
3. Cover, S. A.; Ezquerra, N.F.; O'Brien, J.F.; et. al.; "Interactively Deformable Models for Surgery Simulation", IEEE: Comput. Graph. and Apps, Vol 13, No 6., pp. 68-75, Nov 93.
4. Frisken-Gibson, S.F.. "Using linked volumes to model object collisions, deformation, cutting, carving and joining", IEEE Transac. on Visualization and Computer Graphics, v. 5, n. 4, 99.
5. Kühnapfel, U.; Çakmak, H.K.; Maaß, H.; "3D Modeling for Endoscopic Surgery", Proc. IEEE Symposium on Simulation, Delft University, Delft, NL, Oct. 13, 1999, pp 22-32, ISBN: 90-804551-7-2 (1999).
6. Cotin, S.; Delingette, H.; Ayache, N.; "Volumetric Deformable Models for Simulation of Laparoscopic Surgery", Computer Assisted Radiology (CAR'96), Paris, France, 1996.
7. Sherman, KP; Ward, JW; Wills, DPM; Mohsen, AMMA;"Incorporation of a Scoring System based on a Validated Method of Evaluating Performance at Knee Arthroscopy into a Virtual Reality Knee Arthroscopy Training System", SICOT'99 Conf. (Sydney, Australia), April 99.
8. Cotin, S., Laparosc. Surg. Simul., http://www-sop.inria.fr/epidaure/AISIM/simulateur/sim-frameset.html
9. Monserrat, C.; Meier, U.; Alcañiz, M.; Chinesta, F.; Juan, M.C.; "A new approach for the real-time simulation of tissue deformation in surgery simulation", Comput. Met. and Prgs. in Biomed., v. 64, pp. 77-85.

1. Monserrat, C. et al., "A fast Real Time Tissue Deformation Algorithm for Surgery Simulation", CAR'97, Elsevier Publishers.
2. Blanquer, I.; Hernández, V.; Alcañiz, M.; Monserrat, C.; Grau, V.; Juan, M.C. "Parallel segmentation and rendering using clusters of PCs", Medicine Meets Virtual Reality 2000.
3. Cohen L, Cohem I; "A Finite Element Method Applied to new Active Contour Models and 3D Reconstruction from Cross Sections" June 1990, INRIA Rapports de Recherche Num. 1245.

Image Guided Neurosurgery

CARS 2002 – H.U. Lemke, M.W. Vannier; K. Inamura, A.G. Farman, K. Doi & J.H.C. Reiber (Editors)
©CARS/Springer. All rights reserved.

Acquisition of 3D ultrasound images during neuronavigation

Marloes MJ Letteboer [a], Peter WA Willems [b], Pierre Hellier [c], Wiro J Niessen [a]
[a] Image Sciences Institute, University Medical Center, Utrecht, The Netherlands
[b] Department of Neurosurgery, University Medical Center, Utrecht, The Netherlands
[c] Projet VISTA, IRISA-INRIA, Rennes, France

Abstract

Intraoperative brain deformation is the most important cause affecting the overall accuracy of image guided neurosurgical procedures. One option for correcting this deformation is to acquire 3D ultrasound images during the operation and use these to update the information provided by the preoperatively acquired MR data.
For 8 patients 3D ultrasound images have been reconstructed from a freehand sweep during neurosurgical procedures. The 3D ultrasound data have been qualitatively compared to the preoperatively acquired MR data. Before opening the dura, no brain deformation was measured. After opening the dura the maximum shift measured was 8 mm parallel to the direction of gravity and 6 mm perpendicular to this direction, showing the additional value of 3D ultrasound acquisition compared to 2D ultrasound.

Keywords: 3D ultrasound, image guided neurosurgery, surgical navigation

1. Introduction

In neurosurgery, determining the position of the tumour during interventions by navigation based on preoperatively acquired data (MRI) is a common approach. In current systems that allow for navigation on preoperative data, it is assumed that no intraoperative tissue deformation occurs. However, in neurosurgical procedures, intraoperative brain deformations up to 10 mm have been reported [1,2] making the intraoperative deformation the most important cause affecting the overall accuracy of image guided neurosurgery. Intraoperative imaging is an alternative, however information provided only by intraoperative imaging devices is generally less complete and less detailed. One option for solving the problem of brain deformation is the use of intraoperatively acquired ultrasound [3,4] in combination with preoperative image data, to correct these preoperative images for deformations that have occurred during surgery.

In the commercially available navigation system used, it is already possible to compare 2D ultrasound images, acquired intraoperatively, with the corresponding preoperative MR plane. The deformation of the brain is not restricted to one direction, however. In this article a system to intraoperatively acquire 3D ultrasound using a freehand scanning technique, which is required to obtain insight in the deformation of the brain in all directions, is reported. From the preliminary results from 8 interventions, which have been performed with the system, it can be concluded that brain shift during intervention can be

©CARS/Springer. All rights reserved.

estimated by comparing a preoperative MR volume with an intraoperative US volume. The maximum shift measured over all 8 cases was 8 mm.

2. Methods

2.1 Data acquisition

For planning neuronavigational procedures images from a 0.5 Tesla MRI scanner (Philips Medical Systems, Best, the Netherlands) were acquired. All images are 3D contrast-enhanced, T1 weighted acquisitions, scanned with a slice thickness of 2.2 mm and reconstructed at 1.1 mm. The MR datasets consist of a 256 x 256 matrix, with 120 to 150 slices. The voxel size is 1.0 x 1.0 x 1.1 mm in all cases.

The datasets were transferred from the MRI scanner to the neuronavigation workstation (Stealthstation TREON System with Sononav software, Medtronic Inc., Minneapolis, USA). A camera system and ultrasound machine (Aloka SSD-5000 with 7.5 MHz neuroprobe, Tokyo, Japan) were connected to the neuronavigation workstation.

2.2 Pre-operation

Prior to MRI data acquisition, seven adhesive markers were applied to the patient's head, as widely distributed as possible. During the operation the location of these markers with respect to the reference arc was determined with the aid of the camera system and a trackable pointer. As the patient's head was fixed with respect to the reference arc and since the markers were also visible on the MR scan, it was possible to relate the patient's three-dimensional space to that of the MR scan. This relation between the MR image and patient was expressed in a transformation matrix T_{MR-pat}.

2.3 Intra-operation

During the operation at least two freehand ultrasound sweeps were acquired, one before opening the dura and one after opening the dura but before inducing other structural changes. The position of the ultrasound probe, with respect to the reference arc, is continuously monitored by optical tracking of the probe in the operating field. Thus it is possible to relate the 2D ultrasound image to the patient's three-dimensional space, $T_{2DUS-pat}$.

2.4 Post-operation

After surgery the 2D ultrasound images, the corresponding positions with respect to the reference arc and the MR image with T_{MR-pat} were transferred to a Silicon Graphics station. The 2D ultrasound images were converted from Medtronic to StradX format [5], and reconstructed using the Stacksx software (Cambridge University Engineering Department, England).

©CARS/Springer. All rights reserved.

The Stacksx software constructs a voxel array either using a simple nearest neighbour algorithm (each voxel is set to the value of the nearest B-scan pixel), or using bi-linear interpolation of the four nearest pixels on the closest B-scan. The interpolation resolution can be set manually.

The transformation matrix from 3DUS to 2DUS space can be described by: $T_{3DUS-2DUS}$. Thus the complete transformation from the intraoperative 3DUS space to the preoperative MR space can be described by: $T_{3DUS-2DUS} \cdot T_{2DUS-pat} \cdot T_{pat-MR}$.

After registration the brain shift between the preoperative MR and the intraoperative US before and after opening the dura can be estimated, which is important for navigated neurosurgery.

3. Results and discussion

The method for acquiring 3D ultrasound data during neuro-interventions has been tested on 8 patients, between October and December 2001.

3.1 Number of B-scans during one sweep

In the first study of seven patients, to assess the feasibility to reconstruct 3D ultrasound data using our system, the standard settings for ultrasound acquisition of the neuronavigation system were used. This implied that a maximum of 40 B-scans could be used during a sweep of 4 seconds. This freehand sweep was a combination of translating and tilting the probe over the brain surface, with an average movement of 5 cm. Thus, this leads to a resolution of about 1.2 mm. When comparing this to the resolution of the 2D ultrasound plane, which is about 0.25 mm, it can be concluded that the resolution in the direction of the probe motion is not sufficient for a detailed 3D reconstruction, although these measurements already give an insight in the deformations that have occurred.

To get an isotropic resolution for the 3D ultrasound volume, 200 to 250 B-scans have to be acquired during one sweep. Currently the image buffer of the used navigation system is not large enough to store this many B-scans and also the reconstruction time increases with the number of scans. So a trade-off has to be made between optimal resolution and minimal computation time. In the last intervention the number of B-scans was increased to 120. This leads to an acceptable resolution and a not too excessive increase in reconstruction time.
The total process from acquisition until final transformation from US to MR space requires in the order of 10 minutes in total, so this process is not real time yet.

©CARS/Springer. All rights reserved.

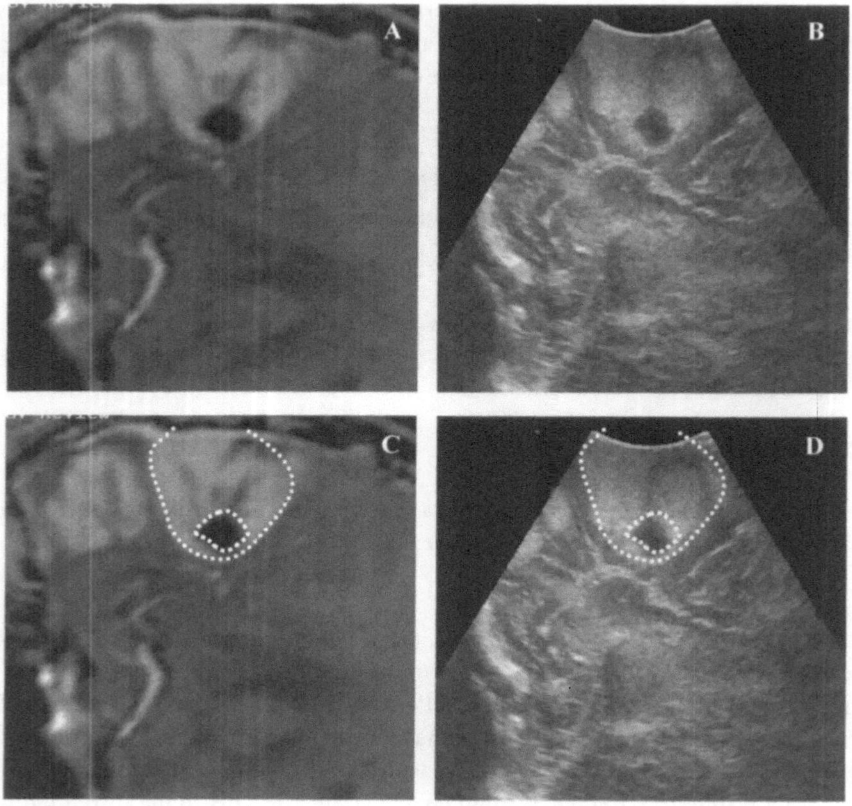

Figure 1: Comparison of an MR and a 3D ultrasound plane recorded before opening the dura. A) MR image. B) Corresponding US plane. C) Segmentation of tumour tissue in the MR image. D) Corresponding US plane with overlay of MR tumour contour

3.2 Measured brain shift

Using 40 B-scans, it is already possible to give an indication of the brain shift. When comparing the preoperative MR and the US volume before opening the dura it can be concluded that in all cases the brain has not shifted significantly (Figure 1). This was as expected because in several articles it is reported that, before opening the dura, the brain will not move significantly.

When comparing the two ultrasound volumes acquired before and after opening the dura a maximum shift of 8 mm has been measured parallel to the direction of gravity (Figure 2) and 6 mm perpendicular to this direction (Figure 3). This shows that large errors can be made when navigating on the preoperatively acquired MR image. And it also shows that 3D ultrasound acquisition has an additional advantage compared to 2D ultrasound

©CARS/Springer. All rights reserved.

imaging because it can detect movement in both directions perpendicular to the direction of gravity at the same time.

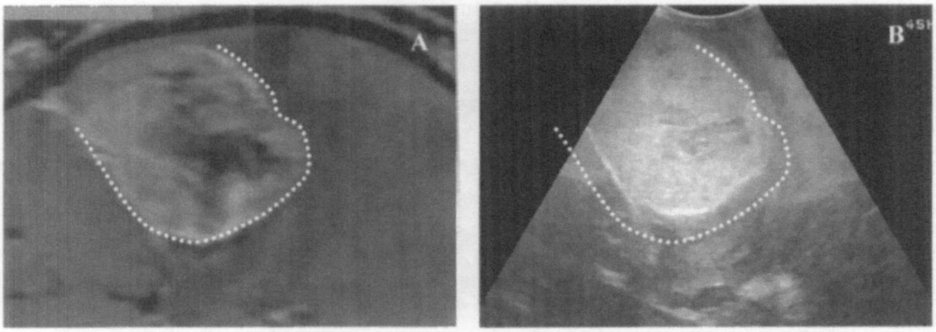

Figure 2: Comparison of an MR and a 3D ultrasound plane recorded after opening the dura. A) MR image with segmentation of tumour (dotted line). B) Corresponding US plane with overlay of MR tumour contour. This shows a shift of the tumour parallel to the direction of gravity.

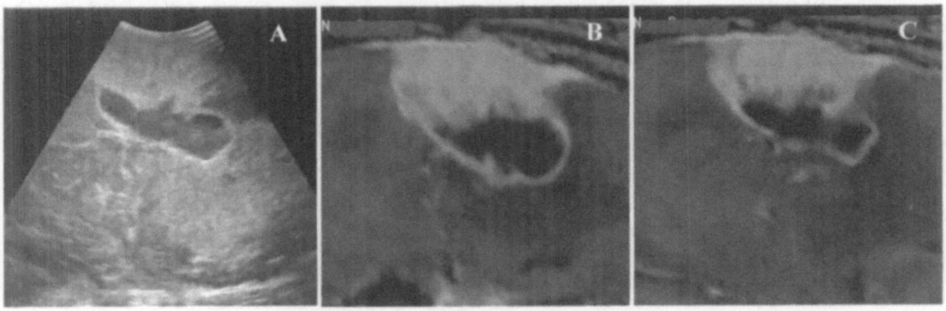

Figure 3: Comparison of an MR and a 3D ultrasound plane recorded after opening the dura. A) US image. B) Corresponding MR plane according to $T_{MR-3DUS}$. C) Actual corresponding MR plane (determined manually). This shows a shift of the tumour perpendicular to the direction of gravity.

4. Conclusions

A method to reconstruct 3D ultrasound images using free hand scanning during neurosurgical procedures has been presented and compared to preoperative MR data.

The quality of the 3D ultrasound volumes is mostly dependent on the number of B-scans that can be acquired during a sweep. The maximum number of B-scans acquired using the standard settings, 40, is sufficient to give an indication of the shift, although 200 to 250 B-scans are necessary for isotropic resolution. The number of 120 B-scans used during the last sweep gives a satisfactory resolution, so this will be used in further experiments.

©CARS/Springer. All rights reserved.

The brain shift before opening the dura is negligible, as was expected. The maximum brain shift after opening the dura measured is 8 mm parallel to the direction of gravity and 6 mm perpendicular to this direction. This shows that 3D ultrasound will give additional information when comparing it to 2D ultrasound.

References

1. Maurer CR, Hill DGL, Truwit CL, "Investigation of intraoperative brain deformation using a 1.5 T interventional MR system: Preliminary results", *IEEE transactions on medical imaging*, Vol. 17 No. 5, p817-826, 1998.
2. Roberts DW, Hartov A, Kennedy FE, Miga MI, Paulsen KD, "Intraoperative brain shift and deformation: a quantitative analysis of cortical displacement in 28 cases", *Neurosurgery*, Vol. 43 No. 4, p749-758, 1998.
3. Buchholz RD, Yeh DD, Kessman P, "The correction of stereotactic inaccuracy caused by brain shift using an intraoperative ultrasound device", *MICCAI Proceedings – Lecture notes in computer science 1496*, Editors: Wells WM, Colchester A, Delp S, p. 459-466, Publisher: Springer-Verlag, Cambridge, 1998.
4. Comeau RM, Sadikot AF, Fenster A, Peters TM, "Intraoperative ultrasound for guidance and tissue shift correction in image-guided neurosurgery", *Medical Physics*, Vol. 27 No. 4, p787-800, 2000.
5. Prager RW, Gee A, Berman L, "StradX: real-time acquisition and visualization of freehand three-dimensional ultrasound", *Medical Image Analysis*, Vol. 3 No. 2, p129-140, 1999.

CARS 2002 – H.U. Lemke, M.W. Vannier; K. Inamura, A.G. Farman, K. Doi & J.H.C. Reiber (Editors)
©CARS/Springer. All rights reserved.

Neuronavigation with intraoperative 3D ultrasound; multimodal 2D and 3D display techniques and interactive stereoscopic visualisation for guiding surgical procedures

T A Nagelhus Hernes[a], F Lindseth[a,b] , T Langø[a] , S Ommedal[a], G Unsgård[c]
[a]SINTEF Unimed, Trondheim, Norway
[b]Dept. of Computer and Information Science, NTNU, Norway
[c]Dept. of Neurosurgery, University Hospital and Medical Faculty, NTNU,Norway

Abstract

We have developed a 3D ultrasound based neuronavigation system that also reads MR and CT images. This raises a need for more advanced 2D and 3D display solutions for presenting essential information. We have integrated a stereoscopy volume visualization module with the navigation system, which makes it possible to control the stereoscopic view using surgical tools, pointers or ultrasound probes. We have also developed an image fusion module that integrates 3D ultrasound and MRI/CT visualization. 3D images from both MR and ultrasound are visualized simultaneously in the same scene by overlay, compositing or splitting visualisation techniques, which makes perception of information easier as compared to displaying images in different scenes. Results from feasibility studies show that the new image visualisations may be useful for planning the operation as well as for guiding surgical procedures. By orientating the stereoscopic projections in accordance to the position of the patient on the operating table, it is easier to interpret complex 3D anatomy and to directly take advantage of 3D information for planning and surgical guidance. In the clinical case studies, we also experienced that by combinding 2D and 3D display, interpretation of both detailed and geometric information may easily be achieved simultaneously.

Keywords: Multimodal imaging, stereoscopy, intraoperative 3D ultrasound

1. Introduction

Computer assisted systems as neuronavigation technology is now growing on the market [1]. These systems have shown to be powerful since the surgical tools may be tracked by positioning systems and the surgeon may hence navigate the tools into the brain based on image information only. However, many of the commercially available neuronavigation systems frequently present only 2D slices of preoperative 3D volumes, a technique that may have limitations for interpreting and understanding the complex 3D geometric anatomy and pathology of the brain during surgery. 3D display techniques may, however, also be considered as more user friendly than 2D display, more convenient and have potential of improving the planning and outcome of surgery. Rendered 3D medical image data and virtual reality visualizations have earlier been reported to be beneficial in diagnosis of cerebral aneurysms as well as in preoperative evaluation, planning and

©CARS/Springer. All rights reserved.

rehearsal of a various of surgery approaches [2,3,4,5,6,7]. Another important feature needed in neuronavigation system, is updated 3D images, ensuring that the surgeon is navigating the surgical tool based on a map that reflects the patient true anatomy during surgery. Imaging technologies as MR, CT and ultrasound are increasingly being introduced intraoperatively in conjunction with navigation technology in order to cope with the brain shift problem. We have developed a neuronavigation system with high quality intraoperative 3D ultrasound capabilities, which makes it possible to update the 3D map 4-8 times during surgery, hence improving the safety and accuracy of the surgical procedure [8,9]. 3D ultrasound has been used in our clinic for guiding surgical procedures in more than 200 brain operations (tumours, AVM, aneurysms) using various display techniques such as orthogonal, anyplane and/or stereoscopic display techniques. We have also developed a multimodal post processing visualisation module for simultaneous display of information from ultrasound and MR imaging modalities using overlay, compositing and/or splitting techniques. The purpose of the present paper is to summarize our experiences in using various 2D and 3D visualisation techniques of both MR and ultrasound images for preoperative planning, for guiding surgical procedures and for post operative evaluation.

2. Materials and Methods

2.1 Preoperative 3D MRI and intraoperative 3D ultrasound acquisition

Preoperative 3D MR images were acquired by a 1.5T MRI scanner (Picker). Fiducials were put on the patient prior to MR scanning and the 3D MRI volumes were registrated to the patient in the operating room using a standard patient registration procedure using the SonoWand neuronavigation system (MISON AS, Trondheim, Norway). Conventional navigation and planning based on the preoperatively acquired 3D MRI images could then be performed. High quality 3D ultrasound maps (5 MHz FPA ultrasound probe) were acquired 4-8 times during surgery. The position and orientation of the ultrasound probe was tracked using an optical positioning system (Polaris, Northern Digital) during free-hand probe movement. A pyramid-shaped volume of the brain was acquired by tilting the probe typically 90 degrees during 15 seconds. The digital images were reconstructed into a regular volume and used for navigation purposes the same way as the MRI and CT volumes. The overall accuracy of ultrasound based navigation system is in the range of 1.4 mm [10].

2.2. 2D and 3D display techniques and interactive stereoscopic visualisation

Surgical tools, as the CUSA and biopsy forceps, were calibrated and used for navigation similarly as the pointer. The positions of the tools or the pointer were tracked by the positioning system and hence decided which images to be displayed on the monitor. Various display techniques as orthogonal slicing, "anyplane" slicing as well as stereoscopic display of the 3D volumes were used during the surgical procedures, as illustrated in figure 1. Our stereoscopic visualisation technique makes it possible for the surgeon to interactively virtually be inside the patient during the surgical procedure. Both the orientation and position of the projection view are decided by a pointer or a surgical tool. The tip of the pointer is displayed as a point in the stereoscopic projection, representing a useful tool for localizing vessels and other anatomy during surgery. The

©CARS/Springer. All rights reserved.

stereoscopic projection is displayed on the screen and realized using red/blue glasses in the operating theatre. The stereo module may also be modified for shutter-glasses, polarization-glasses or "closed up head display".

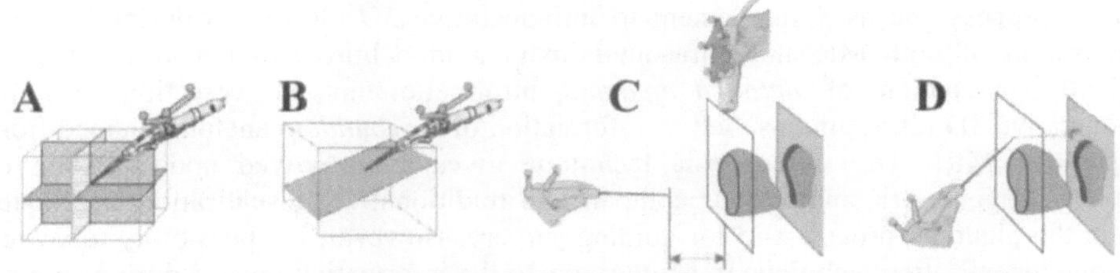

Figure 1. Various display techniques used in the navigation system. A. Orthogonal slicing B. Anyplane slicing. C. Interactive stereoscopic display controlled by pointer or probe. D. Stereoscopic display for navigation of a surgical tool. The projection is frozen and the tip of the tool is interactively displayed in the projection due to movement of the tool.

2.3. Preoperative image data and intraoperative ultrasound image fusion

Postoperatively, an image fusion visualization module [11] reads the preoperative data sets, the patient registration information as well as the intraoperative 3D ultrasound images that are acquired during surgery. Our image fusion visualisation module supports three different ways to fuse corresponding orthogonal (axial, coronal and sagittal) or oblique slices from MRI/CT and ultrasound:

Overlaying: Preoperative MRI/CT slices are overlayed the intraoperative grey level ultrasound slices as a color code. The color overlay used can either be the raw slices itself, an edge enhanced version of the slice or a segmented one. In the first two cases the threshold level may be determined by a slider deciding when to show a pixel as a color overlay on top of the grey-level image.

Compositing: This is similar to the first method, but instead of being either from the ultrasound or the MRI/CT slice, here every pixel in the fused image is a mixture of the two. A slider determines the percentage that each modality contributes to the final image, i.e. the degree of transparency in the overlay.

Splitting: In this display method the image window is split in two, either vertical or horizontal, and one half is filled with half of the MRI/CT slice and the other half is filled with the corresponding other half of the ultrasound slice. The window can also be split in four, filling one, or the two diagonal quadrants with data from the ultrasound slice and the rest with preoperative data. Other splitting algorithms exist, for example filling a rectangular or arbitrary region in the middle of the window with ultrasound and the rest with MRI/CT. Due to the fact that ultrasound does not cover as much of the operational field as MRI/CT, another fusion technique is to fill the window with ultrasound and fill preoperative data around. The ultrasound mask is found in a robust manner using mathematical morphology.

©CARS/Springer. All rights reserved.

3. Results

Experiences gained from the clinic show that preoperative image data is useful in the planning process and as a supplement to intraoperative 3D ultrasound during surgery. Visualisation of both MR and ultrasound imaging modalities simultaneously ensures efficiently perception of *detailed updated* information in the resection area by intraoperative 3D ultrasound as well as information of *surrounding* anatomy gained from preoperative MRI. The stereoscopic technique gives an improved understanding of complex 3D geometric anatomy as compared to traditional 2D visualisation techniques both in the planning process and for guiding surgery. However, the possibility to switch from one visualisation technique to another due to the information needed during surgery seems to be important. Also by orientating the stereoscopic view due to the position of the surgeon and patient as well as to interactively update the stereoscopic view using the surgical tool give new possibilities that may increase the user friendliness of navigation systems. Examples from the clinic, controlling the stereoscopic display using the ultrasound probe or a pointer, is given in figure 2. Also, the feature of navigating the tool down to the lesion based on stereoscopic projection, seems to be advantageous, especially for locating abnormal anatomy, such as aneurysms and feeders of AVMs during surgery.

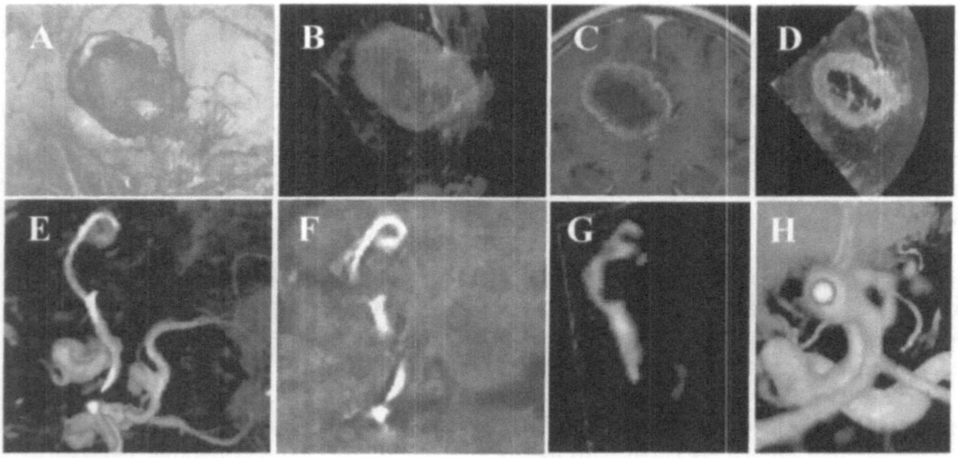

Figure 2: Stereoscopic display of 3D ultrasound and MRI in the operating room. A-D is from a tumour resection (metastasis). A. stereoscopic projection of preoperative MRI with a cut plane in the middle of the tumour. B. Corresponding stereoscopic cut plane visualisation based on intraoperative 3D ultrasound images. Stereoscopic projection from MRI gives a nice overview and the projection from ultrasound gives updated information during surgery. C and D show corresponding tissue planes from MR and ultrasound respectively. These tissue images give more detailed information in the cut plane of the projection. E-H are from two aneurysm surgeries. E. Stereoscopic projection of MR angiography of an aneurysm (top in image). The stereoscopic view gives a nice overview of surrounding anatomy. F and G show corresponding 2D plane from 3D MR angiography and 3D ultrasound power Doppler, respectively, as the cut plane in the stereoscopic projection in E. H. In another aneurysm operation, the stereoscopic view was "frozen" and the pointer was located at one of two aneurysms before clipsing. The sphere shows the location of the tip of the pointer on the aneurysm. True 3D vision is experienced using red/blue glasses (color print).

©CARS/Springer. All rights reserved.

By integrating both ultrasound and MRI information in one multimodal window, the interpretation of information from both imaging modalities simultaneously is improved considerably as compared to displaying ultrasound and MR images in separate windows (figure 3). This is experienced to be useful for interpreting potential brain shift occurred between the image acquisations and any discrepancies or supplementary information gained from MR and ultrasound imaging modalities.

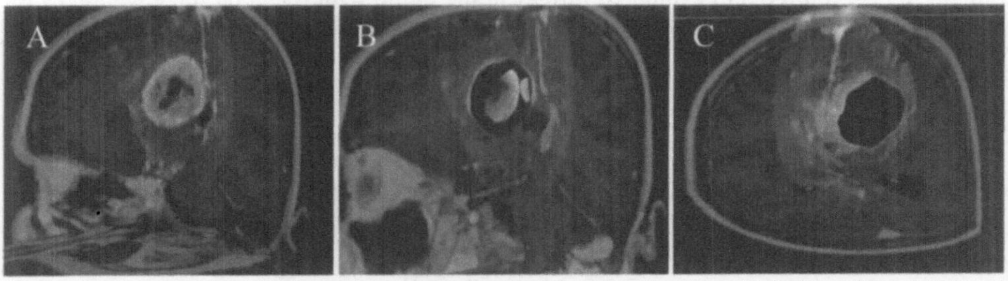

Figure 3: Compositing display of corresponding axial, coronal and sagittal slices from MRI and ultrasound demonstrated post operatively. A. Ultrasound slices on top are made transparent, ensuring that MRI slices can be seen. The transparency may be adjusted. MRI is useful for interpreting surrounding anatomy and ultrasound ensures updated image information during surgery. B. Segmented tumour from MRI overlaid ultrasound in the middle. C. Mismatch between MRI and ultrasound may easily be interpreted.

4. Discussion and Conclusion

In this paper, we have demonstrated technology that integrates navigation systems, interactive 3D stereoscopic display, multimodal imaging and intraoperative 3D ultrasound imaging for improved image guided neurosurgery. We have presented new technology for 3D display that is integrated with navigation technology. The clinical advantages of both navigation technology as well as intraoperative imaging have earlier been explored and outlined by others, as also, the advantages of 3D display technologies. The results from the feasibility case studies presented in this paper are promising. Especially, the stereoscopic visualisation seems to give many advantages due to improved perception of complex 3D anatomy and easy access of information inside the 3D volume. The interactive 3D display module is also fast and makes stereoscopic projections of intraoperative 3D ultrasound data immediately after 3D acquisition has been performed, without any need for post processing of the acquired image data. This is important due to the time constraint during surgery and the need for easily and fast 3D presentation of intraoperatively acquired 3D image data. 3D display seems to be useful both for planning and guidance of tumour resections as well as for guidance during cerebrovascular surgery. 3D visualisation techniques improve the understanding of complex 3D geometric anatomy as compared to traditional 2D slicing, both in the planning process and in image guided surgery. A potential useful application of the stereoscopy module may hence be to interactively locate the feeding artery in artery venous malformations (work in progress) as well as for locating smaller arteries nearby aneurysms that should be avoided when clipsing the aneurysm. Stereoscopic projection of 3D ultrasound power Doppler may also

©CARS/Springer. All rights reserved.

have advantages for evaluating blood flow in normal vessels after an aneurysm has been clipsed. By integrating more information in the 3D display the surgeon may also interact with a multi-informational 3D scene using surgical tools or pointers, hence being able to perform even more advanced image and "information" guided surgery. We experienced, however, that conventional 2D display still is important to get detailed information in the resection area in order to ensure safe and accurate image guided surgery. The potential benefits of combined 2D and 3D display as well as multi-informational display techniques remain to be explored and evaluated further in the clinic with focus on the advantages for both the surgeon as well as for the patient (work in progress).

Acknowledgements

This work was supported by grants from the Research Council of Norway through the Strategic University Program in Medical Technology at the Norwegian University of Science and Technology (NTNU), the Strategic Institute Program at SINTEF Unimed, and the Norwegian Ministry of Health and Social Affairs.

References

1 Reinhardt H., Trippel B, Westermann B and Gratzl: Computer aided surgery with special focus on neuronavigation, Computerized Medical Imaging and Graphics 23, 237-244, 1999.

2 Harbaugh RE, Schlusselberg DS Jeffrey R, Hayden S, Cromwell LD, Pluta D, English RA.:Three-dimensional computer tomograpic angiography in the preoperative evaluation of cerebrovascular lesions. Neurosurgery, 36: 320-326, 1995.

3 Nakajima S, Atsumi H, Bhalerao AH, Jolesz FA, Kikinis R, Yoshimine T, Moriarty TM, Stieg PE: Computer-assisted surgical planning for cerebrovascular neurosurgery. Neurosurgery, 41:403-409, 1997.

4 Muacevic A, Steiger HJ: Computer-assisted resection of cerebral arteriovenous malformation. Neurosurgery, 45:1164-1171,1999.

5 Kato Y, Sano H, Katada K, Ogura Y, Hayakawa M, Kanaoka N, Kanno T: Application of three-dimensional CT angiography (3D-CTA) to cerebral aneurysms, Surg Neurol, 52:113-22, 1999.

6 Masutani Y, Dohi T, Yamane F, Iseki H, Takakura K: Augmented reality visualization system for intravascular neurosurgery, Computer aided surgery 3:239-247, 1998.

7 Vannier MW: Evaluation of 3D imaging, in Critical reviews in diagnostic imaging 41:315-378, by CRC press LLC, 2000.

8 Gronningsaeter A, Kleven A, Ommedal S, Aarseth TE, Lie T, Lindseth F, Langø T, Unsgård G: SonoWand, an ultrasound-based neuronavigation system. Neurosurgery 46: 1373-1379, 2000.

9 Unsgaard, G., Ommedal S., Muller T., Gronningsaeter, A, Nagelhus Hernes, TA: Neuronavigation by intraoperative three-dimensional ultrasound: Initial experience during brain tumor surgery. Neurosurgery, 50, no 4, April 2002.

10 Lango T, Bang, J, Lindseth, F, Nagelhus Hernes, TA: Accuracy evaluation of a 3D ultrasound-based neuronavigation system. Proc of the 16th International Congress and Exhibition in Computer Assisted Radiology and Surgery, (CARS2002) Paris June 27-30, 2002.

11 Lindseth F, Ommedal S, Bang J, Unsgård G, Hernes TAN: Image fusion of ultrasound and MRI as an aid for assessing anatomical shifts and for improving overview and interpretation in ultrasound guided neurosurgery. Proc of the 15th International Congress and Exhibition in Computer Assisted Radiology and Surgery, (CARS2001) Berlin, June 27-30, 2001.

CARS 2002 – H.U. Lemke, M.W. Vannier; K. Inamura, A.G. Farman, K. Doi & J.H.C. Reiber (Editors)
©CARS/Springer. All rights reserved.

Neurosurgical biopsies guided by 3D ultrasound - comparison of image evaluations and histopathological results

Tormod Selbekk[a], Geirmund Unsgård[b,c], Steinar Ommedal[a], Tomm Muller[c], Sverre Torp[b,c], Gunnar Myhr[b,c], Jon Bang[a], Toril A. Nagelhus Hernes[a]
[a] SINTEF Unimed Ultrasound, Trondheim, Norway
[b] Norwegian University of Science and Technology, Trondheim, Norway
[c] University Hospital of Trondheim, Trondheim, Norway

Abstract

The imaging of gliomas and metastases by 3D ultrasound has been evaluated by comparing image findings and histopathological results. Biopsies have been taken prior to resection and close to the tumour border as shown in the ultrasound images. The tumour border shown in the ultrasound images was verified by an edge detection algorithm using the Sobel method. Ultrasound images, with the biopsy position indicated, have been evaluated and compared to the histhopathology of the corresponding biopsy. The degree of match between image evaluations and histopathology should reflect the ability of 3D ultrasound to image size and location of tumours correctly. The image slices of intraoperative 3D ultrasound are also compared to corresponding image slices of preoperative MR data (T1 and T2). The preliminary results show that intraoperative 3D ultrasound provides accurate information about tumour border and location and may accordingly be used for guiding surgical procedures. For gliomas the histopathologic match for the intraoperative 3D ultrasound is better than the corresponding match for the preoperative MR data.

Keywords: 3D ultrasound, neuronavigation, histopathology

1. Introduction

Intraoperative imaging methods have been developed to overcome the limitations of conventional neuronavigation systems. The intraoperative use of MR, CT or ultrasound (US) technology allows acquisition of updated images of the brain during resection, thus compensating for brain shift effects. The use of intraoperative imaging has proven to lead to a more radical resection of the lesion [1-4] that can increase patient survival time [5]. An ultrasound based neuronavigation system, SonoWand (MISON AS, Trondheim, Norway), capable of rapid acquisition and processing of 3D US volumes, has recently been presented on the market [6]. As the ultrasound volumes will serve as the basis for image-guided resection, it is of vital importance that the ultrasound images show the extent and localization of the tumour correctly. The present study was initiated to investigate whether 3D ultrasound could adequately image the tumour border and location for gliomas and metastases. Biopsies were taken prior to resection, using a biopsy forceps equipped with a positioning sensor. The position of the biopsies was electronically

©CARS/Springer. All rights reserved.

marked in the image volumes displayed on the SonoWand system. In this study the evaluation of intraoperative 3D ultrasound data as displayed on the neuronavigation system has been compared with the respective histopathological diagnosis of the biopsy. The image slices of the intraoperative ultrasound volume are also compared with corresponding image slices of preoperative T1 and T2 weighted MR volumes. Biopsies taken close to the tumour border as seen in the intraoperative 3D US images were investigated in the present study.

2. Materials and methods

2.1 Patient data

Patients who were believed to benefit from being operated assisted by ultrasound-based neuronavigation were selected due to the size and location of the tumour. All patients were informed about the methodology and accepted to be included in the study. The lesions were located in the supratentorial region of the brain and were primarily deep-seated tumours with diameter 1-5 cm. A total of 19 operations are included in the study so far; low-grade astrocytoma (n=7), anaplastic astrocytoma (n=6) and metastases (n=6) tumours.

2.2 Preoperative preparations and planning

The patients were scanned by MR technology (Picker or Siemens 1.5 T), and high-resolution 3D MRI volumes with slice thickness 1.5 mm were acquired. The 3D MRI volumes were registered to the patients using standard fiducial markers, followed by planning of the surgical procedures in the operating room. The position of the craniotomy, and in some cases an additional mini craniotomy for the ultrasound probe, was planned based on the preoperative MR images.

2.3 Intraoperative 3D ultrasound imaging

Initially in the study we used a two-rack prototype consisting of a high-end System FiVe ultrasound scanner (GE Vingmed Ultrasound, Horten, Norway), and navigation software developed in our group integrated to an optical tracking system. From 2000 a high-end ultrasound scanner and a Polaris optical tracking system (Northern digital, Waterloo, Ontario, Canada) were integrated with the navigation software into one single rack navigation system, a prerelease version of the final product, SonoWand (MISON AS, Trondheim, Norway). The neuronavigation system is able to track the position of ultrasound probes, pointers and surgical instruments like biopsy forceps and CUSA. The 3D US volumes are acquired by tilting the handheld ultrasound probe for 15-20 sec, thus accumulating a set of 2D ultrasound sector scans that are merged with the corresponding positioning data into a 3D volume. Lango *et al.* have in a comprehensive study regarding the imaging accuracy of 3D ultrasound data acquired by the SonoWand system found the average accuracy to be 1.4 (± 0.45) mm [7].

The systems used in the study supported several methods for volume visualization. Both the 3D US and MR image data could be conventionally displayed as coronal, sagittal and axial image slices. A simplified display mode annotated as the “anyplane view”, in which

©CARS/Springer. All rights reserved.

a single image slice is selected based on the position and orientation of the surgical instrument was used extensively in the present study.

2.4 Image-guided biopsy acquisition

The image slices of the intraoperative 3D ultrasound volume were displayed on the monitor along with corresponding image slices of the preoperative MR data (T1 and T2). The ultrasound based neuronavigation system would select the proper image slices according to the position and orientation of the biopsy forceps that was equipped with a positioning sensor. The tip position of the biopsy forceps was electronically marked in the respective image slices. The surgeon used the biopsy forceps to acquire 3 to 8 biopsies prior to resection, using the MR and ultrasound image slices for guidance. The biopsies were acquired from various parts of the tumour, however most biopsies were taken near the tumour border as defined in the ultrasound images. Biopsies were also taken in the transition zone between tumour and normal brain. As the biopsy was taken, a graphical screen dump of the neuronavigation system monitor was performed in order to document the tip position of the biopsy forceps.

2.5 Image interpretation and histopathological analysis

After the operation, all image material and information documenting the biopsy position and histopathology were entered in a project database. A group consisting of a senior neurosurgeon and 2-3 research scientists evaluated and categorized the images on a regular basis during the study. The tumour border shown in the ultrasound images was verified by an edge detection algorithm using the gradient of the intensity in the images. The ultrasound images were pre-processed by applying a 2D median filter with a Hamming profile. The effect of this filter is a slight smoothing, or low-pass filtering, of the image. The pre-processing suppresses speckle and high frequent noise in the ultrasound images, thus improving the output of the edge detection algorithm. The Sobel method implemented in Matlab 5.2 was used for the edge detection analysis. The shortest distance between the tip of the biopsy forceps and the tumour border detected in the ultrasound images was calculated.

For each of the MR T1, MR T2 and 3D US images the biopsy position was classified by visual inspection either as "tumour", "not tumour" or "uncertain", respectively. The analyses have been performed without prior knowledge of the histopathological diagnoses. The biopsies were prepared for histopathological evaluations either by freeze sections or by paraffin embedding. The histopathological diagnoses were classified in the same groups as used in the image evaluation of the malignancy, i.e. "tumour", "not tumour" or "uncertain". Diagnoses classified as "not tumour" included reactive tissue, edema and gliosis in addition to all normal brain cells. If the histopathological analysis revealed any infiltration of tumour cells in the tissue, the biopsy was categorized as "tumour".

3. Results

As of January 2002 a total of 113 biopsies in 19 operations were acquired prior to resection, of which 63 were taken close to the tumour border and thereby included in the study. The qualitative interpretation of a tumour border in the ultrasound images was

©CARS/Springer. All rights reserved.

verified by the edge detection algorithm. The quality of the output from the edge detection was dependent on the quality of the ultrasound image. However, the slight smoothing of the images improved the output of the edge detection algorithm, creating more continuous edges and reducing scattered noise. Figure 1 shows an ultrasound image of a metastasis before and after pre-processing and the same image with the detected edges overlaid.

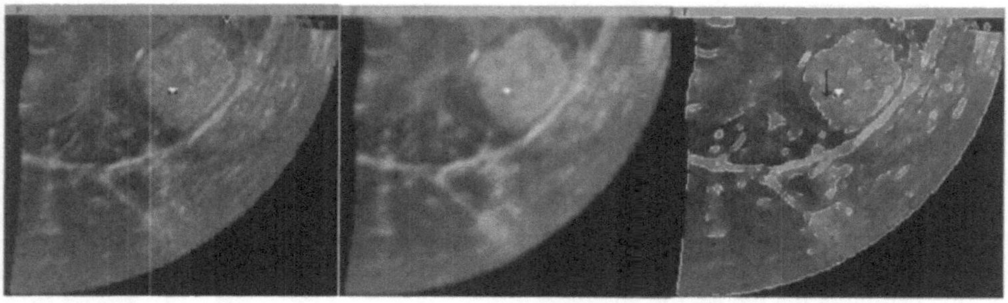

Figure 1: Ultrasound image slice of a metastasis (left), after smoothing the image with a median filter (middle) and the original data with the edges detected by the Sobel method overlaid (right). The calculated distance between the biopsy position and the detected tumour border is indicated by a thin bright line in the right image (indicated by black arrow). The tip position of the biopsy forceps is marked as a triangle in the images.

By comparing the image findings and the respective histopathological diagnoses a number reflecting the ability of intraoperative 3D US to visualize tumour material was found. The preliminary results presented in this paper include biopsies positioned close to the tumour border as shown in the ultrasound images. The distance between the tip of the biopsy forceps and the detected tumour edge was in the range of about 1.5 - 7 mm for the biopsies included in the analyses. Biopsies positioned directly at the tumour border as verified by the edge detection algorithm were excluded from the analyses, due to the potential error in position caused by the imaging resolution of the SonoWand system.

Figure 2 shows corresponding image slices of the ultrasound and MR volumes for a patient with low grade astrocytoma, as displayed on the SonoWand system during biopsy collection. The histopathologic result of the biopsy was low grade astrocytoma, thus matching the image findings for the MR and ultrasound data. The shortest distance between the biopsy position and the tumour border detected in the ultrasound image was in this case calculated to 3.5 mm. Figure 3 shows the same images as in the previous figure, but for an anaplastic astrocytoma. The histopathologic result of the biopsy documented in the figure was anaplastic astrocytoma. The distance between the biopsy position and the tumour border as shown in the ultrasound image was calculated to be 2.9 mm.

The preliminary results for low-grade astrocytoma shows that the US images match the histopathological diagnoses in 26 of 34 cases (76%), while for anaplastic astrocytoma the respective match is obtained in 12 of 14 cases (86%). The corresponding results for metastases, although limited in numbers, are a match in 8 of 8 cases. Work is in progress to evaluate ultrasound imaging of glioblastomas and tumours with radiation induced changes.

©CARS/Springer. All rights reserved.

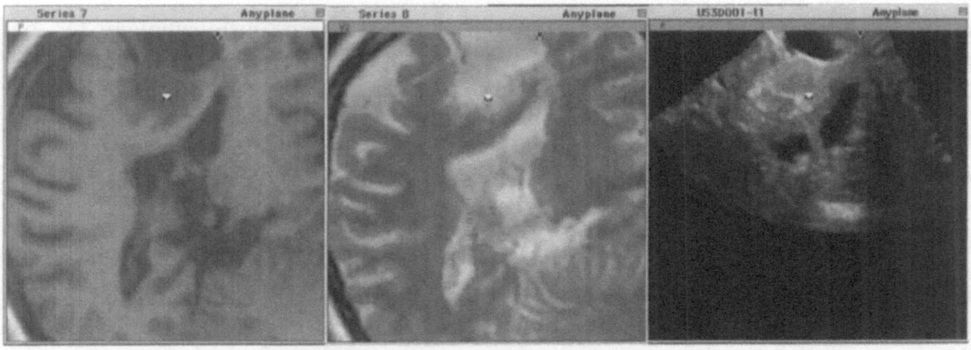

Figure 2: Corresponding image slices of MR T1 (left), MR T2 (middle) and ultrasound (right) volumes for a low grade astrocytoma, as displayed on the SonoWand system. The tip position of the biopsy forceps is indicated as a bright triangle.

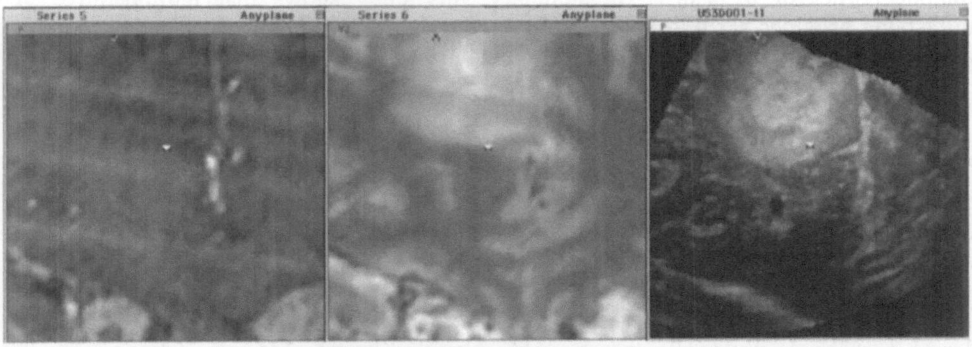

Figure 3: Corresponding image slices of MR T1 (left), MR T2 (middle) and ultrasound (right) volumes for an anaplastic astrocytoma, as displayed on the SonoWand system.

For the corresponding MR T1 images the number of histopathologic matches are 12 of 37 cases (32%) for low-grade astrocytoma, 6 of 10 cases (60%) for anaplastic astrocytoma, and 7 of 8 cases for metastasis. For the MR T2 images the corresponding numbers are 17 of 32 cases (53%) for low-grade astrocytoma, 8 of 12 cases (67%) for anaplastic astrocytoma, and 5 of 6 cases for metastasis.

4. Discussion

The results indicate that in neuronavigation intraoperative 3D ultrasound will give a more correct image of tumour border and localisation as compared to preoperative MRI data. However, this result is affected by the expected difference in imaging accuracy between preoperative data, which have to be registered to the patient using fiducial markers, and the intraoperative 3D ultrasound data. Due to the imaging accuracy of about 1.4 mm for the 3D ultrasound data [7], we expect the US images to more accurately describe the true position of the biopsy as compared to preoperative image data that has been registered to the patient prior to surgery. The accuracy of the preoperative data will be affected by any minor brain shifts occurring during exposure of the dura. This might further bias the results, even if the biopsies were taken immediately after opening of the dura to minimize

©CARS/Springer. All rights reserved.

brain shift. The relatively low match between US images and histopathology for low grade astrocytoma (76%) is mainly due to scattered tumour cells in biopsies taken outside the tumour border shown in ultrasound. These biopsies are histopathologically classified as tumour, because our classification does not discriminate scattered tumour cells from solid tumour. Work is in progress to differentiate the histopatologic evaluations with respect to the degree of tumour infiltration in the biopsy sample.

5. Conclusion

For low-grade astrosytoma and anaplastic astrocytoma the interpretation of the ultrasound images correlates well with the histopathological diagnoses for biopsies acquired close to the tumour border. For these two types of tumours the number of correlating matches for the intraoperative 3D ultrasound is at least as high, or higher, than the number of matches for the preoperative MR data. Our study also indicate that ultrasound depicts well the tumour border of metastasis. In summary, this study shows that intraoperative 3D ultrasound provides accurate information about the tumour border and location and may accordingly be used for guiding surgical procedures.

Acknowledgements

This work was supported by grant from the Research Council of Norway through the Strategic University Program in Medical Technology at the Norwegian University of Science and Technology (NTNU), and the Norwegian ministry of Health and Social Affairs.

References

1. 1. Knauth, M., Wirtz C.R., Tronnier V.M., Aras N., Kunze S., Sartor K., *Intraoperative MR Imaging Increases the Extent of Tumor Resection in Patients with High-Grade Gliomas.* AJNR Am J Neororadiol, 1999. **20**: p. 1642-1646.
2. 2. Le Roux, P.D., Berger M.S., Wang K., Mack L.A., Ojemann G.A., *Low grade gliomas: comparison of intraoperative ultrasound characteristics with preoperative imaging studies.* Journal of Neuro-Oncology, 1992. **13**: p. 189-198.
3. 3. Woydt, M., Krone A., Becker G., Schmidt K., Roggendorf W., Roosen K., *Correlation of Intra-operative Ultrasound with Histopathologic Findings After Tumour Resection in Supratentorial Gliomas.* Acta Neurochir (Wien), 1996. **138**: p. 1391-1398.
4. 4. Unsgaard, G., Ommedal S., Muller T. Gronningsaeter Aa., Nagelhus Hernes T.A., *Neuronavigation by three-dimensional ultrasound: Initial experience during brain tumor surgery.* Neurosurgery, 2002, **50,** April
5. 5. Wirtz, C.R., Knauth M., Staubert A., Bonsanto M., Sartor K., Kunze S., Tronnier V.M., *Clinical Evaluation and Follow-up Results for Intraoperative Magnetic Resonance Imaging in Neurosurgery.* Neurosurgery, 2000. **46**(5): p. 1112-1122.
6. 6. Gronningsaeter, Aa., Kleven A., Ommedal S., Aarseth T.E., Lindseth F., Lango T., Unsgaard G., *SonoWand, an Ultrasound-based Neuronavigation System.* Neurosurgery, 2000. **47**(6): p. 1373-1380.
7. Lango T., Bang, J., Lindseth F., Nagelhus Hernes, T.A., *Accuracy evaluation of a 3D ultrasound-based neuronavigation system.* Proc of the 16th International Congress and Exhibition in Computer Assisted Radiology and Surgery, (CARS2002) Paris June 27-30, 2002

©CARS/Springer. All rights reserved.

How to implement high-field intraoperative magnetic resonance imaging

Ch. Nimsky[a], O. Ganslandt[a], R. Fahlbusch[a]
[a] Department of Neurosurgery, University Erlangen-Nuremberg, Schwabachanlage 6, 91054 Erlangen, Germany

Abstract

The purpose of this study is to develop a new setup for intraoperative imaging that combines the benefits of high-field magnetic resonance (MR) imaging with microscope-based neuronavigation, providing anatomical and functional guidance. Our concept is based on this combination of intraoperative MR imaging evaluating the extent of a resection, while the simultaneous use of functional neuronavigation with integrated data from magnetoencephalography and functional MR imaging, allows to localize eloquent brain areas in the operative field. Thus, preventing increased neurological deficits, which could otherwise result from extended resections, if they were based only on the evaluation by intraoperative MR imaging.

Keywords: Functional data, intraoperative magnetic resonance imaging, neuronavigation.

1. Purpose

In the last 5 years we performed intraoperative MR imaging using a low-field 0.2 Tesla scanner in 330 patients [1-3]. The main indications were the evaluation of the extent of resection in gliomas, pituitary tumors [4], and in epilepsy surgery [5]. The initial concept provided three different operating setups directly in the scanner for interventional procedures, at the 5G-line, the patient still placed on the movable MR tray, or in an adjacent operating room, necessitating intraoperative patient transport. This cumbersome intraoperative patient transport on an air-cushioned OR-table was abandoned when microscope-based neuronavigation could be performed in the fringe-field of the scanner using a new navigation microscope [2]. We performed surgery at the 5 G line in 164 patients, while intraoperative patient transport was applied in 166 patients. In 167 patients neuronavigational guidance was used, while additionally functional data from magnetoencephalography or fMRI were integrated in 65. The simultaneous use of functional navigation prevented additional neurological deficits [6-10]. Intraoperative MR imaging offered the possibility of further tumor removal during the same surgical procedure in case of tumor remnants, increasing the rate of complete tumor removal. Furthermore, the effects of brain shift could be compensated for by updating neuronavigation with intraoperative image data [11-13].
Compared to routine pre- or postoperative imaging, being performed with high-Tesla machines, intraoperative image quality and sequence spectrum could not compete with those. This lead to the development of a new concept to adapt a high-field MR scanner to

CARS 2002 – H.U. Lemke, M.W. Vannier; K. Inamura, A.G. Farman, K. Doi & J.H.C. Reiber (Editors)
©CARS/Springer. All rights reserved.

our operating environment, preserving the benefits of using standard microsurgical equipment and microscope-based neuronavigational guidance with integrated functional data. Active magnetic shielding of modern high-field MR systems results in a steep decrease of the magnetic field, so that the 5 G-line is in close vicinity of the scanner, facilitating the intraoperative application of these high-field MR scanners.

2. Methods

A 1.5 Tesla Magentom Sonata scanner (Siemens Medical Solutions, Erlangen, Germany) is placed in a radiofrequency (RF)-shielded operating theatre (Fig. 1).

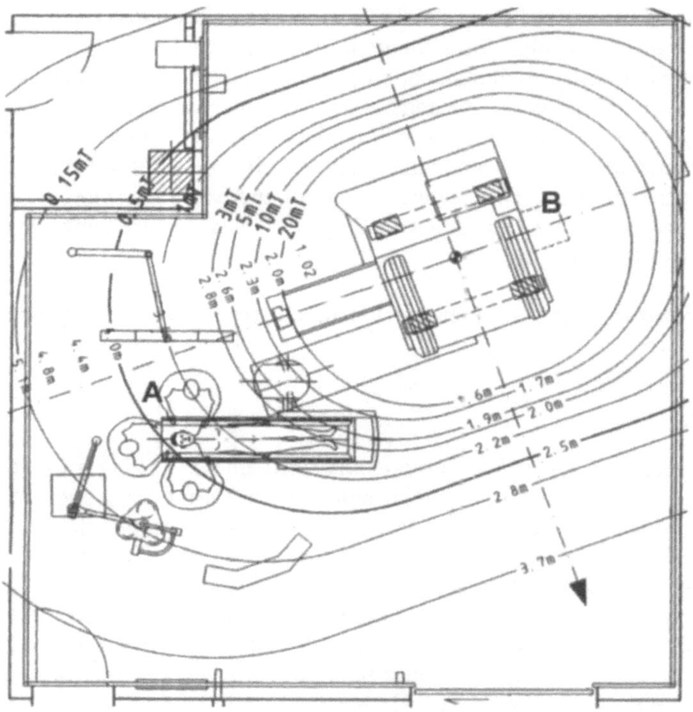

Fig. 1 Placement of the 1.5 Tesla Magnetom Sonata scanner in the radiofrequency-shielded operating room. The thick line depicts the 5G (0.5mT)-line. There are two main operating positions possible, A: at the 5G-line using the rotating OR-table (locked in a position of 160° in this figure), B: in the high-field, the patient directly located in the scanner, e.g. for biopsy procedures.

This operating theatre is equipped with a laminar air-flow field ensuring optimal hygiene requirements. MR-compatible anesthesia monitoring (wireless 2.4 GHz monitoring by Invivo Research, Orlando, USA) and respirator equipment (Servo 9000 C, Siemens Medical Solutions, Erlangen, Germany) are provided. As well as, all standard gaseous support is available in the RF-shielded cabin. Furthermore, glass fiber adapters allow ethernet connections to the intra- and internet at various points of the operating theatre.

©CARS/Springer. All rights reserved.

Electrical support is adjustable from outside so that in case of artifacts during measurements, designated equipment can be shut off.

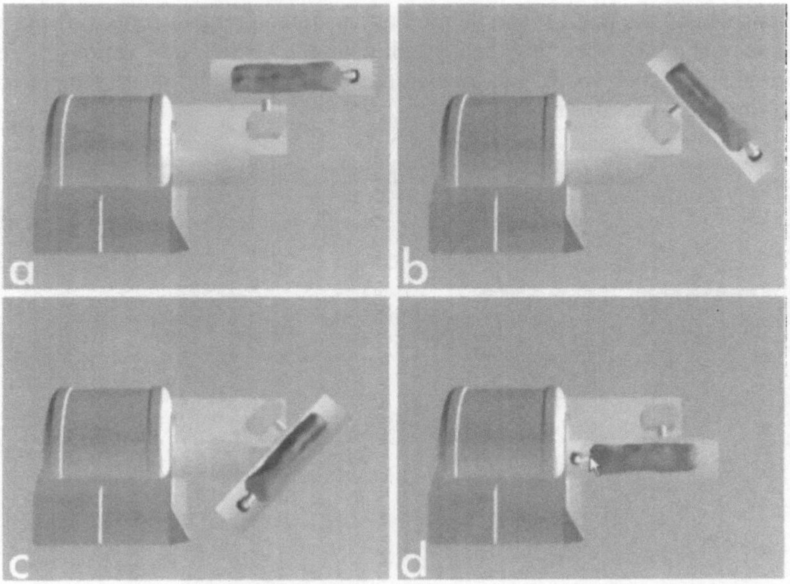

Fig. 2: A rotating OR table is adapted to the scanner, for surgery the patient's head is placed at the 5 G line (a), for scanning the table turns 180° (b-d), all anesthesia lines are going over the pivoting point of the OR table.

A rotating OR table (Trumpf, Saalfeld, Germany) is adapted to the 1.5 Tesla scanner serving as operating table and MR tray (Fig. 2). It permits free adjustments of the head position, also elevation and side rotation are possible. During surgery the head is placed at the 5 G line, for scanning the table is turned around and the patient is placed in the center of the scanner in less than 2 minutes. The head can be fixed in a MR compatible headholder, which is integrated in the standard head coil (Siemens Medical Solutions, Erlangen, Germany). The NC4-Multivision microscope (Zeiss, Oberkochen, Germany) is placed on the left patient side in the fringe-field (Fig. 3). Extensive testing at the Siemens labs did not show any artifacts generated by the microscope during scanning, as well as navigation was not influenced at the 5 G line by the magnetic field. For scanning, the microscope is switched off. Neuronavigational guidance is provided by the VectorVisionSky navigation system (BrainLab, Heimstetten, Germany). The camera tracking the position of the microscope in space and the touch-screen for operating the navigation system are ceiling-mounted (Ondal, Hünfeld, Germany). Neuronavigational accuracy is not impeded by the fringe-field. At the main operating position, functional microscope-based neuronavigation with integrated data from magnetoencephalography or functional MR imaging is available.
An alternative operating position, with the patient body placed in the scanner during surgery, is possible (Fig. 1 position B). There, stereotactic burr hole procedures using full

©CARS/Springer. All rights reserved.

MR-compatible operating equipment can be performed, while intraoperative MR imaging allows an online monitoring of the stereotactic procedure.
Two ceiling-mounted 17.4'' flat-screens (AS4431D, Iiyama, Nagano-shi, Japan) display the MR-console and the microscope video. Furthermore, a remote console is placed in the radiofrequency-shielded operating theater, allowing the operation of various PC-hardware from inside the operating room, e.g. for intraoperative functional measurements or neuro-electrophysiological monitoring [14].

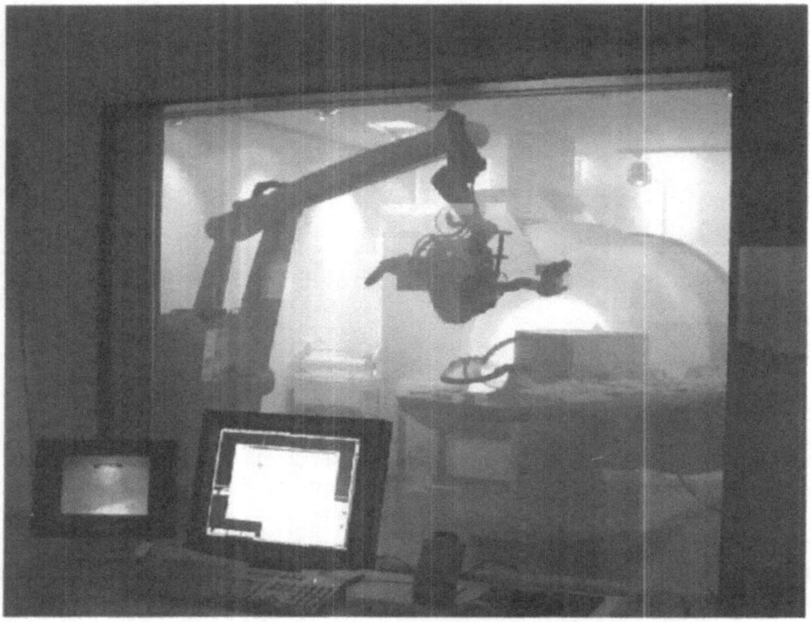

Fig. 3: Placement of the NC4 microscope at the 5 G line.

3. Conclusion

The development of high-field MR systems with active magnetic shielding results in a steep decrease of the magnetic field, so that the 5 G-line is in close vicinity of the scanner, facilitating an intraoperative application [2]. The adaptation of a high-field scanner into an operating room environment is now possible. The concept of a rotating OR-table results in two operating positions, while at the position at the 5 G-line microscope-based neuronavigational guidance using pre- and intraoperative anatomical and functional data is integrated. At the second operating position, the operative field is localized in the high-magnetic field. This setup can be used for stereotactic procedures with fully MR-compatible equipment, here intraoperative MR imaging serves as online control of the stereotactic procedure.
Besides enhanced image quality compared to low-field intraoperative systems, intraoperative high-field imaging offers further modalities, such as functional imaging,

©CARS/Springer. All rights reserved.

angiography, spectroscopy, and diffusion weighted imaging, all contributing to an advanced neuronavigational setup.

Acknowledgements

We acknowledge continuing support by Dr. A. Oppelt and Dr. T. Vetter (Siemens Medical Solutions, Erlangen, Germany), as well as by T. Bauch and A. Dombay (BrainLab, Heimstetten, Germany).

References

1. C. Nimsky, O. Ganslandt, M. Buchfelder and R. Fahlbusch, "Intraoperative Magnetresonanztomographie - Erfahrungen beim Einsatz in der Neurochirurgie", *Nervenarzt*, 71, 987-994, 2000.
2. C. Nimsky, O. Ganslandt, H. Kober, M. Buchfelder and R. Fahlbusch, "Intraoperative magnetic resonance imaging combined with neuronavigation: a new concept", *Neurosurgery*, 48, 1082-1091, 2001.
3. R. Steinmeier, R. Fahlbusch, O. Ganslandt, C. Nimsky, M. Buchfelder, M. Kaus, T. Heigl, G. Lenz, R. Kuth and W. Huk, "Intraoperative Magnetic Resonance Imaging with the Magnetom Open Scanner: Concepts, Neurosurgical Indications, and Procedures. A Preliminary Report", *Neurosurgery*, 43, 739-748, 1998.
4. R. Fahlbusch, O. Ganslandt, M. Buchfelder, W. Schott and C. Nimsky, "Intraoperative magnetic resonance imaging during transsphenoidal surgery", *J Neurosurg*, 95, 381-390, 2001.
5. M. Buchfelder, O. Ganslandt, R. Fahlbusch and C. Nimsky, "Intraoperative magnetic resonance imaging in epilepsy surgery", *J Magn Reson Imaging*, 12, 547-555, 2000.
6. O. Ganslandt, R. Fahlbusch, C. Nimsky, H. Kober, M. Möller, R. Steinmeier, J. Romstöck and J. Vieth, "Functional neuronavigation with magnetoencephalography: outcome in 50 patients with lesions around the motor cortex", *J Neurosurg*, 91, 73-79, 1999.
7. H. Kober, M. Möller, C. Nimsky, J. Vieth, R. Fahlbusch and O. Ganslandt, "New approach to localize speech relevant brain areas and hemispheric dominance using spatially filtered magnetoencephalography", *Hum Brain Mapp*, 14, 236-250, 2001.
8. H. Kober, C. Nimsky, M. Möller, P. Hastreiter, R. Fahlbusch and O. Ganslandt, "Correlation of sensorimotor activation with functional magnetic resonance imaging and magnetoencephalography in presurgical functional imaging: a spatial analysis", *Neuroimage*, 14, 1214-1228, 2001.
9. M. Möller, H. Kober, O. Ganslandt, C. Nimsky, J. Vieth and R. Fahlbusch, "Functional Mapping Speech Evoked Brain Activity by Magnetoencephalography and its Clinical Application", *Biomed Eng*, 44, 159-161, 1999.
10. C. Nimsky, O. Ganslandt, H. Kober, M. Möller, S. Ulmer, B. Tomandl and R. Fahlbusch, "Integration of functional magnetic resonance imaging supported by magnetoencephalography in functional neuronavigation", *Neurosurgery*, 44, 1249-1256, 1999.
11. C. Nimsky, O. Ganslandt, S. Cerny, P. Hastreiter, G. Greiner and R. Fahlbusch, "Quantification of, visualization of, and compensation for brain shift using intraoperative magnetic resonance imaging", *Neurosurgery*, 47, 1070-1080, 2000.
12. C. Nimsky, O. Ganslandt, P. Hastreiter and R. Fahlbusch, "Intraoperative compensation for brain shift", *Surg Neurol*, 56, 357-365, 2001.
13. M. Wolf, T. Vogel, P. Weierich, H. Niemann and C. Nimsky, "Automatic transfer of preoperative fMRI markers into intraoperative MR-images for updating functional neuronavigation", *IEICE T Inf Syst*, E84-D, 1698-1704, 2001.
14. J. Romstöck, R. Fahlbusch, O. Ganslandt, C. Nimsky and C. Strauss, "Localisation of the sensorimotor cortex during surgery for brain tumors: feasibility and waveform patterns of somatosensory evoked potentials", *J Neurol Neurosurg Psychiatry*, 72, 221-229, 2002.

©CARS/Springer. All rights reserved.

Development of Hitchcock stereotactic frame for intraoperative open MRI

Hiroki Taniguchi [a,c], Hiroshi Iseki [a,b], Takaomi Taira [b], Hiroshi Shirakawa [c], Hideaki Iwano [d], Yoshihiro Muragaki [a,b], Madoka Sugiura [a,e], Etsuko Kobayashi [f], Kiyoshi Naemura [a], Tomokatsu Horri [b], Kintomo Takakura [a]

[a] Faculty of Advanced techno-surgery, Institute of Advanced Biomedical Engineering and Science, Graduate school of Medicine, Tokyo Women's Medical University, 8-1 Kawada-cho, Shinjuku-ku, Tokyo 162-8666, Japan. {htaniguchi@abmes.twmu.ac.jp}

[b] Department of Neurosurgery, Neurological Institute, Tokyo Women's Medical University, 8-1 Kawada-cho, Shinjuku-ku , Tokyo 162-8666, Japan.

[c] Hitachi Medical. 2-1, Shintoyofuta, Kashiwa, Chiba, 277-0804, Japan

[d] Mizuho. 30-13, Hongo Bunkyo-ku Tokyo, 113-0033, Japan

[e] Hitachi Ltd. 1-5-1, Marunouchi, Chiyoda-ku, 100-8220, Japan

[f] Tokyo University. 7-3-1, Hongo, Bunkyo-ku Tokyo, 113-8656, Japan

Abstract

We have introduced open MRI into the operating room. When taking intraoperative open MR (iMR) images conventionally, since it was impossible to have used a conventional head coil for diagnosis because of need of space, we used to wrap the body coil around the patient' head to get signal. However, the body coil was less sensitive, wrapping the coil was very rough. Then we have developed Hitchcock Coil for intraoperative open MRI (iMRI). Hitchcock Coil works not only as more sensitive receiving coil than conventional one, but also as iMRI-guided Hitchcock stereotactic device (Hitchcock device), that is to say Navigation System using markers for iMRI. This time we confirmed that Hitchcock Coil were more excellent than the conventional receiving coil in respect of contrast and space resolution, and were acceptable to iMRI.

Key words: Intraoperative open MRI (iMRI), iMRI-guided Hitchcock stereotactic device (Hitchcock device), Hitchcock Coil

1. Introduction

Intraoperative open MRI (iMRI) has been introduced into much institution to perform neurosurgery checking brain shifts in recent years [1-5]. Since our open MRI [6] (Airis II ®: Hitachi Medical Corp) has a narrow magnetic leakage field (5 gauss line) and few restrictions of the instruments for surgery in the operating room, it is possible for conventional surgery. Now, when taking intraoperative open MR (iMR) images conventionally, after once interrupting surgery and covering a patient with a surgical drape, the procedure of taking iMR images is completed. Here, since it was impossible to

©CARS/Springer. All rights reserved.

have used a conventional head coil for diagnosis because of need of space by the head fixation and the surgical drape at that time, we used to wrap the body coil around the patient' head to get signal. This was why we substituted less sensitive body coil for the head coil.
By the way, real-time update navigation uses positional information of iMR images in real time, which has been highlighted in the world as a method of solution for brain shifts. On the contrary, since it is important for neurosurgery to approach to tumors simply and easily and to acquire trajectories and target points accurately, there are many cases that the stereotactic approach enables more accurate surgery. Then we have developed Hitchcock Coil for iMRI to strike a balance between coil function and surgical use. Hitchcock Coil works not only as more sensitive receiving coil than conventional one, but also as iMRI-guided Hitchcock stereotactic device (Hitchcock device), that is to say Navigation System using markers for iMRI. This time we evaluated the performance of Hitchcock Coil using phantoms and confirmed its validity before applying to clinical.

2. Methodology

2.1. Hitchcock Coil

In the case of iMRI-guided stereotactic surgery, we used to wrap the receiving coil around the stereotactic device which consists of the quality of the material of the nonmetallic nature, and thus it is natural that the conventional receiving coil (body coil) becomes less sensitive than the head coil.
It is indispensable to make the receiving coil for surgery establish when iMRI gets into stride. To combine the receiving coil with iMRI-guided stereotactic device is also exactly simplifying and optimizing procedure in iMRI. Then we have developed Hitchcock Coil as one means to solve the above-mentioned problem (Fig.1). Hitchcock Coil consists of Hitchcock stereotactic frame (Hitchcock Frame) in the upper part which fixes 3-dimensional position measuring equipment such as biopsy device and 4-pins fixation frame in the lower part. Both use aluminum of high conductivity. Hitchcock Frame and the 4-pins fixation frame themselves are formed into the receiving coil by means of constituting a parallel resonance circuit in the relay connectors parts connecting their frames. Frequency characteristic is adjusted according to the form of the receiving coil to realize the resonance circuit (Static magnetic field intensity : 0.3T, Resonance frequency : 12.7MHz).

©CARS/Springer. All rights reserved.

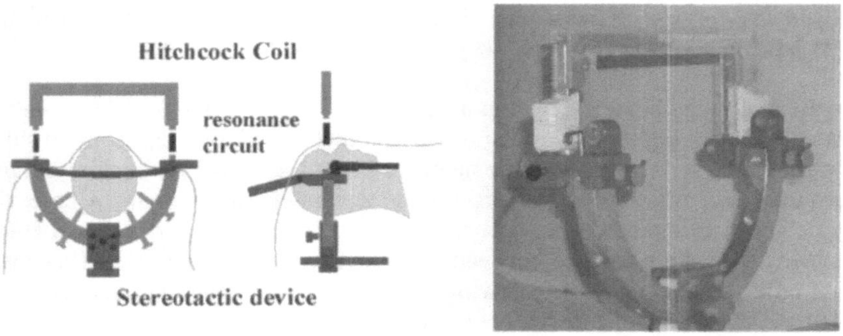

Fig.1: (left) Illustration showing the system of Hitchcock Coil. the coil consists of 3 parts; Hitchcock Frame, 4-pins fization frame, relay connectors, and resonance circuit. (right) Photograph showing the Hitchcock Coil for iMRI in neurosurgery.

2.2 Navigation System

In order to realize Navigation System for iMRI-guided Hitchcock stereotactic surgery, it is indispensable to measure the coordinates of a target point correctly. However, because of the distortion resulting from nonuniformity of magnetic field in open MRI, there is a risk of the measurement errors. Moreover it has been well known that distortion in open MRI becomes large according to separate from the centre of open MRI gantry. Therefore, we must set a reference point of coordinates measurement to the centre of open MRI gantry as much as possible. Furthermore, since Hitchcock Frame is not necessarily set at transversal planes by patient's postures, it is also important to set the transversal planes easily. As procedures of measuring 3-dimensional positions by Navigation System, first, we arrange markers around Hitchcock Frame and set the section which markers is always displayed in the sagittal image or the coronal image of scanogram image. Second, we set the photography range of the transversal image by the sagittal image and the coronal image. In that case, the position of the transversal plane shown on the sagittal and the coronal image is on the line connecting markers. Even if the position of Hitchcock Frame is set at any angles, the transversal image parallel to Hitchcock Frame is obtained. Therefore, when detecting the actual position of ROI in iMR images, the coordinates on Z-axis are estimated by the slice number and the slice interval on the basis of the transversal image parallel to Hitchcock Frame, the coordinates on XY-axis are estimated by the reference point in iMR images. Namely, the world coordinate system on Hitchcock Frame is constituted.

©CARS/Springer. All rights reserved.

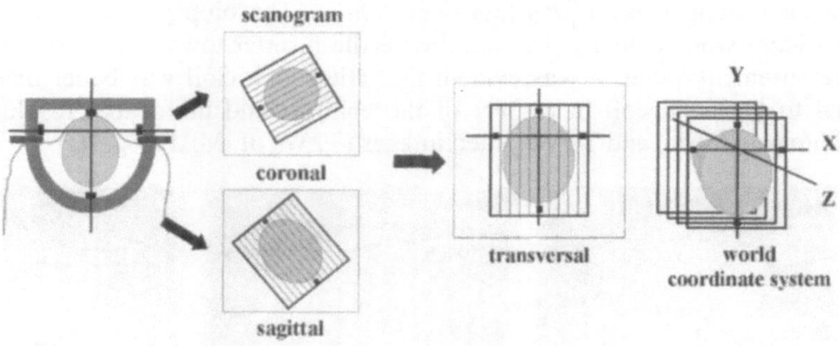

Fig.2: Method of measuring 3-dimensional positions by Navigation System

2.3 Experimental methods

We estimated coil performance (i.e., S/N as a sensitivity index, image size, and distortion). We compared S/N of Hitchcock Coil with that of the conventional receiving coil (body coil) using a standard phantom as sensitivity evaluation. FOV phantom in which the internal marker is arranged was used as evaluation of image size and distortion. As to the image size, the distance of AB on Y-axis and that of CD on X-axis (truth: 100mm respectively) were measured. The image size on Z-axis was also measured by changing the position of the FOV phantom. As to distortion, the Angle across AB and CD was measured. Tolerance was made within 1.5mm and 2 degrees respectively. In addition, we did a biopsy experiment. First, we take the marker images on Hitchcock Frame and measure an actual 3 dimension-position in iMR images. Photography conditions are set to 220mm FOV, 3mm slice thickness, and 1 5mm slice interval respectively. Second, we search for the measurement error between the marker positions by Hitchcock Frame and measurement values. Here, Y-axis coordinates are set to 20mm. we measure the markers arranged to 30mm, 45mm, and 60mm on X-axis coordinates when changing Z-axis coordinates with 30mm, 45mm, and 60mm. An upper frame is arranged 155mm from the centre of Open MRI gantry. Here, Y-axis coordinates of the measurement positions are equivalent to 135mm from the centre of Open MRI gantry.

3. Results

From the experimental result of the performance, S/N of the body Coil is from 60 to 70, whereas that of Hitchcock Coil is from 90 to 100. Therefore sensitivity has advanced from 30% to 40%. The maximum measurement errors in X, Y, and Z-axis about the image size were within 0.8mm, 0.5mm and 1.1mm of truth 100mm respectively. The maximum cross-angle errors of the two straight lines on XY-plane and YZ-plane about distortion were 0.8 degrees and 0.4 degrees respectively. Each data didn't go beyond the tolerance.
From the experimental result of the biopsy, the measurement errors increased on X-axis and Z-axis according to separate from the centre of open MRI gantry. Since the measurement errors on Z-axis depend on the slice thickness and the slice interval, the accuracy was more than 1.5mm. It can be solvable if the reference point is set near the target point (i.e., less than 45mm from the centre of Hitchcock Frame). Therefore, the

©CARS/Springer. All rights reserved.

maximum measurement error was less than 3.0mm. The biopsy measurement was also less than 3.0mm when actually piercing the needle inserter toward the target point based on the measurement value. It was evident that Hitchcock Coil was better than the body coil, equal to the head coil in respect of the contrast and the spatial resolution of T1 weighted images (T1W) and T2 weighted images (T2W) of iMRI (Fig.3).

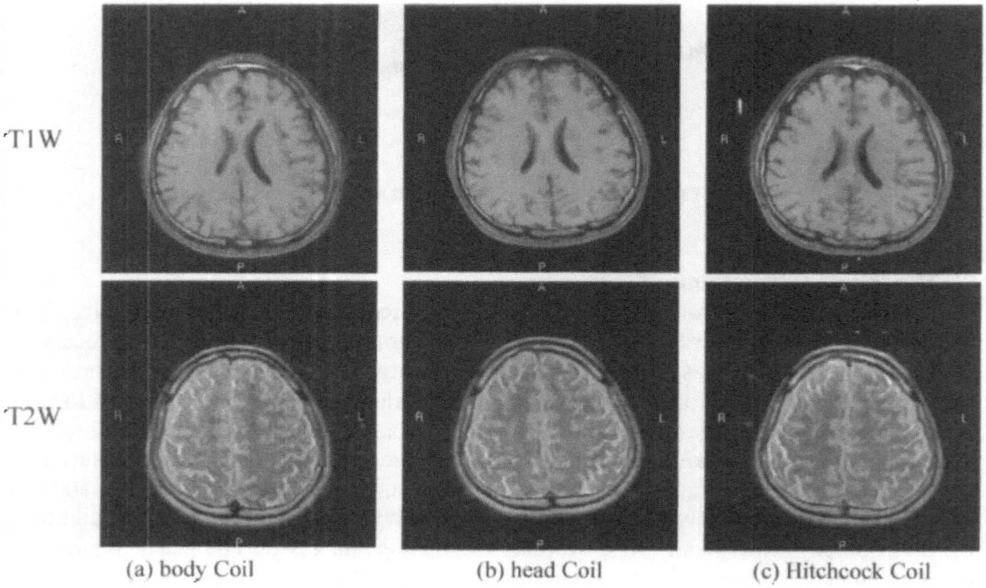

Fig. 3: T1 weighted images and T2 weighted images comparison by each receiving coil.

Table.1: Measurement error between truth and measurement value by Navigation System

	point1(Z:30mm)			point2(Z:45mm)			point3(Z:60mm)		
	x	y	z	x	y	z	x	y	z
X:30mm	0.5	-1.2	-1.5	0.2	-1.2	-3.0	-2.0	-1.1	-3.0
X:45mm	0.5	-1.0	-1.5	0.1	-0.5	-3.0	-1.7	-2.0	-3.0
X:60mm	-0.6	-1.4	-3.0	-1.1	-0.8	-3.0	-2.5	-1.0	-4.5

4. Conclusions

Hitchcock Coil formed by the Hitchcock Frame, the 4-pins fixation frame, the relay connectors, and the resonance circuit consisted of a non-magnetic body and high conductivity has suppressed the sensitivity fall by arranging the receiving coil in the position near a patient. We are sure that Hitchcock Coil is more excellent than the body coil in respect of contrast and space resolution, and are acceptable to iMRI as well. Besides, since preparatory time to attach and remove the receiving coil without moving

©CARS/Springer. All rights reserved.

patients is omitted when taking open MRI images conventionally, the optimization of the process in iMRI can be attempted. Furthermore, Hitchcock Coil will become possible the surgery approaches as Navigation System because of the measurement accuracy of less than ±3mm. Therefore, we will be able to make cost downed to Navigation System, and we will be able to shift to the conventional surgery easily and perform reasonable and flexible surgery instead of the hindrance of the surgery.

Acknowledgements

This study was supported by Industrial Technology Research Grant Program in 2001 from the New Energy and industrial Technology Development Organization (NEDO) of Japan.

References

1. Hadani M, Spiegelman R, Feldman Z, Berkenstadt H, Ram Z.Novel, compact, intraoperative magnetic resonance imaging-guided system for conventional neurosurgical operating rooms. Neurosurgery.2001 Apr ; 48(4) : 799-807 ; discussion 807-9.
2. Schulder M, Liang D, Carmel PW. Cranial surgery navigation aided by a compact intraoperative magnetic resonance imager. J Neurosurg. 2001 Jun; 94(6) : 936-45.
3. Nimsky C, Ganslandt O, Kober H, et al: Intraoperative magnetic resonance imaging combined with neuronavigation: a new concept. Neurosurgery 48:1082-1089; discussion 1089-1091, 2001
4. Black PM, Moriarty T, Alexander E, et al: "Development and implementation of intraoperative magnetic resonance imaging and its neurosurgical applications." *Neurosurgery* 41:831-842; discussion 842-835, 1997
5. Wirtz CR, Tronnier VM, Bonsanto MM, et al: "Image-guided neurosurgery with intraoperative MRI: update of frameless stereotaxy and radicality control." *Stereotactic & Functional Neurosurgery* 68:39-43, 1997
6. Muragaki Y, Iseki H, Maruyama T, et al: "New system of glioma removal using intraoperative MRI combined with functional mapping." *Computer Assisted Radiology and Surgery.* Proceedings of 15th international congress and exhibition 1143. Springer-Verlag, Berlin Heidelberg New York, 2001

©CARS/Springer. All rights reserved.

Intra-operative brain deformation using non-rigid image registration on a shared-memory multiprocessor computer

T. Rohlfing[a], C. R. Maurer, Jr.[a], D. L. G. Hill[b], T. Hartkens[b], W. A. Hall[c], C. L. Truwit[c], H. Liu[c], A. J. Martin[d], R. Shahidi[a]

[a]Image Guidance Laboratories, Department of Neurosurgery, Stanford University, 300 Pasteur Drive, Room S-012, MC 5327, Stanford, CA 94305-5327, USA

[b]Computational Imaging Science Group, Division of Radiological Sciences, Guy's Hospital, King's College London, UK

[c]Departments of Neurosurgery and Radiology, University of Minnesota, Minneapolis, MN, USA

[d]Department of Radiology, University of California San Francisco, CA, USA

Abstract

One major problem with non-rigid image registration techniques is their high computational cost. Because of this, these methods have found limited application to clinical situations where fast execution is required, e.g., intra-operative imaging. This paper applies a parallel implementation of a non-rigid image registration algorithm to pre and intra-operative MR images and quantitatively analyzes its scaling properties. The method computes the intra-operative brain deformation in about one minute using 64 CPUs on a 128-CPU shared-memory supercomputer (SGI Origin 3800). The serial component is no more than 2 percent of the total computation time, allowing a speedup of at least a factor of 50. In most cases, the theoretical limit of the speedup is substantially higher (up to 132-fold in the application examples presented in this paper). Our parallel algorithm is therefore capable of solving non-rigid registration problems with short execution time requirements and may be considered an important step in the application of such techniques to clinically important problems such as the computation of brain deformation during cranial image-guided surgery.

Keywords: Non-rigid image registration, parallel computing, brain deformation.

1. Introduction

Image-to-image registration is a common task in biomedical image processing [1]. The problem of registration arises whenever images acquired from different scanners, at different times, or from different subjects need to be combined for analysis or visualization. Several fast, robust, and accurate intensity-based rigid (with or without scaling) image registration algorithms have been reported and validated [2] and are commonly used for applications where a rigid transformation is appropriate. Non-rigid image registration is an active research area. Non-rigid methods are important for applications where the anatomy deforms or changes over time. Examples include computation of brain deformation during cranial image-guided surgery [3-5], correction of artifact due to patient motion during contrast-enhanced subtraction imaging [6-8],

©CARS/Springer. All rights reserved.

kinematic modelling of abdominal organ motion during respiration [9], and correction of geometric distortion in MR images [10].

One major problem with non-rigid image registration techniques is their high computational cost. Because of this, these methods have found limited application to clinical situations where fast execution is required, e.g., intra-operative imaging. This is disappointing since some of the most interesting and important problems involve intra-operative imaging, e.g., computation of brain deformation during cranial image-guided surgery. Other groups have published results of high-performance computing hardware to similar problems, including rigid registration on a cluster of symmetric multiprocessors [11], non-rigid registration on a massively parallel architecture [12], and non-rigid registration and segmentation on a multi-processor workstation [13]. In this paper, we address the problem of high computation cost using a parallel implementation that takes full advantage of modern large-scale shared-memory multiprocessor computer architectures. We parallelize an algorithm based on free-form deformations using B-spline interpolation [8] and demonstrate how the execution time of a non-rigid image registration algorithm can be dramatically reduced. To illustrate the benefits of parallelization, we perform an experimental analysis of the scaling properties of our parallel implementation.

2. Materials and Methods

2.1 Image Registration Algorithm

Our image registration algorithm computes normalized mutual information (NMI) [14] using a two-dimensional (2-D) joint histogram [15,16]. The transformation model and optimization strategy are independent and modified implementations of the method introduced by Rueckert et al. [8]. Our algorithm adds to the original technique a multiresolution deformation strategy [9] with adaptive grid refinement [6].

2.2 Parallel Implementation

We implement and evaluate the algorithm described below on an SGI Origin 3800 shared-memory computer with 128 MIPS R12K processors running at 400 MHz (Silicon Graphics, Mountain View, CA). The operating system is Irix 6.5 with a single kernel image architecture. Our algorithm is coded entirely in C++ and compiled using version 7.3.1.2 of the MIPSpro compiler suite. Parallelization is achieved using multithreading [17], a programming paradigm that takes full advantage of the shared-memory architecture. Threads are implemented using the POSIX threads library.

The key steps of the non-rigid registration algorithm involve computing the similarity measure between reference and floating image as well as an estimate of its gradient with respect to the transformation parameters. These are the two steps accounting for the bulk of the algorithm's computational cost, although for very different reasons. Computation of image similarity involves processing large amounts of data, in particular evaluating the non-rigid coordinate transformation for every single voxel in the reference image. On the other hand, due to the local effect of all transformation parameters, the gradient computation step deals with relatively small chunks of data only and thus has to evaluate the non-rigid transformation only for a small numbers of voxel at a time. However, the number of these chunks is equal to the number of parameters of the coordinate

©CARS/Springer. All rights reserved.

transformation, which is typically very large. So while evaluation of the global image similarity measure is a single expensive task, gradient computation is a repetition of many tasks, each single one of which is rather inexpensive. It is for this difference that two different strategies are applied in order to parallelize the two computations.

Evaluation of the similarity measure is a global operation that involves the complete image. We parallelize this step by breaking the data into equally sized partitions. Each thread is assigned one of these partitions and computes its contribution to the similarity measure. The voxel pairs encountered by each thread are stored in separate 2-D histograms. After finishing its part of the computation, each thread adds the entries of the histogram it created to the global histogram. This step needs to be kept mutually exclusive and is therefore protected by a mutex lock.

Estimation of the gradient of the image similarity measure is achieved by means of the common finite-difference approximation. Due to the compact support of the B-spline functions (moving any control point affects only its $4 \times 4 \times 4$ neighborhood), the computation of $f(\mathbf{x} + \boldsymbol{\delta}_i)$ and $f(\mathbf{x} - \boldsymbol{\delta}_i)$ is identical to the computation of $f(\mathbf{x})$ outside that neighborhood of the control point controlled by the i-th parameter. One can therefore precompute the 2-D histogram corresponding to $f(\mathbf{x})$ and substitute only the voxel pairs that are affected by moving the current control point. Hence, computing any particular element of the gradient Δf is a local operation that needs to consider only a small fraction of the image data per parameter. It therefore makes no sense to assign parts of the image data to multiple threads as the computational cost of gradient computation is caused by the large number of parameters (up to several hundreds of thousands frequently occur in practically relevant cases). This step is instead parallelized by assigning an equal number of the parameters to each of the threads, which then compute the respective components of the gradient. We do not start a new thread for each parameter as this would cause substantial computational overhead. For the same reason, and because the algorithm would not scale for more than two CPUs, we do not let one thread compute the $+\delta$ contribution while another thread computes the $-\delta$ part. Instead, we create the given number of threads and have each work on a subset of parameters.

2.3 Run Time Analysis

The real time $T(n)$ required to complete a task on n parallel processors can be approximated as

$$T(n) = A + \frac{B}{n},$$

where A is the serial (non-parallelizable) portion of the computation and B is the parallel portion [18]. The parameters A and B can be determined by linear regression of measured CPU times versus the inverse number of CPUs $1/n$.

©CARS/Springer. All rights reserved.

Table 1. Execution times for different numbers of processors and performance parameters of parallelization for non-rigid registration of pre- and intra-operative 3-D MR head images. Regression coefficient was $R > 0.9995$ for all four cases. Units of $T(\cdot)$, A and B are time in seconds.

Patient	$T(1)$	$T(4)$	$T(16)$	$T(64)$	A (serial)	B (parallel)
1	1477	381	107	50	17	1459
2	1759	450	125	60	19	1740
3	1776	458	125	55	18	1758
4	3311	845	227	102	25	3286
Mean	2081	533	146	67	20	2061
SD	832	210	55	24	3.2	717

3. Results

We applied our parallel algorithm for non-rigid image registration to pre- and intraoperative MR images of patients previously used for quantitative analysis of brain deformation under craniotomy [3-5]. We selected four patients for whom we performed parallelized non-rigid registrations as part of the present study.

All non-rigid registrations were performed starting with an initial control point grid spacing of 30 mm that was refined to 15 mm. The original image data was resampled to 2 mm voxel size at the first deformation level and 1 mm at the second level. Visual inspection of subtraction images such as those illustrated in Fig. 1 suggests that the resulting deformation transformations are relatively accurate. Using 64 CPUs, computing the non-rigid coordinate transformation between the pre- and intra-operative images shown in Fig. 1 took about 60 seconds. For the three other image data sets we used, the computations took between 50 and 102 seconds (mean 67 seconds). The theoretical lower bound for the computation time of all four cases was below 30 seconds; the theoretical upper limit for the parallel speedup was between 87 and 132 (mean 104). Table 1 gives all computation times and the performance parameters A and B determined using linear regression.

4. Conclusion

The work presented in this paper addresses one of the major problems of clinical application of non-rigid image registration, that is, high computational cost. By using a currently available shared-memory multiprocessor computer, we reduced execution times from hours to about one minute. Given the rapidly increasing availability of high-speed networks with guaranteed quality of service, e.g., the Internet2, the computational power of supercomputers is becoming available for clinical applications, e.g., computation of brain deformation during cranial image-guided surgery.

©CARS/Springer. All rights reserved.

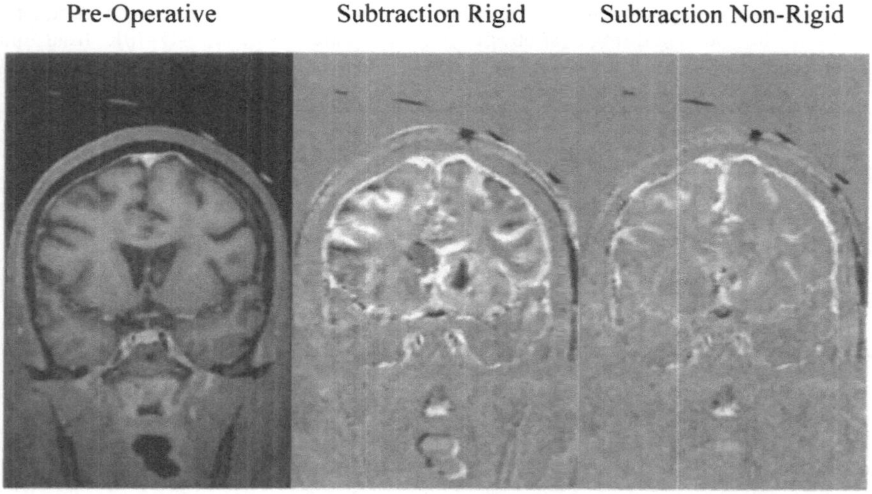

Figure 1. Combined visualization of pre-and intra-operative brain MR images. *Left:* Original coronal MR image; *center:* subtraction of corresponding pre- and intra-operative image after rigid registration; *right:* subtraction after non-rigid registration. Note that after non-rigid registration, the sign of almost all non-zero pixels in the subtraction image is positive. This is the result of contrast applied during surgery; it does not indicate misalignment of the pre- and intra-operative images.

Acknowledgements

TR was supported by the National Science Foundation under Grant No. EIA-0104114. TR, RS, and CRM acknowledge support for this research provided by CBYON, Inc., Mountain View, CA. Computations were performed on an SGI Origin 3800 in the Stanford University Bio-X core facility for Biomedical Computation. The authors thank Bil Lewis for his generous help and expert advice on thread programming.

References

1. JM Fitzpatrick, DLG Hill, CR Maurer Jr. Image registration. In: *Handbook of Medical Imaging, Volume 2: Medical Image Processing and Analysis.* M Sonka, JM Fitzpatrick, eds. Bellingham, WA: SPIE Press, pp 447-513, 2000.
2. JB West, JM Fitzpatrick, MY Wang, et al. Comparison and evaluation of retrospective intermodality brain image registration techniques. *J Comput Assist Tomogr* 21: 554-566, 1997.
3. T Hartkens, DLG Hill, CR Maurer Jr, et al. Quantifying the intraoperative brain deformation using interventional MR imaging. *Proc Int Soc Magn Reson Med* 8: 51, 2000.
4. DLG Hill, CR Maurer Jr, AJ Martin, et al. Assessment of intraoperative brain deformation using interventional MR imaging. *Medical Image Computing and Computer Assisted Intervention*, pp 910-919, 1999.
5. CR Maurer Jr, DLG Hill, AJ Martin, et al. Investigation of intraoperative brain deformation using a 1.5 Tesla interventional MR system: Preliminary results. *IEEE Trans Med Imaging* 17: 817-825, 1998.

©CARS/Springer. All rights reserved.

6. T Rohlfing, CR Maurer Jr. Intensity-based non-rigid registration using adaptive multilevel free-form deformation with an incompressibility constraint. *Medical Image Computing and Computer-Assisted Intervention*, pp 111-119, 2001.
7. T Rohlfing, CR Maurer Jr, J Beier. Correction of motion artifacts in three-dimensional CT-DSA using constrained adaptive multi-level free-form registration. *Computer Assisted Radiology and Surgery*, pp 350-355, 2001.
8. D Rueckert, LI Sonoda, C Hayes, et al. Nonrigid registration using free-form deformations: Application to breast MR images. *IEEE Trans Med Imaging* 18: 712-721, 1999.
9. T Rohlfing, CR Maurer Jr, WG O'Dell, et al. Modeling liver motion and deformation during the respiratory cycle using intensity-based free-form registration of gated MR images. *Medical Imaging: Visualization, Display, and Image-Guided Procedures*, Proc SPIE 4319: 337-348, 2001.
10. C Studholme, RT Constable, JS Duncan. Accurate alignment of functional EPI data to anatomical MRI using a physics-based distortion model. *IEEE Trans Med Imaging* 19: 1115-1127, 2000.
11. SK Warfield, F Jolesz, R Kikinis. A high performance approach to the registration of medical imaging data, *Parallel Comput* 24: 1345-1368, 1998.
12. GE Christensen, MI Miller, MW Vannier, et al. Individualizing neuroanatomical atlases using a massively parallel computer. *IEEE Computer* 29: 32-38, 1996.
13. SK Warfield, A Nabavi, T Butz, et al. Intraoperative segmentation and nonrigid registration for image guided therapy. *Medical Image Computing and Computer Assisted Intervention*, pp 176-185, 2000.
14. C Studholme, DLG Hill, DJ Hawkes. An overlap invariant entropy measure of 3D medical image alignment. *Pattern Recognit* 33: 71-86, 1999.
15. F Maes, A Collignon, D Vandermeulen, et al. Multimodality image registration by maximisation of mutual information. *IEEE Trans Med Imaging* 16: 187-198, 1997.
16. C Studholme, DLG Hill, DJ Hawkes. Automated three-dimensional registration of magnetic resonance and positron emission tomography brain images by multiresolution optimization of voxel similarity measures. *Med Phys* 24: 25-35, 1997.
17. B Lewis, DJ Berg. *Threads Primer: A Guide to Multithreaded Programming*. Upper Saddle River, NJ: Prentice Hall, 1996.
18. GM Amdahl. Validity of the single-processor approach to achieving large scale computing capabilities. *AFIPS Conference Proceedings* 30: 483-485, 1967.

CARS 2002 – H.U. Lemke, M.W. Vannier; K. Inamura, A.G. Farman, K. Doi & J.H.C. Reiber (Editors)
©CARS/Springer. All rights reserved.

Real time three-dimensional image rendering in suboccipital approaches to the skull base

Rosahl SK, Gharabaghi A, Liebig T, Dalle-Feste C, Samii M
International Neuroscience Institute, Alexis-Carrel-Str.4, D-30625 Hannover, Germany

Abstract

The neurosurgeon's orientation in approaches to the skull base depends on mental reconstruction of complex anatomical structures from tri-axial images with few visible landmarks. The study was carried out to define a protocol for intraoperative 3D navigation for the standard retrosigmoid approach.
A CT sequence was combined with an intravenous CT angiography in a total of 82 patients suffering from a variety of tumors in the posterior cranial fossa. Volumetric image rendering was employed to reconstruct the intracranial vasculature and the skull bone. By fine-tuned opacity modulation of the bone it was possible to gradually "look through" the bone on dural venous structures in 3D images (CBYON® suite). The transverse-sigmoid transition and its relation to the asterion on the surface of the skull could be visualized in a single image.
The location of these key structures was drawn to the skin to custom-tailor the incision. Major emissary veins could be followed in 3D images. The asterion proved to be as far as 13 mm off the transverse-sigmoid transition.
Our current protocol provides real-time 3D images that closely match individual patient anatomy. For the retrosigmoid approach, this technology offers a small but significant improvement in safety, speed and quality.

Keywords: Retrosigmoid approach, 3D volume-rendering, intraoperative navigation

1. Introduction

The retrosigmoid approach is the most frequently used avenue to pathologies in the posterior cranial fossa. Its most critical challenge remains the exposure of the transverse and sigmoid sinus transition.[5,6] Damage to these complex vascular structures may result in a situation threatening the patients life. On the other hand, a failure to expose the edge of the sinus complicates surgery in the cerebellopontine angle and places cranial nerves and the brainstem at an undue risk. Unfortunately, the venous complex structures are hidden behind the skull bone. This situation prompted surgeons to search for visible landmarks that may relate to the individual course of the transverse-sigmoid complex as soon as the approach had been introduced in clinical practice.
One of these landmarks is the meeting point of the lambdoid, occipitomastoid and parietomastoid sutures – the asterion (Fig. 1). There is proof from anatomical studies, however, that the asterion is not always located over the transverse-sigmoid transition (TST).[1,2,3,7,8]

©CARS/Springer. All rights reserved.

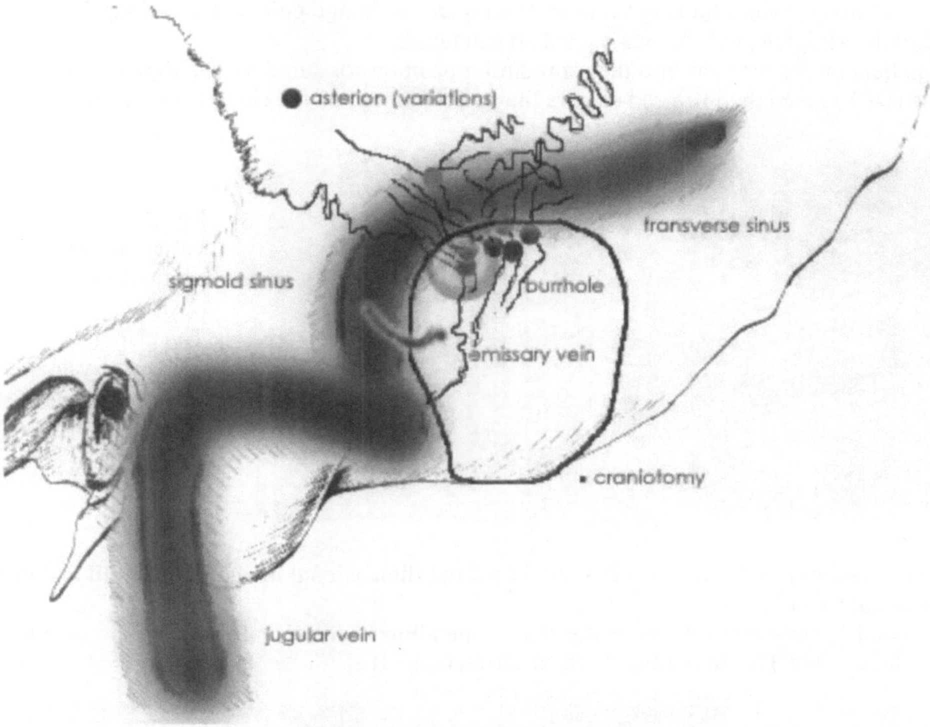

Fig. 1 Schematic drawing of the anatomical relationship of vascular and bony landmarks in the retrosigmoid approach. The location of the asterion in the vicinity of the transverse-sigmoid transition varies considerably among individual patients.

The goal of this study was to employ a surgical image guidance system to obtain a real-time three-dimensional radiographic image of the TST in order to use the sinus themselves as a landmark during the entire retrosigmoid approach, i.e. from the skin incision on. In addition, the position of the asterion should be recorded in relationship to the TST.

2. Procedure

48 patients (24 male, 24 female) with pathologies located in the posterior cranial fossa have participated in the study during from June 2001 through January 2002. Pathologies included 33 vestibular schwannomas, 8 meningiomas, 3 astrocytomas, 2 jugular foramen neurinomas, one hemifacial spasm and one trigeminal neuralgia.
Seven adhesive fiducial skin markers were placed at the forehead, at the mastoid tips, and in the retroauricular area of each patient. To visualize the intracranial vasculature along with the skull bone in a single image, a spiral computed tomography (CT) sequence of the posterior fossa (2mm interslice distance) was performed with rapid intravenous contrast application (intravenous CT angiography, CTA).

©CARS/Springer. All rights reserved.

The axial images were transferred to an intraoperative image guidance system (CBYON® suite, Palo Alto, CA, U.S.A.) via a local area network.
The patients were brought into the semi-sitting position for surgery. The digital reference frame (DRF) faced the infra-red camera that was mounted on the side of surgery (Fig. 2).

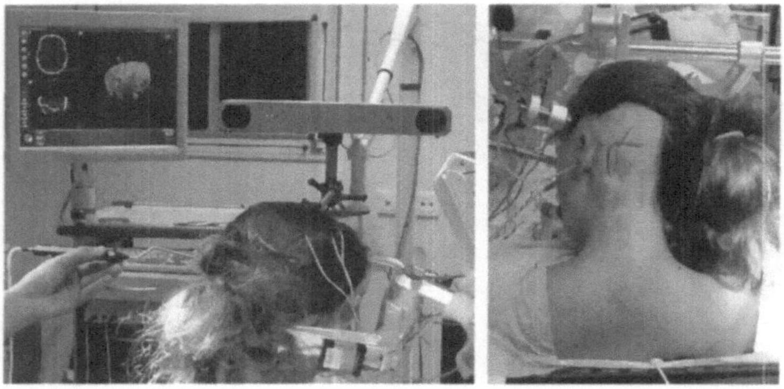

Fig. 2
Patient in the semi-sitting position.
The camera of the guidance system was always placed at the side of surgery.

Volume-rendering was employed to obtain a three-dimensional image of the skull and the intracranial vasculature.
Fine-tuned opacity modulation of the skull bone allowed for visualization of the location and course of the TST in relation to the asterion (Fig. 3).

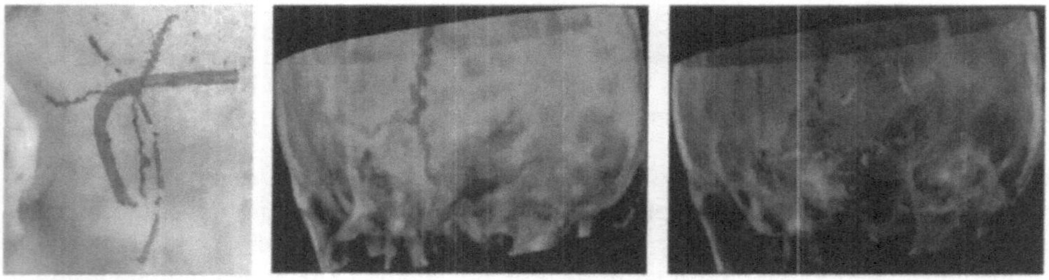

Fig. 3 By decreasing the opacity of the skull (right two panels) it is possible to visualize the relationship between the asterion and the transverse-sigmoid transition. The landmarks can be drawn on the skin to custom-tailor the skin incision (left panel).

In most cases, after skin incision and soft tissue preparation, a craniectomy was carried out and the gap was refilled with methymethacrylate at the end of surgery. When an osteoplastic procedure was performed in young patients the first burrhole was placed close to the TST with a safety margin of about 5 mm (Fig. 4).
Following rough bone preparation, the accuracy of the system was always re-evaluated to exclude errors due to drf dislocation or shifting of the patient's head before the more delicate dissection of emissary veins and sinus edges.

©CARS/Springer. All rights reserved.

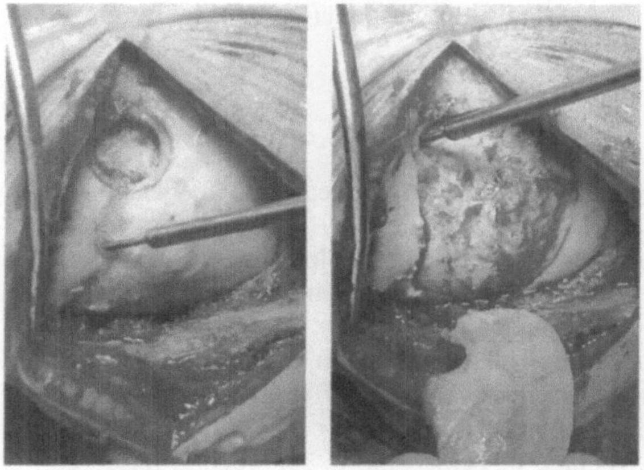

Fig. 4
The burrhole was placed at the level of the TST with a safety margin of about 5mm in this case. An emissary vein is followed with the stylus of the guidance system (left). After an osteoplastic craniotomy has been carried out, the accuracy of the system is re-checked to exclude shifting errors before the delicate sinus edges are dissected (right).

3. Results

Minute bone sutures and the asterion as well as their relationship to the transverse-sigmoid sinus complex could in single volume-rendered 3D images in 44 of the cases. In three cases the sutures were completely ossified and invisible in high-resolution CT scans. In one case, the intravenous contrast filling was insufficient.

System setup time in the OR varied around 15 minutes including physical registration.
With the location of the landmark structures drawn to the skin, the incision could be custom-tailored to the patient's individual anatomy (Fig. 3). The real-time display of the transverse and sigmoid sinus complex by the guidance system matched the operative situs with a precision of +/- 2 mm in 45 cases. Failures included DRF dislocation in 2 and a software error in 1 case.

During surgery, the quality of three-dimensional image rendering of the CBYON system allowed for fast and easy assessment of complex structures hidden behind the bone such as the major intradural vessels, emissary veins and the mastoid cell system. Especially the perception of the tortuous course of vessels was considerably faster with 3D volumetric images than with mental reconstruction of conventional tri-axial images that mainly served as an additional reliability control in this study.

The location of the asterion varied considerably around the inner edge of the TST. There were cases in which it was located as far as 13 mm this point and up to 9 mm laterally.
The asterion was not identifiable in 9 cases in vivo, even though it was clearly visualized by the guidance system.

The TST and the edges of the sinuses were precisely exposed in all 48 patients.
There were no surgical complications related to the approach throughout this series.
Intradurally, navigation was rarely used. Structures inside the petrous bone, such as the jugular foramen, the internal auditory canal and the semicircular canals could be located in 3D images. An accuracy of +/- 2mm, however, was found to be less helpful in drilling

©CARS/Springer. All rights reserved.

at the internal auditory canal since it necessitates the introduction of a safety corridor to the vestibular system.[4]

4. Discussion

Three-dimensional volumetric image rendering may provide real-time images that closely match individual patient anatomy.

The possibility to visualize hidden vascular structures along with minute surface anatomical landmarks in a single, volumetric three-dimensional image with high resolution represents a new quality in neuronavigation.

Our results confirm the large variability of the asterion described by cadaveric studies.[1,2,3,8] This point at the surface of the skull which often is not even visible does not qualify as a surgical landmark.

In the retrosigmoid approach, the advantage of being able to see beyond tissue barriers before actually dissecting them speeds up the surgical procedure and provides additional safety for the patient by ready localization of the transverse-sigmoid sinus complex.

Acknowledgements

The International Neuroscience Institute Hannover participates in an international trial to assess the clinical reliability of the CBYON Suite image guidance system (CBYON® suite, Palo Alto, CA, U.S.A.).

References

1. Day JD, Kellogg JX, Tschabitscher M, Fukushima T: Surface and superficial surgical anatomy of the posterolateral cranial base: significance for surgical planning and approach. Neurosurgery 38(6): 1079-1083, 1996.
2. Day JD, Tschabitscher M: Anatomic position of the asterion. Neurosurgery 42(1): 198-199., 1998.
3. Lang J, Jr., Samii A: Retrosigmoidal approach to the posterior cranial fossa. An anatomical study. Acta Neurochir (Wien) 111(3-4): 147-153., 1991.
4. Samii A, Brinker T, Kaminsky J, Lanksch WR, Samii M: Navigation-guided opening of the internal auditory canal via the retrosigmoid route for acoustic neuroma surgery: cadaveric, radiological, and preliminary clinical study. Neurosurgery 47(2): 382-387, 2000.
5. Samii M, Draf W: *Surgery of the skull base.* Berlin-Heidelberg-New York: Springer, 1989.
6. Samii M, Matthies C: Management of 1000 vestibular schwannomas (acoustic neuromas): surgical management and results with an emphasis on complications and how to avoid them. Neurosurgery 40(1): 11-21; discussion 21-13., 1997.
7. Seeger W: *Planning Strategies of Intracranial Microsurgery.* Berlin-Heidelberg-New York: Springer, 1986.
8. Uz A, Ugur HC, Tekdemir I: Is the asterion a reliable landmark for the lateral approach to posterior fossa? J Clin Neurosci 8(2): 146-147., 2001.

CARS 2002 – H.U. Lemke, M.W. Vannier; K. Inamura, A.G. Farman, K. Doi & J.H.C. Reiber (Editors)
©CARS/Springer. All rights reserved.

The NASA Smart Probe project for real-time multiple microsensor tissue recognition: automating stereotactic brain biopsy and other procedures

R. Andrews[1], R. Mah[1], S. Jeffrey[1], K. Freitas[1], M. Guerrero[1], R. Papasin[1], C. Reed[1]

[1]Smart Systems Lab, NASA Ames Research Center, Moffett Field, CA, USA

Abstract

Automating the sensor, effector, and sensor-effector communication aspects of surgery is essential to perform opera-tions at a site remote from the surgeon, e.g. in Space. Real-time tissue recognition can be combined with image-guidance to augment the sensor component; a robot can be the remote effector component. The NASA Smart Probe uses neural networks to combine data from multiple microsensors in real-time to provide a unique tissue "signature". The concept has been demonstrated in both animal models and clinical trials with women undergoing breast "biopsy" (optical followed by histological). Minimally-invasive multiparameter real-time tissue recognition should improve (1) cancer diagnosis, (2) localization (e.g. functional neurosurgery), and (3) tissue monitoring (e.g. cerebral or cardiac ischemia). The Smart Probe can become the sensor component of a self-contained robotic surgical device.

1. Introduction

Surgery at a site remote from the surgeon presents issues of (1) sensors at the operative site, (2) effectors at the operative site, and (3) the communication between sensors and effectors. In the traditional Operating Room, the surgeon is the "device" that accomplishes all three issues. Depending on the "remote site", these 3 issues may be very different. In image-guided stereotactic brain biopsy, the "remote site" is but a few centimeters away - within the patient's skull. The surgeon uses imaging data as the "sensor", a biopsy needle as the "effector", and is the "communicator" between sensor and effector. For surgery in Space, the Earth-bound surgeon is handicapped by (1) being remote from both sensors and effectors, and (2) time delays in communicating between sensors, surgeon, and effectors (minutes, rather than the milliseconds in which the surgeon's nervous system integrates "sensing" and "effecting"). During the September, 2001, cardiac surgery performed in Strasbourg by a surgeon in New York, the transmission delays were at the upper limit to perform intricate procedures (e.g. cardiac/neurosurgery) in real-time.

Regarding effectors for remote surgery, surgical robots are evolving rapidly. Robots initially were aids to the surgeon, e.g. AESOP (Computer Motion, Santa Barbara, CA), or performed strictly-defined, automated tasks such as reaming out the femur under CT-guidance for artificial hip surgery, e.g. RoboDoc (Integrated Surgical Systems, Davis, CA). Robots have now become effectors guided by the surgeon, allowing minimally-invasive remote cardiac surgery, e.g. DaVinci (Intuitive Surgical, Mountain View, CA) and Zeus (Computer Motion, Santa Barbara, CA). Image-guidance and robotics have been

©CARS/Springer. All rights reserved.

joined in neurosurgery to automate procedures such as brain biopsy and deep brain stimulation for movement disorders, e.g. NeuroMate (Integrated Surgical Systems, Davis, CA).
Regarding communication between sensors and effectors for surgery in Space, given the transmission delay of minutes each way even to Mars, it is not feasible for the surgical "communicator" to be an Earth-bound surgeon. An alternative (with potential for surgery on Earth as well) is to have the "surgeon" be a device which incorporates sensors, effectors, and the communication between sensors and effectors. This device (dubbed "Astrosurgeon") travels with the Astronauts on the Spacecraft, and performs the diagnostic and therapeutic aspects of surgery relatively autonomously (i.e. with only limited input from the Astronauts, who will not have a surgical background).
Regarding sensors for remote surgery, tactile feedback and visual information can be provided to the surgeon. Since transmission delays make this impractical for extraterrestrial surgery, the NASA Smart Probe Project (NSPP) has focused on developing sensing capabilities that provide information directly to the effector (surgical robot). The NSPP premise is that multimodality data from multiple microsensors – integrated in real-time with advanced data processing (neural networks and fuzzy logic) – can resolve the issue of sensor data collection for remote surgery.
The limitations of CT/MR image-guidance for stereotactic brain biopsy, tumor excision, and functional neuro-surgery are well recognized: (1) brain shift and/or fiducial movement may render the pre-operative scan invalid [8,12]; (2) blood vessels may be violated on the trajectory [7,10]; (3) no information is provided about the target when it is presumably reached [3]. Intraoperative MRI, cumbersome and expensive, provides only limited data regarding deep brain (or neoplastic) tissues [13], and is not feasible for remote sites either on Earth or in Space.
To overcome these limitations, the Smart Probe combines image-guidance with data from multiple microsensors as the probe approaches a target - data processed in real-time by neural network/fuzzy logic algorithms [2,4]. The choice of sensor modalities is application-specific. For neurosurgery, we have chosen optical spectroscopy (OS), pressure/resistance, electrophysiology (spontaneous, evoked, impedance), laser-Doppler cerebral blood flow (CBF), pH-PO2-PCO2-temperature, and data from a 1 mm diameter fiberoptic neuroendoscope as the sensors whose data provide a unique signature for each tissue. Various situations can be distinguished: (1) tissue type (e.g. gray matter vs. white matter); (2) tissue status (e.g. normal vs. neoplastic); (3) tissue condition (e.g. normal vs. ischemic).
The most powerful sensor technique for real-time tissue recognition is optical spectroscopy (OS). OS can distinguish neoplastic and pre-neoplastic from normal or inflammatory gastrointestinal tissue and breast tissue, as well as brain gray matter from white matter, *in vivo* [6,9,11]. The NASA Smart Probe combines OS with the other sensors noted above to enhance real-time tissue identification (e.g. tumor vs. normal brain) and characterization (e.g. ischemic vs. non-ischemic brain). Tumor tissue has lower oxygen concentration and increased vascularity in comparison with normal tissue; measures of oxygenation and blood flow can thus improve the identification of tumor tissue.

2. Methods

The Smart Probe configuration is application-specific. For stereotactic brain biopsy, it consists of an outer cannula (2.7 mm diam) with three inner cannulas (each 1.0 mm diam)

©CARS/Springer. All rights reserved.

(Figure 1) [4]. Each of the inner cannulas houses a microsensor or microsensor cluster. The microsensors tested to date (each < 1 mm diam) include a silicon chip pressure sensor (Entran, Fairfield, NJ), a laser-Doppler cerebral blood flow probe (Vasamedics, St. Paul, MN), a standard fiberoptic neuroendoscope (Codman, Raynham, MA), a standard microelectrode, a multiparameter tissue monitor (NeuroTrend, Codman, Raynham, MA), and an OS probe (PC2000, Ocean Optics, Dunedin, FL). The Smart Probe attaches to a standard stereotactic frame and can be advanced precisely by a computer-controlled stepper-motor for stereotactic applications (Figure 1) [2]. Other configurations include an 8-microsensor probe 2.5 mm in diameter, and - for breast biopsy - multiple OS sensors in a "needle" less than 2 mm in diameter.
Animal data were collected from rats of approximately 300 g weight, both normal and with subcutaneously im-planted mammary gland tumors, under protocols approved by the NASA Ames and Stanford University Institutional Review Boards [1,2,4]. Data collection, analysis, and display software are both proprietary (NASA: neural-network/ fuzzy logic) and commercial (e.g. MATLAB, MathWorks, Natick, MA). Data analysis/display hardware utilizes a laptop running Windows NT (Microsoft, Redmond, WA), with a NASA-developed user-friendly graphics interface.

In November, 2001, clinical trials (using a < 2 mm diameter multisensor probe) began at the University of California, Davis, Medical Center. Breast "biopsies" in 8 women with suspected breast cancer have been performed to date (March, 2002) using Smart Probe technology licensed from NASA, and further developed in conjunction with the Lawrence Livermore National Laboratory (Livermore, CA) by the company BioLuminate (Dublin, CA).

3. Results

The optical spectra (350 to 900 nm) for various tissues (including brain, muscle, fat, liver) are plotted as a mean of 10 or more repetitions (Figure 2). These include spectra from 1 mm above, in contact, and 1 mm within the tissue, which are very similar in all 3 positions for a given tissue [4]. The OS spectra from several tissues are plotted in a three-dimensional space (Figure 3). Also plotted are data on tissue density, mean color analysis (red) from the neuroendoscope, and OS (Figure 4). Hyperspectral analysis of more than three parameters can be performed to demonstrate the greater tissue differentiation obtained with specific additional sensor modalities (not illustrated).

Regarding clinical studies, for 8 patients with suspected breast cancer, differences have been found between the blood volume and oxygen concentration in normal breast tissue or benign lesions in comparison with breast carcino-ma. Consistent with the literature, blood volume is increased and oxygen content decreased in breast carcinoma compared with the levels in normal breast tissue or benign breast lesions (BioLuminate data currently proprietary).

4. Conclusions

4.1 NASA's Near-Term Goal

The Smart Probe combines multiple microsensor data to provide real-time cancer diagnosis, with cancer of the breast and brain under study at present. The Smart Probe can complement image-guidance in (1) stereotactic brain biopsy, (2) localization during functional neurosurgery (e.g. deep brain stimulation for Parkinson's disease), and (3)

©CARS/Springer. All rights reserved.

distinguishing tissues (e.g. disc vs. nerve in endoscopic spinal surgery). A hand-held version can identify residual tumor during resection; an implanted version can provide multiparameter monitoring of ischemic brain tissue.

4.2 NASA's Long-Term Goal [3]

The NASA Mars mission (*circa* the year 2020) will last 2 years – 9 months' travel time each way plus 6 months on Mars. The 4 astronauts (no physicians) will undergo pre-mission total body high-resolution MRI scanning (including MR spectroscopy). A body-conforming space suit is worn which incorporates continuous multiparameter monitoring (e.g. blood pressure, temperature, EKG, blood gases, electrolytes). The helmet incorporates multiple (64 or more) high-resolution ultrasound and near-infrared spectroscopy sensors, plus electrodes for EEG monitoring. The suit and helmet permit continuous correlation of the astronaut's medical status on the mission with his/her pre-mission status.

Also on the mission is a compact robot ("Astrosurgeon ') with multiple microsensors for gathering data non- or minimally-invasively in real-time and a databank established over years for various conditions from appendicitis to stroke to myocardial infarction to subdural hematoma. The robot's effectors (lasers, aspirators, device implanters) – guided by the data gathered from the microsensors and compared to the databank (including the Astronaut's own data) in real-time – treat the vast majority of conditions without additional input from Houston Space Center.

If one doubts this scenario is feasible by 2020, merely consider advances in the last quarter of the 20th century: beginning in the pre-CT era and ending with robots that can perform neurosurgery (NeuroMate) or cardiac surgery (DaVinci, Zeus) thousands of miles away from the operating surgeon.

Acknowledgments

Funding has been provided by NASA. Equipment has been provided by Codman/Johnson & Johnson (Raynham, MA), and Vasamedics (St. Paul, MN). NASA has been assigned US Patent #6,109,270 on behalf of the Smart Probe inventors R. Mah and R. Andrews. Information on the licensee for breast cancer diagnosis – BioLuminate, Inc. – is available at www.bioluminate.com. The information and opinions expressed here are those of the authors, and do not necessarily represent official NASA policy.

References

1. Andrews RJ, Bringas JR, Alonzo G: Cerebrospinal fluid pH and pCO2 rapidly follow arterial blood pH and pCO2 with changes in ventilation. *Neurosurgery* 34:466-470, 1994.
2. Andrews R, Mah R, Galvagni A, *et al*: Computerized multimodality stereotactic brain biopsy. *Stereotact Funct Neurosurg* 68:72-79, 1997.
3. Andrews RJ: Neuroprotective 'agents' in surgery: secret 'agent' man, or common 'agent' machine? *Ann New York Acad Sci* 890:59-72, 1999a.
4. Andrews R, Mah R, Freitas K, Guerrero M, Papasin R, Stassinopoulos D: Multimodality stereotactic brain tissue identification: the NASA Smart Probe project. *Stereotact Funct Neurosurg* 73:1-8, 1999b.
5. Andrews RJ: Opportunities for optical technologies in neurology/neurosurgery. *Report of the Advisory Coun-cil on Optical Technologies* (eds IJ Bigio, F Shtern, SM Ascher). *Acad Radiol 6 (Suppl 3):S189-S191, 1999c.*

©CARS/Springer. All rights reserved.

6. Bigio IJ, Bown SG, Briggs G, *et al*: Diagnosis of breast cancer using elastic-scattering spectroscopy: preliminary clinical results. *J Biomed Opt* 5:221-228, 2000.
7. Deep-Brain Stimulation for Parkinson's Disease Study Group: Deep-brain stimulation of the subthalamic nucleus or the pars interna of the globus pallidus in Parkinson's disease. *N Engl J Med* 345:956-963, 2001.
8. Dorward NL, Alberti O, Velani B, *et al*: Postimaging brain distortion: magnitude, correlates and impact on neuronavigation. *J Neurosurg* 88:656-662, 1998.
9. Gillet CA, Johns M, Liu H: Use of a near-infrared probe for localization during stereotactic surgery for movement disorders. *J Neurosurg* 93:498-505, 2000.
10. Kulkarni AV, Guha A, Lozano A, Bernstein M: Incidence of silent hemorrhage and delayed deterioration after stereotactic brain biopsy. *J Neurosurg* 89:31-35, 1998.
11. Mourant JR, Bigio IJ, Boyer J, *et al*: Elastic scattering spectroscopy as a diagnostic tool for differentiating pathologies in the gastrointestinal tract. *J Biomed Opt* 1:192-199, 1996.
12. Roberts D, Hartov A, Kennedy F, Miga M, Paulsen K: Intraoperative brain shift and deformation: a quantitative analysis of cortical displacement in 28 cases. *Neurosurgery* 43:749-760, 1998.
13. Steinmeier R, Fahlbusch R, Ganslandt O, *et al*. Intraoperative magnetic resonance imaging with the Magnetom open scanner: concepts, neurosurgical indications, and procedures: a preliminary report. *Neurosurgery* 43:743-748, 1998.

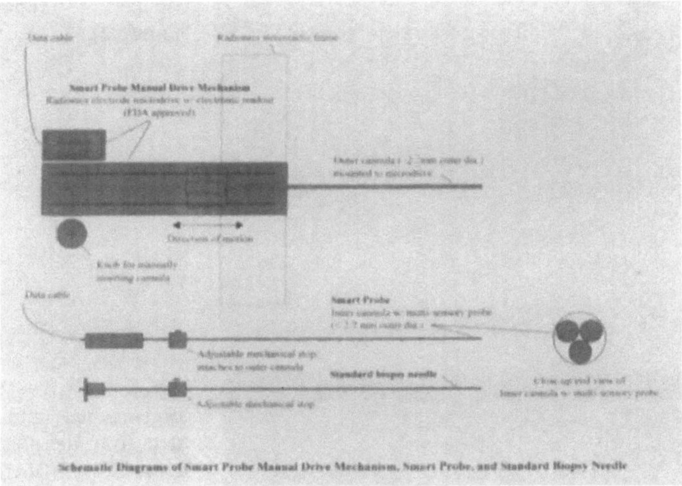

Figure 1. Schematic of Smart Probe for Neurosurgery: 3 microsensor clusters in 2.7 mm diameter cannula.

©CARS/Springer. All rights reserved.

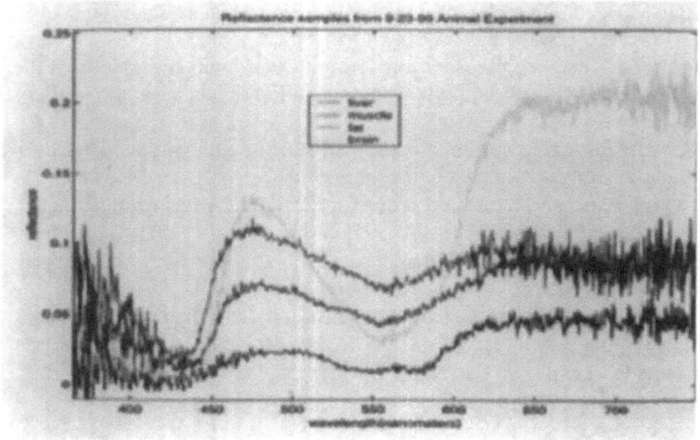

Figure 2. Optical Spectroscopy spectra (mean of ten recordings per tissue) for liver, muscle, fat, and brain. Note the clear differentiation of tissues over the 400 to 600 nm band.

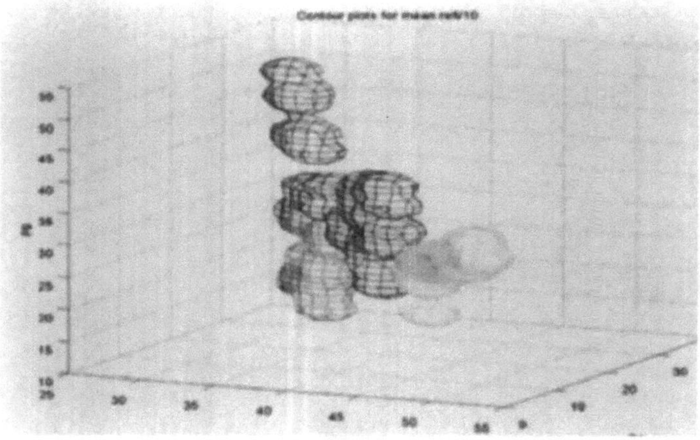

Figure 3. Three-dimensional plot of OS spectra from various tissues (compare Figure 2).

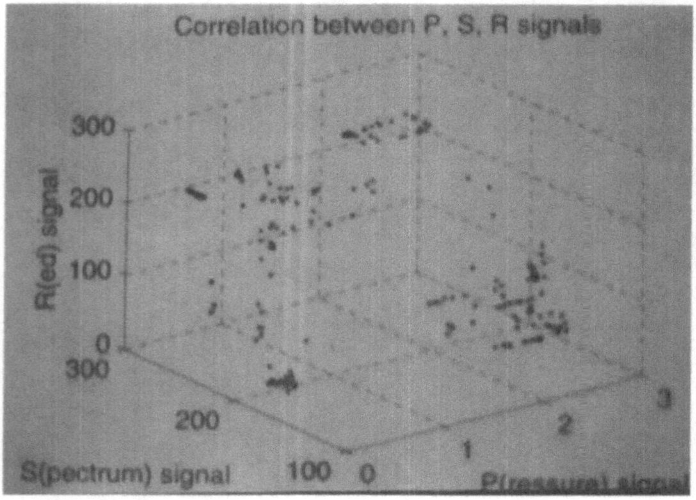

Figure 4. Three-dimensional plot of data from the pressure, color (fiberoptic neuroendo-scope – red), and optical spectroscopy sensors. Spatial separation is apparent.

CARS 2002 – H.U. Lemke, M.W. Vannier; K. Inamura, A.G. Farman, K. Doi & J.H.C. Reiber (Editors)
©CARS/Springer. All rights reserved.

The application accuracy of the NeuroMate robot - a quantitative comparison with frameless and frame-based surgical localization systems

Qing Hang Li, Lucía Zamorano, Abhilash Pandya, Jianxing Gong, and Fernando Diaz
Department of Neurological Surgery, Wayne State University, Detroit Medical Center, Detroit, Michigan 48201 USA.
qli@neurosurgery.wayne.edu

Abstract

The NeuroMate™ robot System ISS (Integrated Surgical Systems, Davis, CA) is an image-guided, robotic-assisted system for brain surgery, which is a commercially available system used today for stereotactic procedures in neurosurgery. In this paper we describe an accuracy studies for the NeuroMate system. We present a quantitative comparison of the application accuracy of the NeuroMate to standard frame based and frameless stereotactic techniques. The study discusses a five-way application accuracy comparison study. The variables of our comparison and their mean errors are: 1) In the robot in a frame-based configuration, the RMS was 0.86 ± 0.32mm; 2) In the robot in the frame-less configuration, the RMS was 1.95 ± 0.44mm; 3) In a Standard Stereotactic (ZD) frame-based approach, the RMS was 1.17 ± 0.25mm; 4) In an infrared tracking system (IR) using the frame for the fiducial registration, the RMS was 1.47 ± 0.45mm; 5) In an infrared tracking system using screw markers as the registration, the RMS was 0.68 ± 0.26mm. The study was done with 2mm sections of CT scans. These results showed that the application accuracy of the frame-based NeuroMate robot is comparable to standard localizing systems whether they are frame-base or infrared tracked.

Keywords: Application accuracy, robotics and robotic manipulators, tracking systems

1. Introduction

Medical robotic systems are beginning to have an increasing role in different image-guided surgical procedures. The key advantages are that robots can effectively position, orient and manipulate surgical tools in 3D space with a high level of accuracy. Several medical robots or robotic arms have been reported for clinical applications.[1-3] This paper presents the NeuroMate (Integrate Surgical Systems, Inc. Davis, CA, USA), an image-guided, computer controlled robotic system for brain surgery that has been specifically designed for surgical applications. [1] The NeuroMate™ includes a five-degree-of-freedom robotic arm assembly and a PC based kinematical positioning software system. The system software (VoXim™, IVS Software Engineering) allows precise image-based planning and visualization of multiple trajectories. During surgery, the system provides interactive 3-dimensional visualization of anatomical structures and brain targets as the various planned trajectories are achieved. The images used for visualization

©CARS/Springer. All rights reserved.

are derived from Computed Tomography (CT) or Magnetic Resonance Imaging (MRI) scans. The robot can be used either with a stereotactic frame or in a frameless mode.

Application accuracy of the techniques and technology being used for image guided surgical interventions is a very important clinical factor to be considered. The application accuracy of a surgical localization system is a function of its mechanical accuracy interacting with the selected parameters of the imaging studies chosen to visualize the lesion and its related anatomy. The overall accuracy of a system is a sum of the individual accuracy of each of these components.[4,5,7] The application accuracy is different from factory calibration (mechanical accuracy) in that it includes the compounded errors when used in a clinical setting. It includes errors like image errors, digitization errors, registration errors and computation errors. Hence, it is critical to evaluate these robots on how accurately and effectively they can position, orient and manipulate surgical tools in 3-dimentional space. The purpose of this study was to quantitatively determine the application accuracy of this system and compare it with commonly used frameless infrared and frame-based surgical localization systems.

2. Materials and Methods

In this section we will discuss a five-way application accuracy comparison study for the NeuroMate system. The variables of our comparison include 1) The robot in a frame-based configuration; 2) The robot in the frame-less configuration; 3) A Standard Stereotactic (ZD) frame-based approach; 4) An infrared tracking system (IR) using the frame for the fiducial registration; 5) An infrared tracking system using screw markers as the registration.

2.1 The application accuracy of the NeuroMate system

The purpose of this study was to quantitatively determine the application accuracy of the NeuroMate system (in both frame-based and frameless configurations) and compare it with, frameless infrared, frame-based infrared and frame-based surgical localization systems. For completeness, we also include the results that compare all five methods with every other method for localization. What follows are the details of the experimental setup for this study.

2.2. Phantom preparation

This five-way comparison was performed using a phantom. This phantom was mounted with five implantable frameless markers (Fischer-Leibinger, Freiburg, Germany) randomly distributed on the surface (which were used for infrared registration). It was also mounted with a ZD stereotactic ring (Fischer-Leibinger, Freiburg, Germany). In addition, a specially designed fixation device was mounted on the top of the phantom, which was used to mount the ultrasound markers for the NeuroMate system (Figure 1). A specially designed mechanical measuring device (Fischer-Leibinger, Freiburg, Germany) was also rigidly mounted to the phantom with a ZD ring and was used for very accurately measuring the location of the probe tips as placed by each of the frame based methods (Figure 2). This measurement device is a very accurate 3 dimensional ruler which allowed the measurement of points in space. For the actual comparison points, three semi-invasive screws markers were mounted into the phantom as target points in the frame less system.

CARS 2002 – H.U. Lemke, M.W. Vannier; K. Inamura, A.G. Farman, K. Doi & J.H.C. Reiber (Editors)
©CARS/Springer. All rights reserved.

The Phantom was imaged using a Siemens Somatom-Plus-S CT scanner (Siemens, Eriangen, Germany). Scan thickness was set at 2 mm and the image resolution used was pixel size 1.18 x 1.18 mm. The images were transferred to two stereotactic computers.

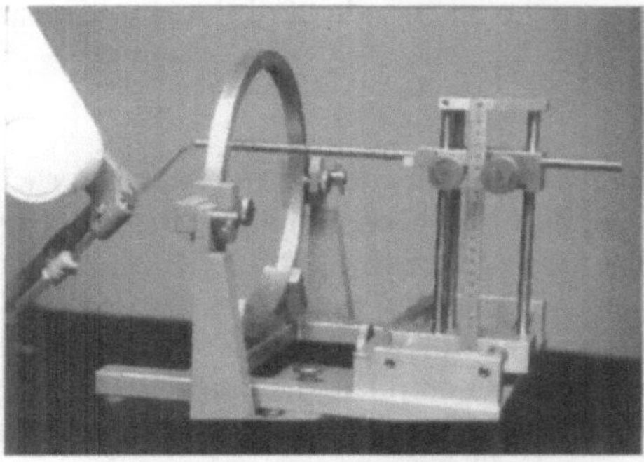

Figure 2. Mechanical measuring device.

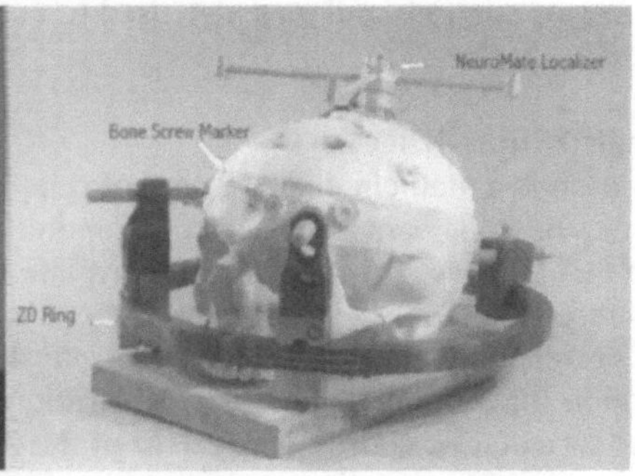

Figure 1. Phantom set-up

2.3 . Experimental procedure

For each system the repeatability and variability of the system were checked. The target point coordinates were accurately measured and compared with the corresponding reference points. The 10 selected measurement points represented a volumetric cube of 100mm within the phantom's 2mm (slice thickness) CT scan. A specially designed mechanical measuring device (Fischer-Leibinger, Freiburg, Germany) was used to determine the deviations from the target points for the frame-based methods. The root mean square (RMS) was calculated to show the differences between the actual points and the measured points for each of the 5 different methods of localization.

A systematic error analysis was performed by comparing the coordinates of target points on the medical images and the coordinates of digitized target points based on registration from each surgical localization system. Statistical analysis was performed on the experimental data. A comparison of the 3-D measurements (x, y, z) of the coordinates of the target point from each experimental data with the fiducial markers to absolute image coordinates was performed. There were repeated measurements for each experiment on each of the methods. This allowed for testing of internal consistency of the measurements for each method. Statistical analysis pertaining to various comparisons among methods was performed.

The mean deviation from the absolute image coordinates were calculated from all 3-D mean measurements (x, y, z) of all experimental data for each system. Also, the deviation from the target point in three directions of each experimental data between the various systems was calculated. Therefore, to assess differences between the systems per each of the x, y, and z measurements a root mean square (RMS) representing the sum of the vectors (representing the maximum distance between the coordinates) of the reference point and the coordinates of the digitized point was calculated. For each group of data, it was calculated as follows:

©CARS/Springer. All rights reserved.

$$\text{distance}_{ijk} = \text{SQRT}\left((X_{ij}-X_{ik})^2 + (Y_{ij}-Y_{ik})^2 + (Z_{ij}-Z_{ik})^2\right)$$
where j,k= 1,2,3.

A paired t-test was applied to test for the significance of the mean deviation among the five different methods and was also used to compare the magnitude of difference of mean distances.

2.4. Registration procedures

Registration is a mathematical process of relating two different coordinate systems to each other by selecting common specially marked points in both coordinate systems. This method can be used, for instance, to correlate the image space (CT, MR, PET etc.) to the patient reference frame. Coordinate matching ensures that any point seen in a medical image corresponds to an actual point in the real world. There were two steps of registration for this study. The first registration step was to correlate the image space (CT) with the stereotactic coordinate system of the ZD frame. The next step was to register the newly formed ZD coordinates of the image to the coordinates of the patient (phantom) using common points between these two coordinate systems. The goals were to match and correlated data from the medical images to the 'real world' (the coordinate space of the surgical instruments).

The Neurosurgical Planning System (NSPS), software developed at Wayne State University, was used for image registration [6]. The NSPS executes on a SUN ULTRASPARC 60 station (Sun Microsystems, Mountain View, California), and was used to achieve fast calculations and to reconstruct volumes from imaging studies. The workstation was connected to the Detroit Medical Center's central computer network, from which images derived from CT and MRI can be transferred. It allows image viewing and manipulation in real-time during preplanning and phantom testing. The coordinates of the target points were recorded and saved into a file as reference points. VoXim Robotic software used to do the registration for the robot executes on a Compaq PC with Window NT (550mHz, 256Mb).

2.5. Tracking technology for registration

There are several methods to capture the common points needed for registration. The two methods used in this study were infrared and ultrasound.

1) Infrared System Registration. The FlashPoint infrared tracking system (FlashPoint Model 5000, Image Guided Surgery Technology Inc. Boulder, CO 80301, USA) was used for this study. Three high-resolution linear infrared sensors are used to measure the location in space of infrared light emitting diodes (LED). The X-Y-Z location of a given point can be determined with the data returned from all of the sensors [8]. For this experiment a contact-style probe with three LEDs was used to take precise and accurate measurements from the objects of interest.

Three infrared sensors track target points defined by several miniature LEDs mounted on the surgeon's operative instrument, which were mounted in a predefined relationship. This combination is referred to as a "surgical rigid body or pointer". Another similar rigid body is mounted to the head holder or patient's ring (patient's rigid body). The patient's “rigid

©CARS/Springer. All rights reserved.

body" is used to tell the system where the real patient is, and the surgical rigid body tells the system the position of the surgical instrument.

2) Ultrasound Registration. For the frameless robotic system, an ultrasound system was used to capture the required common points for registration. For the frame-based procedure, there is no need for registration because the NeuroMate hardware is already setup and calibrated within the ZD ring coordinate system. For the frameless procedure, an ultrasound probe was used to determine the position of fiducial markers on the phantom. The frame-less localizing unit features an implantable base that allows insertion of a helicopter-shaped ultrasonic localizing device and corresponding CT and MRI localizers. The localizer used in the image-space provides markers (which can be clearly identified in the image) that define the points of commonality between the image and the real space. These markers are first located and digitized in the image using the Voxim software. In the intraoperative situation, an identical ultrasound localizer system is used to capture the points in real space. The ultrasound receiver and transmitter system mounted on the robot and patient capture the same points as was marked in the image space. The ultrasound system collects position data from which the system can compute the patient registration parameters. After the capture process, a registration is done to match the image space with the patient space.

3. Results:

In order to determine whether the NeuroMate™ is accurate enough for clinical application, three commonly used stereotactic localization systems (ZD stereotactic ring, infrared tracking system registered with bone screw markers and with ZD ring) were used to carry out a quantitative comparison. Application accuracy of the various methods of localization were tested and measured with the methods described in the methods section. The Infrared bone (screw) marker condition had the lowest mean error (0.68) with the frame-based robot at a close second (0.86mm), however, the t-test result indicated that there was no significant difference between them. The robotic frameless option had the highest error (1.95mm). The t-test results showed that there was a significant difference between the frame-based robotic system and the frame-less robotic system ($p<0.001$). Our results indicate that the frame-based robotic system has the same level of the application accuracy as the best standard surgical localization system (bone screw markers using infrared tracking). In order to check whether different arm position of NeuroMate™ influence the application, two different arm positions were used for each target. A paired t-test was used to compare the results. There was no significant difference.

4. Conclusions

This preliminary study demonstrates that

1) The application accuracy of the frame-based NeuroMate™ robotic system is comparable to other commonly used surgical localization system. The frame-based NeuroMate™ is statistically better than frame-based infrared. But there is no difference between the frame-based NeuroMate™, the ZD frame and the infrared tracking system with bone screw markers.

©CARS/Springer. All rights reserved.

2) There is a significant difference between the NeuroMate™ frame based and frameless registration. Although the manufacturer reports the ultrasound accuracy (the measurement of transducer to receiver distance determination) to be 0.2 mm, this is only in the ideal case. In our study, our positioning of the ultrasound device was setup as it would be in the OR environment. The external noise and non-ideal position that can be expected in normal operations results in significantly more error. This indicated that the ultrasound tracking technique may need to be further improved.

Medical robotics brings a new revolution in this traditional field. The purpose is not to replace the surgeon but to augment his skills, improve patient safety and reduce the cost. Further studies are needed to quantitatively determine the feasibility of robotic systems to safely assist in surgical procedures. We believe that further development of the software and hardware of NeuroMate™ system along with better ergonomics will improve its usability and clinical application. Future potential developments include robotic drawing of optimized craniotomy and robotic augmentation.

Acknowledgements

This work is partially funded by NASA Grant 99-HEDS-01-079.
Patrick Pittet, M.S., Fernand Badano, Ph.D,Vincent Robert, M.S. (Intergrated Surgical System, Inc. France) for hardware and technical support.
Joerg Fischer, IVS Solutions- for robotic software supports.

References

1. Benabid AL, Lavallée S, Hoffman D, Cinquin P, Demongeot J, Danel F : Computer-driven robot for stereotactic neurosurgery : Computer in strereotactic neurosurgery , Kelly and Kall Eds, Blackwell Scientific publication, Cambridge, 1992
2. Damiano RJ Jr, Ehrman WJ, Ducko CT, Tabaie HA, Stephenson ER Jr, Kingsley CP, Chambers CE.: Initial United States clinical trial of robotically assisted endoscopic coronary artery bypass grafting. *J Thorac Cardiovasc Surg* 2000 Jan;119(1):77-82.
3. DiGioia AM 3rd, Jaramaz B, Colgan BD.: Computer assisted orthopaedic surgery. Image gided and robotic assistive technologies. *Clin Orthop* 1998 Sep;(354):8-16.
4. Li, Q, Zamorano L, Jiang Z, F., Diaz F: The Application Accuracy of the Frameless Implantable Marker System and Analysis of Relating Affecting Factors: Lecture Notes in Computer Science 1496. Eds by William M. Wells, Alan Cohchester and Scott Delp, page 253-260, 1998.
5. Li, Q, Zamorano L, Jiang Z, Gong J, Pandya A, Perez R, Diaz F: Effect of Optical Digitizer Selection on the Application accuracy of a Surgical Localization System A Quantitative Comparison between the OPTOTRAK and FlashPoint Tracking Systems: Computer Aided Surgery 4:314-321. 1999.
6. Zamorano L, Nolte L, Jiang C, Kadi M.: Image-guided neurosurgery: Frame based versus frameless approaches. Neurosurgical Operative Atlas 3: 402-422, 1993.
7. Maciunas R, Galloway R, Latimer J: The Application Accuracy of Stereotactic Frames: Neurosurgery, Vol. 35, No. 4 – October 1994.

Robotics and Telesurgery

CARS 2002 – H.U. Lemke, M.W. Vannier; K. Inamura, A.G. Farman, K. Doi & J.H.C. Reiber (Editors)
©CARS/Springer. All rights reserved.

Interactive robots for medical applications

Jocelyne Troccaz, Peter Berkelman, Philippe Cinquin, Adriana Vilchis-Gonzales
TIMC/IMAG Laboratory
Faculté de Médecine - Domaine de la Merci - 38706 La Tronche cedex - France
jocelyne.troccaz@imag.fr

Abstract

Over the last two decades, medical robotics has evolved from the adaptation of industrial robots to medical tasks to a specific domain of robotics requiring the development of innovative architectures and control modes. In particular, robots enabling cooperation with the physician are being developed. We name them interactive robots. In this paper, we will present three examples of such robots: PADyC is a passive system which constrains the motions of the surgical tool held by the clinical operator in function of the surgical task; TER and PER which are two low weight, compliant robots respectively dedicated to tele-echography and endoscopy.

Keywords: Robotics, man/machine cooperation, computer-aided medical interventions

1. Introduction

Classical taxonomies in medical robotics distinguish three categories of guiding systems for computer-aided surgery: active, passive and semi-active systems. In this division, the degree of passivity corresponds to the type of interaction between the human and the device.

- Passive systems such as [1,2] display information to the surgeon about the position of the surgical tool relative to anatomical data or to a pre-planned strategy. The surgeon is totally responsible for the execution of the surgical action.
- Active systems realize a part of the intervention autonomously. A robot may machine a bone, or hold a sensor or a surgical tool without the need for interaction with a human operator who generally supervises the action. See for instance [3].
- A semi-active system involves a combined action with the human operator for the complete realization of the task. A mechanical guide brought in position by a robot [4] or manually [5] may align a linear drilling trajectory that the surgeon will execute. This type of systems allows an ergonomic, direct and accurate transfer of the surgical planning to the operating site. Nevertheless, they are restricted to rather elementary tasks such as linear motions and planar cuts. Moreover, this transfer is implemented using task-specific hardware; this hardware may be considered as the implementation of a *mechanical constraint.*

Two other types of systems have been introduced more recently :

- *Synergistic systems* are intended for direct physical guidance of a surgical tool, a tool that is also held and controlled directly by a surgeon [6]. The concrete objective is to build general-purpose mechanical devices to be held by the surgeon's hand which allow him to feel the virtual world of patient data (including safety regions around

©CARS/Springer. All rights reserved.

anatomical obstacles to be avoided) and of surgical strategies, while moving in the real world. This is a generalization of semi-active systems which allows to make mechanical constraints not limited to simple mathematical objects and programmable.

- *Tele-robotic systems* for which the surgeon remotely controls a surgical tool held by a robot (see for instance [7]) are also somewhat difficult to classify in the three categories listed below since the master and slave manipulators involve different types of interaction.

Since our goal is to develop robotic systems which enable tight cooperation between man and machine, we focused on the three types of systems allowing this cooperation, namely semi-active, synergistic and tele-operated robots and we will call them in the following *interactive robots*. In this paper, examples of interactive robots developed in the TIMC laboratory are presented.

2. PADyC: a passive arm with dynamic constraints

2.1 Basic principle of synergy

Both the surgeon and the synergistic device hold the tool, apply forces to it and to each other, and impart motions. Under computer control, the synergistic device may allow the surgeon to have control of some degrees of freedom (DOF) while the device controls the others. The system filters the motions proposed by the surgeon to keep only those which are compatible with the surgical plan. For instance, during the pre-planning stage, an orthopaedic surgeon selects a cutting plane for machining a bone before placing a knee prosthesis. In such a case, the synergistic system guarantees that the motions of the cutting tool are strictly limited to the pre-planned plane while the surgeon is in charge of the selection of the motions within the plane. There exist several implementations of this approach. The different technologies allow to feel different types of constraints: viscous constraints for programmable brakes, rigid constraints for systems based on mechanical constraints (PADyC, Cobot [8]), visco-elastic constraints for actuated systems such as ACRobot [9].

2.2 PADyC principle

The actuation of PADyC comes exclusively from a human operator. Meanwhile, in order to help the operator in the execution of a pre-planned strategy, each joint may turn only at an angular velocity which falls between the limits established by two reference clutch plates. The angular velocities of these two reference plates are controlled by a computer. An overrunning clutch offers no restriction when a joint is turning slower than the reference plate of the clutch, but limits the angular velocity of the joint to the speed of the reference plate. The control of PADyC basically consists in determining, at each instant, the vector of dynamic constraints - i.e. angular velocity windows - that guarantees that the configuration of the arm will be compatible with the task and more, will help its completion. For example, when the task is to stay inside an authorized region and the current configuration is far from the limits of the region, the angular velocity windows of all joints are set wide open, and the device allows unrestricted freedom of motion naturally. As a constraint surface is approached, however, the angular velocity windows are made narrower in some directions, such that, ultimately, the only velocities available

©CARS/Springer. All rights reserved.

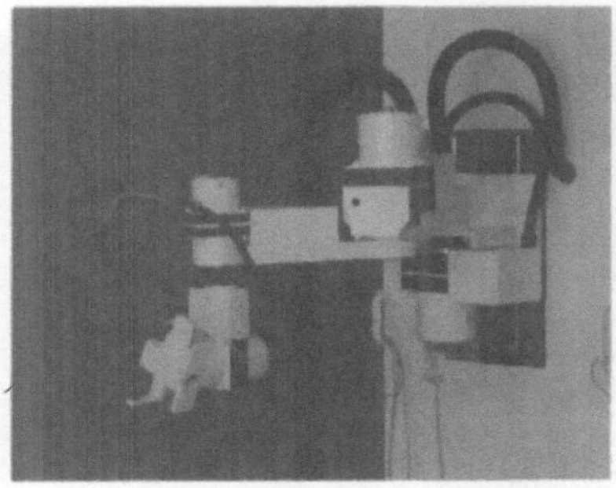

Fig. 1: PADyC : 6 DOF prototype for computer-aided pericardial puncture.

to each joint are the one which move the device away from, or parallel to the constraint surface. The system is kept in stable position when un-powered. PADyC allows to execute "free", "position", "trajectories" and "region" tasks smoothly and without friction. Experiments on prototypes were very promising [10]. A 6 dof PADyC (see figure 1) for computer-aided puncture of the heart is under development [11].

3. TER: a robot for tele-echography

3.1 TER objectives

Among many types of medical equipment, ultrasound diagnostic systems are widely used because of their convenience and safety. Performing an ultrasound examination involves good eye-hand coordination and the ability to integrate the acquired information over time and space; the physician has to be able to mentally build 3D information from both the 2D images and the gesture information and to put a diagnosis from these information. Some of these specialized skills may lack in some healthcare centres or for emergency situations. Tele-consultation is therefore an interesting alternative to conventional care. Development of a high performance remote diagnostic system, which enables an expert operator at the hospital to examine a patient at home, in an emergency vehicle or in a remote clinic, may have a very significant added value. Several robot-based echography projects have been launched worldwide (see [12,13] for instance).

3.2 TER principle

The tele-operated TER system [14] allows the expert physician to move by hand a virtual probe in a natural and unconstrained way and safely reproduces this motion on the distant robotic site where the patient is. The physician located in the master site moves the virtual probe placed on a haptic device to control the real echographic probe placed on the slave robot. The slave robot (see figure 2) is a parallel uncoupled one. It includes two independent parallel structures having two independent groups of pneumatic artificial muscle actuators. Thin and flexible cables are used to position and orient the echographic probe. The cables are connected to the pneumatic artificial muscles. The haptic control station in the master site is developed to give a realistic environment of what remotely occurs. It integrates a PHANToM device (from SensAble Device Inc) which has 6 DOFs and renders 3D-force information to the expert operator [15]. The obtained ultrasound image is continuously sent from the slave site to the operator that has to perform the examination and to provide a diagnosis. A non-expert operator is located close to the patient and supervises the procedure that he can interrupt in an emergency case. The patient can at all times communicate with the operator or with the expert. Two IDSN 128kb/s connections are used; one is for the Visio-phonic data and echographic images and the other one is for the transmission of the control information for the slave-robot.

©CARS/Springer. All rights reserved.

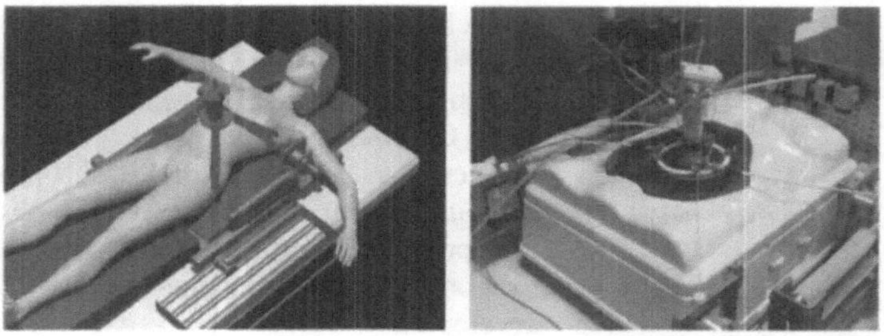

Fig. 2 The TER slave robot (left: general sketch - right: prototype used with a phantom)

Experiments have been performed with an echographic phantom. The objective of the test consisted in identifying the internal structures and in following them like in a real examination. The phantom was unknown to the medical experts. Experiments demonstrated that the use of the TER system is very intuitive; there is a short adaptation time of 5 to 10 minutes necessary to the medical expert to feel comfortable when moving the virtual probe using the haptic device. The quality of images and robot controllability are considered as good. The medical experts were able to recognize the internal structures of the echographic phantom and to follow them. Clinical validation is the next stage of this project.

4. PER: a robot for endoscopy

4.1 PER objectives

In conventional minimally invasive surgery, surgeons operate with long, thin instruments through 'keyhole' incisions approximately 10 mm in diameter in the abdomen of the patient. An endoscope, a thin optical tube which is inserted through one of the incisions and connected to an external video camera, is used to visualise the internal organ structures and instrument tips. The endoscope video camera image is displayed on a monitor during surgery. Since a single surgeon generally has both hands occupied with surgical instruments (for example, one for grasping and one for cutting), an assistant is necessary simply to hold the endoscope steady in a desired position. For practical use in an operating room environment, the endoscope manipulator must be unobtrusive, safe, simple to set up and use, and easily sterilizable. Several robot systems such as [16,17] have previously been developed for laparoscopic endoscope manipulation during surgery. Commercially available robotic surgical endoscope manipulators are included in the Da Vinci™ [7] system from Intuitive Surgical Systems and Aesop™ [17] and Zeus™ from Computer Motion. These manipulators are typically elements of large, heavy, complex and expensive systems and resemble conventional industrial robot manipulators. We have taken a simple, lightweight, low cost approach instead.

4.2 PER principles

Our current endoscope manipulator prototype is pictured in figure 3 attached to a training model abdomen. Thin, flexible cables are used to position and orient the endoscope. The cables are connected through flexible sleeves to pneumatic artificial muscle actuators as the ones used for the TER robot. This means of actuation is simple, lightweight, and has

©CARS/Springer. All rights reserved.

the added benefit of passive compliance. The positioning mechanism is fixed to the endoscope and strapped to the patient at the incision location, so no rigid base is necessary and the manipulator moves with the patient during breathing, repositioning by the surgeon, motions of other instruments, or any other displacement of the abdomen wall.

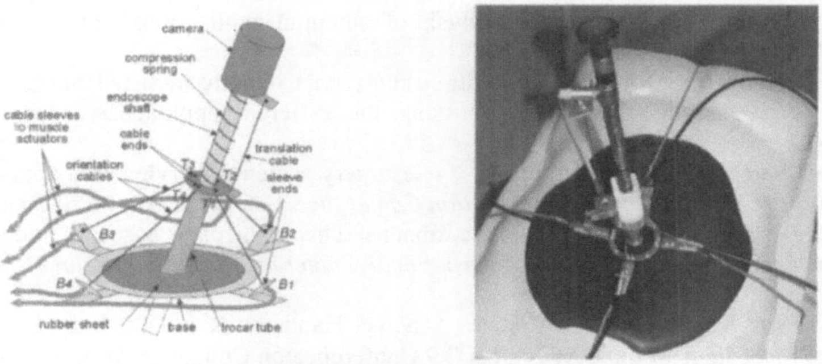

Fig. 3 The PER system: principle and prototype

The endoscope manipulator has been demonstrated with a simulated abdomen and good experimental performance results were obtained [18]. We plan to proceed towards clinical testing and validation, progressing from the current simulated abdomen to animal models.

5. Conclusion

Medico-surgical robotics requires the development of systems enabling a natural interaction with the clinician. Guiding systems including interactive robots take the best advantage of (1) the robot and its computer-based model of the surgical action, and (2) the surgeon and his knowledge, know-how, sensing capabilities and ability to react to unexpected or non-modeled events. In this paper, we have presented work in progress in the TIMC laboratory concerning this domain.

Acknowledgements

These projects are supported by the French Ministry or Research and Technology, ANVAR, France Telecom R&D.

References

1. Mosges R. et al. Computer assisted surgery. an innovative surgical technique in clinical routine. In *Computer Assisted Radiology, CAR 89*, pp. 413-415, H.U. Lemke, editor, Springer-Verlag, 1989
2. Lavallée S., Sautot P., Troccaz J., Cinquin P. and Merloz P. Computer Assisted Spine Surgery: a technique for accurate transpedicular screw fixation using CT data and a 3D optical localizer. In *Proceedings of the First International Symposium on Medical Robotics and Computer Assisted Surgery (MRCAS'94)*, pp 315-322, Pittsburgh, 1994

©CARS/Springer. All rights reserved.

3. Paul H., Bargar W., Mittlestadt B., Musit B., Taylor R., Kazanzides P., Williamson B., Hanson W.. Development of a surgical robot for cementless total hip arthroplasty. In *Clinical Orthopaedics and related research*, (285) :57-66, December 1992
4. Lavallée S., et al. Image guided robot: a clinical application in stereotactic neurosurgery. In *IEEE Int. Conf. on Robotics and Automation*, pp. 618-625, Nice, 1992
5. Radermacher K., Staudte H.W. and Rau G. "Computer assisted orthopaedic surgery by means of individual templates - aspects and analysis of potential applications". In Proceedings of MRCAS'94, pp 42-48, Pittsburgh
6. Troccaz J., Peshkin M., Davies B. Guiding systems for Computer-assisted Surgery (CAS) : introducing synergistic devices and discussing the different approaches. Medical Image Analysis, 2(2), pp101-119, 1998
7. Guthart G.S., Salisbury J.K. The Intuitive™ telesurgery system: overview and application. In *Proceedings of IEEE Robotics and Automation Conference*, San Francisco, Avril 2000
8. Colgate J.E., Peshkin M., Moore C.. Passive robots and haptic displays based on nonholonomic elements. In *Proceedings of the IEEE International Conference on Robotics and Automation*, 1996
9. Davies B., Harris S., Jakopec M., Cobb J. A Novel Hands-on Robot for Knee Replacement Surgery. In Proceedings of the CAOS USA '99 Conference on Computer Assisted Orthopaedic Surgery, pp 70-74, UPMC, Shadyside Hospital, Penn. USA June 1999
10. Troccaz J., Delnondedieu Y. Semi-active guiding systems in surgery. A two-dof prototype of the passive arm with dynamic constraints (PADyC). Mechatronics, 6(4):399--421, June 1996
11. Schneider O., Troccaz J. A Six Degree of Freedom Passive Arm with Dynamic Constraints (PADyC) for Cardiac Surgery Application: Preliminary Experiments Computer-Aided Surgery, Special issue on medical robotics, Ed. K. Cleary, to appear, 2002
12. S. Salcudean, G. Bell, S. Bachmann, W.H. Zhu, P Abolmaesumi and P.D. Lawrence (1999). Robot-assisted diagnostic ultrasound-design and feasibility experiments. *Lecture Notes in Computer Science. Medical Image Computing and Computer-Assisted Intervention* (MICCAI'99). pp. 1062-1071
13. K. Masuda, E. Kimura, N. Tateishi and K. Ishihara. Three dimensional motion mechanism of ultrasound probe and its application for tele-echography system. *Proceedings of the IEEE/RSJ International Conference on Intelligent Robots and Systems*. Maui, Hawaii, USA, Oct 29-Nov 03 2001. pp 1112-1116.
14. A. Vilchis et al. "TER: a system for Robotic Tele-echography". *Fourth International Conference on Medical Image Computing and Computer Assisted Intervention,* Utrecht, the Netherlands 14-17 October 2001, pp 326-334.
15. A. Guerraz, A. Vilchis, J. Troccaz, P. Cinquin, B. Hennion, Franck Pellisier and Pierre Thorel, "A Haptic Virtual Environment for tele-Echography". *10th Annual Medicine Meets Virtual Reality Conference*, Newport California January 23-26 2002.
16. Taylor R.H., et al. Telerobotic assistant for laparoscopic surgery. In Computer Integrated Surgery: Technology and Clinical Applications, (Taylor, Lavallée, Burdea, Mosges, Eds.), pp581-592, MIT Press, 1995
17. Sackier J.M., Wang Y. Robotically assisted laparoscopic surgery: from concept to development. In Computer Integrated Surgery: Technology and Clinical Applications, (Taylor, Lavallée, Burdea, Mosges, Eds.), pp577-580, MIT Press, 1995
18. Berkelman P., Cinquin P., Troccaz J., Ayoubi J.M., Letoublon C., Bouchard F. A Compact, Compliant Laparoscopic Endoscope Manipulator, Proceedings of the IEEE Conference on Robotics and Automation, 2002

Surgical Robotics and Instrumentation

CARS 2002 – H.U. Lemke, M.W. Vannier; K. Inamura, A.G. Farman, K. Doi & J.H.C. Reiber (Editors)
©CARS/Springer. All rights reserved.

A dual-view endoscope with image shift

Y. Yamauchi [a], J. Yamashita [a], Y. Fukui [a,b], K. Yokoyama [c], T. Sekiya [d], E. Ito [d], M. Kanai [d], T. Fukuyo [e], D. Hashimoto [f], H. Iseki [g] and K. Takakura [g]
[a] National Institute of Advanced Industrial Science and Technology (AIST), Tsukuba Central 6, Tsukuba 3058566 Japan, y.yamauchi@aist.go.jp
[b] Institute of Information Sciences and Electronics, University of Tsukuba, Tsukuba, Japan
[c] ENT Clinic @ Tsukuba South Avenue, Tsukuba, Japan
[d] Research & Development Center, Asahi Optical Co., Ltd., Tokyo, Japan
[e] Shinko Optical, Tokyo, Japan
[f] Saitama Medical Center, Saitama Medical School, Kawagoe, Japan
[g] Dept. of Neurosurgery, Tokyo Women's Medical University, Tokyo, Japan

Abstract

We present a new endoscopic system that provides two different views simultaneously, one is a wide view (120 degrees) and the other is a zoomed view with image-shift mechanism. A Porro prism (II) is used to shift the zoomed image vertically and horizontally. With this endoscope, surgeons can observe throughout the surgical field without moving or rotating the endoscope itself. We have evaluated and confirmed the operationality and image quality of the endoscope by an in-vivo experiment on two pigs.

Keywords: dual-view endoscope, image shift, Porro prism (II)

1. Purpose

Endoscopic surgery is becoming popular in neurosurgery and general surgery. One of the most important points in endoscopic surgery is the smooth, adequate and safe manipulation (moving and zooming) of the endoscope to acquire the best view.
We have developed a new type of rigid endoscope with following features: a) moving the field of view (FOV) without moving or bending the endoscope itself ("image-shift mechanism"), and b) simultaneous display of both wide and zoomed views ("dual-view mechanism").

The wide view continuously provides the extensive observation of the surgical field, and the zoomed view is focused on the point of the surgical operation.
Safety issue is very important in designing endoscopic systems. Many researchers have developed and evaluated robotic systems for endoscopic operations [1-3]. Although they achieve the safety by the virtue of the software or mechanism, the potential risk is not low as long as the systems has some moving parts. Therefore, non-robotic endoscopes as our system achieve intrinsic safety, avoiding the accidental hitting. OR-time can be shortened because the set-up time is potentially less than that of robotic systems.

©CARS/Springer. All rights reserved.

2. Methods

At present, our endoscopic system is designed for a laparoscopic surgery. It consists of a lens tube attached to an optical unit outside the body (Fig. 1). As other rigid laparoscopes, the lens tube is a straight-view scope with an objective lens, a series of rod lenses and a set of fibre bundles to transmit light inside. The diameter of the lens tube is 10 mm and the length is 360 mm. Whole of the FOV of the objective lens (120 degrees) is illuminated almost uniformly. The "Fogless" technology designed by Shinko Optical prevents the objective lens from fogging that leads to low visibility.

The optical unit consists of an image-shift system, two mirrors, a relay lens and a zoom lens with a zoom ratio of 3 times (Fig. 2). Color CCD cameras are attached to the relay lens and the zoom lens. The whole size of the optical unit is 40 mm by 50 mm by 176 mm, and it weights about 500 grams. It realizes two novel mechanisms as follows:

a) Image-shift mechanism

The “image-shift” is to move the zoomed view without moving the endoscope itself. There are two types of endoscopic systems that alter the FOV. One is to electrically or optically trim the FOV, and the other uses wedge prisms [4]. In the former systems, the displacement of the FOV is quite limited. The latter, although it is a very smart system, cannot coexist with the dual-view mechanism, because prisms are set in front of the objective lens.

We use a Porro prism (II) as the image-shift system (Fig. 3). A Porro prism (II) is commonly used in binoculars to invert image. The prism situated just behind the lens tube, can be manually moved vertically and horizontally (perpendicular to the optical axis) by rotating two screws. The zoom lens is laid behind the prism, and thus its FOV moves in conjunction with the prism. Displacement of the prism in 1 mm causes the movement of FOV in 60 degrees. The range of the movement of FOV is 120 degrees vertically and horizontally.

b) Dual-view mechanism

The “dual-view” is to observe both the wide view and the zoomed view at a time. One common solution is to magnify a part of the FOV by image processing, but rack of spatial resolution is inevitable. Another solution is to bundle two lens tubes for the wide view and for the zoomed view. Technically it is difficult to attenuate the entire diameter of the tubes less than 10 mm.

In our system we split the image from the lens tubes at the image-shift system. The first reflective surface of the Porro prism is used as a beam splitter. About half of the light passes through the reflective surface to the first mirror, while the rest is transmitted through the prism, shifted and zoomed in the zoom lens. The maximum magnification of zooming is 10 times on a 20-inch monitor (70mm in object distance).

©CARS/Springer. All rights reserved.

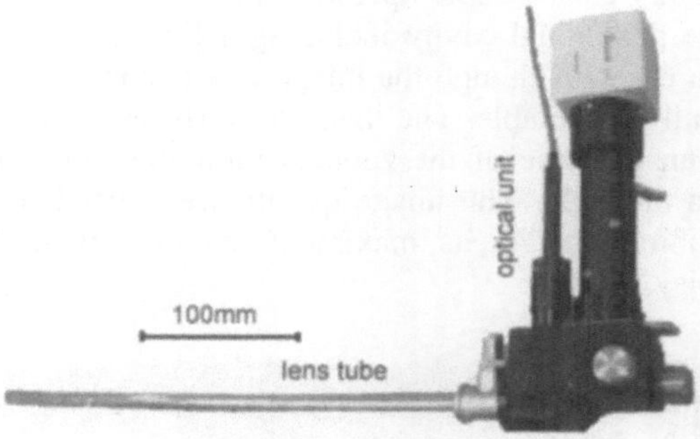

Figure 1. Dual-view endoscope. The optical unit is attached to the lens tube perpendicularly, to avoid interfering with the surgeon's operation.

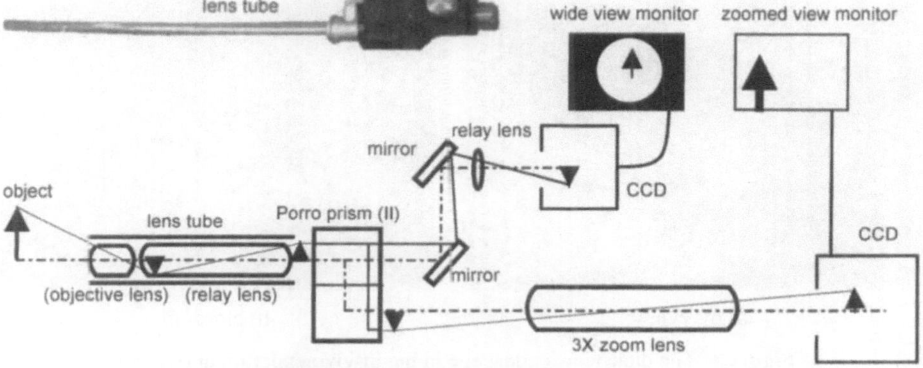

Figure 2. Optical system in the dual-view endoscope.

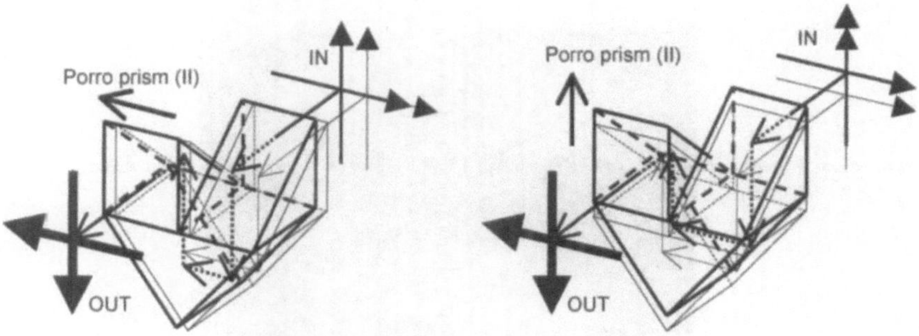

Figure 3. Image-shift mechanism by a Porro prism (II). The FOV of the endoscope shifts horizontally (*left*) and vertically (*right*) according to the displacement of the prism.

3. Results

We performed an in vivo laparoscopic observation on two anesthetized pigs, to evaluate the dual-view, image-shift mechanisms and its image quality. The abdominal walls of both pigs were lifted, one was with gasless (subcutaneous wiring) method and the other was with pneumoperitoneum. The endoscope was mounted and fixed at the end of the surgical bed, then was inserted through a trocar to observe inside (Fig. 4). The setup-time

©CARS/Springer. All rights reserved.

of the endoscope was as short as the ordinary laparoscopic operations. Figure 5 shows an example of the wide view. Whole of the abdominal cavity including a liver and a gall bladder was sufficiently observed in both cases. Although the image was distorted at the periphery of the wide view, it was clinically acceptable. The light was distributed almost uniformly to the view. Figure 6 shows an example of the zoomed view that smoothly moved from the left edge of the liver to the right. The image quality was sufficient to operate forceps, at medium magnification ratio. At its maximum magnification, the brightness was low and the image was noisy, though.

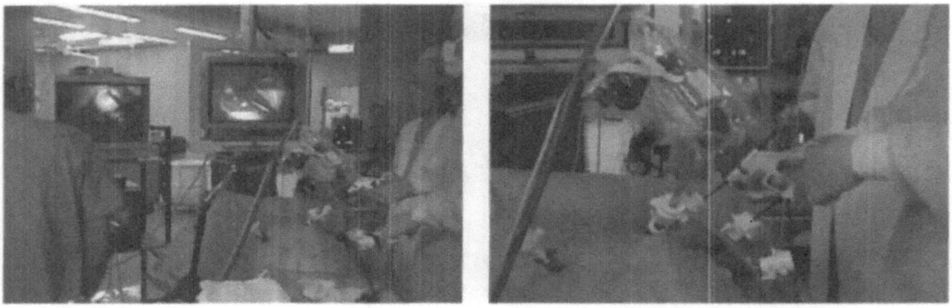

a) overview b) close-up

Figure 4. The dual-view endoscope in the in-vivo experiment of a pig.
a) Both the wide (*right*) and zoomed (*left*) views are displayed at a time.
b) The endoscope is fixed, and the surgeon does not need to move or rotate it.

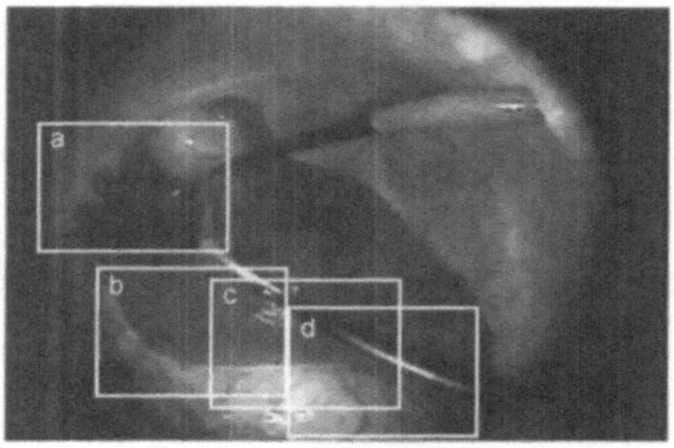

Figure 5. Wide view (120 deg.) in the pig's abdomen.
Forceps, liver and gallbladder can be observed in one scene.

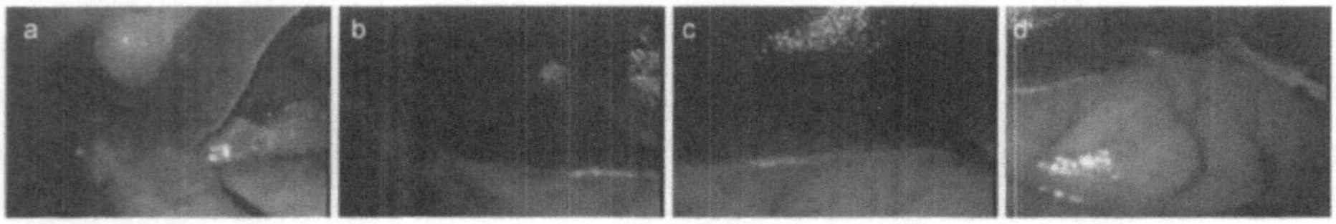

Figure 6. Zoomed view in figure 5's scene, shifted from left to right.

©CARS/Springer. All rights reserved.

4. Conclusion

This paper presented an improved endoscopic system with dual-view and image-shift mechanisms. In vivo experiment confirmed the performance of the proposed system. Future work includes 1) image quality of the zoomed view, that should be solved by the optimization of the whole optical system and 2) surgeon interface to move the zoomed view, which is also important in the field of robotic surgery.

Acknowledgements

This is a part of "Advanced Support System for Endoscopic and Other Minimally Invasive Surgery" project of the New Energy and Industrial Technology Development Organization (NEDO) for 2000-2004.

References

1. M. E. Allaf, S. V. Jackman, P. G. Schulam, J. A. Cadeddu, B. R. Lee, R. G. Moore and L. R. Kavoussi. "Laparoscopic visual field. Voice vs foot pedal interfaces for control of the AESOP robot", *Surg Endosc*, Vol. 12, No. 12, pp. 1415-1418, 1998.
2. B. Poulose, M. Kutka, M. Mendoza-Sagaon, A. Barnes, C. Yang, R. Taylor and M. Talamini. "Human Versus Robotic Organ Retraction During Laparoscopic Nissen Fundoplication", *MICCAI'98*, W. C. Delp, Lecture Notes in Computer Science Vol. 1496, pp. 197-206, Springer-Verlag, Berlin, 1998
3. M. Tomikawa, E. Kobayashi, F. Nakamura, I. Sakuma, M. Hashizume, M. Shimada, N. Gotoh, K. Konishi, T. Dohi and K. Sugimachi. "Usefulness of a newly-developed laparoscope manipulator during laparoscopic splenectomy", *CARS 2001*, H. U. Lemke et al., International Congress Series Vol. 1230, p.1164, Elsevier Science B. V., Amsterdam, 2001
4. E. Kobayashi, K. Daeyong, I. Sakuma and T. Dohi. "A new wide-angle view endoscopic robot using wedge prisms", *CARS 2001*, H. U. Lemke et al., International Congress Series Vol. 1230, pp.150-153, Elsevier Science B. V., Amsterdam, 2001

©CARS/Springer. All rights reserved.

Head tracking of a surgical robotic scopeholder - a user involvement test of the system

O.J. Elle[a], M.G. Gulbrandsen[a], E. Samset[a], G. ten Cate[a], L. Aurdal[a], A. Austad[b], T.K. Lien[c] , E. Fosse[a].
[a] Interventional Centre, National Hospital of Norway
[b] Dept. of Eng. Cybern., Norwegian University of Science and Technology
[c] Dept. of Prod. and Qual.Eng., Norwegian University of Science and Technology

Abstract

This paper addresses the concept, development and testing of a new head-tracking system and a user involvement test for comparison between the proposed system and two other control techniques to control the scope - either voice control of Aesop from ComputerMotion (ComputerMotion Inc., Goleta, California) or HeadControl of EndoAssist from Armstrong (Armstrong Healthcare Limited, High Wycombe, England). The average time to complete the task using HeadTracking in both 3D and 2D -mode was shorter than the times for the two other control modes. The average task time using HeadTracking were 39,9% shorter, using 3D with head-mounted display (HMD) and 54,1% using 2D screen compared to HeadControl with EndoAssist. These results were found to be statistical significant ($p<0.05$). In order for robotic devices to be introduced successfully into surgical practice, the development of transparent surgeon/machine interface is critical. This user involvement test showed that our HeadTracking system with it's ability to follow the head movements in an intuitive manner, is transparent in functionality to the surgeons which found the system to be the best suited to control the scope in laparoscopic surgery.

Keywords: Endoscopic surgery, robotic surgery, head tracking

1. Introduction

Endoscopy, as a minimally invasive technique, is associated with less patient trauma, less risk for infections and reduced overall cost related to the convalescence of the patient. However, the introduction of endoscopic surgery has some disadvantages compared to open surgery. The loss of depth perception using 2D-videoscopes makes the endoscopic skills and experience of the surgeons very important. This drawback has led to the development of 3D-videoscopes, cameras and Head Mounted Displays (HMD). HMD's lets the surgeon be immersed in the video images. However it has been observed that many surgeons, using head-mounted displays on 3D-vision systems, turn their head into awkward positions during the procedure in order to change the direction of view. Development of motion sickness while using the head mounted displays has also been reported [1]. Intuitively the field of view should change according to the movement of the head and body.

©CARS/Springer. All rights reserved.

Conventionally, an assistant holds the scope while communicating directly with the laparoscopic surgeon during the procedure. Since the early 90's robotic scope holders have been developed to eliminate the need for an assistant and thus eliminating possible misunderstandings between surgeon and assistant. This does also provide a more stable image on the screen, which reduces the wear of the surgeon and allows for a better quality of tele-transferred video-images where the transmission rate is a limiting factor.

We have developed a prototype of a Head-Tracker to overcome the problems related to the use of Head Mounted Displays in videoscopic surgery as presented at CARS2000 in San Francisco [2]. The proposed system tracks the head movements of the surgeons and directs the resulting signals to a robot that holds the camera. Thus, the camera movement is coupled to the head movement, which gives the expected change of view. This concept is well known in weapons control systems where fore instance fighter pilots uses head tracking to control their view and eye tracking to identify the target [3].

ComputerMotion (ComputerMotion Inc., Goleta, California) has developed a robotic scope holder, called Aesop, which is voice-controlled. Hand-control and foot-control is also provided by this system. EndoAssist from Armstrong (Armstrong Healthcare Limited, High Wycombe, England) has a robotic scope-holder which is head controlled. The head control uses infrared cameras above the monitor and an infrared emitter attached to the head to verify whether the head is turned right, left, up or down which results in a camera movement in the detected direction. Others have also reported on the performance of similar robot systems used for holding the camera [2,4-9].

This paper will address the concept, development and testing of the new head-tracking system and a user involvement test for comparison between the proposed system and other control techniques to control the scope either by voice control of Aesop [7,8] or HeadControl of EndoAssist [9].

2. Materials and Methods

2.1 Development

The camera holding robot, Aesop3000DS (Computer Motion) was used. This robot can be controlled by a computer through a serial interface. A stereoscopic camera and a head mounted display system, Vista (Vista Medical Technologies, Boston, Massachusetts, USA), was also used.

Based on experience with previously developed prototypes [2], a new prototype HeadTracker was developed (fig. 1). The control algorithm was written in C++. Two one-dimensional piezo-electric gyro-sensors from Grand Wing Servo-Tech Co. (Grand Wing Servo-Tech Co. Ltd., Taiwan) were used as motion sensors. The gyro-sensors were mounted perpendicular to each other to sense angular velocity around the actual axis (right/left and up/down) and assembled together into a small box attached to the head mounted displays. A foot pedal activates the system. The head movements were tracked only while the pedal was enabled.

©CARS/Springer. All rights reserved.

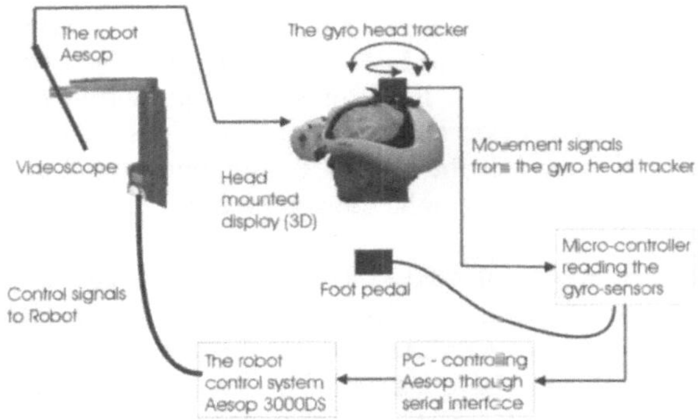

Figure 1 : The HeadTracking system based on piezo-electric gyro-sensors and Aesop3000DS

2.2 User test

Based on [2,4-10] a user test protocol was made for comparison of the prototype Gyroscopic HeadTracker [2] with different commercially available control techniques for robotic scope control.

The HeadTracking system was compared to three other control modalities in a user involvement test.

The control modalities subject for comparison was:

1. HT-3D: Head tracking (HT) of Aesop3000DS through a serial interface using a 3D camera and head mounted stereoscopic display
2. HT-2D: Head tracking (HT) of Aesop3000DS through a serial interface using the same 3D camera but looking at a 2D screen
3. VC-2D: Voice control (VC) of Aesop3000DS
4. HC-2D: Head control (HC) of EndoAssist

The test set-up (fig. 2) include an OR table, a laparoscopic trainer box, two laparoscopic needle holders, two robotic scope holders – Aesop and EndoAssist and the stereoscopic video system. The Vista system consists of a Head Mounted Display (HMD), a 3D camera, a 3D scope and a 2D screen. The planar horizontal floor in the laparoscopic trainer box was provided with 5 pins mounted in a sinusoidal path with a line drawn between them.

©CARS/Springer. All rights reserved.

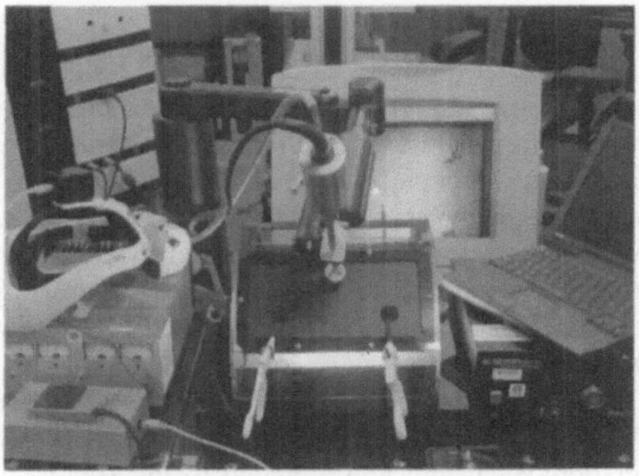

Figure 2 : Set-up for the User Involvement and Laboratory testing of HeadTracking.

Three different tasks were designed for this test:

- Task 1 – Move the scope along the path by letting pin 1 to 5 being in the centre of the image.
- Task 2 – Move the scope along the path from pin 1 to pin 5. At each pin, grip the pin by the right and left instruments simultaneously.
- Task 3 – Move a red rubber cylinder along the path from pin 1 to pin 5.

9 persons (6 surgeons, 2 engineers and 1 other) participated in the test. The participants used task 1 and 3 as training, before task 2 was performed as the evaluated test. The time for each of the 5 trials was recorded. Some of the trials were recorded with a video camera for later analysis. A questionnaire was performed to track the user impression of the system.

3. Results

The average time to complete task 2 using HeadTracking in both modes was shorter than the times for the two other control modes. The average task times using HeadTracking were 39,9% shorter using 3D with head-mounted display (HMD) and 54,1% shorter using 2D screen, compared to HeadControl with EndoAssist (table 1). The "Univariate Analysis of Variances" test was performed on the test-data using the program SPSS (SPSS Inc., Chicago, Illinois, www.spss.com) for statistical analysis. The analysis showed significant differences of means between method 1 and 3 and also between method 1 and 4 ($p<0.05$). The difference between control method 1 and 2 is not statistically significant.

Control Method		Mean-Time	Std. Dev.	% red. rel. HC	Mean val. Quest.
1	**HT-3D**	45,24	16.88	39,9	2.33
2	**HT-2D**	34,60	13.29	54,1	2.50
3	**VC-2D**	61,11	25.59	18,9	2.56
4	**HC-2D**	75,33	25.12	0	2.36

Table 1 : Results from both the performance tests and the questionnaires for each control mode – HeadTracking (HT), VoiceControl (VC) and HeadControl (HC).

©CARS/Springer. All rights reserved.

4. Discussion

A HeadTracker that makes it feel as if the camera is attached to your nose when turning your head is intuitively a more natural motion control system for the camera than voice control, especially since it can be controlled in a continuous manner. Actual frequencies when controlling the camera with head movements are about 1Hz. A direct interface to the control system was needed to make the proposed system succeed. The gyroscopic HeadTracker has shown a very good response and is a promising concept for robotic control of the scope and camera. The last version of the HeadTracker using the robot system Aesop3000DS with a serial interface to a computer running a customised control program, resulted in a bandwidth of about 4,8Hz. Thus the HeadTracker in combination with the Aesop3000DS can achieve the response needed. A test with the HeadTracker coupled to the Aesop3000DS system and attached to the Head Mounted Display of the Vista 3D system showed a sufficient performance, the camera view was easily directed to the desired position.

It was expected that scope control with HeadTracking would be most beneficial when used in conjunction with 3D vision using head-mounted displays. But the test data showed that the HT system in conjunction with a 2D display gave even shorter task times. Since HeadTracking with 3D always was tested before 2D, the learning effect may be the cause for some of this difference. To prevent learning effects from favouring the HT systems, the tests with VC and HC were the two lasts to be performed.

The results for the HC and VC systems can partly be attributed to some technical problems. A voice command possibility of the VC method, “move_right move_up” giving a diagonal movement up to the right, was not used during the test. However, the difference in performance can not be explained by these problems alone.

The questionnaires showed the same ranking of the different control modalities as with the performance test with the exception of HeadTracking under 3D and 2D where the head mounted 3D display in combination with the HeadTracker now showed the best score. The scores were close to each other, and the participants have not used the whole scale ranging from 1 to 5 when differentiating between the different systems. Even though the HeadTracking system with Head Mounted Display showed the worst score on “physical comfort” compared to the other systems, the high score on “control ability”, “cognitive comfort (intuitive)”, “effectiveness” and “efficiency”, more than compensated for this.

5. Conclusion

In order for robotic devices to be introduced successfully into surgical practice, the development of transparent surgeon/machine interface is critical. This user involvement test showed that our HeadTracking system with it’s ability to follow the head movements in an intuitive manner, is transparent in functionality to the surgeons which found the system to be best suited to control the scope in laparoscopic surgery. Both the performance test and the questionnaires showed the same results where HeadTracking

©CARS/Springer. All rights reserved.

was fastest, most intuitive and effective for controlling the scope. The HeadControl of EndoAssist, where the head is used to indicate separate movement commands and the VoiceControl where the different commands are given by voice is quite closely related to each other. The difference between them and HeadTracking, where the actual head movements are tracked and followed by the scope in an intuitive manner, is by this found to be crucial for the transparency of the system.

References

1. P. A. Howarth and P. J. Costello, The occurrence of virtual simulation sickness symptoms when an HMD was used as a personal viewing system, Displays, 18, 107-116, 1997.
2. O. J. Elle, E. Samset, J. O. Høgetveit and E. Fosse. Head-tracking in scopic surgical procedures using Robot-held camera and head-mounted stereoscopic display, CARS 2000, Proceedings of the 14th International Congress and Exhibition, 121-127, Elsevier Science B.V., Amsterdam, 2000.
3. M. Walker, A. Leger, B. Hudgins, P. Dauchy, D. Pastor, H. Pongratz, G. Rood, A. South, K. Carr, D. Jarrett, T. Anderson, J. Borah, and C. Wientjes, Head based control. RTO Technical report 7. Alternative control technologies, 29-59, NATO : Research and Technology organization, CASI, Neully-sur-Seine, 1998, ISBN 92-837-1009-6.
4. M. E. Allaf, S. V. Jackman, P. G. Schulam, J. A. Cadeddu, B. R. Lee, R. G. Moore and L. R. Kavoussi, Laparoscopic visual field. Voice vs foot pedal interfaces for control of the AESOP robot. Surg Endosc 12, 1415-1418, 1998.
5. L. R. Kavoussi, R. G. Moore, J. B. Adams and A. W. Partin, Comparison of robotic versus human laparoscopic camera control. J Urol 154, 2134-2136, 1995.
6. A. Nishikawa, T. Hosoi, K. Koara, A. Hikita D. Negoro, S. Asano, F. Miyazaki, M. Sekimoto, Y. Miyake, M. Yasui and M. Monden. A laparoscope positioning system with the surgeon's face image-based human-mashine interface, CARS 2001, Proceedings of the 15th International Congress and Exhibition, 165-170, Elsevier Science B.V., Amsterdam, 2001.
7. J. M. Sackier and Y. WANG, ROBOTICALLY ASSISTED LAPAROSCOPIC SURGERY - FROM CONCEPT TO DEVELOPMENT. Surgical Endoscopy-Ultrasound and Interventional Techniques 8, 63-66, 1994.
8. J. M. Sackier, C. Wooters, L. Jacobs, A. Halverson, D. Uecker and Y. L. Wang, Voice activation of a surgical robotic assistant. Am J Surg 174, 406-409, 1997.
9. Y. Yavuz, B. Ystgaard, E. Skogvoll and R. Marvik, A comparative experimental study evaluating the performance of surgical robots aesop and endosista. Surg Laparosc Endosc Percutan Tech 10, 163-167, 2000.
10. W.S. Green, P.W. Jordan (eds.), Human Factors in Productdesign; Current Practice and Future Trends, Taylor & Francis, 1999, ISBN 0-7484-0829-0

CARS 2002 – H.U. Lemke, M.W. Vannier; K. Inamura, A.G. Farman, K. Doi & J.H.C. Reiber (Editors)
©CARS/Springer. All rights reserved.

Application of image tracking for positioning scope in the robotic assisted laparoscopic surgery

Shahram Payandeh and Annie Zhang
Experimental Robotics Laboratory
School of Engineering Science
Simon Fraser University
Burnaby, BC, Canada, V5A 1S6

Abstract

Utilization of a scope facilitated the success of Minimally Invasive Surgery (MIS), hence the name, endoscopic or laparoscopic surgery. The scope can be fed through a small incision hole offering the surgeon a two-dimensional view of the surgical site. In general, the (laparo-) scope is hand-held by the assistant surgeon, thereby offering an unsteady image of the viewing area. The authors proposed the use of image processing to enhance the resulting image. This paper presents some of the preliminary results. In particular, the paper presents models for lens distortion and a calibrating approach as well as an image tracking method. It is shown that it is possible to track a especially designed marker located at the tip of laparoscopic instruments. Experimental results are presented to show the feasibility of the method.

Keywords: Laparoscopic surgery, image analysis, image tracking.

1. Introduction

With the improved development of various tools and techniques; laparoscopic surgery is becoming increasingly popular. This is mainly due to the minimal invasive nature of such surgery that allows operations to be performed on patients through small incisions. Compared to the traditional surgeries, this technique can greatly reduce the pain and provide a more rapid recovery for patients [1].

Surgeons can access the surgical site, which is inside the inflated 3-dimensional abdominal cavity, through incision points (shown in Figure 1). Accessing is done using long-stem graspers, while viewing 2-dimensional images. Currently, the images are only supplied without any pre-processing. In addition, an assistant to the surgeon is needed to hold the laparoscope where consistent and steady orientations of the images are not always guaranteed. This paper proposes to extend the imaging capability of the current practice through processing of the images for visual diagnostics and tracking in robotic applications.

This paper is organized as follows: section 2 presents models for the distortion of the laparoscopic lens; section 3 presents a camera model; section 4 gives an application of the

©CARS/Springer. All rights reserved.

camera model to the design of tracking system. This notion is then used in the context of the image-guided surgery using robotic devices.

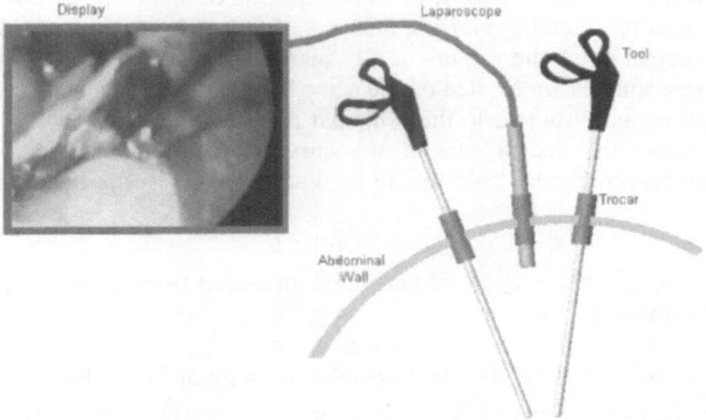

Figure 1 – Laparoscopic tools and 2D image from the surgical site.

2. Distortion Model

As it is well known, no lens can produce perfect images. Common imperfections are aberrations that degrade the quality or sharpness of the image or lens distortions that deteriorate the geometric quality (or positional accuracy) of the image. In this section, we mainly concerned about the lens distortion [2][3]. Radial distortion, as its name implies, causes image position to be distorted along radial line from the optical axis. Faulty grinding of the lens elements is the major cause. Tangential distortion due to imperfect centering of the lens components and other manufacturing defects in a compound lens; it is also called decentering. That is the optical center and the lenses are not strictly collinear. The pixel shift is away from the optical center and the new position lies at a new angle location as measured from the optical center.

Tangential lens distortions are generally very small and are seldom corrected for. Three different methods of correcting for radial distortion are: 1) Corrections from a radial-lens distortion property; b) Interpolating corrections from a table and c) Numerical methods in which the redial-lens distortions curve are approximated by a polynomial.

In this paper, the last method was followed to obtain the model of the laparoscope. We assume radial distortion to be symmetric about the optical axis. Symmetric radial distortion can be universally represented as an odd-ordered polynomial series:[4]

$$\Delta r = k_1 r + k_2 r^3 + k_3 r^5 + k_4 r^7 + \ldots..$$

Δr is the radial lens distortion at a radial distance r from the principal point (interception of the image plane with the optical axis). The coefficients define the shape of a curve. They can be obtained through a least square curve fitting computation, which matches a

©CARS/Springer. All rights reserved.

curve to known radial distortions. These data are obtained at various radial distances as determined through camera calibration.
In our experiments, a black-and-white grid with spacing of 8mm was used for determining the model. Images representing viewing distance of 50mm to 80mm were obtained. After finding the principal point and centers of all squares, the distance of the Center Square is calculated. These squares are located on the same line that intersects at the principal point. In the distorted image distances to the principal point as a function of r are obtained in order to determine the coefficients of the curve. For example, using the following equation which represents the least square method, we can get the required coefficients, say X :[4]

$$X = (A^T A)^{-1} A^T L$$

For example, suppose that r is the distance that measured from the image plane while r' is the corrected distance. Then

$$r' = \Delta r + r$$

Two methods were used to get the pixel value for each point (x, y). Here (x, y) represents pixel points in the image plane while (x', y') represents corrected image points.

Method 1:
$$x' = x + \Delta x = x + k_1 x + k_2 x^3$$
$$y' = y + \Delta y = y + k_1 y + k_2 y^3$$

The result of using this approach to obtain the undistorted image is shown in Figure 2. As it can be seen from this Figure, the image is stretched along its axes. The problem is that the distortion Δr is only concerned with the distance of the pixel point from the principle point.

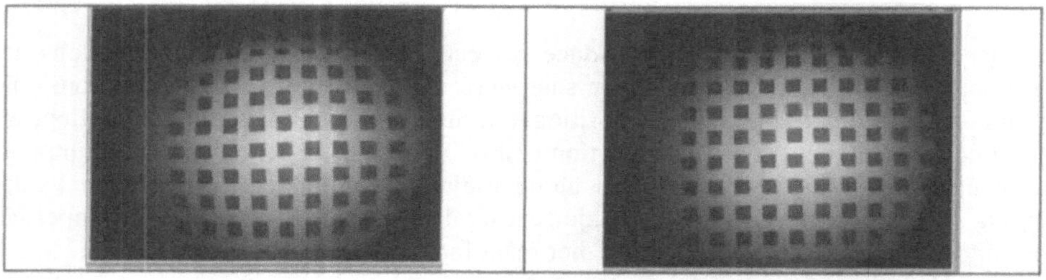

Figure 2 – An undistorted image using Method 1 and Method 2.

Method 2: Since $\frac{r}{\Delta r} = \frac{x}{\Delta x} = \frac{y}{\Delta y}$, we can use the following equations for undistorting the image:
$$x' = x + \Delta x = x(1 + \Delta r / r) = x(1 + k_1 + k_2 r^2)$$
$$y' = y + \Delta y = y(1 + \Delta r / r) = y(1 + k_1 + k_2 r^2).$$

This method considers the relationship between distortion and the distance from the principle center.

3. Camera Model

Typical parameters used for calibration can be classified into two classes: extrinsic parameters and intrinsic parameters [5]. In order to get meaningful measurement results

©CARS/Springer. All rights reserved.

from the laparoscopic images, our approach focuses on getting the intrinsic parameters: the effective focal length, the real image center and the scale factor.

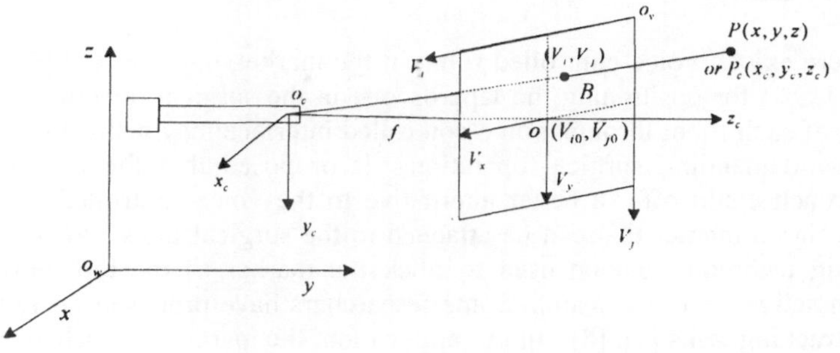

Figure 3 - Camera geometry with perspective projection.

Figure 3 illustrates the basic geometry of the camera model. (x,y,z) is the world coordinate system. In robotic systems, this coordinate frame can be placed at the robot base. (x_c,y_c,z_c) is the camera coordinate system, (x,y,z) is the 3D coordinates of a object P in the world coordinate system, (x_c,y_c,z_c) is the coordinate of point P in the camera coordinate system with the z_c axis the same as the optical axis. Here the camera coordinate frame is defined at the tip of the laparoscope. (x_d,y_d) (not shown in figure 3) is the image coordinates of $P(x_c,y_c,z_c)$ projected into the image plane if a perfect pinhole model assumption is used. (V_i,V_j) is the coordinates used in the image buffer. Additional scale factors need to be specified that relates the image coordinate in the front image plane to the image buffer coordinate system.

For example one of the intrinsic parameters to be calibrated is the real focal length. As shown in figure 3.1, transforming from 3D camera coordinate (x_c,y_c,z_c) to image coordinate (V_i,V_j) based on the perspective projection with pinhole camera geometry, we can get the following equation:

$$\frac{oo_c}{z_c}=\frac{f}{z_c}=\frac{(V_i-V_{i0})S_x}{x_c}=\frac{(V_j-V_{j0})S_y}{y_c}$$

$$x_c=\frac{z_c(V_i-V_{i0})S_x}{f},\ y_c=\frac{z_c(V_j-V_{j0})S_y}{f}$$

where oo_c is the distance between the center of the image buffer to the center of the camera coordinate frame, (V_{i0},V_{j0}) are rows and column numbers of the image center, S_x,S_y are the scale factors that map the real image coordinate (x_d,y_d) to image buffer coordinate (V_i,V_j). When V_i,V_j,X_c and Z_c are known parameters the effective focal length can

©CARS/Springer. All rights reserved.

be calculated from the above equation. Also, when f, V_i, z_i and x_c, y_c are known parameters, we can get the depth information z_c of an object in the field of view.

4. Image Tracking

Currently, there exist a voice-controlled robot in the market, e.g. AESOP [6] (Computer motion, CA, USA) for positioning the laparoscope in the surgical operation. In general, the operation of such robot through voice-controlled interface may distract the surgeon in already highly demanding surgical operations. It proposed that the automatic image tracking approach could offer a better alternative to the voice-controlled interface. We propose to design a marker that can be attached to the surgical tools. When needed, the image tracking technique can be used to track the marker as the tool moves. Image tracking is an active area of research. Some researchers have proposed many techniques for different tracking tasks [7], [8]. In our application, the marker is attached to the tip of the tools, and then identified for the tracking task.
Figure 4 shows the experimental results of the marker tracking. Figure to the left show the actual image of what camera can see with the marker in the field of view and figure to the right shows the kinematic model of a laparoscope holding mechanism (SFU-LapHolder). When the marker moves in the actual field of view, the tracking spatial parameters are pass to the simulated robotic device.

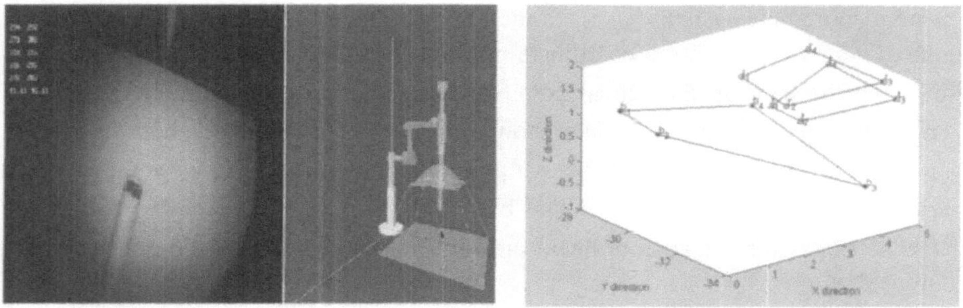

Figure 4 - The actual image of the marker and the tracking simulation.

Figure 4 also shows some experimental comparison of the tracking algorithm. Here, the results were evaluated for four given known points in the workspace. Three methods of measurements were followed: a) our proposed tracking algorithm (t); b) using a 3D sensing transducers (PcBird) (p) and c) real physical measurements (r). It was found that our tracking results follow very closely the actual physical measurements.

©CARS/Springer. All rights reserved.

5. Conclusions

This paper presents an alternative method for positioning the laparoscope in the robotic assisted surgery. Previously proposed methods involved voice controlled systems or master-slave operations. Our proposed method has many advantages. First it uses the available images of the surgical site through addition of an image-processing unit. Second, the information obtained through the proposed method can be used both for positioning the scope which can offer a desired field of view and it can be used for further 3D reconstruction of the surgical site.

The results of this paper were compared with the actual true values of some calibration points in the workspace. It was found that for this initial comparison of the results, the accuracy of the proposed method is justified for the purpose of the application.

For example, the objective is for the surgeon to obtain a proper field of view for the specific surgical task. When in the tracking mode, the surgeon can move the designated laparoscopic tool with the marker in the field of view. When activated, the robot will pivot the scope about the incision point and/or translate the scope inside or outside of the abdominal cavity. If not satisfied, the tracking continues until the desired field of view is obtained.

The tracking is accomplished in the master/slave mode where the Laparoscopic tool with the marker is the master and the scope holder robot is the salve. Although the accuracy of the tracking system was determined to be within 2-3mm, such inaccuracy can be further compensated by the salve part of the system which is controlled by the surgeon.

References

1. Faraz, A. and Payandeh, S., *Engineering approaches to mechanical and robotic design for minimally invasive surgery (MIS)*, Kluwer Academec Publisher, 2000
2. Kopparapu, K. and Cork, P., *Effect of lens distortion on camera calibration parameters,* hhtp://www.cat.csiro.au/automation.staff/nil/csiro/publications/
3. Poliner, J. and Wilimington, R., *Evaluation of lens distortion errors in video-based motion analysis*, NASA Technical Paper, 3266, 1993
4. Asari, K., Kumar, S. and Radhakrishnan, D., A new appraoch for nonlinear distortion correction in endoscopic images based on least squares estimation, IEEE Transaction on Medical Imaging, Vol. 18, No. 4, pp. 345-354, 1999
5. Tasi, R., *A versatile camera calibration technique for high-accuracy 3D machine vision metrology using off-the-shelf TV cameras and lenses,* IEEE Journal of Robotics and Automation, Vol. RA-3, No. 4, pp. 323-344, 1987
6. Mettler, L., Ibrahim, M. and Jonat, W., *One year of experience working with the aid of a robotic assistant in the voice-controlled optic holder AESOP in gynecological endoscopic surgery, Human Reproduction,* Vol. 13, No. 10, pp. 2748-2750,1998
7. Papanikolopulos, N., Khosla, P. and Kanada, T., *Visual tracking of a moving target by a camera mounted on a robot: a combination of control and vision,* IEEE Transactions on Robotics and Automation, Vol. 9, No. 1, pp. 14-20, 1993
8. Reddi, S. and Loizou, G., *Analysis of camera behavior during tracking,* IEEE Transaction on Pattern Analysis and machine Intelligence, No. 8, pp. 127-134, 1995

©CARS/Springer. All rights reserved.

The implementation of an intuitive man-machine interface in robot-aided endoscopic laser surgery

Hsiao-Wei Tang[a], Hendrik Van Brussel[a], Philippe Koninckx[b], Jos Vander Sloten[c]
[a] Division PMA, Dept. of Mechanical Engineering,
[b] Dept. of Obstetrics and Gynecology, University Hospital Gasthuisberg,
[c] Division BMGO, Dept. of Mechanical Engineering,
Katholieke Universiteit Leuven, Belgium

Abstract

The precision of laser endoscopic surgery mainly depends upon the skill of the surgeon i.e. the accuracy of movement and the coordination between firing and speed of movement, which determines the depth of vaporisation. We implemented an intuitive drawing interface to control a robot in order to facilitate manual skills and enhance precision. The accuracy of the robot system was evaluated by assessing its performance with sinusoid test signals; the enhanced precision in comparison with classic surgery was demonstrated by cutting characters on an apple. In addition, we monitored the speed of the laser movement and the focal distance of the laser by tracking the laser spot on the screen. This is used to generate continuously a high quality cut of constant depth.

Keywords: Intuitive interface, minimal invasive surgery, endoscopic robot, CO_2 laser

1. Introduction

Minimal invasive surgery (MIS) has become increasingly popular on recent years [1]. In MIS procedures surgeons acquire visual information of the operative site by an endoscope and manipulate instruments through small apertures to perform surgery. Endoscopic surgery has the advantages of less pain and morbidity for the patient while possibly enhancing precision through the enlarged view [2]. Endoscopic surgery on the contrary, requires additional skills and training of the surgeon, in order to prevent complications. The main difficulties are the hand-eye coordination, the lack of depth of vision and the instruments used. Lasers are widely applied in MIS procedures, especially in gynecology [3]. It is an ideal cutting instrument because of its precision having coagulating properties for vessels up to 1mm. During CO_2 endoscopic surgery a red He-Ne laser spot indicates the impact point of the invisible CO_2 laser on the TV screen. Since the laser is coupled to the endoscope, the laser spot is moving simultaneously with the endoscope. Thus, surgeons perceive the visual information from the TV screen and steer the endoscope with one hand to cut with the laser. It is as drawing on the screen by the laser. The focal distance of the laser, speed of movement and the accuracy of the movement are essential for the cutting performance since power density is highest at the focal distance and since depth of cutting depends on the speed of movement. In comparison with open surgery CO_2 laser surgery required from the surgeons a new style of control. The motion command is opposite to the desired motion as perceived, and the scale is arbitrary and

©CARS/Springer. All rights reserved.

unknown. Indeed, there are no direct indications for the focal distance. Surgeons only approximately estimate the distance to the tissues by referencing the size of the organs or the spot position on the screen [4]. In addition, the foot pedal used to activate the laser can distract the surgeon. Accidents were reported by accidentally activating the laser. It is physical demanding to manipulate the endoscope with camera and laser for a long time, maintaining precision and safety. Thus, taking all difficulties into account, it is not easy to achieve high quality performance during long periods. Therefore, specific training and improved man-machine interface by the aids of robotics and advanced technology, such as stereovision or voice command were introduced [5].

We improved an existing endoscopic robot to manipulate the endoscope and laser. An intuitive and ergonomic wireless pen and drawing interface are introduced to control the laser tip. The pen button replaces the foot pedal. A real-time DSP controller represents the commands from the surgeon to robot. The spot moving speed is monitored and the distance to the tissues is estimated by image processing techniques.

2. Methods

The modified endoscopic robot is the FIPS system from KARL STORZ GmbH & Co (Tüttlingen). This robot has only 4 degrees of freedom (DOF), 3 revolute and 1 prismatic joints, (Figure 1). Its fixed rotational point that coincide with the trocar insertion through the abdominal wall made it possible to limit the robot to 4 DOFs. The original 8 buttons control commanding the 4 DOFs is sufficient to position the endoscope. The robot was developed to hold the camera, not to perform surgery. The scale between the drawing movement input to the laser spot output is adjustable to switch between fine or fast cutting situations.

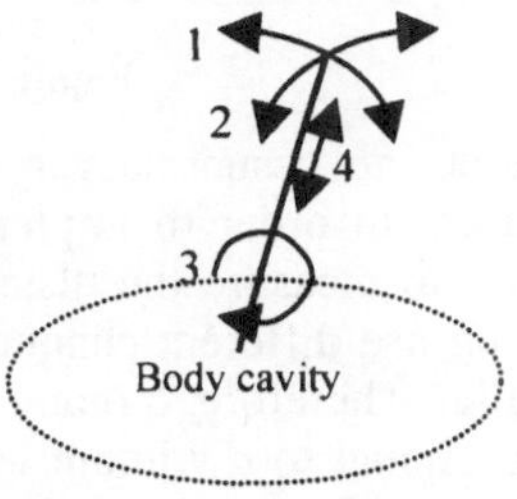

Figure 1. The 4 DOFs of FIPS system: 1,2,3 are revolute joints; 4 is prismatic joint

A digitizer tablet and a wireless pen that are commonly used in Computer Aided Design (CAD) were implemented to replace the button control interface in order to take advantage of humans' drawing skill. The tablet is known to be a better interface for continuous tracking and drawing [6]. The relative position on the 2D tablet is translated to the endoscope's orientation by the two rotation axes. A low pass filter is installed to eliminate the tremor of the surgeon to improve the stabilisation of the robot.

The laser trigger is put on the pen instead of the commonly used foot pedal. By pressing the button on the pen when drawing on the tablet, surgeons can easily control laser firing without affecting the stability. It is simple, intuitive and ergonomic for both novice or experienced surgeons. They can look on the screen and draw/cut/ablate tissues by the intuitive drawing interface as if drawing on the screen. In figure 2, the set up of the whole system is shown. With this system, surgeons can operate, using the intelligent robot and intuitive interface.

©CARS/Springer. All rights reserved.

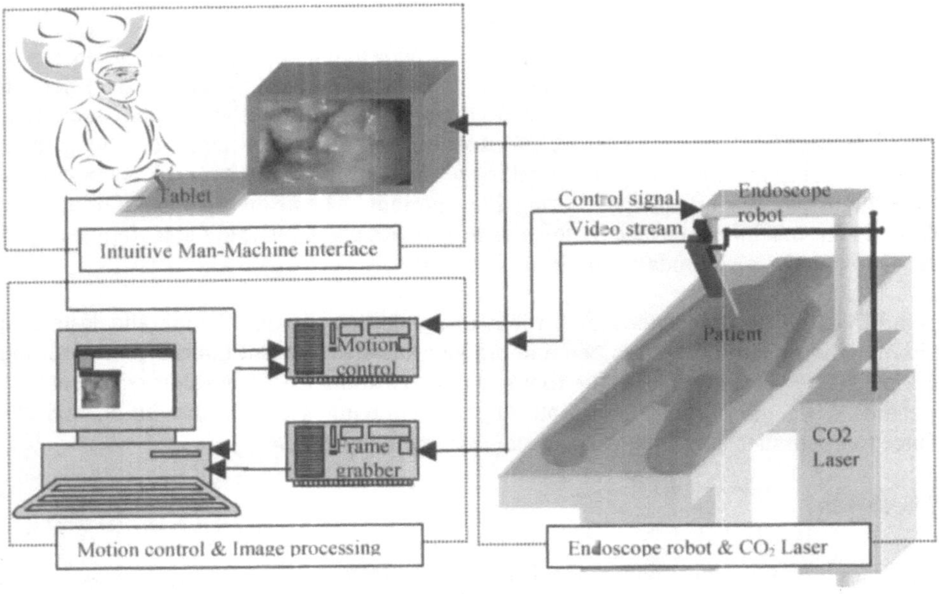

Figure 2. The intuitive operating robot system

Distance to tissues is very important in laser cutting since the laser should always be focused. In order to implement an auto focus function on the system, we must have a sensor to measure the distance to the tissues. As illustrated in figure 3, vision and laser cutting use different channels. We can adjust the center of lens and the laser beam to be parallel. Therefore, δ remains constant. By using simple optics theory, we assume that s is proportional to d without considering the distortion of lens. However, the size of images shows on the screen s_s is constant. Thus, we can get the relation between d and δ_s is inverse proportional. We use this algorithm to obtain the approximate d to use in our auto focus function. Since δ_s can be measured manually or by image processing techniques. At first, we acquired the reference δ_s from the image when the laser is focus on the tissues. Then, image-processing techniques are implemented to track the laser spot on the screen continuously where the distance d can be evaluated. By this information, we can control the prismatic joint to focus the laser automatically. Moreover, by accessing the information of distance and of orientation of the laser beam, the movement speed of the laser contact point can be estimated and shown. It could be further extended to display the profile of the surface inside human body.

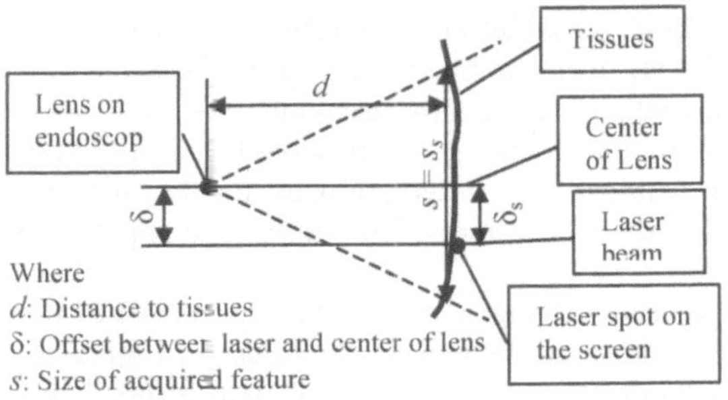

Where
d: Distance to tissues
δ: Offset between laser and center of lens
s: Size of acquired feature
s_s: Size shown on the screen
δ_s: distance on the screen between laser spot and center
Since $d \propto s$........(1) and $s_s \propto 1/\delta_s$........(2)
From (1), (2) we can get $d \propto 1/\delta_s$........(3)

Figure 3. The relation between distance to tissues and laser spot on the screen

CARS 2002 – H.U. Lemke, M.W. Vannier; K. Inamura, A.G. Farman, K. Doi & J.H.C. Reiber (Editors)
©CARS/Springer. All rights reserved.

3. Results

The system was made operational successfully. The accuracy was tested by applying sinusoid input signals to the two revolute axes. They were used to handle the orientation of the endoscope and laser to cut on the tissues. Two sinusoid signals with 90-degree phase lag were applied from the DSP itself to both axes simultaneously. Then, the robot will draw a circle on a surface. Afterward, we use the tablet to measure the output of the tip of the endoscope where we coupled the wireless pen as the extension of the endoscope. It is put perpendicular to and contacts the tablet at the center of the circle. The amplitude of the sinusoid signal is 5° in each direction and the frequency is 0.25 Hz. The distance from the rotation point (trocar) of the robot to the tablet is set fixed at 21cm for easy calculation. As shown in figure 4, the output of the x-y plot on the tablet does not fit perfectly to the input circular trajectory but the repeatability of the robot is quite good. In figure 5, from the separate results of both axes in time series, we can see the maximum error of both axes is around 0.7°, occurring at maximum speed. The backlash-induced error is relatively small.

The intuitive interface robot is mainly designed as an instrument to be manipulated by surgeons. To demonstrate the feasibility, we applied a second test, which used the interface to write some characters on the surface of an apple. This illustrates the idea and achievement of this development. The test is performed in a simulated operating situation. The user looked at screen and wrote the characters by hand. The result can be seen in figure 6. The reference scale indicates that each character is about 3 mm high × 3 mm wide.

A simple linear model was built to estimate distance to tissues. We acquire the images of the endoscope sequentially from a frame grabber. The image-processing algorithm for laser spot tracking is implemented in

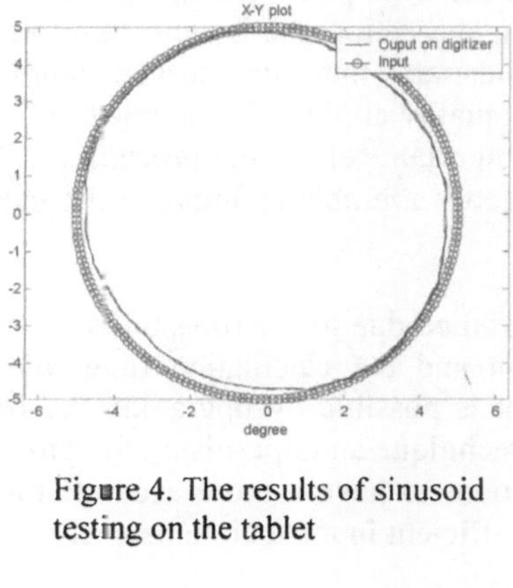

Figure 4. The results of sinusoid testing on the tablet

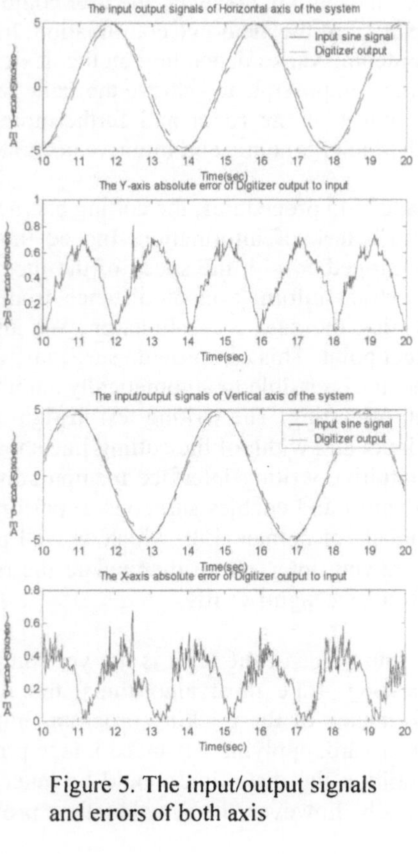

Figure 5. The input/output signals and errors of both axis

©CARS/Springer. All rights reserved.

the program. It can calculate the distance between laser spot and center of the lens on the image and evaluate the distance to tissues. The frequency of the measurement is about 5 Hz. The estimated distance is shown on the screen and feedback to the controller to calculate the speed of movement. The image processing is not very fast and robust due to the time needed by the frame grabber card and the image-processing algorithms.

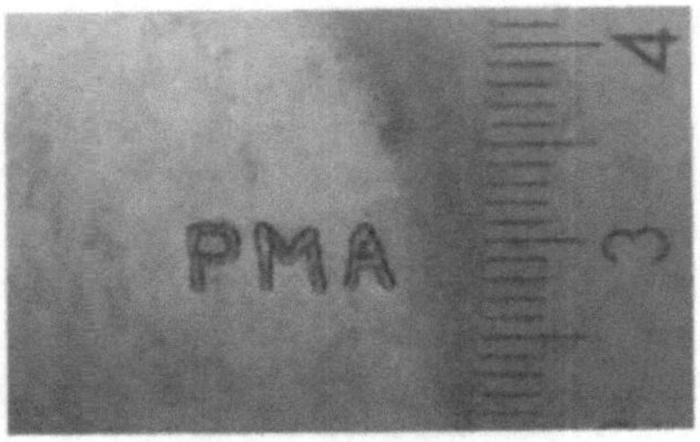

Figure 6. The PMA apple

4. Discussion

A medical robot for endoscopic surgery should have the following characteristics: accuracy, stability, mobility, lightweight, easy sterilizing, back-drivability, small, high safety, simple manipulation and easy installation. Initially, the data from the first test suggested that the accuracy of our robot was not very good. The errors came from many sources such as the time delay between the input and output signal, the vibration of the structure that supports the robot, the deviation when installing the tablet, the dynamic friction in each axis and so on. In the second writing test shown in figure 6, however, the user could write characters smoothly and easily due to the adaptation of the hand-eye coordination. In conventional manual endoscopic laser surgery, the outcome varies depending on the dexterity and skill of the surgeon. It is obvious that it is almost impossible to achieve the same results as using the robot. The 4 DOFs simplified the control of the robot and furthermore the implementation of the drawing interface resulted in ergonomic and intuitive accurate manipulation of the cutting using a laser.

In hand held procedures, the cutting characteristics of the laser are only roughly controlled due to a lack of information. Indeed the focal distance determines the power density, which together with the speed of the movement of laser determines the energy per area. We extract information of distance from the video stream by tracking the laser spot, providing the auto focus function. We also estimated the movement speed of the laser contact point. This can provide surgeons with a sense of the desired movement. Moreover it becomes possible to automatically smoothen laser speed in order to maintain a constant depth of cutting. The writing test in figure 6, where the absorption rate is represented by the depth and width of the cutting line shows that the absorption rate is almost uniform by the intuitive writing interface manipulation. This illustrates that our interface simplified the control and enables surgeons to perform a high quality cutting. Our application takes advantage of human skill, which as well plays an important role in the procedures. With our drawing interface to manipulate the robot, surgeons are able to improve the cutting performance significantly.

The auto focus of the laser is not yet completely installed due to the robustness of image processing. Like most algorithms, the illumination and the calculation time rule the performance of the tracking program. Improvement is possible by upgrading the frame grabber card, applying advanced image processing technique and optimising the program. In addition the distortion should be taken into account to have a more accurate model. Clinically, however, the actual method probably is sufficient in most circumstances.

©CARS/Springer. All rights reserved.

Because the FIPS system is originally designed for holding the camera, not for precise cutting, it still requires further enhancement or redesign to improve repeatability, accuracy, stability and back-drivability. Since this system only acts as one hand of the surgeon, a second robot could be developed to enhance the other hand's ability. Finally, the most important issues in medical robotic application are the safety requirements, which includes: hardware, software and redundant sensors. The robot system must perform fail-safe operation and should have the ability to predict errors not only to perform safely but also to prevent human mistakes. Therefore, the development of specific intelligent monitoring system is crucial in the future. Firing accidents could be prevented by linking firing to movement.

5. Conclusions

This paper describes the ideas and realization of converting the navigation endoscope robot into an advanced intuitive operating instrument. By implementing the acquainted intuitive man-machine interface and replacing the foot pedal with a pen button, surgeons can achieve comfortably more accurate operation with less training. The relationship between the spot and the screen is used to obtain the distance from the laparoscope point to the tissues and the speed of movement. This is used to automatically focus the laser by fixing the distance to the surface and to monitor the speed of movement in order to obtain a constant high quality char-free cut of the spectacular CO_2 laser.

Acknowledgements

The financial support from Fonds voor Wetenschappelijk Onderzoek –Vlaanderen (FWO) was gratefully acknowledged. We thank KARL STORZ GmbH, Tüttlingen Germany for providing the robot and the endoscopic instruments, and Nova Medica NV Belgium/Lumenis Inc. for supplying the CO_2 laser.

References

1. L. Cravello, R. de Montgolfier, C.D'Ercole V. Roger and B. Blanc, "Endoscopic Surgery: The End of Classic Surgery?", European J. of Obstetrics & Gynecology and Reproductive Biology, Vol.75, page 103-106, 1997
2. http://www.patient-info.com/laser.htm
3. R. Garry, D. Shelley-Jones, P. Mooney and G. Phillips, "Six Hundred Endomentrial Laser Ablation", Obstetrics & Gynecology, Vol. 85, No. 1,page 24-29, 1995
4. J.Donnez and M. Nisolle, An altas of laser operative laparoscopy and hysteroscopy, The Parthenon publishing group, chapter 2, London, 1994
5. M.Degueldre, J.Vandromme, P.T. Huong and G.B. Cadière, "Robotically assisted laparoscopic microsurgical tubal reanastomosis: a feasibility study",Fertility and sterility,Vol.74, No.5, page 1020-1023, 2000
6. H.Martin, Handbook of human-computer interaction, North Holland, page 1344, Amsterdam, 1988

CARS 2002 – H.U. Lemke, M.W. Vannier; K. Inamura, A.G. Farman, K. Doi & J.H.C. Reiber (Editors)
©CARS/Springer. All rights reserved.

Motion estimation in minimally invasive beating heart surgery

Tobias Ortmaier, Martin Gröger, Gerd Hirzinger
German Aerospace Center (DLR)
Institute of Robotics and Mechatronics
82234 Wessling, Germany, E-mail: Tobias.Ortmaier@dlr.de

Abstract

Motion estimation is a prerequisite for autonomous functions in robotic surgery. In beating heart surgery it allows motion compensation of the heart surface and thus a safe and secure operation. Algorithms for a short-term prediction of the heart motion are presented. Prediction increases the reliability of the motion estimation scheme, because short disturbances of the underlying tracking framework can be compensated.

Keywords: Beating heart surgery, motion estimation, robotic surgery

1. Introduction

Conventional techniques for coronary artery bypass surgeries contain severe risks and a significant morbidity for the patient, caused by the splitting of the sternum and the use of the heart-lung machine to sustain the circulation. TECAB (Totally Endoscopic Coronary Artery Bypass) at the beating heart plays an important role to reduce these risks. Mechanical stabilizers (Fig. 1) are widely used to restrict the motion of the heart. The surgery itself is performed with MIRS (Minimally Invasive Robotic Surgery) systems (see [1]). The remaining motion of the stabilized heart complicates safe and secure surgery. This disadvantage leads directly to the demand of measuring and compensating the organ movement. If the MIRS system is able to estimate and compensate the motion of the heart reliably, the surgeon can work on a virtually stabilized beating heart and gains back the safety he was used to in on-pump coronary artery bypass surgery. In [2] it is shown, that the motion can be reliably estimated by exploiting natural landmarks (see Fig. 1). The tracking scheme yields quasi-periodic trajectories as presented in Fig. 2. This periodic behaviour results from the patient's respiration (low frequency) and the heart beat (high frequency). Tracking works well, if no disturbances (e.g. occlusions by a surgical instrument) occur. In this case the tracking scheme can not provide any reasonable information and a robust motion compensation is not possible. To

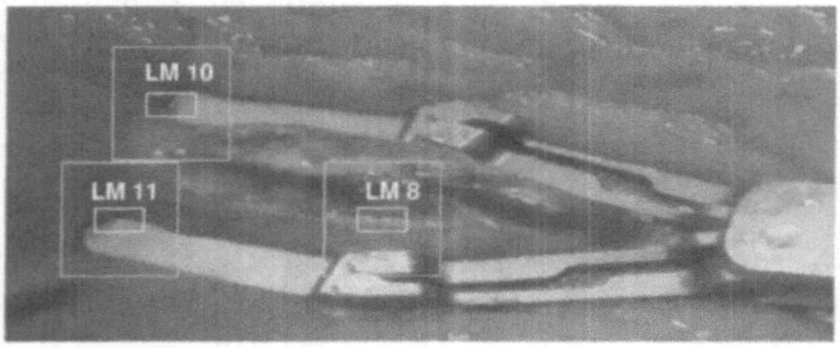

Figure 1: Beating Heart with Stabilizer.

©CARS/Springer. All rights reserved.

handle this problem, a motion estimation scheme is presented in Sec. 2, which uses the quasi-periodicity of the trajectories. Section 3 summarizes the results and gives directions for further research.

2. Robust Motion Estimation

This section presents local prediction (Sec. 2.2) as well as global prediction (Sec. 2.3) schemes. Here *local* means that information of only one trajectory is used to predict its position one or several steps ahead. This algorithm was developed to detect outliers reliably or to position the search area of the tracking algorithm. Additionally, this method can be extended to more-step prediction easily, although prediction accuracy degrades with increasing prediction interval *s*. The *global* scheme avoids this drawback by exploiting the trajectories of several landmarks simultaneously.

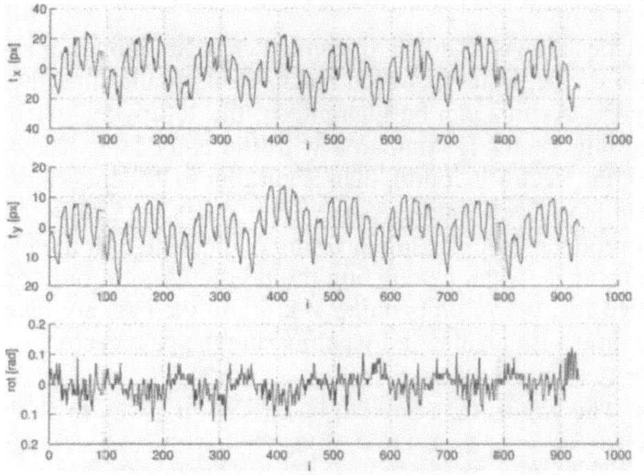

Figure 2: Detected Trajectories.

The prediction schemes presented here are model free, i.e. no explicit models (e.g. differential equations) are used. Model parameters which might vary over time as well as being patient-dependent do not need to be determined. Furthermore, it is very difficult to gain an explicit model for the heart surface trajectories (HST), which describe the translational displacement of the patterns over time. The first section (Sec. 2.1) gives the preliminaries for both the local and the global prediction schemes.

2.1 Algorithm

A sequence of measurements, called *time series*, is used to capture the unknown inner states of the underlying dynamical system producing the measured output y_k. A time series y can be written as:

$$y = [y_n, y_{n-1}, \ldots, y_1]^T, \qquad (1)$$

with y_k being a scalar-valued measurement at time t_k. The variable $x_k \in \Re^d$ represents the inner states of the dynamical system at time t_k and F the unknown system: $x_{k+1} = F(x_k)$. As the inner states x_k and the function F are unknown and therefore cannot be used to predict the next y_k (with $k > n$), one has to find an alternative description of the dynamical system, based on the known measurements y_k only. If F is smooth (at least C^2), then this can be achieved with the help of Takens Theorem [3]: Taking a sufficiently long vector built of past values of a time series enables the reconstruction of the underlying structure of the system dynamics which produced the sequence. The sufficiently long vector is called

©CARS/Springer. All rights reserved.

embedding vector D_k and is made of p past measurements with lag h between two subsequent measurements:

$$D_k = \left[y_k, y_{k-h}, \ldots, y_{k-(p-1)h}\right]^T . \quad (2)$$

According to Takens, p has to satisfy the following condition $p > 2d$.
Unfortunately, the dimension d is unknown. Additionally, the embedding (time) lag h has to be chosen carefully [4]. Before an algorithm to determine optimal values for p and h is presented, the prediction algorithm itself is introduced. Therefore, it is assumed that p and h are chosen appropriately.

Prediction algorithm It has to be shown that the dynamical system moves on an attractor (a subset of the state space of the system), which means in particular that there are no transient inner states any more. As this can be guaranteed, the following scheme can be applied: The current embedding vector is compared with the embedding vectors lying in the past. If a similar embedding vector is found, then according to Takens, similar inner states of the dynamical system have been found. As the inner states are similar and $F \in C^2$, the dynamical system will produce outputs similar to the one detected in the past (see also [4]). To be less sensitive to noise when calculating the prediction, not only one similar embedding vector is searched for, but M embedding vectors in the past are taken into account: A s-step prediction at time k is calculated, by comparing the past vectors

$$D_{k-i} \in \Re^d \text{ with } i \in \Im , \quad (3)$$

with the actual reference vector D_k. The values for i have to be chosen in a way to fit the borders of the known time series ($\Im = \{s, s+1, ..., k-1-(p-1)h\}$). The past vectors D_{k-i} are also called memory of the prediction algorithm. Depending on the Euclidean distance

$$\delta_i = \left\| D_k - D_{k-i} \right\|_2 \text{ with } i \in \Im \quad (4)$$

the prediction $y'_{k+s} = y'_{k+s}(s, M)$ is calculated by the M best fitting vectors $\{\widetilde{D}_j\}_{j=1,\ldots,M}$ from $\{D_{k-i}\}_{i \in \Im}$ found at the positions f_j with $j = 1,\ldots, M$. The $\{\widetilde{D}_j\}_{j=1,\ldots,M}$ corresponding to the best M matches (M smallest δ_i) can be written as $\widetilde{D}_j = D_{k-f_j}$. The distances are:

$$\widetilde{\delta}_j = \left\| D_k - \widetilde{D}_j \right\|_2 = \delta_{k-f_j} . \quad (5)$$

The estimation y'_{k+s} for y_{k+s} is calculated as

$$y'_{k+s} = \sum_{j=1}^{M} w_j y_{k-f_j+s} . \quad (6)$$

The weights w_j are determined according to:

$$w_j = \frac{1}{N} \frac{1}{\widetilde{\delta}_j} \text{ with } N = \sum_{j=1}^{M} \frac{1}{\widetilde{\delta}_j} . \quad (7)$$

Determination of p and h In [4] several algorithms for calculating p and h are proposed, such as mutual information or autocorrelation. Both are, according to [4], theoretically well-founded for $p = 2$ only; so other solutions have to be found: Since D_k is used for prediction the prediction quality is taken into account to decide if appropriate

©CARS/Springer. All rights reserved.

values for p and h were chosen. To evaluate the prediction quality m predictions are considered. The mean μ_{err} and the standard deviation σ_{err} of the prediction errors $e_l = \left\| y'_l - y_l \right\|_2$ are calculated to evaluate the prediction. Keeping in mind, that $\mu_{err} = \mu_{err}(p,h,\ldots)$ and $\sigma_{err} = \sigma_{err}(p,h,\ldots)$, the parameters p and h are varied to find the best parameters p_{opt} and h_{opt} corresponding to the smallest μ_{err}.

2.2 Local Prediction

The prediction algorithm has to detect and replace outliers reliably. As a result, prediction accuracy is increased, because outliers are removed from the memory D_{k-i} and from the embedding vector D_k. The following scheme detects and replaces outliers reliably: If the prediction error e_k is larger than a threshold C, then y_k is regarded as an outlier and replaced by the predicted value y'_k. An appropriate value for C is the standard deviation (a measure for the variability of HSTs) of the past tracking results. Prediction itself can be seen in Fig. 3, with μ_{err}=1.048 px and σ_{err}=0.974 px. The sensitivity of the prediction quality μ_{err} is, within a certain range for p and h, very low and almost all parameter combinations lead to small prediction errors. It is possible to predict HSTs for more than one step only but as the prediction interval s increases, prediction quality degrades. This happens because the correlation between the last valid point y_k and the point y_{k+s} to be predicted degrades. Results for a five-step prediction ($s = 5$) with $p_{opt} = 12$ and $h_{opt} = 2$ providing the minimal prediction error are μ_{err}=1.49 px and σ_{err}=1.31 px.

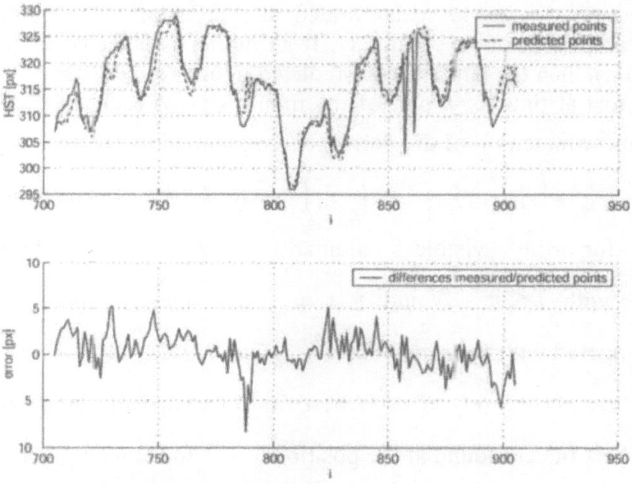

Figure 3: Prediction of HST.
Parameters f_{sample} = 25 Hz, s = 1, M = 1, p = 7, h = 4.

2.3 Global Prediction

As the quality of local prediction degrades with increasing prediction interval s, other solutions to bridge longer occlusions have to be found. Usually, not the entire workspace is occluded (e.g. by an instrument), but only parts of it. Whereas one or a few landmarks are not visible other landmarks still are. The motion of the visible landmarks can be used to estimate the unknown motion of the occluded ones.

The algorithm presented here has two prerequisites: The conditions shown in Sec. 2.1 have to be fulfilled for each landmark. Additionally, the phase (relative motion) between

©CARS/Springer. All rights reserved.

the motion of two landmarks has to remain constant over time. As all landmarks are located on the same organ and move with the same frequencies, this is fulfilled, too.
Instead of one landmark as in Sec. 2.1, N landmarks are considered simultaneously. Their time series' can be written as $y^r = \left[y_n^r; y_{n-1}^r, \ldots, y_1^r\right]^T$ with $1 \le r \le N$. For each landmark the embedding vector D_k^r with $D_k^r = \left[y_k^r, y_{k-h}^r, \ldots, y_{k-(p-1)h}^r\right]^T$ can be built. As before, p denotes the embedding dimension and h the embedding lag. Prediction quality is not very dependent on the embedding parameters p and h (Sec. 2.2), so they are chosen equal for all N landmarks. The measurements y_i considered here, are not scalar-valued any longer, but contain x-position ($t_{x,i}$) and y-position ($t_{y,i}$) of the tracked landmark $y_i = [t_{x,i}, t_{y,i}]^T$. The prediction algorithm presented in Sec. 2.1 can be extended to vector-valued measurements easily and is applied in the same way as to scalar-valued measurements. The outlier detection is applied on each component of y_i separately. If an outlier is detected in one direction (either x- or y-direction), then the landmark is predicted in both directions.
Assuming that landmark a is lost at time k_0, a part of the time series of each landmark which is sufficiently long to allow matching of the corresponding embedding vector D_k^r (see Sec. 2.1), has to be saved: $y_{k_0}^r = \left[y_{k_o-1}^r, y_{k_o-2}^r, \ldots, y_{k_o-1-l}^r\right]^T$, with $l < k_0 - 1$. The actual embedding vectors D_k^r for the visible landmarks have to be built: $D_k^r = \left[y_k^r, y_{k-h}^r, \ldots, y_{k-(p-1)h}^r\right]^T$, with $1 \le r \le N$ and $r \ne a$. As in Sec. 2.1 these embedding vectors have to be compared with their memory $D_{k_0-i}^r$ with i=1,2,…,1-(p-1) h+1, built from the corresponding time series' $y_{k_0}^r$. The M best fits for each valid landmark have to be searched. These M best fits are found at the positions f_j^r and can be given as $y_{k_0-f_j^r}^r$. Their weights w_j^r are computed as shown in Eq. 7. Since some landmarks might be more useful for estimation than others (e.g. closer to the lost landmark), weights u^r for each valid landmark are introduced: $\sum_{r=1, r\ne a}^{N} u^r = 1$ and $u^r \in \Re$. Finally, the estimation for $y_{k_0+s}^a$ with $s \ge 0$ can be calculated by: $y_{k_0+s}^a = \sum_{r=1, r\ne a}^{N} u^r \left(\sum_{j=1}^{M} w_j^r y_{k_0-f_j^r}^a \right)$.

This estimation is based on current values contained in the embedding vectors D_k^r of the valid landmarks, no estimation error accumulates. Therefore, this method is suitable for long-term estimations. Of course, not only one landmark might be lost; the scheme presented here works also if several landmarks are disturbed simultaneously.

Experiments Experimental results of the above presented algorithm are given for landmarks LM10, LM11, and LM8 (Fig.1). As the stabilizer is a rigid body, an affine motion model is well suited and thus tracking of LM10 and LM11 is quite robust and accurate. Landmark 8 is disturbed by three subsequent outliers at $i_{\text{OUT}} \in \{825,826,827\}$

©CARS/Springer. All rights reserved.

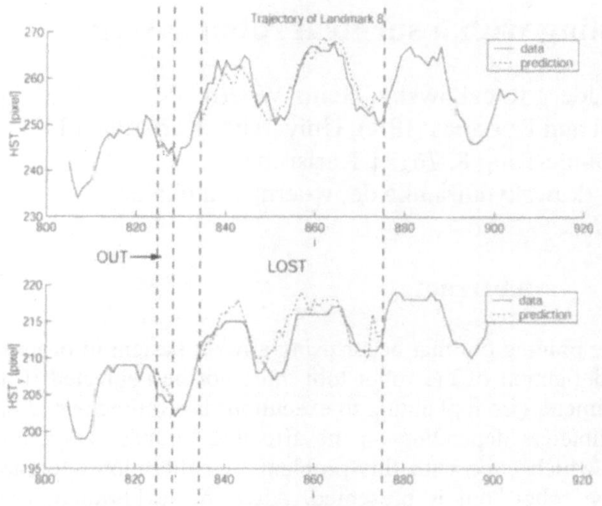

Figure 4: Prediction of Landmark 8.
Parameters: f_{sample} =25 Hz, M =3, p =22, h =13.

and during $i_{LOST} \in \{835,...,875\}$ the trajectory is disturbed for almost two seconds (41 frames), as with short occlusions by surgical instruments. Estimation for LM8 is given in Fig. 4. The weights $u^1 = u^2 = 1/2$ are chosen equally, both landmarks have the same influence on the prediction of LM8. The estimation in x-direction ($\mu_{err,x}$=1.59 px and $\sigma_{err,x}$=1.56 px) is better than in y-direction ($\mu_{err,y}$=2.20 px and $\sigma_{err,y}$=1.83 px).

3. Conclusion and Perspectives

Motion estimation is a highly desirably capability, because it allows autonomous functions as well as motion compensation (Sec. 1). Robust motion estimation in beating heart surgery is possible: Outliers and short occlusions which disturb the underlying tracking scheme can be detected and compensated. This is a first step towards reliable motion compensation allowing new and safe surgery techniques. Additional development is necessary to increase the reliability of the tracking scheme further, by taking other sources of information (e.g. ECG) into account.

Acknowledgement

The authors thank Dr. D. Böhm from the Department of Cardiac Surgery at the University Hospital Hamburg-Eppendorf for providing the video sequences.

References

1. G.S. Guthart and J.K. Salisbury, "The intuitive telesurgery system: Overview and application",in *Proc. IEEE Int. Conf. on Robotics and Automation*, 2000
2. M. Gröger, T. Ortmaier, W. Sepp, and G. Hirzinger, "Tracking local motion on the beating heart", in *SPIE Medical Imaging Conference*, San Diego, February 2002
3. F. Takens, "Detecting strange attractors in turbulence", *Lecture Notes in Mathematics*, vol. 898, pp. 366-381, 1981
4. H. Kantz and T. Schreiber, *Nonlinear Time Series Analysis*. Cambridge University Press, 1997

CARS 2002 – H.U. Lemke, M.W. Vannier; K. Inamura, A.G. Farman, K. Doi & J.H.C. Reiber (Editors)
©CARS/Springer. All rights reserved.

Sensor-aided milling with a surgical robot system

Dirk Engel, Joerg Raczkowsky, Heinz Woern
Institute for Process Control and Robotics (IPR), Universität Karlsruhe (TH)
Engler-Bunte-Ring 8, 76131 Karlsruhe
dengel@ira.uka.de, rkowsky@ira.uka.de, woern@ira.uka.de

Abstract

In this paper sources of errors are pointed out that occur using a robot system in order to cut bones. It is shown that the deflection of the robot tool must not be neglected if an accuracy in the range of one millimeter (from planning to execution) is required, since the tool deflection is up to 1.5 millimeters depending on the affecting torques. Therefore, special focus is set on methods which cope with this problem. A calibration approach considering the deflection of the robot tool is presented. After this calibration, it is possible to consider the tool deflection during the registration procedure (ball-in-cone strategy) as well as during the intervention. Furthermore, a discrete feed control algorithm is outlined.

Keywords: Robot-assisted surgery, sensor control

1. Introduction

The main purposes of a surgical robot system are on the one hand the support for the surgeon and on the other hand the improvement of the surgical result. Thereby, the safety of the patient, the surgeon, and the medical staff are presumed [1, 2]. Unlike the surgeon, the robot controller has direct access to the planning data. Further, the robot arm provides high repeat accuracy and high precision independent of the progress of operation time. Hence, the greatest benefit of a robot system in the operating theater is the gain in quality. The presented methods and implementations are part of the surgical robot system "RobaCKa" for craniofacial surgery, which has been developed at our institute. The robot assistance in craniofacial surgery is reasonable because of the vicinity to vital parts and the great impact of bone repositionings at the human skull to the later appearance of the patient. In the following sections, sources of errors, which have to be considered developing an accurate surgical robot system as well as our methods of solution are discussed.

For the measurement of process data and for system surveillance the robot system is equipped with several sensors (Fig. 1). The robot tool consists of: pneumatic collision protection (CP), force-/torque sensor (FTS), rigid body equipped with infrared LEDs to be tracked by an optical navigation system, and surgical milling cutter. The CP is a fail safe electrical/mechanical system without any data measurement. Additionally, the FTS acquires the exact forces and torques which are transmitted to a sensor data processing computer. This serial arrangement, CP followed by FTS, and the resulting elasticity are the main sources of the occurring tool deflection. A CP with a trigger sensibility of 0.2°

©CARS/Springer. All rights reserved.

causes an excursion of up to 1 mm at the tool tip (given tool length 300 mm), for example. Since the patient position is determined during the registration procedure using the robot as measuring device, the deflection error impairs not only the quality of the trajectory execution, but also the quality of registration.

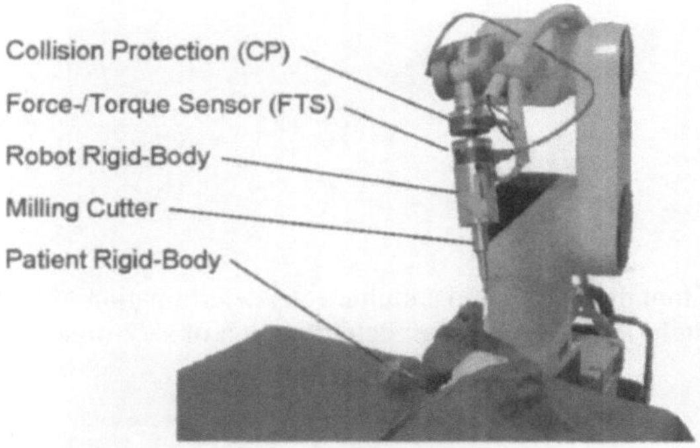

Fig.1: RobaCKa system set-up, robot and sensors

2. Determination of tool deflection

The determination of the tool deflection is performed at the same time when the physical tool dimension is calibrated. In order to compute the tool length, the robot has to be guided above a calibration body (e.g. a metal cube), from where the robot moves down until a contact state was reached. This procedure is conducted in three steps:

1. Tool is in perpendicular configuration
2. Tool is -45° angled around x-axis
3. Tool is +45° angled around x-axis

The tool length can be computed as: $l = (2+\sqrt{2})\Delta h$, $\Delta h = h_{90^\circ} - 0.5(h_{-45^\circ} + h_{+45^\circ})$. Δh is the difference of height in the different contact states, measured along the robot z-axis (Fig. 2, left). The moment of contact of the perpendicular configuration is detected by the increase of the total force. To avoid a bending of the tool in the angled configurations the contact state is assumed when the torque around the x-axis is equal zero, $T_x = 0$.

For the calibration of the tool tip offset along the x- and y-axis, the robot tool is guided to the left side of the calibration body (Fig. 2, right). In the following, the robot moves its tool to contact the calibration body with the tip, detaches after contact and turns its tool 90° around the z-axis. This procedure is repeated four times until the calibration body was contacted in positive and negative x-/y-direction. Afterwards, the physical tool dimension is known. For the determination of the tool deflection d_x and d_y, the robot continues moving its tool after a detected x-/y-contact in the same direction until a previously adjusted maximal torque is reached. In this way, to each measured torque a corresponding deflection can be assigned. The change of the tool length d_z can be neglected because of $d_{x,y} \ll l$. Fig. 3 depicts the correlation of the measured torques $T_{x,y}$ and the corresponding

©CARS/Springer. All rights reserved.

tool deflection $d_{y,x}$. The graph shows also that the corre ation can be linear approximated by $d_x = c_{xy}\,T_y$ and $d_y = c_{yx}\,T_x$ (c_{xy}, c_{yx}: constant factors).

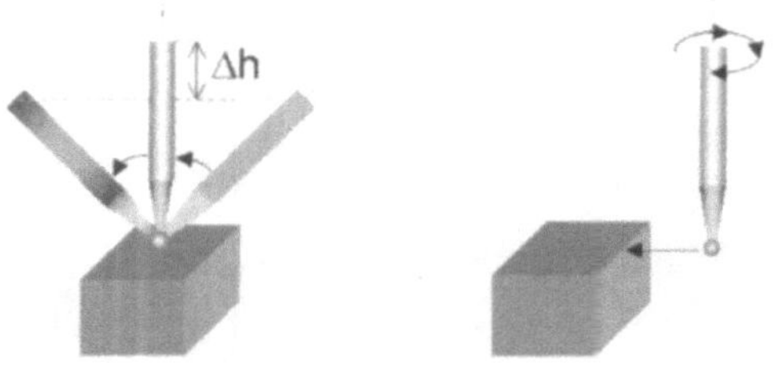

Fig.2: Calibration of tool dimension and simultaneous determination of tool deflection. First step: calculation of tool length (left). Second step: determination of x-/y-offset and tool deflection (right)

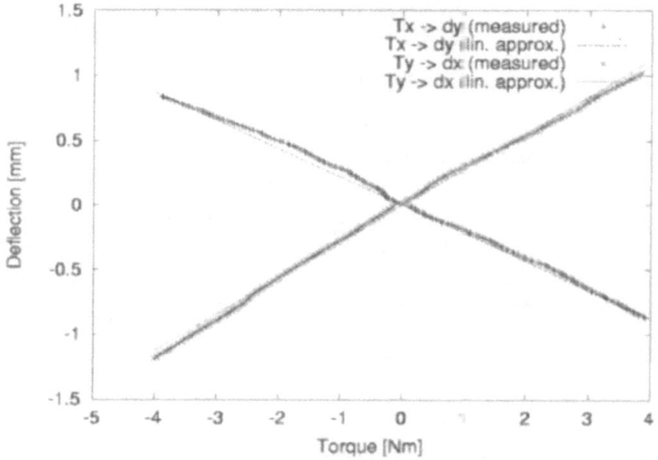

Fig. 3: Correlation of affecting torque and tool deflection. The correlation can be linear approximated by $d_x = c_y\,T_y$ and $d_y = c_x\,T_x$ ($c_{x,y}$: constant factors)

3. Registration

The role of registration is to establish the spatial relationship (via a transformation matrix) registration) between the planning data and the real patient [3]. Therefore, four titanium screws are implanted preopratively into the patient skull before the CT scans are taken. The positions of these four fiducial landmarks are preoperatively determined in the 3D-patient-model based on CT slices; and also intraoperatively by guiding the robot tool to the screw positions (ball-in-cone strategy) [4]. The calculation of the transformation matrix is done by "Least-Squares Fitting" [5]. After the registration, the intraoperative robot pathways of the planned cut trajectories are known, because the planning was performed in relation to the same coordinate system which was used for the preoperative screw position determination.

©CARS/Springer. All rights reserved.

As aforementioned, the position of the landmarks are determined intraoperatively by guiding the robot force-controlled to the screw positions. However, the robot follows the user who pushes and pulls the robot tool - in order to be safe against tremor and unintended hitches - very slowly and only if the forces exceed lower limits. Because of this matter of fact, a remaining bending stress is possible between the FTS and the tool tip placed in the screw cone. Such a stress causes an error while measuring the landmark position using the internal robot resolvers. In order to compensate this error, an offset vector **d** = $(d_x, d_y, 0)^T$ corresponding to the remaining torques is added to the measured landmark position. An example for the compensation of a registration error caused by the tool deflection is depicted in Fig. 4.

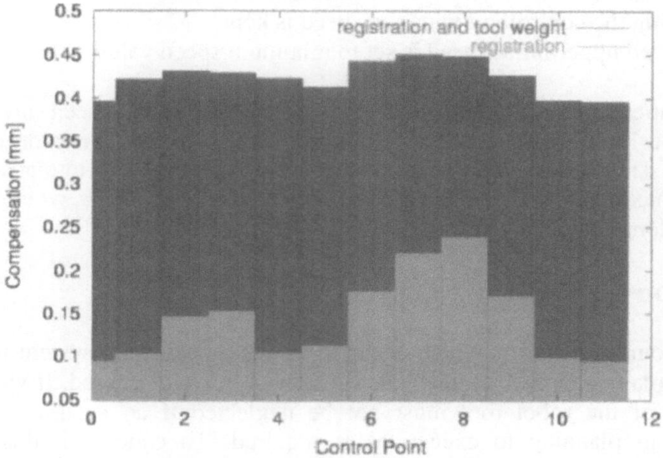

Fig. 4 Correction distances to compensate the tool deflection during registration procedure (light grey) and additional compensation of tool deflection caused by tool weight (dark grey). Data refer to cut trajectory depicted in Fig. 5

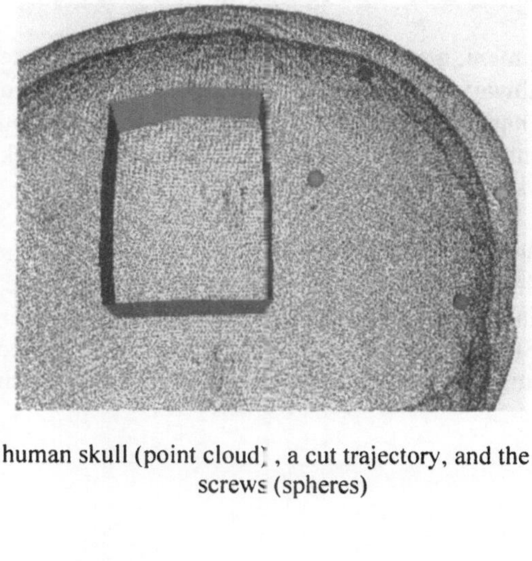

Fig. 5 3D-model of a human skull (point cloud), a cut trajectory, and the positions of the titanium screws (spheres)

©CARS/Springer. All rights reserved.

4. Execution of a cut trajectory

After the registration, when the patient position in relation to the robot base is known, the robot tool orientation can be calculated in every point of the planned trajectory. Hence, it is possible to consider the deflection caused by the weight of the tool before the actual execution of the cut trajectory starts (Fig. 4, Fig. 5). During the cutting process the feed of the robot tool is controlled with a discrete controlling algorithm. The forces are kept in a controlling window with a lower and an upper limit. This controlling algorithm knows three states:

1. Torques less than lower limit, speed is increased.
2. Torques within the controlling window, speed is kept
3. Torques exceed upper limit, speed is set to minimum speed value

Furthermore, the tool acceleration and the cutting depth has been investigated. An acceleration too high causes a sidewise tool deflection into the direction of the milling cutter rotation. The successive increasing speed takes this behavior into account. In order to reduce the maximal forces, a cut can be performed in several steps, whereby the milling cutter is lead along the planned trajectory in different depths.

5. Conclusions and future work

In this paper sources of errors which occur using a surgical robot system in order to cut bones were explained as well as methods of solution were discussed. It was shown, that the deflection of the robot tool must not be neglected if an accuracy of about one millimeter (from planning to execution) is required. To cope with this problem the calibration of the robot tool, a discrete feed control and a method which takes the deflection of the robot tool into account were presented. The consideration of the tool deflection increases the accuracy of the registration as well as the execution of the planned trajectory. Additionally, the feed control of the milling cutter is an important factor to reduce the tool deflection and to act with consideration for the patient fixation.

In a next step of development, a real-time compensation of the tool deflection is intended. Therefore, the robot pathway should be adapted respectively to the occurring torques by an online control mechanism. Furthermore, it is planned to counterbalance micro-movements of the patient by simultaneous consideration of the tracking data yielded by the optical navigation system.

The overall system was tested with dummies, in animal experiments, and also in a preliminary test with a human test subject using a pen instead of the milling cutter. This subject test took place in an operating theater of our research partner, the Department of Oral and Maxillofacial Surgery - University of Heidelberg, and proved the applicability of the robot system. First surgical interventions will be performed later this year.

©CARS/Springer. All rights reserved.

Acknowledgements

This research has been performed at the Institute for Process Control and Robotics headed by Prof. Dr.-Ing. H. Woern at the University of Karlsruhe, Germany. The work has been funded by the German Research Foundation (Deutsche Forschungsgemeinschaft), as it is part of the collaborative research center SFB 414: "Information Technology in Medicine – Computer and Sensor Aided Surgery".

References

1. Davies, B. L.: "A Discussion of Safety Issues for Medical Robots", *Computer-Integrated Surgery – Technology and Clinical Applications*, pp. 287-296, The MIT Press, 1996.
2. Engel, D., Raczkowsky, J., Woern, H.: "A Safe Robot System for Craniofacial Surgery", *IEEE International Conference on Robotics and Automation*, pp. 2020-2024, Seoul, Korea, 2001.
3. Simon, D.: "What is 'Registration' and Why is it so Important in CAOS?", *Proceedings of the First Joint CVRMed / MRCAS Conference*, pp. 57-60, June, 1997.
4. Kazanzides, P., Zuhars, J., Mittelstadt, B., Taylor, R. H.: "Force Sensing and Control for a Surgical Robot", *IEEE International Conference on Robotics and Automation*, pp. 612-617, Nice, France, 1992.
5. Arun, K. S., Huang, T. S., Blostein, S. D.: "Least-Squares Fitting of Two 3-D Point Sets", IEEE Transactions on Pattern Analysis and Machine Intelligence, pp. 698-670, Vol. PAMI-9, No. 5, 1997.

©CARS/Springer. All rights reserved.

Software architecture for robotically assisted and image-guided minimally invasive interventions

Kevin Cleary[a], Alexandru Patriciu[b,c], Sheng Xu[c],
Mihai Mocanu[a,d], Dan Stoianovici[b,c]
[a]Imaging Science and Information Systems (ISIS) Center, Radiology Department, 2115 Wisconsin Avenue, Suite 603, Georgetown University Medical Center, Washington, DC, USA
[b]URobotics Laboratory, Urology Department, Johns Hopkins Medical Institutions, Baltimore, MD, USA
[c]NSF-funded Center for Computer Integrated Surgical Systems andTechnologies, Johns Hopkins University, Baltimore, MD, USA
[d]Department of Software Engineering, University of Craiova, Romania

Abstract

Although more sophisticated software and hardware components are becoming available, technology for the operating room and interventional suite can be slow to change. The integration of vendor specific software and hardware components remains difficult, and the resulting systems are limited in reuse, flexibility, interoperability, and maintainability. One potential solution to this problem is to develop open software architectures as a platform for rapidly integrating new technologies into the operating room. In an ongoing effort to develop modular software architectures for systems designed to assist in minimally invasive interventions, two systems are outlined here: a "needle driver" robot and an image-guided surgery system based of magnetic tracking of internal organ motion. To date, the robot system has been used to complete a cadaver study of nerve and facet block placement under joystick control of the interventionalist. The image-guided surgery system has been used in phantom studies of liver needle placement. Potential future developments include fluoroscopy servoing in which the robot will automatically align the needle along the C-arm trajectory and the integration of the robot and tracking systems.

Keywords: Medical robotics, image-guided surgery, minimally invasive interventions

1. Introduction

Minimally invasive procedures are rapidly growing in popularity, due to the substantially reduced trauma for the patient. As part of these procedures, there are many clinical situations where precise manipulation of instruments is important. Novel integrated systems incorporating tracking, visualization, and robotics, may enable the physician to more accurately target hard-to-reach anatomy as well as target the anatomy directly from the images themselves.

Image guidance has been used in one form or another in various medical procedures since the first applications of ionizing radiation. However, during the last decade there has been

©CARS/Springer. All rights reserved.

a continuous and marked increase in interest in this field, which can be largely attributed to developments in imaging algorithms and increased computer power [1]. Percutaneous needle and instrument placement has also become an essential part of diagnostic and therapeutic modalities. However, software architectures for the integration of imaging, localization, and robotic instrumentation have not been investigated except in a very few research centers. For example, current surgical navigation systems usually employ proprietary software interfaces with fixed instrument types.

The goal of software architectures for these systems is to facilitate the development of applications for the interventional environment. The long-term goal of the research program at Georgetown is to develop an integrated system to enable the next generation of minimally invasive interventions. Within this project, a flexible, component-based software framework plays a central role. Since its development is a cooperation between medical imaging and robotics experts at Georgetown and Johns Hopkins Medical Centers, a systematic process for software development is needed. This includes software development based on formal specifications, advanced methods for software design (UML), source code control (SourceSafe), rapid application development in high-level object-oriented languages (C++), and use of documentation tools (Doxygen).

A related effort is the 3D Slicer for surgical planning and intraoperative visualization [4]. The 3D Slicer is freely available, open-source software for visualization, registration, segmentation, and quantification of medical data. The Slicer is an ongoing collaboration between the MIT Artificial Intelligence Lab and the Surgical Planning Lab at Brigham & Women's Hospital, an affiliate of Harvard Medical School. The Center for Computer Integrated Surgical Systems and Technologies at Johns Hopkins University has also been working to extend Slicer to include robot control, among other functionality.

2. Specifications and Methods

Large software applications are typically built in layers. At the lowest level, our architecture includes proprietary, vendor-specific software levels for individual hardware components such as a motion control card and watchdog timer. On top of this level, we build a higher level application programming interface (API). At the highest level is the user interface. Our application is built on C and C++ based libraries including the Motion Engineering Incorporated (MEI) DSP-Series Motion Control Library, the Matrox Imaging Library (MIL), and the Visualization ToolKit (VTK) from Kitware [2].

2.1. Robot Control Library

An object-oriented software library for robot control, denoted URoboticsLib, has been designed and implemented by the URobotics Laboratory at Johns Hopkins. This library was built on the MEI Motion Control Library and is meant for high-level control of a new generation of robots such as the one in Figure 1. The library was defined and tested as a API using object oriented methodologies including the uniform modelling language (UML) tool Visual Modeller for design and Visual C++ for coding. When developing this library, attention was paid to portability (the core part of the library does not use Microsoft Foundation Classes (MFC)), flexibility and ease of use (all functions are based on engineering units such as millimeters), ease of progress towards a wide range of

©CARS/Springer. All rights reserved.

applications, an efficient and simple user interface, and support for calibration and use in clinical studies.

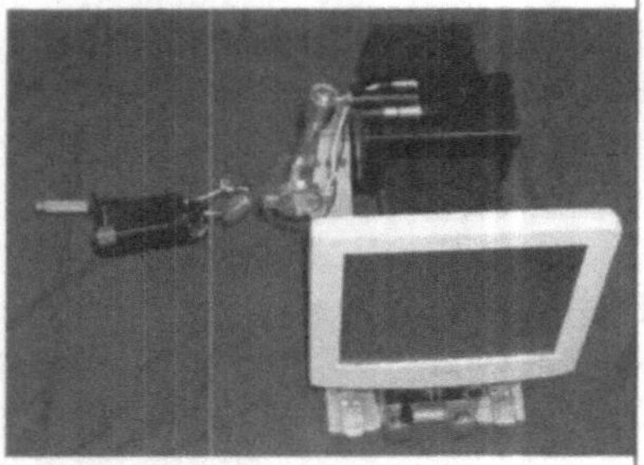

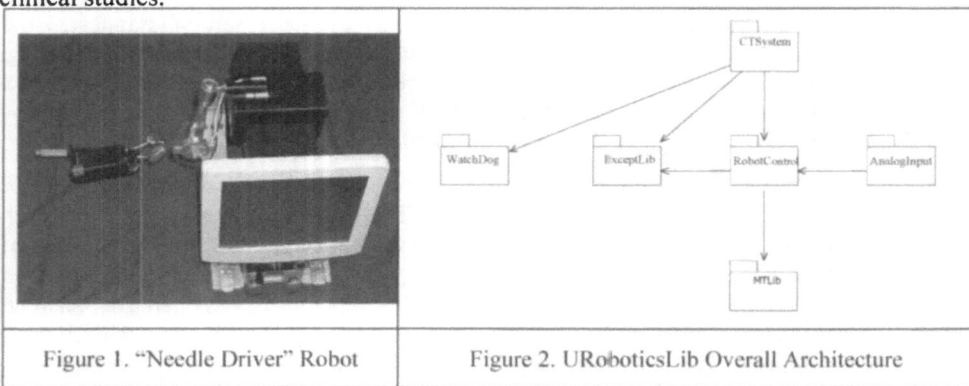

Figure 1. "Needle Driver" Robot

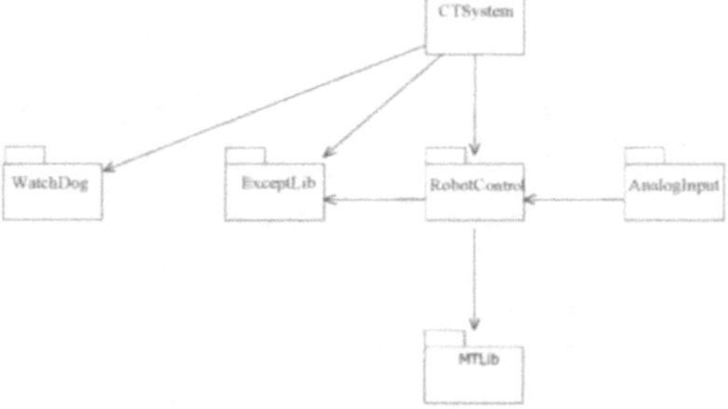

Figure 2. URoboticsLib Overall Architecture

The overall architecture of the URoboticsLib library is shown in Figure 2. Packages include classes for basic robot control, safety features (WatchDog), real-time control (CMEICard), support classes for error reporting and handling (ExceptLib) or for multithreading and access synchronization (MTLib). The overriding goals were that

1) the library must not be tied to a specific motion card; and
2) the library has to be easy to reconfigure and extend.

There were several other key requirements including platform independence, parallel execution speed achieved by multithreading, real-time monitoring accomplished through the use of specialized hardware, and the ability to specify a user-defined control loop.

A generic interface to a motion control card was developed as shown in Figure 3. This included generic "disconnected" interfaces such as CMotionControlCard, CAnalogInputCard, and CDigitalIOCard. While the Motion Engineering Inc. card was used in our application, the library is designed so that another card may be easily substitute

2.2. Imaging Libraries

The fact that C code can be combined seamlessly with new C++ code has been a major advantage. Migration from C to C++ has not required us to discard or rewrite functional C code. Many commercial frameworks, and even some components of the Standard Library itself, are built upon legacy C code that is wrapped in an object-oriented interface. We have chosen a similar approach, using both C and C++ libraries in object-oriented imaging applications [3].

The device-independent Matrox Imaging Library (MIL) is a high-level C library with an extensive set of optimized functions for image processing (point-to-point, statistics, filtering, morphology, geometric transforms), pattern matching, blob analysis, gauging, OCR, bar and matrix code recognition, and calibration. We are using MIL to accelerate the development of medical imaging and image analysis applications, such as fluoroscopy servoing for robot control.

The Visualization ToolKit (VTK) is an open source, freely available software system used as a graphics engine for image processing and visualization. VTK consists of a C++ class

©CARS/Springer. All rights reserved.

library, and several interpreted interface layers such as Tcl/Tk. VTK supports a wide variety of visualization algorithms including scalar, vector, tensor, texture, and volumetric methods. Advanced modelling techniques such as implicit modelling, polygon reduction, mesh smoothing, cutting and contouring are also included.

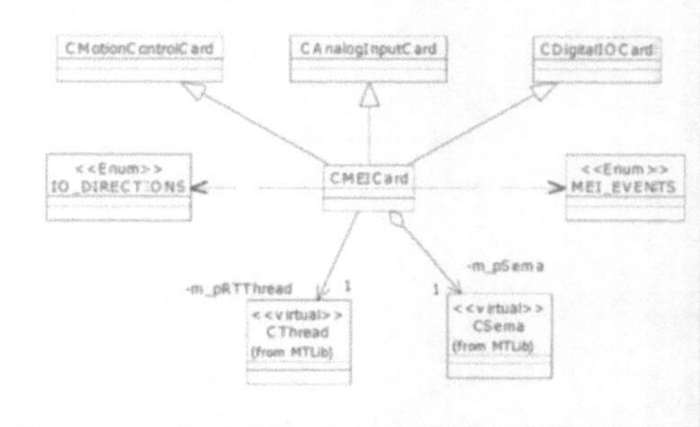

Figure 3. Robot Motion Control

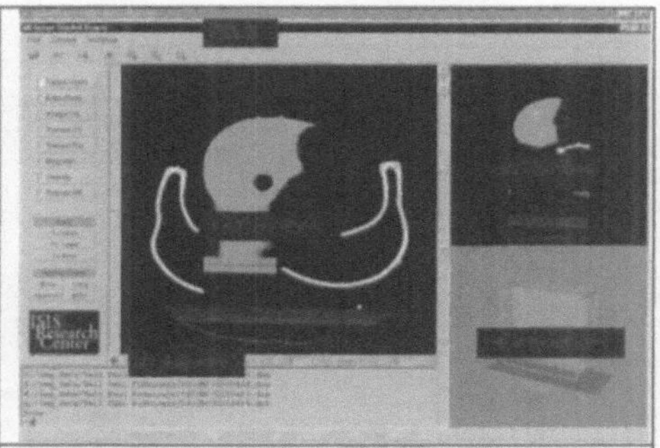

Figure 4. User Interface for IGBiopsy

3. Image-Guided System Architecture

IGBiopsy is a system developed at Georgetown incorporating magnetic tracking for image guidance during minimally invasive abdominal interventions. An image-guided surgery system typically provides a method for registration of pre-operative images to the physical space of the patient, a user interface that display images and the position of instruments, and a computer workstation that runs the application. Unlike image-guided surgical systems based on bony landmarks, the IGBiopsy system is designed to be applied to internal organs such as the liver that move with respiration. This means that some method of tracking and/or modelling respiratory motion is required, as well as a means for targeting the anatomy as it moves during respiration. The IGBiopsy system incorporates a magnetically tracked catheter that is part of the AURORA™ magnetic tracking system from Northern Digital, Inc. Preliminary results to date using a specially designed liver respiratory motion simulator show that this approach may be feasible for future image-guided liver interventions. In the long term, interfacing this tracking system with the robot software described previously could provide a system capable of compensating for respiratory motion and precisely placing a needle in a breathing subject.

The IGBiopsy user interface is shown in Figure 4 which also has labels indicating the major classes. The magnetically tracked catheter indicates the current position of the liver and can also provide the physician with a visual cue to indicate the right time for placing the needle. In the most recent version of the software, a targeting window was added to help the user align the needle based on the skin entry point and angle of approach. A depth control indicator was also added. This grouping of targeting window and depth indicator should help even an inexperienced physician to precisely drive the needle to the target.

©CARS/Springer. All rights reserved.

Key software issues addressed in the design of the IGBiopsy system included portability, platform independence, and parallel execution speed achieved by pipelining. The class levels used in the development are shown in Figure 5.

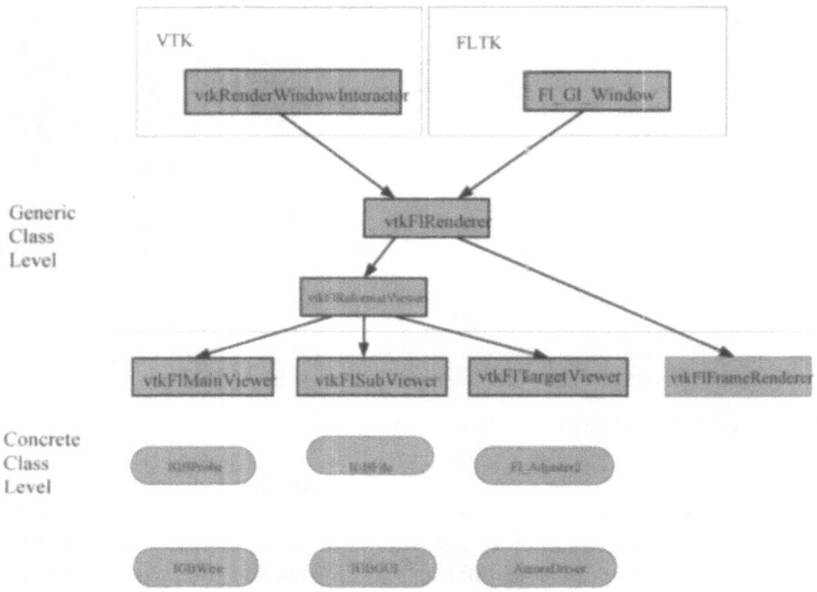

Figure 5. Hierarchy Chart for the Image-Guided Surgery System

The object-oriented design for the system is based on a formal and iterative process of decomposing requirements by objects rather than by functions through multiple design cycles. The generic steps performed are:

- Identification of main objects that describe entities and processes in the environment.
- Definition of views that will be used to present those objects to users.
- Determination of interactions between entity and process objects required to accomplish specific tasks.

This design process was applied from the initial development of the system. This led to a design decision to base the system on software libraries currently in widespread use: OpenGL, Visualization Toolkit (VTK), Fast Light Tool Kit (FLTK), in which:

- Upper entries form the VTK-FLTK (-OpenGL) "basement" of the system, i.e. vtkFlRenderWindowInteractor class used to attach and enable VTK to render to and interact with a FLTK window, or Fl_Gl_Window – the FLTK (-OpenGL) window group class.
- Intermediate entries indicate generic elements supported in an abstract manner in the system, i.e. vtkFlRenderer.
- Lower entries contain concrete elements, their role may be seen in "transforming" the view, i.e. vtkFlReformatViewer – which contains functions for "marching

©CARS/Springer. All rights reserved.

through" the volume, or in "selecting" a view or working with specialized views, i.e. vtkFlMainViewer, vtkFlSubViewer or vtkFlTargetViewer.

- Also at a lower level in the object-oriented design of Image-guided Biopsy System we placed classes like IGBFile (file input/output) and IGBProbe/IGBAurora (acquire probe/catheter data from the magnetic tracker).

4. Conclusion

Minimally invasive image-guided surgery is increasingly popular as it can considerably reduce trauma for the patient. Robotic systems may provide increased precision in performing surgical interventions, and may be integrated with image-guided surgery systems for targeting purposes. The integration of the software parts of such components, similar to those described in this paper, may lead to the development of novel interventional techniques. To date, software testing has shown good robustness and safety performance. Although some preliminary clinical experiments have been completed, more clinical studies are still required to further investigate the advantages and disadvantages of this system for interventional procedures.

The lifecycle of the software system described here is expected to include a short initial development phase (08/01 to 4/02), a longer phase of product support and refinement, and extensive testing from the customer (physician) perspective. A formal software development and change control process is also needed to ensure reliable and usable systems.

Acknowledgements

This work was funded by U.S. Army grant DAMD17-99-1-9022. The content of this manuscript does not necessarily reflect the position or policy of the U.S. Government.

References

1. Viergever, M. A., "Image guidance of therapy", *IEEE Transactions on Medical Imaging*, 17(5), 669-671, 1998.
2. Schroeder W., Martin K., Lorensen B., *The Visualization Toolkit - An Object-Oriented Approach To 3D Graphics*, Prentice Hall, 1998.
3. Elder, M. C., Knight, J. C. "Specifying User Interfaces for Safety-Critical Medical Systems," *Medical Robotics and Computer Assisted Surgery*, Wiley-Liss, 1995, pp. 148-155.
4. Gering, D.T., et al. "An Integrated Visualization System for Surgical Planning and Guidance using Image Fusion and Interventional Imaging", *Medical Image Computing and Computer-Assisted Intervention-MICCAI* 1999, Springer, pp. 809-819.

©CARS/Springer. All rights reserved.

Effect of video streaming delay on telemedicine based on the surgical cockpit system

Kenta Hori[a], Tomohiro Kuroda[ab], Hiroshi Oyama[ab], Yasuhiko Ozaki[b], Takehiko Nakamura[a], Takashi Takahashi[ab]
[a] Department of Medical Informatics, Kyoto University Hospital, 54, Kawara-cho, Shogoin, Sakyo, Kyoto, 606-8507, JAPAN
[b] Graduate School of Informatics, Kyoto University, Yoshida-Honmachi, Sakyo, Kyoto, 606-8501, JAPAN

Abstract

Live video streaming technology is indispensable for collaboration on telemedicine. The live video streaming technology plays important roles for tele-operation and tele-communication between a tele-operating console room and a remote operating room. However, network transmission delay is unavoidable problem in live video streaming technology. The main theme of the research is to evaluate effect of live video streaming delay for robot drivability and mental effect of given view in telesurgery. Target-pointing task was performed via tele-operating master-slave manipulator in the Surgical Cockpit System. The subjects were 27 of 5th grade medical students that had no experience of tele-robot manipulation. Drivability of a robot was measured by physically and sensory evaluation. Mental effect of given view was measured by sensory evaluation. Video-streaming delay declined accuracy of robot motion control and reduced speed of tele-robot operation. The subjects felt incongruous sense of given view, difficulty of robot control, and uneasiness of spatial recognition under video delayed condition. The video presentation with approximately 0.5 seconds of live video streaming delay causes stresses and strains of a tele-operating surgeon for delicate manipulation of a tele-surgery robot.

Keywords: Telesurgery, live video streaming, network delay

1. Introduction

In telesurgery, a tele-operating surgeon to operate a surgical robot placed in a room, called "operator site", is spatially separated from a patient and other surgical staffs in a remote operating room, called "operation site". Information network connecting the two sites enable the surgeon to operate the patient. The surgeon needs to understand motion of surgical instruments, condition of the patient, and other status in the operation site. For faultless collaboration among the surgeon, surgical staffs and surgical robots, communication must include environmental information of the operation site, such as behavior of robots and staffs, vital information of a patient, and so on.

The authors have been developing a telesurgery support system named "Surgical Cockpit System" for surgeons in operator site[1]. The Surgical Cockpit System consists of three fundamental subsystems, operating-field subsystem, robot subsystem, and surgical-

©CARS/Springer. All rights reserved.

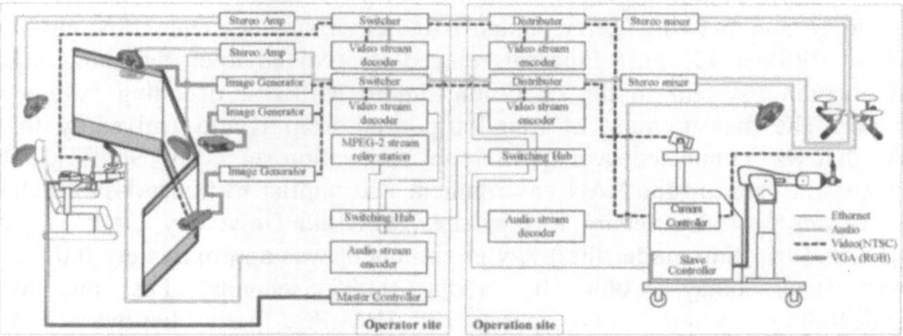

Fig. 1: Prototype of the Surgical Cockpit System

environment subsystem. The operating-field subsystem provides view around operating field and target organs. The robot subsystem supports manipulation of surgical robots, tele-instruction tools and other tools for telesurgery. The surgical-environment subsystem, the peculiarity of the Surgical Cockpit System, provides multi-purpose information display system, which visualizes any kinds of additional information such as panoramic view of the operating room, multi-angle presentation of the target of the patient, virtual surgeon guides, vital information of the patient and so on. This research focuses on information supporting methodologies on the surgical-environment subsystem.

Live video transmission is indispensable for the operating-field subsystem and the surgical-environment subsystem. However, delay of live video transmission is large. Total system delay of tele-robotic surgery consists of delay of robot control command transmission and stream video transmission. Live video streaming delay is larger than delay of robot control command transmission. Therefore, to evaluate effect of video streaming delay on telemedicine is equivalent to evaluation of effect of information network delay.

The purpose of this study is to evaluate effect of video streaming delay on tele-operation via the Surgical Cockpit System. This report discusses effect of live video streaming delay caused by information network transmission and video compression delay for telemedicine.

2. Methods

Effect of video streaming delay was evaluated via pseudo-tele-robotic surgery by using prototype of the Surgical Cockpit System (Fig. 1). To evaluate effect of video streaming delay, the experiment was performed under three conditions of delay time: no-delay condition, wired-suburbs condition, and satellite condition.

In the no-delay condition, live video was presented with no delay. A camera in the operation site and a display system in the operator site were connected directly with a video cable. The no-delay condition assumed that the operator site was in the next room of the operation site.

©CARS/Springer. All rights reserved.

In the wired-suburbs condition, video-streaming delay consisted of MPEG-2 encoding and decoding delay and network delay under LAN environment. The LAN environment consisted of 100Base-TX Fast Ethernet relayed by two ethernet switching hub from MPEG-2 encoding system in the operation site to MPEG-2 decoding system in the operator site. The measurement of round trip time from Kyoto University to Osaka University that was connected over the Internet connection served by SINET[2] showed that transmission delay in the LAN environment was similar to transmission delay over the Internet from Kyoto University, Kyoto, Japan, to Osaka University, Osaka, Japan. The measured round trip time under the LAN environment was approximately 0.01 seconds, and transmission delay would be about 0.005 seconds. For the MPEG-2 encoding/decoding system, two pairs of IBM-PC with hardware MPEG-2 encoding/decoding boards were used. The GOP (Group of Picture) consisted of only I Frames. As the specification of the MPEG-2 encoding/decoding board, the buffer size was decided independently of the GOP pattern. The measurement of MPEG-2 encoding and decoding time shows that the delay of MPEG-2 encoding and decoding is about 0.5 seconds. A camera was connected to the MPEG-2 encoding system. MPEG-2 streaming data output from the MPEG-2 encoding system was transmitted to MPEG-2 decoding system through the LAN. Video image output from the MPEG-2 decoding system was presented by display system. Total delay time of the wired-suburbs condition was approximately 0.5 seconds.

In the satellite condition, satellite-communication delay was appended to the delay of the wired-suburbs condition. The MPEG-2 streaming data was transmitted through a relay station. In the relay station, the MPEG-2 streaming data received from the MPEG-2 encoding system was relayed to the MPEG-2 decoding system after buffered in 0.25 seconds. The measurement of round trip time from Kyoto University, Kyoto, Japan, to Asian Institute of Technology, Pathumthani, Thailand, which was connected over satellite communication served by AI3 project[3] showed that approximate transmission delay over satellite communication was 0.25 seconds. Therefore, the satellite-communication delay was decided to be 0.25 seconds. Total delay time of the satellite condition was approximately 0.75 seconds.

A task scenario of the experiment was a target-pointing task that assumed brain centesis for biopsy. A subject tried to apply the tip of the instrument to a target area. The target area was 1.5 centimeters in diameter. The subject was instructed to adjust the instrument perpendicularly on the target area. Subjects were 27 of 5th grade medical school students in Kyoto University. The conditions were evaluated by comparing location/posture of the instrument at the end of a task (final posture) and time to finish a task (task achievement time), and by sensory evaluation of usability. Final posture was evaluated based on error angle between the normal line on the target area and direction of the instrument at the final posture. Task achievement time was defined as whole process time of the task. Final posture and task achievement time were analysed with non-parametric test (Mann-Whitney test) by using SPSS. The rejection ratio was 0.05.

As sensory evaluation of usability, an incongruous sense of given view, difficulty of robot control, and easiness of spatial recognition were evaluated by cyclic paired comparison [4]. For the cyclic paired comparison, evaluation order of conditions should be in cyclic

©CARS/Springer. All rights reserved.

order. In the experiments, experimented conditions were sequentially occurred in order of no-delay condition, wired-suburbs condition, satellite condition and no-delay condition

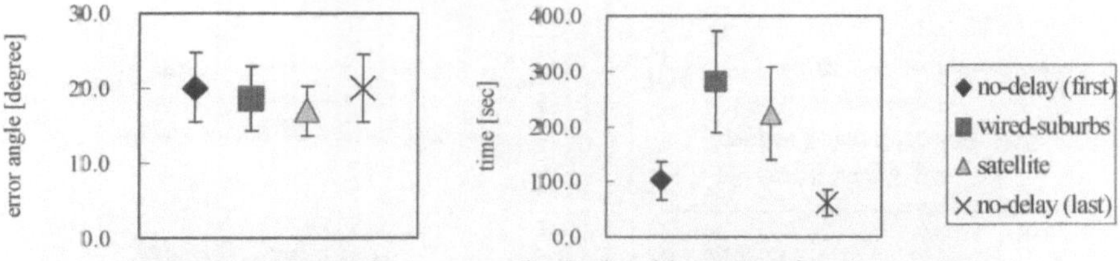

(a) Final posture (b) Task achievement time

Fig. 2: The results of physical evaluation

Conditions	Final posture	Task achievement time
no-delay(first) - wired-suburbs	0.631	0.000*
wired-suburbs - satellite	0.938	0.133
no-delay (first) - no-delay (last)	0.718	0.006*

* significantly different ($\alpha < 0.05$)

Table 1. Significance probablity

for each subject. The last no-delay condition could be used to evaluate the learning effect for evaluation of final posture and task achievement time. The rejection ratio was 0.05.

3. Results

Final posture is shown in Fig. 2(a). All conditions were not statistically different in error angle. The results showed that the accuracy of the final posture was not affected by video streaming delay. However, the standard deviation under large delayed conditions tended to be smaller than the standard deviation under small delayed conditions. The result indicates that delicate control was required in large delay, and a subject should be careful to control the robot. The first and the last no-delayed conditions were not statistically different. Result shows that experience had no effect on the final posture.

Figure 2(b) shows task achievement time. Task achievement time under no-delay conditions was significantly shorter than wired-suburbs conditions and satellite conditions. Wired-suburbs conditions and satellite conditions were not significantly different for task achievement time. The task achievement time of the last no-delay conditions was significantly smaller than the first no-delay conditions. The result shows that learning effect affected for task achievement time.

In sensory evaluation of the experiment, main effect and order effect were estimated. The minimum of estimated unbiased variance was used as an error value. In the experiment, total order effect was minimum and was regarded as an error. Two data were rejected by

©CARS/Springer. All rights reserved.

the large order effect. Sensory evaluation shows that estimated order was significant in

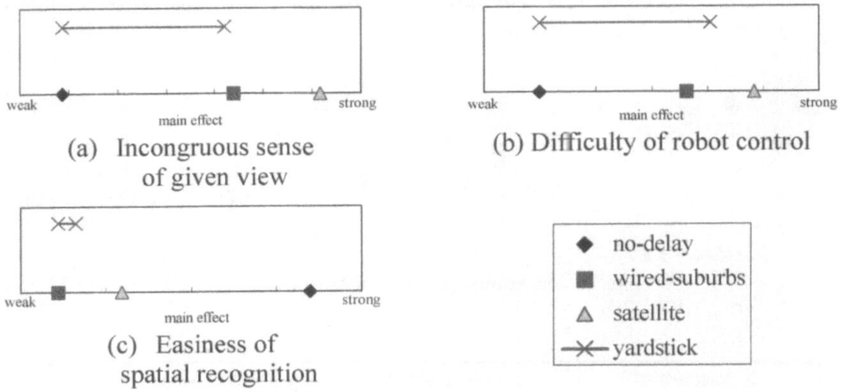

Fig. 3: The results of sensory evaluation

each evaluation of incongruous sense of given view, difficulty of robot control and easiness of spatial recognition. The results are shown in Fig. 3.

Incongruous sense of given view was significantly more incongruous under wired-suburbs conditions and satellite conditions than no-delay conditions. Wired-suburbs conditions were not significantly different from satellite conditions. The estimated degree of incongruous shows wired-suburbs conditions tend to be positioned between no-delay conditions and satellite conditions. The relations were similar for delay time and estimated degree.

For difficulty of robot control, no-delay conditions were significantly better than satellite conditions. Wired-suburbs conditions were not significantly different from no-delay conditions and satellite conditions, but wired-suburbs conditions tended to have worse drivability the no-delay conditions and better than satellite conditions. The results showed that video streaming delay obviously affected for robot drivability

For easiness of spatial recognition, significant difference was confirmed in each pair of the experimented conditions. No-delay conditions were significantly easier for spatial recognition than wired-suburbs and satellite conditions. Wired-suburbs conditions were more difficult for spatial recognition than satellite conditions. The result indicates that different mechanisms would be applied for spatial recognition by given view between small delayed conditions and large delayed conditions.

As the results of the experiment, delay between robot control command and video presentation of the robot motion caused for incongruous sense of given view and speed of robot operation should be reduced. The subjects felt difficult to control the robot by the incongruousness of given view. A subject should concentrate on delicate control of the robot under incongruousness of video presentation and declined robot drivability under delayed video streaming.

©CARS/Springer. All rights reserved.

4. Conclusion

In this research, the effect of delayed video streaming was evaluated. The delay of live video streaming is unavoidable problem in telesurgery. The evaluation of delay effect is required for designing a telesurgery support system, such as multi-angle presentation around operating-field on the surgical-environment subsystem of the Surgical Cockpit System. Effect of video streaming delay was evaluated with final posture of surgical instruments, whole process time of a tele-surgical operation, and sensory evaluation of system usability.

As the results of the experiment, delayed video presentation caused for incongruous sense of displayed image. Image incongruousness declined drivability of the robot. By declination of the robot usability, the surgeon should control the location/posture of surgical instruments delicately under delayed video presentation. To develop telesurgery system for delayed network environment, detailed and precise presentation of relative location/posture should be required to reduce stresses and strains of a tele-operating surgeon.

In this research, the effect of network delay was evaluated. However, other network problems were not evaluated for telemedicine, such as packet loss, connection timeout, bandwidth limitation, and so on. Effect of other network problems, and mixed problems should be evaluated in the future research.

Acknowledgements

This research was supported in part by a grant JSPS-RFTF99I00905 from Japan Society for the Promotion of Science.

References

1. K. Hori, H. Oyama, Y. Ozaki, et al, "Surgical Cockpit System and Effectiveness of its Immersive Environment", Computer Assisted Radiology and Surgery 2001, p.1160, Berlin/Germany, 2001
2. Science Information Network, http://www.sinet.ad.jp/index-e.html
3. Asian Internet Interconnection Initiatives Project, http://www.ai3.net/
4. S. Nagasawa, "Analysis of Cyclic Paired Comparison AHP with Logarithmic Linear Model, Annual Conference of the Operations Research Society of Japan 1994 Autumn, 1994 (in Japanese)

Minimally Invasive Spine Surgery

CARS 2002 – H.U. Lemke, M.W. Vannier; K. Inamurc, A.G. Farman, K. Doi & J.H.C. Reiber (Editors)
©CARS/Springer. All rights reserved.

The new frontier of minimally invasive spine surgery through Computer Assisted Technology (CAT)

John C. Chiu, Thomas J. Clifford, Robert A. Princenthal, Romulo B. Sison
Neurospine Dept. and Digital Imaging Medical/Surgical Planning Laboratory
California Center for Minimally Invasive Spinal Surgery
California Spine Institute
Thousand Oaks (Newbury Park), CA 91320, USA

Abstract

To identify and demonstrate the Minimally Invasive Spine Surgery (MISS) treatment for cervical, thoracic and lumbar disc disease with various techniques and surgical techniques with digital Computer Assisted Technology (CAT) via a seamless computerized digital network. These will aid the precise diagnosis and improved MISS treatment [1] [2].

Keywords: Minimally invasive spinal surgery, computer assisted technology, institution information system (IITS)

1. Introduction

Minimally Invasive Spine Surgery (MISS) has rapidly come of age due to the explosive development of bio-computer technology, [3] [4] digital video imaging, laser application [5] and much better medical/surgical instruments. [3] (Table 1). Medical professionals expect that up to 85% of spinal surgery will soon be done with MISS. [6]

Evolution of MISS (4 generations):

- **1st generation**: Intradiscal procedure **(downstairs technique)** I.e. chymopapain injection, laser spinal discectomy, APLD, IDET
- **2nd generation**: in addition to above method, it moves upstairs, with extra discal, transforamenal and epidural technique for discectomy (**upstairs technique**) with micro instrument, laser, radiofrequency and bipolar probe application
- **3rd generation**: in addition to above methods, it involves bone work for **decompression of spinal stenosis** with rongeur, burr, rasp, curette and laser
- **4th generation**: in addition above methods, it utilizes contemporary **biotechnology**, biocomputer, **image guided surgery**, **robotic aided** instruments, virtual spinal endoscopy, spinal fusion, artificial disc, to further MISS with better precision and accuracy

Table 1: Evolution of minimally invasive spine surgery

©CARS/Springer. All rights reserved.

2. Material and methods

Several computer aided innovations, different endoscopes, [3] (Fig 1, 2) surgical robotics [4] (Fig 3, 4) and MISS systems are introduced. Intra-operative x-ray fluoroscopy, digital video photography, various MISS instruments, laser application, newer endoscopy with better visualization (Fig 5, 6), and thermodiskoplasty (i.e. the use of the laser at low energy levels, to shrink and tighten disc material) [5] are described. MISS techniques used in surgery are demonstrated pictorially. [7]

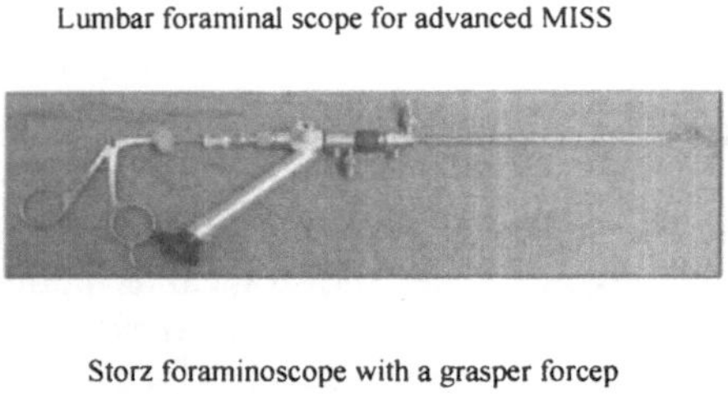

Lumbar foraminal scope for advanced MISS
Storz foraminoscope with a grasper forcep

Fig. 1: Advanced spinal endoscope for lumbar surgery

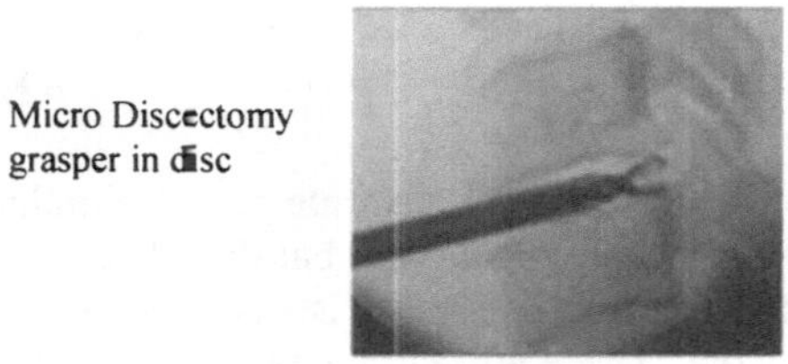

Fig. 2: Fluoroscopic x-ray view of cervical discectomy

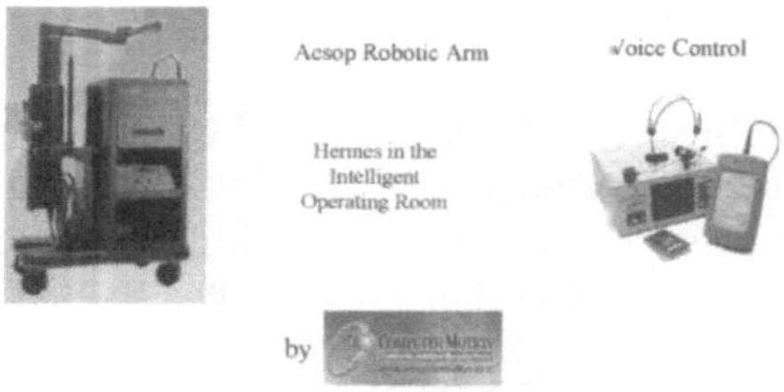

Fig. 3: Surgical robot - AESOP 300 with Hermes Voice Control

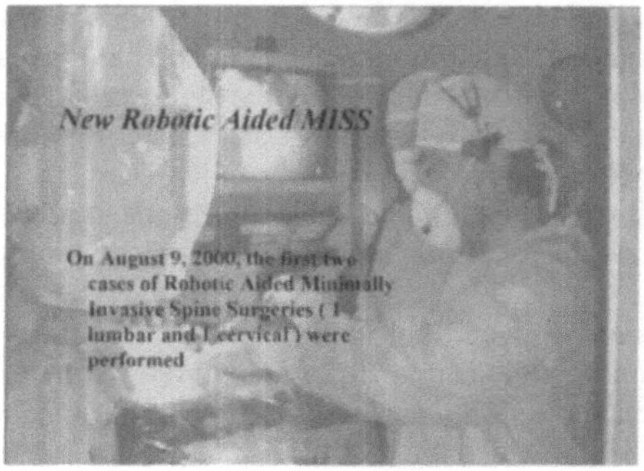

Fig 4: Robotic-aided minimally invasive spinal surgery

©CARS/Springer. All rights reserved.

What the Endoscope Sees

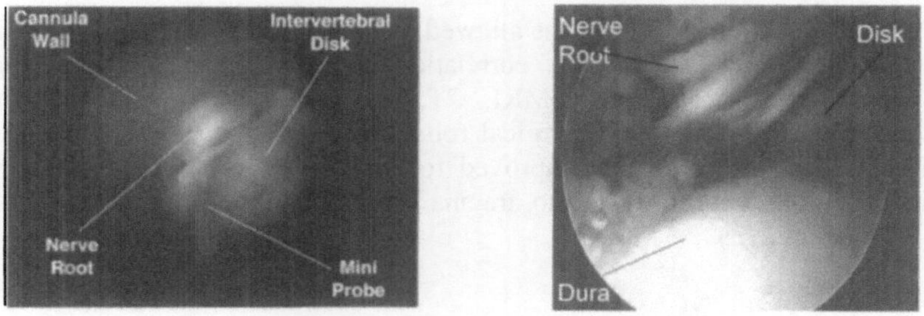

Fig. 5 Endoscopic view of nerv roots

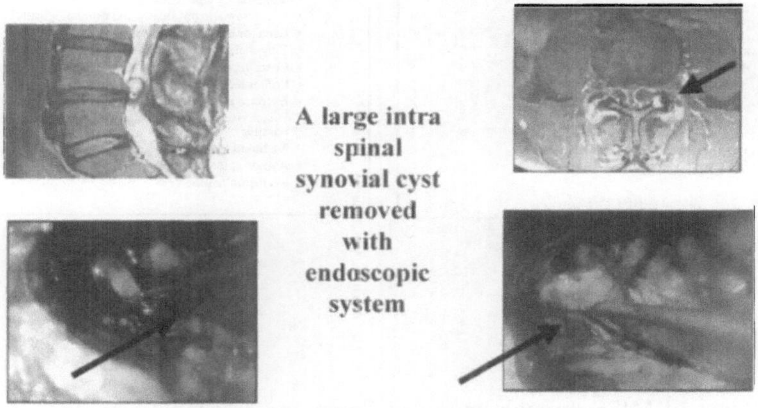
A large intra
spinal
synovial cyst
removed
with
endoscopic
system

Fig. 6 Endoscopic removal of a large spinal cyst

An Institutional Information System (IIS) including an all digital Picture Archiving and Communication System (PACS), [8] a digital 3-D imaging virtual reality system (Fig 7) are included our Medical Surgical Planning Laboratory for better diagnosis and pre-operative surgical planning for MISS. This laboratory is networked with the entire Institutional Information System (IIS) for intramural and extramural connectivity or networking. This establishes the foundation for telemedicine, teleconferencing and telesurgery for improved patient care, education, research and development.

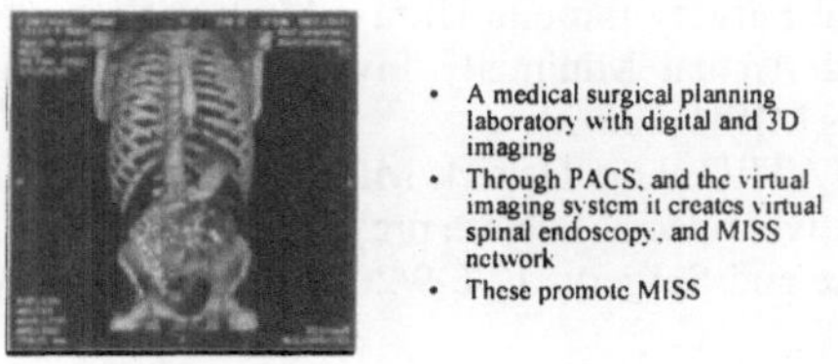
• A medical surgical planning laboratory with digital and 3D imaging
• Through PACS, and the virtual imaging system it creates virtual spinal endoscopy, and MISS network
• These promote MISS

Fig. 7 Virtual reality image assists surgical planning

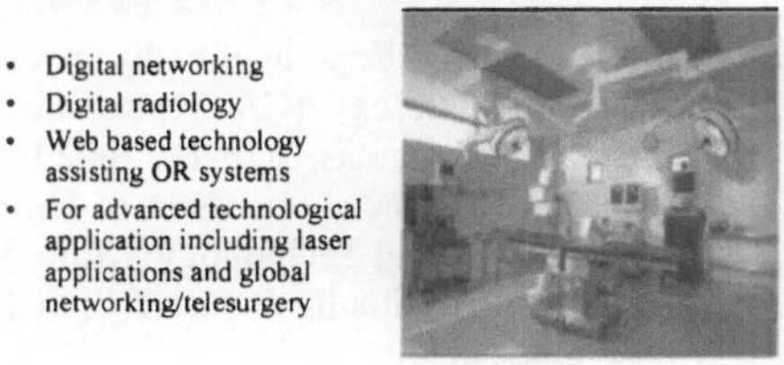
• Digital networking
• Digital radiology
• Web based technology assisting OR systems
• For advanced technological application including laser applications and global networking/telesurgery

Fig. 8 Advanced digital endoscopy surgical suites

©CARS/Springer. All rights reserved.

3. Results

Computer Assisted Technology (CAT) has allowed and promotes rapid progress in MISS technology (Fig 8). There is a definite correlation between clinical findings, digital radiology, neuropsychological studies, MRI, CT, 3D virtual imaging, virtual spinal endoscopy and surgical findings. [9] Surgical robotics adds further precision in MISS. Overall MISS surgical outcome has improved to above 94% or more, patients with symptomatic relief but with little or no trauma and zero mortality from the MISS procedures. 10 (Tables 2, 3)

Result at multi (19)centers: 27,760 cases of MISS [10]

- Patient satisfaction score: 91%
- Most cases were same-day outpatient
- Only 9 of 57 discitis (0.2%) cases had abnormal cultures
- All 41 (0.17%) csf leaks
- Most common complication was sympathetic mediated pain or dysethesia 131 (0.55%); progression to RSD was rare
- Nearly all 89 (0.38%) motor and sensory deficits were transient
- 139 (0.59%) patients required a second surgery
- Zero mortality

Table 2

Advantages of the procedure:

- Same-day, outpatient surgery
- Less traumatic physically and psychologically
- Local or brief general anesthesia
- Tiny incision closed with band-aid
- Costs 40% less than conventional spinal discectomy
- Earlier return to work
- Exercise program begins same day as surgery
- Direct visualization and confirmation of discectomy possible
- No blood transfusion
- Avoids epidural scarring
- No fusion required

Table 3

4. Conclusion

The advantages of MISS through improved Computer Assisted Technology, (CAT) [11] and Institutional Information System (IIS) compared to open spinal surgery for treatment of disc disease are obvious. This less traumatic, easier improved outpatient MISS treatment leads to excellent results, faster recovery, and significant economic savings. Soon further MISS applications will include spinal disk replacement, artificial disk, spine arthroplasty, vertebralplasty, spinal fixation/fusion and perhaps genome therapy.

References

1. Chiu, J., Cutting Edge Minimally Invasive Spinal Surgery through Ultra – Modern Computer Assisted Technology (CAT) presented The 3rd Annual Minimally Invasive Spine Update Nassau, The Bahamas, 2/15-18, 2002 Proceedings MISU p.30-31.
2. Mogel, Greg, Special Assistant to Director of TATRC, Fort Detrick MD, Telemedicine and Advanced Medical Technology: Military Perspective, Special Lecture presented at 2001 World Congress of Minimally Invasive Spinal Medicine and Surgery, 12/6-9/2002, Las Vegas, NV. Proceedings p.53.
3. Chatenever D., Minimally invasive surgical visualization-- past, present and future. J of Minimally Invasive Spinal Technique, 2001; 1(1): 2-7.
4. Wright, J., Clinical pathways for integrating computers and robotics into spine surgery. J of Minimally Invasive Spinal Technique, 2001; 1(1): 22-23.

©CARS/Springer. All rights reserved.

5. Chiu, J., Clifford, T., Greenspan, M., Richley, R., Sison, R., Percutaneous Microdecompressive Endoscopic Cervical Discectomy with Laser Thermodiskoplasty. The Mt. Sinai J of Med, 9/2000; 67(4): 278-282.
6. Chiu, J., Babur, H., Clifford, T. Sison, R., Survey on Minimally Invasive Spinal Surgery, The Practice of Minimal Invasive Spinal Technique, Special Millennium Edition, AAMIMS, Ed. LLC 2001; 219-220.
7. Chiu, J., Clifford, T., Posterolateral Approach for percutaneous thoracic endoscopic discectomy. J of Minimally Invasive Spinal Technique, 2001; 1(1): 26-30
8. Huang, H.K., PACS, informatics, and the neurosurgery command module. J of Minimally Invasive Spinal Technique, 2001; 1(1): 62-67
9. Haller, J., Ryken, T., Vannier, M., Image-guided surgery of the spine - Case Report. J of Minimally Invasive Spinal Technique, 2001; 1(1): 87-92
10. Chiu, J., Clifford, T., Savitz, M., Yeung, A., Batterjee, K., Destandau, J., Hoogland, T., Kambin, P., Knight, M., Lee, S.H., Leu, H., Pedachenko, E., Peterson, R., Felipe-Ramirez, J., Rezaian, A., Reuter, M., Scheffer, S., Schmidt, N., Werner, D., Shang-Li, L., Zhaomin, Z., Multicenter study of percutaneous endoscopic discectomy (lumbar, cervical, and thoracic. J of Minimally Invasive Spinal Technique, 2001; 1(1): 33-37
11. Lemke, H., Internet Based Personal Electronic Medical Records – Digital Informatics presented at 2001 World Congress of Minimally Invasive Spinal Medicine and Surgery, 12/6-9/2002, Las Vegas, NV. Proceedings p.52.

©CARS/Springer. All rights reserved.

Image-guided magnetic surgery

Michael W. Vannier[1]
[1]University of Iowa, Iowa City, Iowa

Abstract

Catheters, magnetic seeds, untethered endoscopes, and slurries of ferromagnetic particles may be moved, guided, and/or steered in living tissue by the shaped field of a repositionable external magnet for minimally invasive surgical procedures. A magnetic surgery system (MSS) consists of a control processor, a pointing device, a magnet assembly generating a magnetic field, a display, and a 3D medical imaging system. Biplane fluoroscopic images of the patient in which the magnetic delivery vehicle is implanted are shown on a screen, each image representing a projection in space of the operating region. The pointing device is operated to move a cursor from a projection of a present location of the magnetic delivery vehicle to a projection of a desired future location. When the locations are completely specified, the currents applied to multiple magnets in the MSS produce a magnetic field and move or orient the magnetic delivery vehicle. Multiple superconducting magnetic coils are activated simultaneously to move a magnetic object to precisely specified locations within the body under command of a physician-operator observing the motion with live fluoroscopic imaging fused with a more detailed preoperative image. A workstation contains the preoperative images and the fluoroscopic images, as well as the means to effect changes in the coil currents and position the magnetic object motion as desired. The control method operates the coils in pairs on opposite sides of the body to minimize the necessary current changes, thus avoiding the quenching of the superconducting coils. Combinations of these pairs can execute motion of the magnetic object in any direction in an impulsive manner and with high precision. The display provides real-time imaging of the implanted magnetic object in comparison to the desired path as the object is moved. This system has applications in neurosurgery, cardiac electrophysiology mapping and ablation, brachytherapy, and endoscopy that are currently under development. The technical features of an MSS and examples of its applications will be presented.

Keywords: Image-guided therapy, interventional neuroradiology

1. Introduction

Image-guided therapy using magnetic control of catheters or intravascular ferromagnetic particles is not new. Hans Tilander described the concept and conducted testing in animals and cadavers in the early 1950s. [1] Progress was made in the 1960s [2-6], but it wasn't until the mid-1970s [7-11] that in vivo human experimentation began to establish feasibility, but not practicality for the methods. [12-13] There are reviews of progress in the 80s [13] and 90s [15], but it has taken until 2002 to bring all of the technologies needed for successful magnetic control of surgical implements into multicenter clinical testing and anticipated commercialisation with eventual widespread use. [16-18]

©CARS/Springer. All rights reserved.

The explosive growth of less invasive procedures has made the cath lab, or interventional suite, a dynamic impetus for most hospitals has fueled the development of sophisticated imaging systems providing accurate visualization of internal organs, as well as specialized catheters and other interventional disposables. More recently, the advent of pre-operative roadmapping using MR or CT, intraoperative 3-D angiography and catheter based localization systems such as Biosense™ have advanced diagnostic visualization into the digital age, allowing for rapid 3D reconstruction of body systems. Despite these advances in imaging clarity and precision, catheters and other surgical instruments have largely remained manually controlled and highly dependent on practitioner dexterity. There has been little or no integrated control of instrument and image, a logical next step in computer-integrated surgical automation. The Stereotaxis Magnetic Surgery System (MSS) facilitates combining information and instrument actuation, allowing development of true interventional workstations - a versatile platform for interventional therapeutics. (Stereotaxis, Inc., St. Louis, MO, http://www.stereotaxis.com)

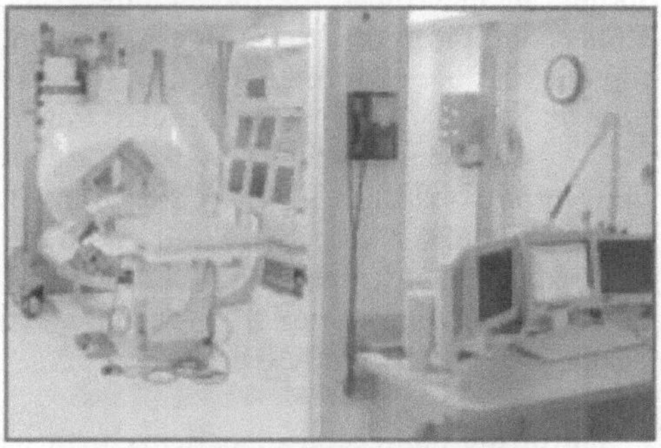

Fig. 1: Magnetic surgery system.

The first generation interventional workstation, TELSTAR, the result of nearly a decade of research and development, TELSTAR has served as the platform for the initial navigational applications under investigation in both interventional neuroradiology (INR) and cardiology. The FDA has given Investigatory Device Exemption (IDE) approval for the first navigational applications, and clin cal trials for these applications are underway.

1.1 Clinical trials

The Stereotaxis Magnetic Navigation System and magnetic catheters and guidewires are presently involved in three clinical trials at major U.S. medical centers including the University of Iowa, in anticipation of subsequent submission to the U.S. Food and Drug Administration [FDA] for marketing clearance and CE marking for European distribution.

2. Interventional neurosurgery

Mechanically controlled devices, even in the hands of the most skilled specialist, are viewed as having inherent functional limitations that are barriers to achieving certain highly desirable clinical interventions. In the case of cerebrovascular disease, for example, there is clear evidence that endovascular (intravascular) treatment methods are, in many cases, the most desirable therapeutic approach for a number of neurovascular defects.

©CARS/Springer. All rights reserved.

Currently, however, there are fewer than 200 INR specialists with the years of intensive training and highly developed technical skills required to carry out these procedures. There are 5,200 neurosurgeons and an even greater number of neurologists practicing in the U.S. who are highly trained in the overall clinical management of cerebrovascular patients; yet only a handful have the extensive additional training required to carry out endovascular procedures. Both areas of Interventional Neurosurgery are under investigation in MSS clinical trials: 1) Interventional Neuroradiology (INR) - Catheter based treatment of neurovascular disease and 2) Minimally Invasive Neurosurgery - Minimally invasive treatment of diseases of the brain. While both areas represent large, expanding patient volumes, each has significant limitations imposed by current manual navigation techniques.

2.1 Neurovascular disease

Neurovascular disease, including stroke, is the third leading cause of death worldwide. These blood vessel disorders include those life threatening events that occlude or block the arteries (ischemic stroke) and those that result in a ballooning of a weakened arterial wall (aneurysm) and rupture and bleeding of the artery (hemorrhagic stroke). Medical science has made significant strides in the endovascular treatment of the first two: a promising new treatment for ischemic stroke involves urgent intra-arterial catheter delivery of clot dissolving (thrombolytic) drugs to the site of the occlusion. This treatment is limited by the need to administer therapy within a few hours of stroke onset, exacerbated by the small number of interventional neuroradiologists (fewer than 200 in the U.S.) able to perform the intra-arterial procedure. Aneurysms are treated percutaneously by transcatheter delivery of micro coils.

Neurosurgeons usually control the admission of patients with neurologic disorders and have demonstrated a reluctance to fully embrace the evolution towards less invasive endovascular aneurysm coiling techniques. Their apprehension is justified, in part, by the potential inherent drawbacks of endovascular coiling resulting from coil compaction and the inability to entirely occlude the aneurysm neck. These constraints result in more than 20% of all endovascular aneurysm patients requiring a repeat procedure because of aneurysm re-growth. A further limitation to endovascular approaches is that more than 20% of all aneurysms have wide necks and are difficult or impossible to occlude using micro-coils. Consequently, in the United States, most aneurysms are still treated by Neurosurgeons, using more invasive open surgical techniques.

2.2 Diseases of the bain prenchyma

Among the many conditions which can affect the brain there are a number of diseases which can be treated, less invasively, through a small hole in the skull (burr hole) by a Neurosurgeon. These include neurodegenerative diseases such as Parkinson's, as well as movement disorders (Essential Tremor) and the Epilepsies (investigational use only) which are currently treated by deep brain electrostimulation (requiring precise targeting of neurostimulator electrodes) and a second category of diseases, including neurodegenerative disorders and brain tumors, which is ultimately expected to yield to precisely contoured delivery of growth factors (neurotrophic factors) or drugs.

©CARS/Springer. All rights reserved.

Neurosurgical access through a burr hole is usually gained via "framed" or "frameless" stereotaxy. The former describes those traditional mechanical devices which are clamped to the skull, pre-operatively, and used to target a straight-line catheter (cannula) inserted through the burr hole. More recently, "frameless" methodologies have emerged, which use computer integrated visualization or trajectory planning technologies to access straight-line targets, without cumbersome mechanical frames.

These methods are used for the delivery of biopsy tools (for sampling tumors), deep brain stimulators (for treatment of Parkinson's or Essential tremor) and infusion catheters (for drug delivery). They have, in common, the inherent limitations of straight-line access, no re-targeting capability, and the need for manual control.

2.3 Aneurysm filling

The "gold standard" for treatment of neurovascular aneurysms involves opening the skull (craniotomy) by a Neurosurgeon so as to access the aneurysm site through parenchymal tissue in order to clip the aneurysm. This clipping procedure permanently blocks the neck of the aneurysm and rarely has to be repeated. It is, however, extremely invasive, often involving the manipulation of sensitive areas. Endovascular procedures have evolved for occluding the aneurysm by accessing it through the neurovasculature, percutaneously; in order to deliver carefully sized platinum micro-coils, which greatly reduce turbulent blood flow within the aneurysm and, in the majority of cases, result in a permanently curative solution. However, in about 20% of the cases, coiling is unsuccessful owing to the width of the aneurysm neck or it's remote location.

A proprietary magnetic embolic was designed to be positioned and held within the lumen of an aneurysm. This technique uses magnetic gradients to overcome any flow induced risk of migration, even under extreme, pulsatile-flow conditions. The magnetic fields are expected to actually solidify and contain the embolic, allowing it to set within the aneurysm.

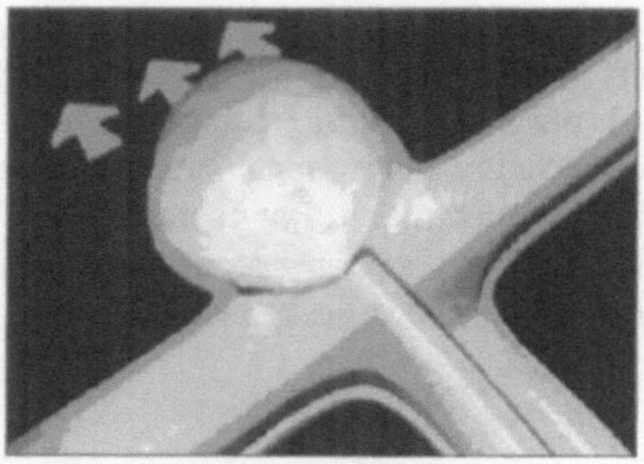

Fig. 2: Illustration of magnetic embolic being pulled by the magnet into a terminal aneurysm.

3. Navigation

3.1 Endovascular navigation

A proprietary guidewire and catheter are being developed for use with workstation to provide simple "point and click" navigation to targets within the neurovasculature. Using

©CARS/Springer. All rights reserved.

an intuitive touchpad interface, the interventionalist will draw the direction in two planes (as shown below), prompting to orient the magnetic field so that the guidewire or catheter enters the desired vessel branch, even if the lumen is as narrow as 1mm and the turn angle well in excess of 90 degrees. While skilled Interventional Neuroradiologists are usually able to manually navigate a guidewire to most targets within the neurovasculature, the effort is often time-consuming and sometimes frustratingly difficult. For most Neurosurgeons, the process remains technically insurmountable. In those emergency situations such as rapid stroke intervention, where the treatment of choice is expected to become intra-arterial targeted delivery of thrombolytics, administered within a few hours of onset, the navigational hurdle could become an obstacle to widespread treatment of "brain-attack", owing to the limited number of trained INR practitioners in the U.S.

3.2 Parenchymal navigation

Nowhere in the body is the need for less invasive procedures more relevant than in the brain, which is largely filled with vitally sensitive "eloquent" tissue. The brain is routinely accessed by Neurosurgeons for treatment of various neurologic diseases with therapies that range from excision and ablation to neurostimulation and infusion. These interventions have in common, the challenge of avoiding the most sensitive areas of the brain while delivering treatment to nearby foci. The least invasive approaches today involve insertion of a straight-line cannula, which is targeted by external means. However, re-targeting requires withdrawal and re-insertion, sometimes through a second burr hole. Under an FDA-approved Investigational Device Exemption (IDE), Stereotaxis pioneered the first human brain surgery procedure to use computer-integrated surgical automation to navigate a flexible catheter along multiple curvilinear paths from a single entry point.

The Stereotaxis System is designed for surgical path planning before the procedure, using imported DICOM pre-operative MR or CT images. The System is designed to manage a complex series of magnetic field changes to automatically drive the catheter along pre-planned, curvilinear pathway to its target site in the brain, with sub-millimetric precision.

Stereotaxis' catheter delivery system for use in the brain will be designed to serve as a minimally invasive general purpose flexible cannula which can be navigated along complex paths, to deliver proprietary instruments such as biopsy tools or "off the shelf" devices such as neurostimulator electrodes. For instance, an "off the shelf" deep brain stimulator (DBS) with a magnetic stylet can potentially be precisely targeted to avoid eloquent tissue and, once positioned, the stylet removed, leaving the DBS in place.

4. Summary

The potential ability of the Stereotaxis System to control and navigate devices within the neurovasculature and the brain parenchyma has been observed in human clinical cases. The workstations and related disposables are designed to provide a computer-integrated surgical automation platform for interventional neurosurgery, combining sophisticated imaging and visualization with preoperative planning and digital instrument control. The system may potentially reduce procedure times, provide new solutions for neurologic challenges and enable a broader universe of practitioners to participate in the rapidly growing field of endovascular neurosurgery.

©CARS/Springer. All rights reserved.

Acknowledgements

This work was supported in part by Stereotaxis, Inc. of St. Louis, MO. Their assistance, both technical and administrative is gratefully appreciated, especially for Peter Werp, Andrew Hall, and Bevil Hogg. The advice and encouragement of Matthew Howard, III, MD, has been most important and helpful to this effort.

References

1. H Tillander, Magnetic Guidance of a Catheter with Articulated Steel Tip, Acta Radiologica, (35):62-64 (1951).
2. GD Summers, Magnetics for Power and Control of Body Implants, Proc 5th National Biomedical Sciences Instrumentation Symposium, (4):293-302 (1967).
3. EH Frei et al. Magnetic Propulsion of Diagnostic or Therapeutic Elements Through the Body Ducts of Animal or Human Patients, U.S. Patent 3,358,676, Dec. 19, 1967.
4. SB Yodh et al. A New Magnet System for Intravascular Navigation, Med and Biol. Engrg. vol. 6, pp. 143-147 (1968).
5. DB Montgomery, RJ Weggel. Symposium on BioEngineering: Magnetic Forces for Medical Applications, Journal of Applied Physics 40:1039-1041, (1969).
6. DB Montgomery et al, Superconducting Magnet System for Intravascular Navigation, Jour of Applied Physics 40:2129-2132 (1969).
7. H Tillander, Selective Angiography with a Catheter Guided by a Magnet, IEEE Transactions on Magnetics, vol. 6, No. 2, 355-358 (1970).
8. J Driller et al., Cerebral Arteriovenous Malformations Treated with Magnetically Guided Emboli, Proc. 25th Ann Conf on Engrg and Biology, vol. 14 (1972), p. 306.
9. SK Hilal et al. Magnetically Guided Devices for Vascular Exploration and Treatment, Radiology, (113):529-540 (1974).
10. JJR Hale, Medical Applications of Magnet Devices. IEEE Transactions on Magnetics, (Mag-11) 5:1405-1407 (1974).
11. R Hale et al. The Design of a 2T Superconducting Solenoid for Magnetic Catheter Guidance, IEEE Transactions on Magnetics, (MAG-11) 2:563-564 (1975).
12. J Barry et al. Ferromagnetic Embolization, Radiology, (138):341-349 (1981).
13. J Driller et al. A Review of Medical Applications of Magnet Attraction and Detection, (11) 6:271-277 (1987).
14. MS Grady, et al. Nonlinear magnetic stereotaxis: Three-dimensional, in vivo remote magnetic manipulation of a small object in canine brain, Med. Phys. 17(3), May/Jun. 1990, pp. 405-415.
15. Howard MA III, Dacey RG, Henegar MM, et al. Review of magnetic neurosurgery research. J Image Guided Surg 1995; 1 (6):295-9.
16. RG McNeil et al. Magnetic-Implant Guidance System for Stereotactic Neurosurgery, IEEE Trans. Biomed. Eng., vol. 42, No. 8, Aug. 1995, pp. 793-801.
17. RG McNeil et al. Improved Magnetic-Implant Guidance System, IEEE Trans. Biomed. Eng., vol. 42, No. 8, Aug. 1995, pp. 802-808.
18. MA Howard, III, et al. Measurement of the force required to move through in vivo human brain tissue. IEEE Trans on Biomed Engrg, 46:891-894, 1999.

Computer Assisted Orthopaedic Surgery

CARS 2002 – H.U. Lemke, M.W. Vannier; K. Inamura, A.G. Farman, K. Doi & J.H.C. Reiber (Editors)
©CARS/Springer. All rights reserved.

Validation of fluoroscopy based navigation in the hip region. What you see is what you get?

N.W.L. Schep[1], Th. van Walsum [2], J.S. de Graaf [1], I.A.M.J. Broeders [1], Ch.van der Werken [1].

[1] Department of Surgery UMC Utrecht, G04-223, P.O. Box 85500, 3508 GA Utrecht, The Netherlands, n.w.l.schep@chir.azu.nl

[2] Image Sciences Institute UMC Utrecht, E 01.335, P.O. Box 85500, 3508 GA Utrecht, The Netherlands

Abstract

Navigation systems can be used for osteosynthesis of femoral neck fractures. The goal of this study was to evaluate the accuracy of a fluoroscopy based navigation system (Medivision, Oberdorf, CH.) in displaying a virtual drill and in measuring the length of a drill channel. To evaluate the position of the virtual reamer an 8 mm Perspex bar was inserted in predefined drill channels in 20 sawbones. AP and AX fluoroscopic images of the sawbones with the Perspex bar were loaded into the workstation. Next, the Perspex bar was exchanged for a navigated dynamic hip screw (DHS) reamer. The position of the Perspex bar in the images represented the true position of the reamer. Subsequently, the difference in position between the virtual reamer and the Perspex bar was measured. Drill channel lengths, measured with the system, were compared with measurements obtained with a digital ruler. The mean difference in position of Perspex bar and reamer was 0.90 mm (0.00-3.21mm) in 360 images. The mean difference in length measurements between the system and the digital ruler was 1.00 mm ($p=0.01$ $SD=1.33$). In conclusion reaming and measuring screw channels of a DHS with this navigation system can be performed with an acceptable error margin.

Keywords: Validation, fluoroscopy based navigation, dynamic hip screw

1. Introduction

The success of closed reduction and internal fixation of intracapsular femoral neck fractures is mainly determined by the quality of reduction and fixation. Among the various treatment options the dynamic hip screw (DHS, AO-Synthes®) is used as the standard implant in our center for osteosynthesis of these fractures. After reduction of the fracture, a K-wire is inserted to guide a reamer for drilling an insertion channel for the DHS.

However, with current fluoroscopy techniques positioning of the K-wire in the femoral neck and head can only be visualized in two-dimensional (2-D) projections. This may lead to repetitive position changes of the C-arm, because both anteroposterior (AP) and axial (AX) images are required and makes the procedure prone to imperfect positioning of the

©CARS/Springer. All rights reserved.

K-wire resulting in malpositioning of the implant. Moreover, interactive fluoroscopic guidance may result in a substantial radiation exposure to both patients and surgical team.

Fluoroscopy based navigation may offer a solution to these problems. With this technique the virtual position and direction of the reamer can be simultaneously superimposed on AP and axial AX fluoroscopic images. Subsequently, the surgeon instantaneously drills the hole for the hip screw under navigation without the use of a K-wire.

Surgeons using this technique have to rely on the accuracy of the navigation system, since the only intraoperative feedback on the "true" position of reamer is the position of a virtual reamer superimposed on the fluoroscopic images. Non correspondence between the virtual position and the true position may lead to complications.

The objective of this study was to evaluate the accuracy of the displayed position of the virtual reamer in relation to the true position of the instrument when using a fluoroscopy based navigation system. Secondary the accuracy of the drill channel measuring tool of the system was analyzed.

2. Materials and Methods

All tests were performed on 20 sawbones (Synbone AG Davos, CH) in a laboratory setting. Drilling was performed directly with a specially developed non-canulated 8 mm DHS reamer, without the setup for plate reaming. A specially designed 135° aiming device was used as a drill guide. During drilling the virtual position of the DHS reamer was superimposed on the AP and AX images of the proximal femur and was displayed on the workstation (Medivision, Oberdorf, CH.).

Position tracking was performed with light emitting diodes and an opto-elektric camera (Optotrak 3020®, Nothern Digital –inc.). The C-arm (Philips BV 300-9 inch, Best, the Netherlands) was equipped with a shield holding 24 light emitting diodes (LEDs). The C-arm images were calibrated to compensate for the elastic deformation caused by the weight of the components of the C-arm under gravity and the fluoroscope's image intensifier distortion. [1] To maintain the relationship between the sawbone and the fluoroscopic images a shield with four LEDs, named the dynamic reference frame (DRF) was rigidly attached to the proximal part of the shaft of the sawbone before image acquisition. LEDs were also attached to a compact air drive to track its position.

First, AP and AX images were made and loaded in the workstation. 'AX' was defined as the projection where the axis of the femoral neck was exactly in line with the axis of the shaft of the femur. Subsequently, the C-arm was rotated 90 degrees and the projection defined as 'AP' was obtained.

Before drilling a length calibration of the non-canulated 8 mm DHS reamer had to be performed, the diameter of the reamer was also defined and stored in the system. During drilling the starting point at the outer border of the femoral cortex and the end point at the preferred position below the femoral head cortex were marked by pressing a footswitch.

©CARS/Springer. All rights reserved.

The drill channel length measurements provided by the navigation system, were compared with true length measurements defined with a digital ruler (Helios, Niedernhall, Germany). This procedure was repeated in all 20 sawbones.

To evaluate the virtual position of the navigated DHS reamer, new AP and AX images were obtained with an 8 mm Perspex bar inserted in the predefined drill channel of each sawbone. The position of the Perspex bar in these fluoroscopic images represented the true position of the reamer and therefore, acted as a reference. These images were loaded in the Medivision workstation. After image acquisition the Perspex bar was removed and exchanged for the navigated DHS reamer. On the workstation the virtual position of the DHS reamer was superimposed on the images containing the Perspex bar.

Next, the AP and AX images with and without the superimposed virtual reamer were transferred to a personal computer (Pentium III, 600 Mhz, 256MB) for measurements. (Figure 1) A dedicated computer program was developed to determine the centerlines and diameters of both Perspex bar and virtual reamer. Differences between the centerline position of the Perspex bar and the virtual reamer were determined in a standardized cutplane, outlined by a radiographic marker placed centrally over the femoral neck. This difference in position was defined as the positional error of the system in this test setup (| D-P |). (Figure 2) Additionally, the angles between the centerlines were determined. Position measurements in AP en AX images were accomplished after 5 different length calibrations, resulting in 200 measurements.

Intraoperatively it may be difficult to obtain accurate AP and AX images. Therefore, the influence of the C-arm orientation, during image acquisition, on the accuracy of the virtual reamer position was also evaluated using the same methods. Eight additional fluoroscopic images with the Perspex bar were obtained in angles of 90° (AX), 80°, 70°, 60°, 30°, 20°, 10° and 0° (AP). Again the difference in the centerline position between the Perspex bar and the virtual reamer was assessed for each angle in 160 images.

All results were evaluated with SPSS 7.5 for Windows (SPSS, Inc, Chicago). First the mean values of length measurements of the drill channels obtained with the Medivision and the digital ruler were evaluated. With a Wilcoxon signed- rank test the hypothesis was tested that no difference could be found between these populations.

The mean difference in position between the centerline position of the Perspex bar and virtual reamer was calculated out of a total of 360 measurements. Additionally the mean angle of the centerlines and the mean focal point was computed in all images.

To evaluate the relationship between the C-arm angles and the error of the system, a scatterplot for X= C-arm angle and Y= | D-P | was drawn to evaluate the relationship between the C-arm angles and the error of the system. Finally, a linear regression test was performed for these variables.

©CARS/Springer. All rights reserved.

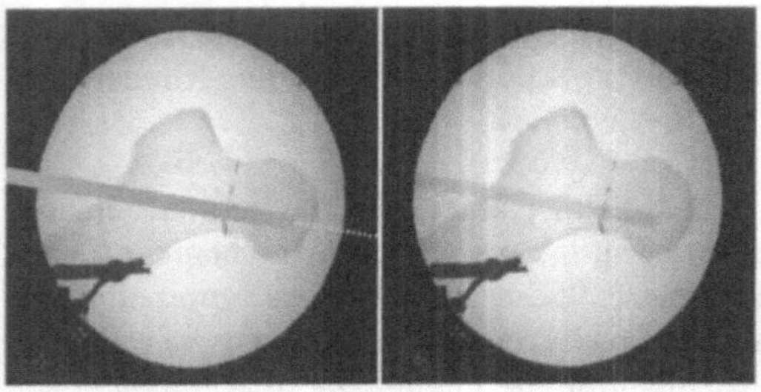

Figure 1: Captured AP images: Right image shows the Perspex bar, left image shows the navigated reamer, superimposed on the fluoroscopic image. Black line on femoral neck is radiographic marker that has been used to determine cut plane

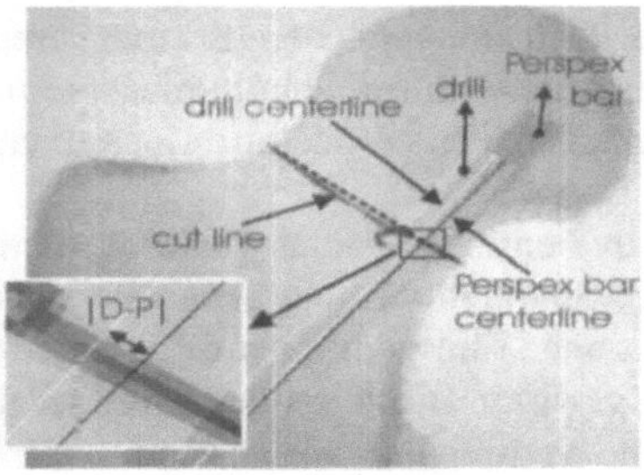

Figure 2: The centerlines of the Perspex bar and reamer are drawn in the images by the computer program. Difference in position of both centerlines is displayed as | D-P |.

3. Results

The mean difference in length measurements of the drill channels between the MediVision system and the digital ruler was 1.00 mm ($p=0.01$, std deviation =1.33). In 4 bones the lengths measured with the system appeared to be longer and in 15 bones the lengths appeared to be shorter than the true situation.

The difference in the position of the centerlines showed a mean difference of 0.90 mm (0.00-3.21 mm) in a total of 360 measurements at the predefined position in the femoral neck. Nine out of 360 measurements (2.5%) showed a difference of more than 2 mm. The mean angle was 0.39° and the mean focal point was 6 cm proximal of the cut line.

Linear regression analysis for the C-arm orientation and | D-P | showed a linear causal association with a regression coefficient –0.01 and $p < 0.01$. The mean difference in centerline position in AP images was 1.17 mm vs. 0.65 mm in AX images. Independent samples T-test comparing the means of | D-P | in the AP and AX images showed a significant difference with $p < 0.01$.

4. Discussion

The objective of this study was to evaluate the accuracy of the Medivision trauma module for drilling the screw channel for a DHS. First the length measuring tool of the navigation system was evaluated. In 75% of the cases virtual drill channel lengths measured with the system were shorter (mean 1mm) than the true channel length. In practice this means that in most cases undersized screws will be chosen. However, a mean difference of 1 mm is of no clinical relevance for this procedure.

©CARS/Springer. All rights reserved.

In addition to length measurements, this study focussed on positional errors of the virtual reamer, projected on single shot AP and AX images. In all experiments the difference in position between the virtual reamer and true position was measured in a predefined cutplane in the middle of the femoral neck We chose the clinically most relevant cutplane at the narrowest point of the calcar. The position of the virtual reamer appeared to be reliable in 97% of cases when considering an inaccuracy of ≤ 2mm as clinically relevant. In nine out of 360 measurements a difference of more than 2 mm was found. In these cases it is most likely that the DRF was moved relative to the femur during the experiment, resulting in a loss of the relationship between the sawbone and the fluoroscopic images. This is an important pitfall in surgical navigation. Intraoperatively the surgeon has to monitor the fixation of the DRF. In case loss of rigid fixation is suspected it is obligatory to discontinue the procedure and to acquire new images.

Obviously, the parameter $|D\text{-}P|$ is dependent of the position of the cutplane chosen, in case the centerline of the Perspex bar and the centerline of the virtual reamer do not run parallel. However, the mean angle between these centerlines was 0.39° with the intersection point at a mean distance of 6 cm ahead of the predefined measurement point. The inaccuracy, due to the deviation of the centerlines from the intersection point at the level of the femoral head did not lead to an unacceptable level in this study.

Surprisingly, the accuracy of the virtual position of the reamer on 2-D fluoroscopy images appeared to be related to the angle of image acquisition. When the C-arm was moved from AX (90°) to AP (0°), mean inaccuracy of the position of the virtual reamer increased.. Navigation based on AX fluoroscopic images appeared to be more accurate compared to navigation based on AP images. The C-arm images are calibrated to compensate for the elastic deformation caused by the weight of the components of the C-arm under gravity and the image intensifier distortion. A possible explanation for the difference in error between AP and AX images could be a difference in accuracy of C-arm calibration in the extreme positions.

In conclusion surgeons working with these systems have to realize that system inaccuracy consists of the sum of multiple errors. Sources of these errors are inaccuracy in position tracking by the opto-electric camera, in calibration of the C-arm, image distortion and in calibration of the drilling tool. However, the fluoroscopy based navigation system validated in this study provides a reliable virtual position of the reamer compared with the true situation when drilling the channel for a DHS.

References

1. Hofstetter, R., Slomczykowski, M., Sati, M., and Nolte, L. P.: Fluoroscopy as an imaging means for computer-assisted surgical navigation. Comput. Aided Surg. 4:65-76, 1999.

©CARS/Springer. All rights reserved.

Realistic haptic volume interaction for petrous bone surgery simulation

A. Petersik[a], B. Pflesser[a], U. Tiede[a], K.H. Höhne[a], R. Leuwer[b]
[a] Institute of Mathematics and Computer Science in Medicine (IMDM)
[b] ENT-Clinic
University Hospital Hamburg-Eppendorf, Germany
petersik@uke.uni-hamburg.de

Abstract

In this paper, a new approach for haptic volume interaction with high resolution voxel-based anatomic models is presented. The haptic rendering is based on a multi-point collision detection approach which provides realistic tool interaction with the models. Both haptics and graphics are rendered at sub-voxel resolution, which leads to a high level of detail and enables the exploration of the models at any scale. Forces are calculated at an update rate of 6000 Hz and sent to a 3-Degree-of-Freedom (3-DOF) force-feedback device. Compared to single-point based haptic rendering, the unique approach of the multi-point collision detection in combination with sub-voxel rendering provides more realistic and very detailed haptic sensations. As a main application, a simulator for petrous bone surgery was developed. With a simulated drill, bony structure can be removed and the access path to the middle ear can be studied in a realistic manner.

Keywords: Haptic, collision detection, volume interaction

1. Introduction

The sense of touch is essential in a wide field of medical applications, like surgery simulators. In contrast to our other senses it allows us to simultaneously explore and interact with our environment. Today most applications concentrate on the simulation of elastic deformations of soft tissue. The simulation of material removal in medical applications is a less developed field and simulation systems either do not include cutting operations at all, or in a simplified manner, which does not provide the 'look and feel' close to a real incision.

Moreover haptic rendering is mostly based on traditional computer graphics methods where objects are represented by polygons only. Creating detailed polygonal models of organs result in a huge number of polygons which increases computation time for collision detection dramatically. However for realistic haptic rendering a collision detection algorithm with a constant computation time is essential. Choosing a volume based model, the computation time for a collision detection is independent of the complexity of the scene. Additionally a volume based model allows the simulation of interactive cutting operations and the display of arbitrary cut planes.

©CARS/Springer. All rights reserved.

Furthermore we realized that today 3-DOF haptic rendering is mostly point-based, i.e. only one point is used to calculate collisions and forces. This induces several problems:

- Discontinuities (e.g. sharp edges) on the surface can lead to discontinuities in the haptic display.
- The virtual tool can reach points which can not be reached by the simulated real world tool. (A large drill could enter a small hole.)

One goal of the work presented in this paper is to develop a haptic rendering algorithm which is able to display arbitrary complex anatomic models with high realism and accuracy. Another goal was to not only enable the haptic exploration of the anatomic models but also to be able to modify those models interactively with simulated real world tools in a realistic manner. Using the developed algorithms, we implemented a petrous bone surgery simulator, where a simulated drill can be used both to explore and to manipulate the anatomic model.

2. Methods

To develop a simulator which allows drilling into the bone the following points concerning haptics had to be considered:

- Haptic rendering should be based on a multi-point collision detection to allow a realistic tool-object interaction.
- To enable a realistic haptic interaction while modifying the models with drill like tools, an algorithm is needed which calculates realistic drilling forces.

2.1 Data representation

The model of the petrous bone is represented by attributed voxels (volume elements) which have a size of $0.33mm^3$. The attributes describe data like density values and associated organ. The associated organ is determined during the semi-automatic, threshold based segmentation process.

Our voxel-based representation does not contain an explicit representation of the object surfaces. The surfaces are calculated based on the segmentation data. This is done by a ray-casting algorithm [6] which renders isosurfaces at sub-voxel resolution based on the partial volume effect and density value of the voxels. The same ray-casting algorithm is used to determine the surface for both graphic and haptic rendering.

2.2 Haptic surface rendering

In our implementation of the petrous bone surgery simulator we are using a sphere-shaped tool, which simulates a drill. To achieve a realistic haptic rendering, collisions between the tool and the static scene must be computed and a collision-free position must be determined. Then a force which pushes the haptic device to the collision-free position must be applied. For a realistic haptic tool-object interaction, a multi-point collision detection algorithm is needed.

To implement the multi-point collision detection, the tool is represented by a number of sample points which are distributed at preferably equal distances over the tool surface. Each of these points is checked whether it collides with the objects or not. Additionally

©CARS/Springer. All rights reserved.

every point has an associated normal vector which is pointing to the inside of the tool. All inward pointing surface normals have the same length.
The inward pointing vectors are used to find the static object's surface. An advantage of this approach is that no computation of surface normals for the voxel-based anatomic object is required. To get a good compromise of adequate tool representation and computation time, we use 26 sample points on the sphere's surface.
Whenever a collision between tool and static objects occurs the following two parameters must be computed:

- Direction and
- Magnitude of collision force

Both variables must be computed with high precision to allow a realistic interaction for e.g. petrous bone surgery. Our multi-point collision detection algorithm was inspired by the work described in [2]. However our approach differs from this work in several points. While our model is also using a voxel representation for the static objects, the exact location of the surfaces is calculated by a ray-casting algorithm at sub-voxel resolution (see 2.1). This leads to a more precise calculation of both force direction and magnitude. The algorithms presented in [2, 4] can not provide the precision which is needed in our case, since the static objects are voxelized in a binary manner. Additionally our sub-voxel approach leads to a stable contact situation, even under sliding motion without having to reduce the device's bandwidth by methods like e.g. "virtual-coupling" or force-averaging.

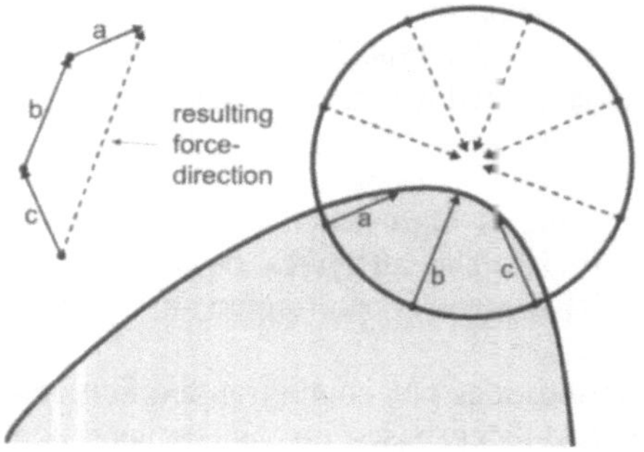

Fig. 1 Calculation of collision forces on the object surface

Another improvement we have made is the representation of the tool. While the dynamic object in [2] is voxelized and the center points of the voxels are used for the collision detection, we are using sample points which are located exactly on the surface of the tool. To calculate the collision force direction, the surface points of the tool are checked, whether they are colliding with the object. All colliding surface points are traced along the corresponding inward pointing normal until the surface of the object is found or the end of the normal is reached. All vectors found are added and the direction of the sum vector is the direction of the force vector which must be applied to the haptic device (fig. 1). As stated in [2], the summation of the vectors found would lead to force instabilities. As more of the tool's contact points collide with the static object, more stiffness is the result which creates a less stable contact situation. To avoid instabilities, we use an improved algorithm which averages the vectors depending on the number of found vectors.

©CARS/Springer. All rights reserved.

2.3 Proxy object algorithm

Any haptic device has a limited maximum force which can be applied to it. When the user pushes harder than this limit, it is possible that the physical position of the tool immerses completely into the virtual model. In this case calculation of the force direction as described above is not possible anymore.

To overcome that limitation a modified proxy object algorithm [7, 5] was implemented. The idea behind the proxy is to store a position where no collision between tool and scene occurs. When the tool moves in freespace, tool and device position are identical. But when the device immerses into an object, the proxy remains on the object's surface.

In order to update the proxy position on the static object's surface while the device is moving, the distance between the device position and the proxy must be locally minimized by regarding the surface constraints. Since searching for the local minimum would be computationally too expensive in our model, a simplified algorithm was implemented. Whenever more than a certain number of surface sample points of the dynamic object are in contact with an object, the path between proxy and new tool position is traced until the object surface is found and the resulting force can be calculated as described above. Since the difference between two successive positions is very small, this approximation gives a realistic feeling of the virtual objects.

2.4 Volume modification

Our freeform volume modification algorithm which is descibed in detail in [3] is working with sub-voxel precision. The parts removed are modeled by simulating the partial volume effect. This produces realistic structures even when using very small tools.

2.5 Calculation of drilling forces

Since the volume modification algorithm updates the volume at a rather low frequency, we can not use the same haptic rendering algorithm as described above to calculate a realistic force while drilling.

An approach to overcome that problem is to use a force which is opposite to the drilling direction and takes several parameters into account to improve the sensation of the drilled structures.

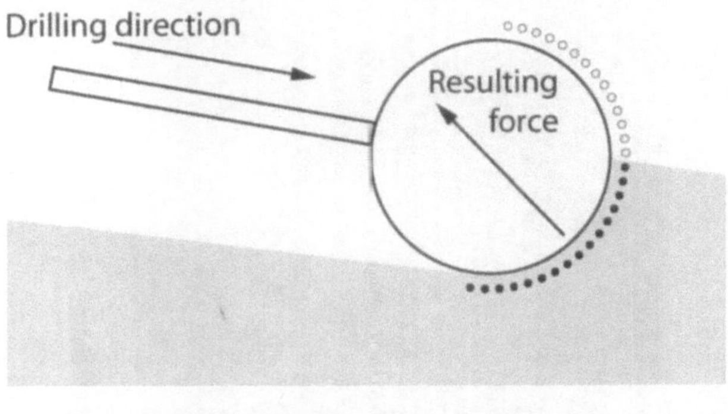

Fig. 2 Adaption of magnitude and direction of the drilling force

©CARS/Springer. All rights reserved.

- The higher the drilling speed, the higher must be the drilling force.
- The more volume is removed, the higher must be the drilling force.
- Depending on the position of the removed structures in relation to the drill, the direction of the drilling force must be adapted (fig. 2).

Additionally a vibration is modulated onto the drilling force to improve the sensation of the drilling procedure. By changing parameters, different types of drills, like diamant and metal drills can be simulated.

3. Results

With our approach we achieve a high quality haptic rendering of non-deformable arbitrary complex anatomic models [1]. The perception of spatial relationships is greatly enhanced with haptic feedback. Even very small surface details or small objects like nerves and vessels can be sensed realistically due to our sub-voxel based approach. The main focus of our work was the interaction with non-deformable material (e.g. bone). With the algorithms presented in this paper we developed a system for the simulation of petrous bone surgery. In this simulator, the haptic device is used to simulate drilling into the mastoid bone to get access to the middle-ear. The monitor of the simulator is mounted above and the haptics device below a mirror which allows the surgeon to work at the location where the scene is displayed (fig. 3). The spatial perception is enhanced by using stereoscopic viewing. The configuration of the simulator provides a position of the surgeon's hands, patient orientation and viewing direction which is similar to the real procedure. The simulator is of great assistance for learning the complex anatomy of the petrous bone.

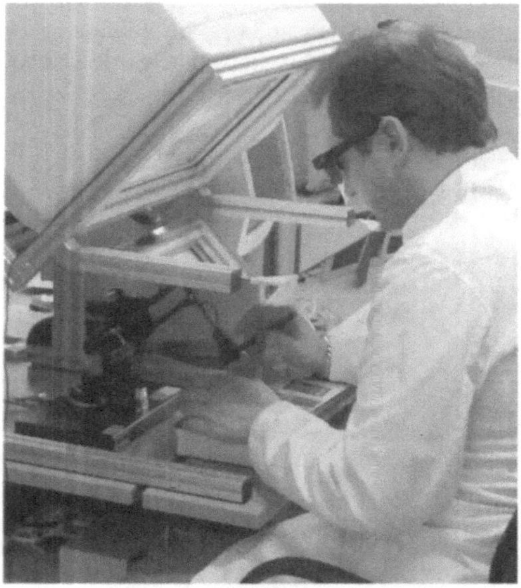

Fig. 3 Training with the simulator

©CARS/Springer. All rights reserved.

4. Conclusions and future work

We presented an approach for realistic haptic rendering and volume interaction with anatomic models. It overcomes several problems of single-point based haptic rendering. The multi-point based collision detection approach makes tool-object interactions more realistic, especially for the use in surgery simulations. Another important advantage is that surface details can be sensed as expected from the graphical representation. Sub-voxel rendering leads to both a graphical and haptic realistic, high detailed and congruent display. The volume interaction uses a sub-voxel based algorithm which allows the use of small tools, like drills used in petrous bone surgery.

While only sphere-shaped tools are realized in the petrous bone surgery simulator, future implementations will extend this to more general shapes. The calculation of the magnitude of the collision force will be investigated further to improve haptic rendering at locations with many tool object intersections as they appear especially in deep clefts.
Other improvements will be done to speed up graphical rendering of the modified structures, to allow for faster movements while drilling.

References

1. K. H. Höhne, B. Pflesser, A. Pommert, M. Riemer, R. Schubert, T. Schiemann, U. Tiede, and U. Schumacher. A realistic model of human structure from the Visible Human data. Meth. Inform. Med., 40(2):83-89, 2001.
2. W. A. McNeely, K. D. Puterbaugh, and J. J. Troy. Six degree-of-freedom haptic rendering using voxel sampling. Computer Graphics (SIGGRAPH99 Proceedings), pages 401-408, 1999.
3. B. Pflesser, U. Tiede, K. H. Höhne, and R. Leuwer. Volume based planning and rehearsal of surgical interventions. In H. U. Lemke, M. W. Vannier, K. Inamura, A. G. Farman, and K. Doi, editors, Computer Assisted Radiology and Surgery, Proc. CARS 2000, volume 1214 of Excerpta Medica International Congress Series, pages 607-612. Elsevier, Amsterdam, 2000.
4. M. Renz, C. Preusche, M. Potke, H.-P. Kriegel, and G. Hirzinger. Stable haptic interaction with virtual environments using an adapted voxmap-pointshell algorithm. Proc. of the Eurohaptics Conference, pages 149.154, 2001.
5. D. C. Ruspini, K. Kolarov, and O. Khatib. The haptic display of complex graphical environments. Proc. of ACM SIGGRAPH, pages 345-352, 1997.
6. U. Tiede, T. Schiemann, and K. H. Höhne. High quality rendering of attributed volume data. In D. Ebert, H. Hagen, and H. Rushmeier, editors, Proc. IEEE Visualization '98, pages 255-262. IEEE Computer Society Press, Los Alamitos, CA, 1998.
7. C. Zilles and K. Salisbury. A constraint-based god object method for haptics display. Proceedings of IEEE/RSJ, 1995.

CARS 2002 – H.U. Lemke, M.W. Vannier; K. Inamura, A.G. Farman, K. Doi & J.H.C. Reiber (Editors)
©CARS/Springer. All rights reserved.

Non-invasive osteotomy using focused ultrasound

Satoshi Ishida [a], Nobuhiko Hata [a], Takashi Azuma [b] Shinichiro Umemura [b], Takeyoshi Dohi [a]
[a] Graduate School of Information Science and Technology, The University of Tokyo
[b] Central Research Laboratory, Hitachi Ltd.

Abstract

Surgical reconstruction of bony defects such as Rotational Acetabular Osteotomy (RAO) in the orthopedics region involves operation of bony cutting using surgical saws or drills. Operators have to incise skin and open muscular system under anesthesia to make the bone visible, and require patients great pain and marks after the operation. So the system of bony cutting using focused ultrasound without incising skin has been developed. The ultrasound energy and the high pressure caused by cavitation generated by the minus vapor pressure ablates the focus area of the bone. The experiment of ablating the surface of a pig's bone by ultrasound was carried out in various irradiational conditions. At high oscillating frequency, in the case of the continuum wave, the mark of ablation without thermal damage was found at the focal point and the size was same as convergence beam area of ultrasonic wave. Besides, the ultrasonic propagation in the living body which consists of multiple organizations was analyzed using the time-domain finite element method. In comparison with the experimental result, the conditions in which ablation occurs without causing thermal damage at the focus on the bone was specified by controlling input power to the transducer and irradiation time.

Keywords: Ultrasound, osteotomy, simulation

1. Introduction

In an orthopedics region, not a few medical treatments involve osteotomy like High Tibial Osteotomy, Rotational Acetabular Osteotomy, and so on. In these operations, in order to avoid damaging the organization like important nerves or blood vessels existing around the bone operators are going to cut, by any means such as a scalpel or a laser, they incise skin and open muscular system greatly under anesthesia to make the bone visible. Consequently, the patient's operation marks are large and the operation time is long, so it is hard for patients to bear the operation mentally and physically. The purpose of this study is to develop the system in order to cut the human bone non-invasively by using focused ultrasound, without incising skin. The reason why we select the ultrasound as an energy source is the characteristic of less-invasion over the human body compared with an electromagnetic wave or radiation, and the small attenuation by distance when focused ultrasound was irradiated at the human body that has the scale of 10mm order. It makes us possible to concentrate high energy from the outside of the body into a very small region inside.

©CARS/Springer. All rights reserved.

In this study we applied the method of ESWL (Extracorporeal Shock Wave Lithotoripsy) [1]. The focused ultrasound irradiated through skin, muscle and fat at the surface of the bone creates high intensified energy in a small area, and then the heat transferred from the ultrasound energy and the high pressure caused by cavitation generated by the minus vapor pressure [2][3] ablates the focus of the bone. By moving the focus almost continuously and automatically, the target bone is cut in a suitable shape non-invasively. However, in the living body there are plural organizations, so complex attenuation and diffusion occurs. Direct measurements of the ultrasound distortion produced by human organization have been made and techniques for the correction of this distortion have been examined [4][5], but the physical cause of ultrasonic wavefront distortion are not well understood and it is difficult to control. Moreover, since the thermal damage over the organization of the cutting part has a bad influence on re-growth of the bone after cutting, occurrence of too much heat must be avoided. In this research we had the experiment of irradiating the focused ultrasound into a pig bone, and also had the simulation reappearing the same experimental system in order to make clear the phenomenon that occurs around the focus.

2. Method

2.1 Experiment of irradiating ultrasound

In this research, the experiment of ablating a bone by ultrasound was carried out. The focused ultrasound was irradiated toward a point on the surface of a pig's bone fixed spatially to the tank with which the degassed water was filled (Fig. 1). The vibrator used for generating of ultrasonic waves is a piezo-electric element, PZT (zircon acid titanium acid barium) element. The element of the curvature radius of 10mm, the focal length of 1.0mm, and the F number 1.0 was used. Oscillating frequency was changed from 1MHz to 3MHz, applied voltage was changed from 10W to 100W, the input waveform to a PZT element was tried both continuation wave and pulse wave. Under these conditions, the change of the situation of a converging point was investigated.

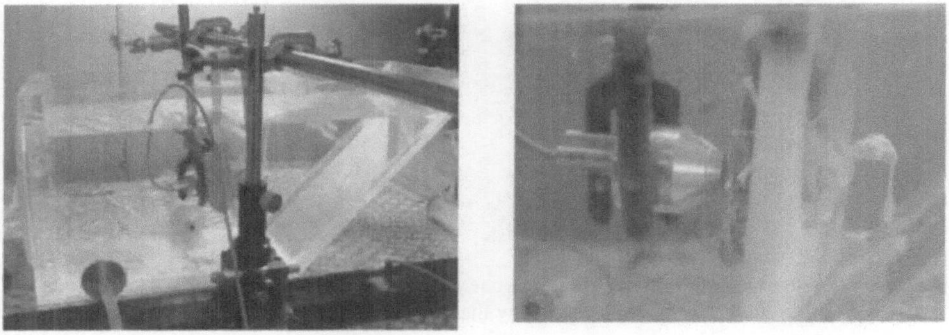

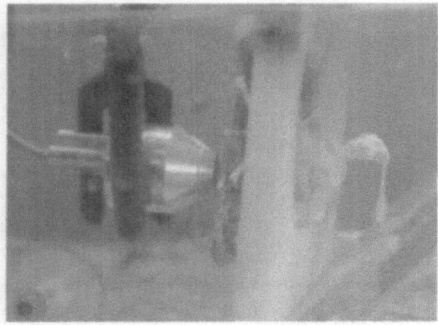

Fig. 1. Experiment of irradiating focused ultrasound toward a pig bone. The ultrasound was focused vertically to the surface of the bone, and the tank was planned to reduce standing wave.

©CARS/Springer. All rights reserved.

2.2 Simulation of ultrasound propagation

Besides, in order to solve the generated phenomenon accurately, the ultrasonic propagation in the living body consists of multiple organizations was analyzed by PZFlex (Weidlinger Associates) solving dynamic wave equation

$$i\hbar \frac{\partial \Psi}{\partial t} = \hat{H}\Psi \tag{1}$$

and using the finite-difference time-domain (FDTD) algorithm that is fourth-order accurate [6][7]. Attenuation of the ultrasonic energy in the soft tissue, such as the muscular system, between the vibrator generating ultrasonic waves and the bone surface as a focus, was measured quantitatively, then comparison with an experimental result was performed. Moreover, the numerical values considered to be related to ablation of bones, such as quantity of heat generated at a converging point, and pressure, share stress, etc., were checked out in various irradiation conditions of ultrasonic waves, such as input voltage, irradiation time to PZT, and the optimal irradiation conditions were examined.

3. Result

As a result of the experiment above, when high oscillating frequency was used, in the case of the continuum wave, the mark of ablation was found at the focal point. The ablation size was same as the convergence beam area of an ultrasonic wave confirmed by Schlieren photography, so it was made clear that only the point planned in advance was ablated. In some irradiation conditions, especially in high input voltage, the protein in a bone carried out organization necrosis with too much heat, therefore the focus turned black, and various changes were seen by changing conditions. Fig.2 shows in some conditions there was no noticeable thermal damage around the focus.

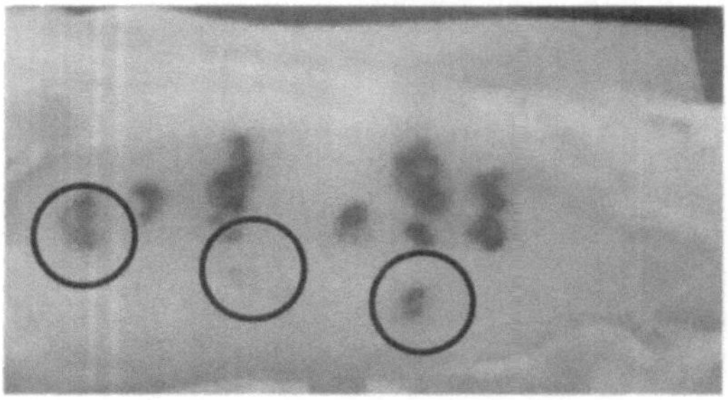

Fig. 2. Ablation marks on the surface of a pig bone. The one in the middle circle scarcely contains cell necrosis by thermal damage.

The simulation using FDTD method reproducing the experimental system above showed that at least 3MHz or more of oscillating frequency was required irrespective of input voltage in PZT, since the focal radius became large and energy hardly focused when oscillating frequency was low. However, absorption of the wave energy in the soft tissue becomes large as oscillating frequency is high. For example, as shown in Fig.3 and Fig.4,

©CARS/Springer. All rights reserved.

in 3MHz the wave energy decreases to 1/4 while passing through the soft tissue with the thickness of 10mm. Therefore, it is very important to grasp composition of the organization in front of the bone. It also turned out that the energy converging into a focus almost linearly depends on the input voltage to a PZT element. In comparison with the experimental result, the conditions in which ablation occurs without causing organization necrosis at the focus on the bone was specified by controlling input voltage and irradiation time.

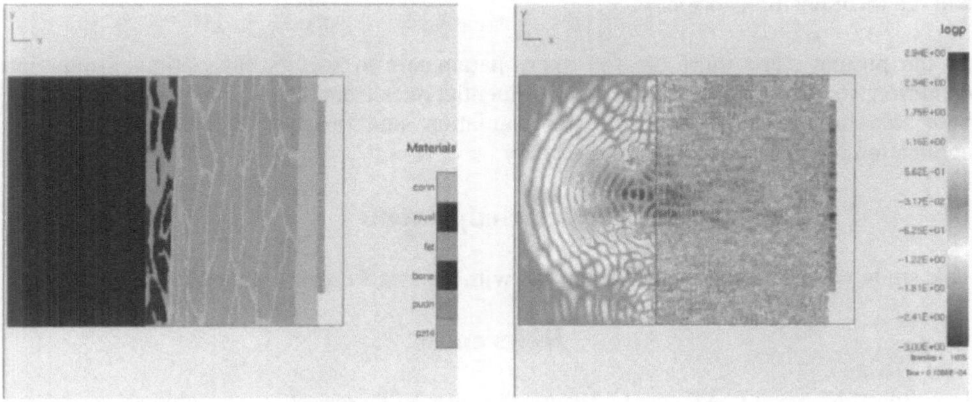

Fig. 3. Propagation of wave energy through the soft tissue between PZT and bone surface. PZT elements are arranged linearly, and create quasi-convex wave by delaying time. Array length and

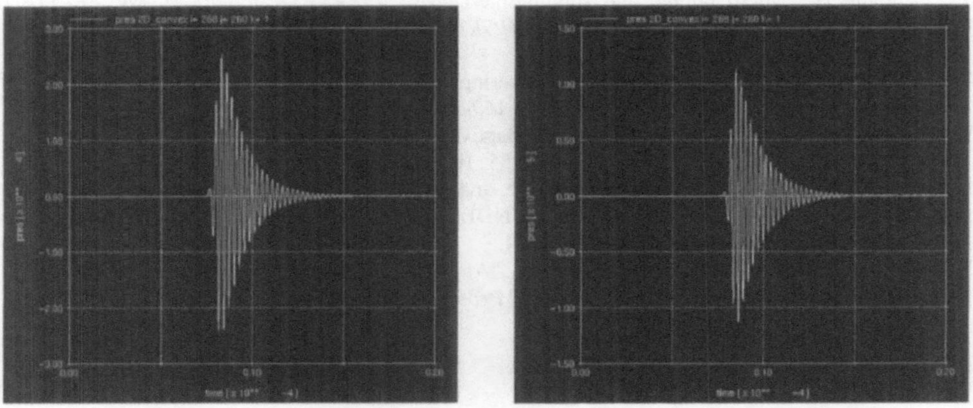

a) b)

Fig. 4. History of pressure energy at the focus in the case of Fig. 3. The material between PZT and bone surface is a) Soft tissue. b) Water.

focal length are both 10mm.

©CARS/Springer. All rights reserved.

4. Discussion

According to the irradiation conditions of ultrasound, or the circumstances of the bone, the phenomenon which happens in a focus was greatly different. Since the absorption coefficient and the refractive index of a wave change with the composition of the organization in front of the bone, it is required to take images of the focal point at any time by CT or MRI, and to update to the simulation, in order to grasp the focal situation and the focal position correctly.

At the present stage there are too many parameters to specify the optimal irradiation condition, so we are going to sort more influential ones from them by carrying forward the both sides of the experiment and the simulation, and finally aim at the final clinical application form of non-invasive osteotomy.

Acknowledgements

This study was performed in collaboration with Central Research Laboratory, Hitachi Ltd.

References

1. Robert M, Segui B, Vergnes C, Taourel P, Guiter J, "Piezoelectric extracorporeal shockwave lithotripsy of distal ureteric calculi: assessment of shockwave focusing with unenhanced spiral computed tomography", *BJU INTERNATIONAL*, 87 (4). 316-321, 2001.
2. Carstensen EL, Gracewski S, Dalecki D, "The search for cavitation in vivo", *ULTRASOUND IN MEDICINE AND BIOLOGY*, 26: (9), 1377-1385, 2000.
3. Mitome H, "Micro bubble and sonoluminescence", *JAPANESE JOURNAL OF APPLIED PHYSICS PART 1-REGULAR PAPERS SHORT NOTES & REVIEW PAPERS*, 40: (5B), 3484-3487, 2001.
4. C.Dorme, M.Fink, "Ultrasonic beam steering through inhomogeneous layers with a time reversal mirror", *IEEE Ultrasonics*, 43(1), 167-175, 1996.
5. S.Krishnan, P.C.Li, M.O'Donnell, "Adaptive compensation for phase and magnitude aberrations", *IEEE Ultrasonics*, 43(1), 44-55, 1996.
6. G. L. Wojcik, D. K. Vaughan, V. Murray*, and J. Mould, Jr., "TIME-DOMAIN MODELING OF COMPOSITE ARRAYS FOR UNDERWATER IMAGING", *IEEE Ultrasonics*, Symposium Proceedings, 1027-1032, 1994.
7. T. Deveze, L. Beaulie, and W. Tabbara, "An absorbing boundary condition for the fourth order FDTD scheme", *IEEE Antennas and Propagat. Soc. Int. Symp.*, vol. 1, 342-345, 1992.

CARS 2002 – H.U. Lemke, M.W. Vannier; K. Inamura, A.G. Farman, K. Doi & J.H.C. Reiber (Editors)
©CARS/Springer. All rights reserved.

Computer assisted arthroscopic anterior cruciate ligament reconstruction

J. Sabczynski[a], E. Hille[b], S. Dries[b], W. Zylka[c], L. Tafler[c], P. Haaker[a], T. Istel[a]
[a] Philips Research, Division Technical Systems,
Röntgenstrasse 24-26, D-22335 Hamburg, Germany
[b] Barmbek/Eilbek General Hospital, Department of Orthopedics,
Rübenkamp 148, D-22307 Hamburg, Germany
[c] University of Applied Sciences Gelsenkirchen, Dept. of Physical Engineering,
Neidenburger Strasse 43, D-45877 Gelsenkirchen, Germany

Abstract

Rupture of the Anterior Cruciate Ligament (ACL) is a common problem, mainly in young and active adults. It may lead to premature degenerative arthritis of the knee joint. The current standard surgical procedure is the endoscopic reconstruction of the ACL using a central-third bone – patellar tendon – bone graft. Correct placement, especially the isometry of the femoral and tibial insertion of the graft, is of primary importance for the stability of the reconstructed ligament. However, planning the correct insertion points and accurately executing the planned procedure is often difficult. In this paper we report on a fluoroscopic navigation system using intra-operative x-ray images to identify the correct position of the insertion points, and to guide the drilling of the tibial and femoral tunnel.

Keywords: Surgical navigation, ACL reconstruction, fluoroscopic navigation

1. Introduction

Reconstruction of the torn ACL is a highly demanding surgical task, since patients that opt for that procedure typically expect their knee joint to be as stable as before the lesion occurred. The patients are mainly young and active adults, who want to continue their sports activities, and prevent early osteoarthritis of the knee joint.
There are four main factors affecting the outcome of ACL replacement surgery: The replacement material, the tensioning of the graft, the fixation devices[1;2] and the positioning of the graft[3;4;5]. The pretensioned bone – patellar tendon – bone graft fixed with interference screws is the standard at our institution ([b]), with regard to the first three points, while the positioning is carried out under control of mechanical guides at present.
Postoperative assessment usually utilizes radiographs[6;7]. Several authors have published correlations between the natural insertion sites in human cadaveric knees and radiographs taken from those specimens [8;9;10] or correlations between graft position and clinical outcome[11;12], so criteria are available for determining the correct positioning of tibial[13;14] and femoral[15;16] graft attachment sites from standard anteroposterior and lateral radiographs. For the tibial insertion, there are also arthroscopically identifiable landmarks [17;18], though this is not true for the femoral origin (excluding mechanical guides).

©CARS/Springer. All rights reserved.

The integration of assessment criteria into planning and execution generally makes the processes more concludent. There is evidence for an increase in positioning reliability and accuracy with imaging aids, if used in preoperative planning as well as if used intraoperatively. Mean deviation of drill hole position from optimum (target based on radiologic criteria) decreases with C-arm control versus "eyeballing"[19], and is reduced again with overlay of a planning sketch tool onto the C-arm monitor[20;21].
In our case, intraoperative C-arm control of the guidewire's position is quite common, although this increases irradiation dose for both staff and patient. Navigational aids enable the surgeon to work with only two (a-p and lateral) C-arm images during the whole procedure. The planning sketch mentioned above is registered to the C-arm images. The computer is used to overlay radiographic target points, to calculate tunnel length and isometry of the graft and to integrate assessment criteria into the procedure.

2. Navigation system

The navigation system consists of a surgical workstation connected to a standard surgical C-arm (BV26, Philips Medical Systems, Best, The Netherlands). An optical position measurement device (Northern Digital Inc., Waterloo, Ontario) determines positions of instruments and tracking devices (trackers). The C-arm is equipped with a tracker in order to measure the position and orientation of the image intensifier. Prior to the operation a calibration phantom is attached to the image intensifier, and a calibration procedure is performed to determine the geometrical imaging properties of the C-arm. The calibration phantom is detached before the operation starts, and need not to imaged together with the patient. Therefore, the images are not degraded by the phantom.
External influences on the imaging properties, like mechanical distortions of the C-arm suspension system or external magnetic fields, are compensated for. The imaging properties of a C-arm x-ray system consist of the geometrical properties of the X-ray generation and detection part, and the properties of the image intensifier.

2.1 Compensation of mechanical variations

The main characteristic of a surgical C-arm system is the 'C'-shaped suspension system. At opposite ends of the 'C' the X-ray tube and at the image intensifier are mounted. This design allows a five degrees of freedom movement around the patient. The weight of tube and image intensifier may change the geometry of the suspension system. This again changes the position of the focus point of the X-ray tube relative to the detector. The effect depends on the orientation of the suspension system, and may reach several millimeters. However, it is reproducible and can thus be calibrated for.
Since the C-arm used is not equipped with angle encoders to determine the current orientation of the suspension system, a triaxial accelerometer (K-BEAM 8390A, Kistler Instrumente AG, Winterthur, Switzerland) was attached to the image intensifier. The accelerometer is used to measure the direction of the gravitation force acting on the image intensifier. This direction uniquely describes the position of suspension system for all surgically relevant positions of the C-arm.
The X-ray imaging properties of the C-arm can be described sufficiently by the coordinates of the focus point of the x-ray tube in the image intensifier coordinate system, as defined by the image intensifier tracker. During the calibration procedure, these coordinates are determined in several positions of the C-arm covering all surgically

©CARS/Springer. All rights reserved.

relevant positions. A look-up table is created including the C-arm positions and the coordinates of the x-ray focus point. During the operation proper, i.e. after removing the calibration phantom, the position of the C-arm is measured, whenever an image is taken. The look-up table is used to determine the corresponding focus coordinates. If necessary, the values are interpolated.

2.2. Compensation of image intensifier distortions

External magnetic fields have an effect on the image produced by an image intensifier. The following characteristic effects may appear [22;23]: (1) pin-cushion distortion due to the curved surface of the image intensifier, (2) shift of the image centre, (3) rotation of the image, and (4) "S"-shaped distortion. These image distortions can be described by a third degree polynomial correction approach. Coordinates of the distorted image (x and y) are transformed to coordinates of an undistorted image [22]:

$$x' = \sum_{i,j=0}^{3} a_{ij} x^i y^j , \qquad y' = \sum_{i,j=0}^{3} b_{ij} x^i y^j . \qquad (1)$$

Since the effect of external magnetic fields depends on the position and orientation of the C-arm, a triaxial magnetometer (HMR2300, Honeywell, Morristown, NJ) is attached to the image intensifier and is used to measure the strength and direction of the magnetic field in its vicinity. A look-up table is produced according to the procedure described in section 2.1.

3. Surgical procedure

The surgical procedure is divided into preparation of the navigation system, planning of tibial and femoral insertion points, checking their position, planning of tunnel directions, and execution of the plans.

3.1 Preparation

After harvesting the central third of the patellar tendon, tracking devices are attached to femur and tibia through small incisions. These trackers define femoral and tibial coordinate systems, which are used later for coordinate transformations. A pointing instrument, e.g. a Stille hook, is prepared by attaching a tracker. In order to make the geometry of the pointing instrument (i.e. the position of its tip relative to tracker) known to the system, a calibration procedure using a learning device with known geometry is performed.

3.2. Planning the tibial insertion

The position of the tibial insertion point of the ACL graft can now be determined arthroscopically: The surgeon simply points to the optimal position under arthroscopic vision. This position is recorded by the navigation system in the tibial coordinate system.

3.2. Planning the femoral insertion

In order to determine the correct placement of the femoral insertion point a strictly lateral fluoroscopic image is produced. Simultaneously with the image the positions and orientations of the C-arm, and of the femoral and the tibial tracker are recorded. Since the

©CARS/Springer. All rights reserved.

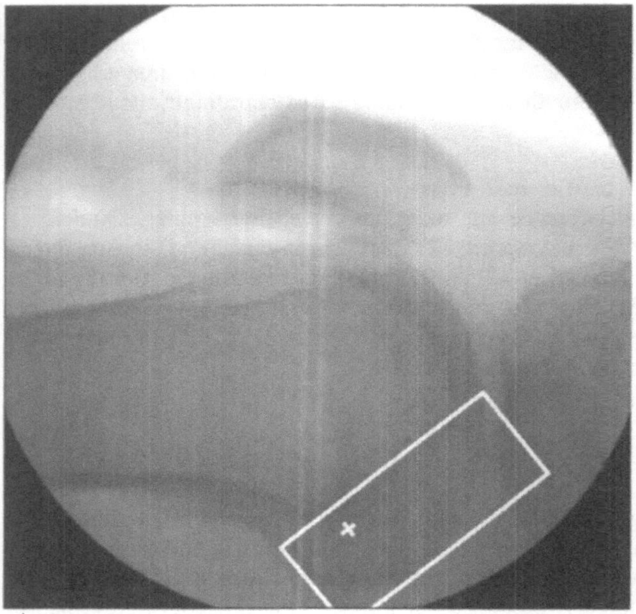

Fig. 1: Strictly lateral X-ray image of a knee phantom. The Blumensaat line and the box surrounding the condyles are drawn by the user. The femoral insertion point of the ACL is calculated and drawn according to [15].

C-arm has been calibrated prior to the operation (see section 2), its geometrical imaging properties are fully known. The radiographic equivalent of the intercondylar roof, the Blumensaat line, is visible in the image. According to the Radiographic Quadrant Method by Bernard et al. [15] the position of the femoral insertion point can be identified in the *image* relative to the Blumensaat line. First the Blumensaat line is drawn in the image, second the size of the box enclosing the condyles is adjusted (see Figure 1). The insertion point is drawn automatically based on the findings of [15].
The image coordinates of this point are recorded by the navigation system. These image coordinates define a unique projection line, i.e. an X-ray beam, in three-dimensional space. The three-dimensional insertion point on the bone-surface is located on this beam. The beam itself is given by two points in space: (1) the position of the X-ray focus point at the time of imaging and (2) the position of the point in the detector plane corresponding to the recorded image point. Once this X-ray beam is known, a graphical overlay is produced on all previously acquired images.
The next step is to transfer the two-dimensional image coordinates of the insertion point to the three-dimensional femoral coordinate system. This is done by touching the bony femoral surface with the pointing instrument. In order to help the surgeon to find the correct insertion point, the current distance of the tip of the pointing device to the x-ray beam is calculated by the navigation system and thus displayed on screen. If the distance is minimal *and* the tip of the pointer is on the femur surface, the position of the pointer is recorded.

3.3 Checking the insertion points

After defining femoral and tibial insertion points of the ACL graft, the isometry of these points is tested by flexing the knee joint. The navigation system measures and displays the distance between both insertion points. If the isometry is sufficient the direction of tibial and femoral tunnels can be determined.

©CARS/Springer. All rights reserved.

3.4. Planning the tunnel directions

Since the tibial tunnel must be drilled first and the femoral tunnel can be drilled through the tibial tunnel only afterwards, strong geometrical constraints apply to the direction of the tunnels. Only drill trajectories, which pass through both tibial and femoral insertion points, are allowed. The remaining degree of freedom for the surgeon is the flexion of the knee. The surgeon can adjust the flexion of the knee until the direction of the tunnels is correct. Since femur and tibia are tracked by the position measurement system, the navigation system can display both tunnels on all acquired C-arm images in the correct position relative to the anatomy.

3.5 Execution of the plans

Once all planned trajectories are known, the drilling proper can begin. A k-wire (2 mm diameter) is used to prepare the drilling of the tibial tunnel. A drill-guide is equipped with a tracker of the optical position measurement system, and its tip position and orientation are calibrated for (see also section 3.1). Then the navigation system displays the drill-guide in all images and a targeting tool can be used to indicate how far the tip and end of the drill-guide are away from the planned trajectory. Once the drill-guide is properly aligned the k-wire is drilled into the tibia. The tibial tunnel is then drilled with a hollow drill over the k-wire. The procedure is repeated for the femoral tunnel. After drilling the tunnels, the bone – patellar tendon – bone graft is introduced, and fixed with interference screws.

4. Conclusion

We have developed an fluoroscopic navigation system for arthroscopic reconstruction of the anterior cruciate ligament. While the tibial insertion of the ACL graft is determined easily under direct arthroscopic control, the femoral origin can be identified in lateral X-ray images. Since the femoral tunnel is drilled through the tibial tunnel, strong geometrical restrictions on the tunnel directions apply. Our navigation system takes these restrictions into account, and allows an easy intra-operative planning of both tunnels.

Acknowledgements

The authors thank Prof. Dr. Höpker, Barmbek General Hospital, for the preparation of the knees. The authors also want to thank the mechanical workshop of Philips Research Hamburg, namely Roman Swiderski, Horst Peemöller, Willi Rohwer, and Walter Schröder, for their continuous support.

References

1. To, J. T., Howell, S. M., and Hull, M. L., "Contributions of femoral fixation methods to the stiffness of ACL replacements at implantation.", *Arthroscopy.*, 15(4): 379-387, 1999.
2. Butler, J. C., Branch, T. P., and Hutton, W. C., "Optimal graft fixation–the effect of gap size and screw size on bone plug fixation in ACL reconstruction.", *Arthroscopy.*, 10(5): 524-529, 1994.
3. Boden, B., Migaud, H., Gougeon, F., Debroucker, M. J., and Duquennoy, A., "Effect of graft position on laxity after ACL reconstruction. Stress radiography in 90 knees 2 to 5 years after autograft.", *Acta Orthop.Belg.*, 62(1): 2-7, 1996.
4. Bylski-Austrow, D. I., Grood, E. S., Hefzy, M. S., Holden, J. P., and Butler, D. L., "ACL replacements: a mechanical study of femoral attachment location, flexion angle at tensioning, and initial tension.", *J.OrthopRes*, 8: 522-531, 1990.

©CARS/Springer. All rights reserved.

5. Djian, P., Christel, P., Roger, B., and Witvoet, J., "Roentgenographic and magnetic resonance imaging of anterior cruciate reconstruction using a patellar tendon graft–correlations with physical findings.", *Knee.Surg.Sports Traumatol.Arthrosc.*, 2(4): 207-213, 1994.
6. Klos, T.-V. S., Harman, M. K., Devilee, R. J., Banks, S. A., and Cook, F. F., "Patellar tendon graft position after ACL reconstruction. Interobserver variability on lateral radiographs.", *Acta Orthop.Scand.*, 70(2): 180-184, 1999.
7. Klos, T.-V. S., Banks, A. Z., Lambregts, K.-A. H., Banks, S. A., Cook, F. F., "Radiographic parameters for ACL reconstruction.", *Proceedings of CAR'96: Computer Assisted Radiology-10th International Symposium*, Ed.: Vannier, M. W., Inamura, K., and Farman, A. G., 832-836. Springer, Paris,France, 1996.
8. Collette, M., Mertens, H., Peters, M., and Chaput, A., "Radiological method for preoperative determination of isometric attachment points of an ACL graft.", *Knee.Surg.Sports Traumatol.Arthrosc.*, 4(2): 75-83, 1996.
9. Feller, J. A., Glisson, R. R., Seaber, A. V., Feagin, J. A. J., and Garrett, W. E. J., "Graft isometricity in unitunnel ACL reconstruction: analysis of influential factors using a radiographic model.", *Knee.Surg.Sports Traumatol.Arthrosc.*, 1(3-4): 136-142, 1993.
10. Lintner, D. M., Dewitt, S. E., and Moseley, J. B., "Radiographic evaluation of native ACL attachments and graft placement for reconstruction. A cadaveric study.", *Am.J.Sports Med.*, 24(1): 72-78, 1996.
11. Khalfayan, E. E., Sharkey, P. F., Alexander, A. H., Bruckner, J. D., and Bynum, E. B., "The relationship between tunnel placement and clinical results after ACL reconstruction.", *Am.J.Sports Med.*, 24(3): 335-341, 1996.
12. Muneta, T., Yamamoto, H., Ishibashi, T., Asahina, S., Murakami, S., and Furuya, K., "The effects of tibial tunnel placement and roofplasty on reconstructed ACL knees.", *Arthroscopy.*, 11(1): 57-62, 1995.
13. Howell, S. M., "Principles for placing the tibial tunnel and avoiding roof impingement during reconstruction of a torn ACL.", *Knee.Surg.Sports Traumat.Arthrosc.*,6(Suppl):S49-S55, 1998.
14. Ikeda, H., Muneta, T., Niga, S., Hoshino, A., Asahina, S., and Yamamoto, H., "The long-term effects of tibial drill hole position on the outcome of ACL reconstruction.", *Arthroscopy.*, 15(3): 287-291, 1999.
15. Bernard, M., Hertel, P., Hornung, H., and Cierpinski, T., "Femoral insertion of the ACL. Radiographic quadrant method.", *Am.J.Knee.Surg.*, 10(1): 14-21, 1997.
16. Cassisa, G., Nasi, M., Peretti, M., and Pappalardo, S., "X-ray evaluation of interferential femoral screw positioning in ACL reconstruction.", *Chir.Organi.Mov.*, 81(3): 257-261, 1996.
17. Berg, E. E., "Parsons' knob (tuberculum intercondylare tertium). A guide to tibial ACL insertion.", *Clin.Orthop.*292: 229-231, 1993.
18. Morgan, C. D., Kalman, V. R., and Grawl, D. M., "Definitive landmarks for reproducible tibial tunnel placement in ACL reconstruction.", *Arthroscopy.*, 11(3): 275-288, 1995.
19. Milankov, M. and Miljkovic, N., "A new positioning device for precise femoral insertion of the ACL autograft", *Knee.Surg.Sports Traumatol.Arthrosc.*, 3(3): 149-153, 2000.
20. Klos, T.-V. S., Habets, R. J., Banks, A. Z., Banks, S. A., Devilee, R. J., and Cook, F. F., "Computer assistance in ACL reconstruction.", *Clin.Orthop.*354: 65-69, 1998.
21. Klos, T.-V. S., Banks, S. A., Cook, F. F., Harman, M. K., Banks, A. Z., Ed, b. S., Morgan, K., Sieburg, H. B., Mattheus, R., and Christensen, J. P. "Interactive fluoroscopic controlled ACL." *InteractiveTechnology and the New Paradigm for Healthcare.Medicine meets Virtual Reality III Proceedings*): 173-174. San Diego, CA, USA, 1995
22. Koppe, R., Klotz, E., Op de Beek, J., and Aerts, H. "3D vessel reconstruction based on rotational angiography.", *Proceedings CAR'95,* H.U. Lemke, K. Inamura, C.C. Jaffe, M.W. Vannier (editors)): 101-107, Berlin, 1995.
23. Grass, M., Koppe, R., Klotz, E., Proksa, R., Kuhn, M. H., Aerts, H., Op, d. B., and Kemkers, R., "Three-dimensional reconstruction of high contrast objects using C-arm image intensifier projection data", *Comput.Med.Imaging Graph.*, 23(6): 311-321, 1999.

CARS 2002 – H.U. Lemke, M.W. Vannier; K. Inamura, A.G. Farman, K. Doi & J.H.C. Reiber (Editors)
©CARS/Springer. All rights reserved.

Fast generation of 3D bone models for craniofacial surgical planning: an interactive approach

Ritter L.[a], Liévin M.[a], Sader R.[b], Zeilhofer H-F.[b], Keeve E.[a]
[a] Surgical Systems Laboratory, Research Center caesar
Friedensplatz 16, 53111 Bonn, Germany
[b] Dept. of Cranio- and Maxillofacial Surgery, Technical University of Munich,
Ismaningerstr. 22, 81675 Munich, Germany

Abstract

A comprehensive image processing pipeline for efficient and accurate construction of 3D surface skull models for computer-aided craniofacial surgical planning is presented. In a pre-processing step, algorithms for noise and artefact reduction enhance initial CT data sets. Next, segmentation is real-time visualized in volume and provides the user with an instant overview of the ongoing segmentation. Finally, a dedicated implementation of the Marching Cube algorithm for bone surface extraction is employed. The pipeline was tested by generation of surface models from ten CT scans acquired for craniofacial surgical planning.

Keywords: Interactive bone segmentation, craniofacial surgery, volume visualization.

1. Introduction

In this paper we describe an original and interactive approach to efficiently and accurately construct patient specific virtual 3D surface models of the skull from CT scans. Computer-aided craniofacial surgery has many applications for patient individual 3D models, e.g. virtual surgical planning of bone realignments, simulation of minimally-invasive distraction osteogenesis or generation of rapid prototyping models [1, 2, 3]. However, accurate generation of these essential 3D models is often cumbersome and commonly achieved by successively performing the following steps: image filtering, segmentation and surface reconstruction. While each processing step is substance to intensive research itself, from a practical point it can be useful to consider these steps as a conglomerate yielding a 3D model as the final product. Therefore each algorithm should be chosen carefully with respect to the following one and interaction between these algorithms should be inspected. According to this approach we encountered several drawbacks in commonly used pipelines by observing clinical users:

- Manual parameterization of filter algorithms is required.
- Unfiltered metal artefacts impair segmentation.
- Segmentation errors are encountered after surface generation.
- Surface generation does not respect grey values of the original image.

To address these problems (while not solving them all) we designed a coherent processing pipeline consisting of an automatic filtering algorithm based on Markov random fields, a

©CARS/Springer. All rights reserved.

statistical algorithm reducing metal artefacts and a 3D interactive segmentation using either region-growing or thresholding algorithms followed by a dedicated implementation of the Marching Cube surface generation algorithm.
The vital step in this pipeline is a real-time segmentation approach providing the user with an instant volume view of the ongoing segmentation. This approach avoids the time-consuming surface generation step when iteratively checking for segmentation errors in volume.
All processing steps are implemented as modules into the software framework Julius [4] that handles essential steps like data management and visualization.
The pipeline was tested with ten different CT scans from actual cases for craniofacial surgical treatment with indications ranging from corrective bimaxillary repositioning osteotomies to complex reconstructions after tumor resection.

2. Methods

In this section we describe the subsequent processing steps, starting with the two image enhancement techniques employed. Next we introduce a new 3D interactive segmentation interface that volume renders the active segmentation process in real-time. Finally we describe the surface generation step.

2.1 Image enhancement

Artefacts from metallic dental fillings of the patient often impair the quality of cranial CT scans. Moreover, CT scans are affected by acquisition noise. In order to reproducibly enhance the initial data and facilitate subsequent segmentation we apply a dedicated algorithm for metal artefact reduction and an automatic image enhancement algorithm based on Markov random fields.
First, metal artefacts on each slice are automatically identified by a statistical noise estimation. Thereby an optimal conservation of the initial image content is achieved since only affected regions on the particular slices are selected for artefact removal. The selected regions then undergo non-linear interpolation in order to diminish artefacts. The proposed algorithm is computationally fast and takes morphological features into account since the complete volumetric spatial domain is considered. Although the original information content of the CT scan is altered by interpolation, the final 3D model justifies this kind of data manipulation.

As a second step the data is filtered by a Markov random fields based algorithm. This theory has been applied for image enhancement [5] as well as for image segmentation [6]. The algorithm is implemented as a regularization process, iterating over the image until the stability or minimum energy is reached. The minimization of the noise, generally modeled as Gaussian additive, produces noise free images. Prior constraints increase the homogeneity and the contrast between anatomical areas. Thanks to the statistical theory, noise estimation allows this algorithm to be automatic, without any user parameter tuning. In parallel implementation, the computation time on a whole volume (e.g. 50 Mbytes) can be reduced to a few minutes.

©CARS/Springer. All rights reserved.

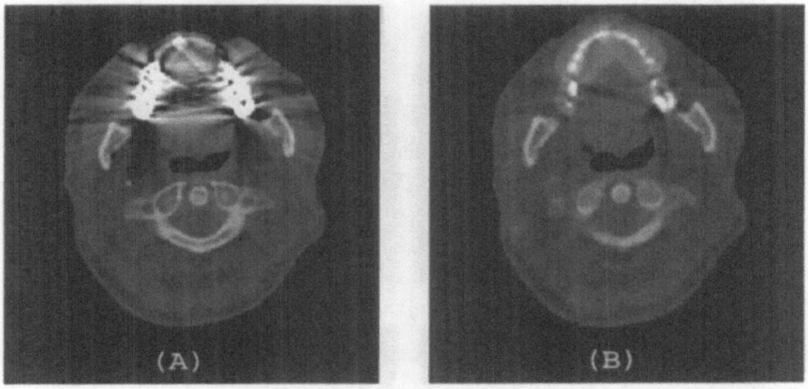

Figure 1: Axial CT slices before (A) and after (B) image enhancement consisting of metal artefact reduction and Markov random field based filtering.

2.2. 3D Interactive segmentation

Volume rendering by 3D texture mapping is used to initially display the CT data set. Compatible with OpenGL 1.2 [7], this technique allows real-time volume rendering: slices of the volume are directly rendered from back to front. An update rate of 10Hz is reached for a display size of 600x600 pixels to visualize a volume-texture data of 512x512x128 voxels on an Onyx 3200 IR3.

Segmentation results are interactively displayed in 3D allowing the user to inspect the whole volume from arbitrary angles (see Figure 2). Additionally, the segmentation is visualized as an overlay plane on the well-known 2-D slices of the CT scan in axial, sagittal and coronal views. This display technique has been applied to two generic bone segmentation methods: region growing and thresholding. These algorithms are integrated into the pipeline as alternative segmentation methods with special attention to visualization, intuitive user interaction and the subsequent surface generation algorithm.

Threshold segmentation is to distinguish pixels or voxels within an image by their grey value. An upper or lower threshold can be defined, separating the image into structure of interest and background. This method works explicitly well for bone segmentation from CT scans since bone tissue attenuates significantly more X-rays during acquisition and is therefore represented by much higher values on the Hounsfield scale compared to soft tissues. Thresholding by hardware color mapping as the first implementation concerns the integration of the segmentation process directly into the visualization pipeline. A lookup table for the color mapping is generated and scaled within two initial thresholds. Since visualization of a dynamic color mapping is hardware accelerated and can be manipulated by the user, the segmentation process is displayed in volume with a real-time update rate. The user can easily change upper and lower threshold values either by moving one of the two sliders or directly enter a specific value.

©CARS/Springer. All rights reserved.

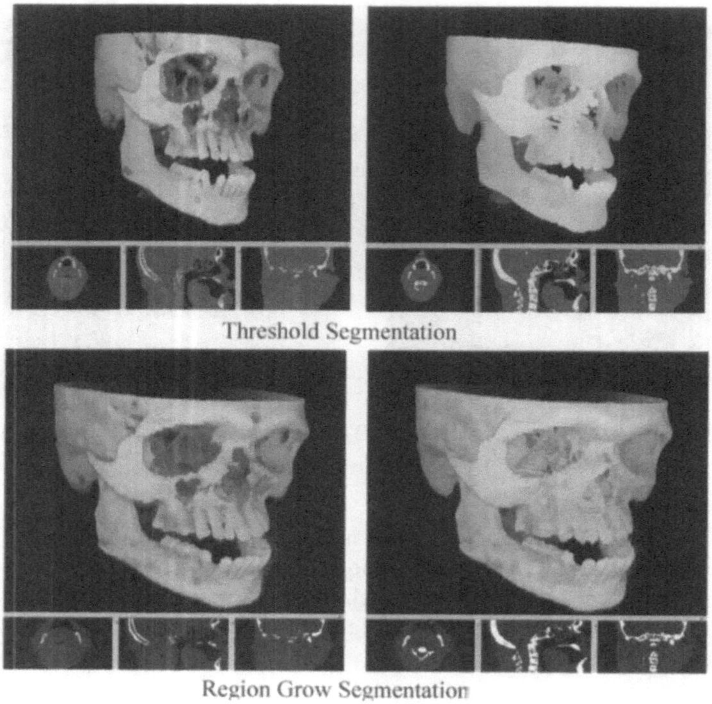

Figure 2: Screenshots of segmentations with the 3D texture mapping view and with the axial, sagittal and coronal slice view below is shown. Note the segmented parts displayed in lighter gray in the 3D scene compared to the yet unsegmented in darker gray. Progress by parameter tuning is shown from left to right for thresholding on the top and region growing on the bottom row.

Whereas thresholding focuses on the difference of pixel intensities, the region growing method looks for regions of voxels with similar intensities. First, seed points are chosen interactively within the region on the image where bone is present: their Hounsfield values correspond to an upper threshold. From these points, the iterative process investigates all neighboring voxels for similarity, up to the value of the lower threshold. To achieve real-time visualization of the region-growing algorithm in 3D, the algorithm is split in two parts. Thereby computational more and less expensive tasks are separated: a computational growing on the original data and an updating module that handles growing for the visualization pipeline are designed. The updating module only sends the areas where the growing is updated to the visualization pipeline. This approach is reasonable because region growing interferes only with a small portion of the anatomy or at least with a reasonable ratio of the initial volume. Updating one subvolume takes an average of 4 milliseconds allowing an update-visualization rate of 5 Hz for a region growing on 10^6 voxels.

2.3. Iso-surface generation

Finally we reconstruct a surface model by a dedicated implementation of the Marching Cube algorithm [8]. Here we apply the algorithm not on a binary volume derived from segmentation but rather on the original volume. For threshold segmentation the iso-

©CARS/Springer. All rights reserved.

surface value for the algorithm is directly taken from the user defined threshold values. For region growing, the iso-surface values associated to the segmented binary volume are computed and used for surface extraction. This allows us to consider the original Hounsfield units for tri-linear interpolation and grey-level gradient shading.

3. Results

The statistical estimation of slices affected by metal artefacts reliably worked for all studied cases. Diminishing detected artefacts improved image quality (see Figure 1) and greatly enhanced final models compared to non-processed data. The Markov random fields image filtering reliably removed noise and enhanced edges. This was found especially helpful for segmentation by region growing where better results were achieved when the data was filtered.

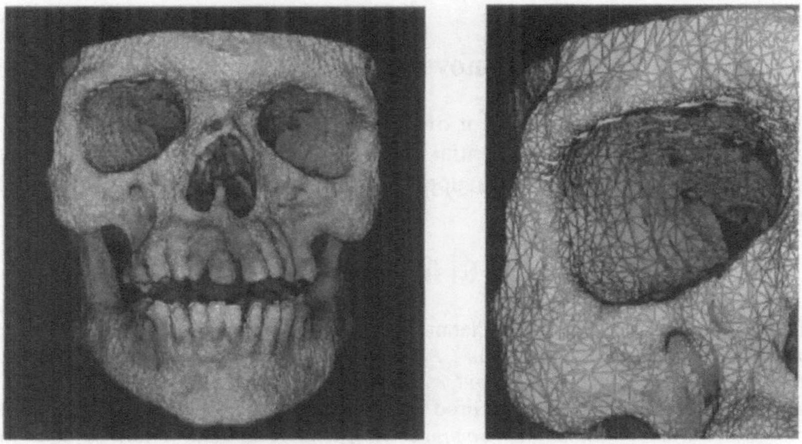

Figure 3: Grid of the 3D surface model as an overlay in blue on the volume rendered segmentation scene in yellow. The left image shows the front view of the whole model while the right image is zoomed on the orbita. Note the small errors on the supraorbital margin.

We were able to achieve interactive segmentation with an update rate of at least 10 Hz for all tested cases. The interactive volume display approach greatly reduced the time required for bone segmentation. Especially the 3D assessment before surface generation helped to efficiently encounter segmentation errors and correct parameters when necessary. To assess the correspondence of the volume visualized segmentation and the final 3D surface model we superimposed the surface mesh over the volume visualized segmentation with the chosen parameter (see Figure 3). Inspection of all models revealed good correspondence of volume visualization and surface model i.e. a reliable impression the final result can be assessed during segmentation in real-time. The additional 2D display of the segmentation results was also helpful for verification, providing the medical professional with a familiar environment.
Finally, our implementation of the Marching Cube algorithm was able to preserve small anatomical details (e.g. foramen mentale) that were lost when applying the algorithm on the binary volume derived from the same segmentation.

©CARS/Springer. All rights reserved.

4. Conclusions

We have presented a dedicated pipeline for the fast and accurate generation of 3D surface models of the skull for computer-aided craniofacial surgical planning. The image pre-processing steps in this pipeline work automatically, however, for future work we plan to further improve performance of these steps by accelerating the filtering and increasing accuracy of the metal-artefact reduction.

An interactive 3D approach of region-growing as well as threshold segmentation was presented accelerating the interactive segmentation. Further segmentation algorithms (e.g. watershed segmentation) will be tested for volume visualized interactive segmentation of MR data sets.

Although avoiding iterative surface generations for error correction seems to obviously accelerate segmentation we plan to assess time and accuracy measurements in a clinical environment.

Acknowledgements

We are very thankful to the department of radiology of the Klinikum rechts der Isar, TU Munich for providing us with the essential data sets. We also like to thank Thomas Jansen and Bartosz von Rymon-Lipinski for supporting the implementation of the pipeline into the Julius software framework.

References

1. Everett et al., “A 3D System for Planning and Simulating Minimally-Invasive Distraction Osteogenesis of the Facial Skeleton,” *Proceedings of Third International Conference On Medical Robotics, Imaging and Computer Assisted Surgery*, pp. 1029-1039, 2000.
2. Keeve E., Girod S., Kikinis R., Girod B., "Deformable Modeling of Facial Tissue for Craniofacial Surgery Simulation," *Computer Aided Surgery*, John Wiley & Sons Inc., New York, Vol. 3, No. 5, pp. 228-238, 1999.
3. Petzold R., Zeilhofer H.-F., Kalender W.A., “Rapid prototyping technology in medicine – basics and applications” *Comput Med Imaging Graph.*, Vol. 23 No. 5, pp. 277-84. 1999
4. Keeve, E., Jansen T., Krol Z., Ritter L., von Rymon-Lipinski B., Sader R., Zeilhofer H.-F., Zerfass P., "JULIUS - An Extendable Software Framework for Surgical Planning and Image-Guided Navigation" *Medical Image Computing and Computer-Assisted Intervention - MICCAI'01*, W.J. Niessen, M. A. Viergever, pp. 1336-37, Springer, Utrecht, 2001.
5. Geman, S. Geman, D. “Stochastic relaxation, Gibbs distributions and the Bayesian restoration of images,” *IEEE Transactions on Pattern Analysis and Machine Intelligence*, Vol. 6, pp. 721-742, 1984.
6. Held K., Rota Kopps E., Krause B., Wells W., Kikinis R., Muller-Gartner H., “Markov Random Field Segmentation of Brain MR Images,” *IEEE Transactions on Medical Imaging, Vol.16*, pp. 878-887,1998.
7. http://www.opengl.org
8. Lorensen W. E., Cline H. E., "Marching Cube: A High Resolution 3D Surface Construction Algorithm," *Computer Graphics*, Vol. 21, No. 4, pp. 163-169, 1987.

CARS 2002 – H.U. Lemke, M.W. Vannier; K. Inamura, A.G. Farman, K. Doi & J.H.C. Reiber (Editors)
©CARS/Springer. All rights reserved.

A virtual fluoroscopy system based on a small and unobtrusive registration / calibration phantom

R Phillips[a], V Peter[a], G-E Faure[a], Q Li[a], KP Sherman[b], WJ Viant[a], MS Bielby[a], AMMA Mohsen[b]

[a] Department of Computer Science, University of Hull, Hull, UK, HU6 7RX

[b] Department of Orthopaedics and Traumatology, Hull Royal Infirmary, Anlaby Road, Hull, UK HU3 2JZ

Abstract

The C-arm fluoroscope is an indispensable intraoperative 2D imaging device for orthopaedic surgery. A recent technique known as virtual fluoroscopy (VF) enhances the fluoroscope's capability for image guided surgery by tracking optically the position of the C-arm, surgical instruments and the patient. Virtuality is achieved by overlay of surgical instruments onto one or more previously captured fluoroscopic images. This paper presents a new technique for determining the position and calibrating the geometry of a C-arm fluoroscope. This technique is based on a small registration phantom that is placed close to the patient whilst imaging. This paper also reports on a VF-based protocol for the placement of the femoral component for an Oxford unicompartmental knee prosthesis. A key benefit of VF is that it reduces considerably the radiation hazard of using a C-arm fluoroscope and it enhances the surgeon's ability to plan intraoperatively and implement surgery.

Keywords: Fluoroscopy, image-guided, calibration.

1. Introduction

The C-arm fluoroscope is an indispensable intraoperative 2D imaging device for orthopaedic surgery but it poses a significant radiation hazard to theatre staff and patients. A technique known as virtual fluoroscopy (VF) enhances the fluoroscope's capability so that it produces virtual images of patient anatomy and surgical instruments during surgery.

Typically in VF a number of fluoroscopic images are taken intraoperatively of the patient just prior to actual surgery. For each such image, the position and geometry of the associated image cone space is recorded. During surgery the position of the surgeon's instrument is tracked optically and this allows the computer to overlay a projection of this instrument onto the previously captured images to produce virtual images. By attaching an optically tracked frame (known as a dynamic reference frame - DRF) to bones involved in surgery, virtual images can be produced even though these bones may have moved since being initially imaged.

This paper presents a new technique for determining the position and calibrating the geometry of a C-arm fluoroscope. This technique is based on a small registration phantom

©CARS/Springer. All rights reserved.

that is placed close to the patient whilst imaging. This paper also reports on a VF-based protocol for the placement of the femoral component for an Oxford unicompartmental knee prosthesis.

2. Methods

To overlay the position of surgical instruments onto previously captured fluoroscopic images requires, firstly, accurate 2D calibration of fluoroscopic images and, secondly, accurate registration of the fluoroscopic image cone space with the coordinate space of an optical tracking system.

2.1 Preoperative calibration of x-ray images

Fluoroscopic images suffer from a number of distortion effects [1]. This image distortion is dynamic both in terms of time and with the position of the C-arm.

Calibration in our VF system involves preoperative imaging of an x-ray translucent plate containing an evenly spaced grid of 64 x 64 balls placed on the x-ray receptor cover of the C-arm. From this image, software calculates a distortion-undistortion map. Intraoperatively, all fluoroscopic images are then displayed with the distortion removed. Sufficient image accuracy for the placement of surgical instruments is obtained by calibrating in just two positions, i.e. with the C-arm vertical and horizontal. Calibration is typically required once a month.

2.2 Intraoperative registration of fluoroscopic image space

Registration of the fluoroscope's image space with the optical tracking system involves accurate localisation of the position of the x-ray source and the image plane of the C-arm. Our registration approach involves placing a small registration phantom in the image space of the C-arm of each image. This phantom consists of an H arrangement of 21 metal balls that measures approximately 2" x 2" by ½" (Fig. 1). The projection of these balls appears in a fluoroscopic image. The phantom is held by an end-effector and a lockable passive arm. The position of the phantom is tracked by an NDI Polaris optical tracking system. When a patient is imaged, software undistorts the image and then automatically detects the position of the phantom in the image. Then knowing the position of the phantom, a registration algorithm calculates the position of the C-arm in the coordinate space of the optical tracking system. It is worth noting that the above registration technique partly compensates for C-arm flex (both position and orientation) and the rotational and translation components of dynamic distortion.

Significant obscuration of the phantom frequently occurs in the image due to shadow of muscles, bone edges, retractors, etc. Furthermore, image contrast varies considerably between images and patients, and varies considerably within an image. Software has been developed that is robust to such problems. The software comprises two distinct algorithms. The ball detection algorithm first detects a candidate set of metal ball projections from the image. The second, the phantom detector algorithm, selects a subset of these metal balls that provide a feasible projection of the phantom. The ball detection algorithm uses contrast gradient in two directions to initially select possible ball

©CARS/Springer. All rights reserved.

projections. It then applies a series of six filters to eliminate less promising projections. These filters include tests for size, shape, proximity, contrast and gradient variation. Robustness of the phantom detection algorithm is achieved by detection requiring a minimum of 14 balls. The algorithm is normally able to detect a limb of the H even when there are 4 neighbouring ball projections missing.

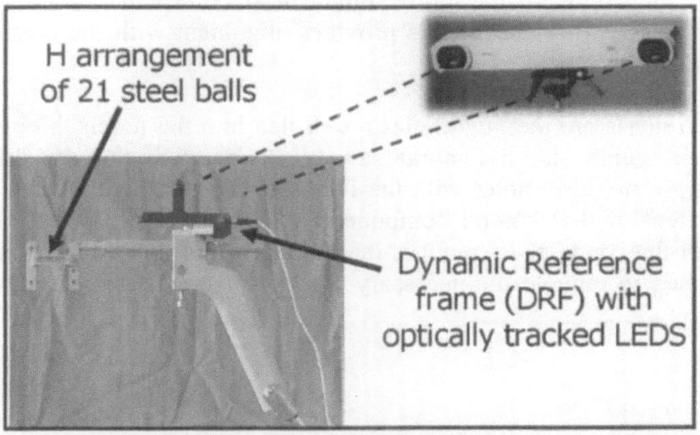

Figure 1. Phantom mounted in end-effector with DRF for optical position tracking.

Computer simulation was used to determine a phantom design that had the best trade-off between reconstruction performance and the clinical need to make the phantom as unobtrusive as possible.

2.3 A VF protocol for unicompartmental knee replacement

Unicondylar knee replacements are used to treat medial compartment osteoarthritis. A unicondylar knee replacement replaces the joint surfaces of the medial compartment of the knee joint. The prosthesis comprises a tibial and a femoral component and a polyethylene bearing completes the prosthetic joint. The approach to the knee is typically through a 5-8 cm incision.

The goal of unicompartmental knee arthroplasty is to create a mechanical axis that is neutral. The joint line of the replaced compartment should be parallel to the floor and perpendicular to the mechanical axis. Thus the femoral and tibial components are aligned to be perpendicular to the mechanical axis. Well-designed instrumentation greatly assists accurate component placement. The paper will focus on using VF for the accurate placement of the femoral component of the prosthesis.

2.4 Existing protocol for unicompartmental knee replacement surgery

Preparing for the femoral component starts by making a femoral drill hole 1 cm anterior to the anteromedial corner of the inter condylar notch of the distal femur. This is the point where the anatomical and mechanical axis typically intersects. An intramedullary rod is then inserted into the femoral intramedullary canal using this starter hole. The axis of this rod represents the anatomical axis of the femur and the intramedullary rod.

©CARS/Springer. All rights reserved.

The femoral drill guide is now positioned in the knee joint using a tibial template and a feeler gauge. The alignment criteria for this guide are as follows.

a) From the front, the guide should be in the middle of the condyle and the handle of the guide should be parallel with the long axis of the tibia.
b) The upper surface of the guide should be parallel with the intramedullary rod.
c) The 7° angled fin of the guide should be parallel with the intramedullary rod when viewed from above (this provides alignment with the mechanical axis of the femur).

When all these criteria are met, two holes are drilled into the femur through the holes in the femoral drill guide and a femoral saw block inserted into the drill holes. The placement of these two drill holes with the femoral drill guide is the critical step for the accurate placement of the femoral component. A flat cut is then made to remove the posterior part of the condyle. A spigot is then inserted into the larger of these two holes and a mill is used to remove the necessary amount of bone from the distal end of the femur.

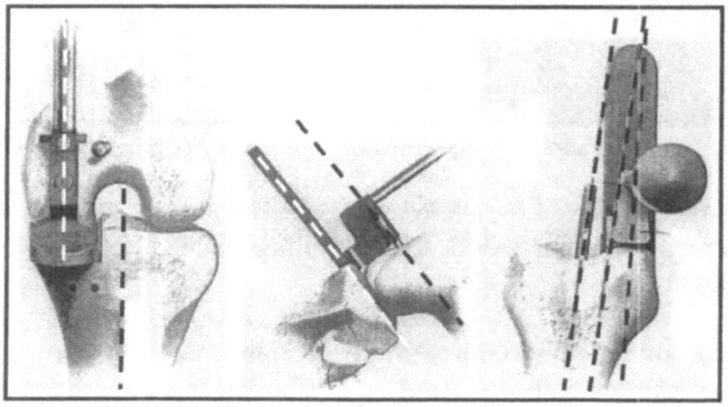

(a (b (c

Figure 2. Alignment criteria for the femoral drill guide.

2.5 A VF-based protocol for unicompartmental knee replacement surgery

In the operating theatre a Polaris optical tracking system is used to track both patient anatomy and surgical instruments. More specifically dynamic reference frames are attached both to the femur and the tibia. This allows the overlay of surgical instruments onto fluoroscopic images to take account of movements of both femur and tibia. A reference frame is also attached to the femoral drill guide.

The following intraoperative fluoroscopic images are taken of the patient: AP view of the femur head, AP and lateral view of the femur shaft, AP and lateral view of the tibia and an AP of the knee in 40° of flexion with a beam view 30° off vertical.

Our VF system provides a number of simple but flexible planning facilities for identification of anatomy on VF images in terms of 3D points, lines and planes. Using these facilities, the surgeon locates the anatomy of interest, namely: the head of the femur, the anatomical and mechanical axis of the femur and the axis of the tibia.

©CARS/Springer. All rights reserved.

As before the femoral drill guide is now positioned in the knee joint. As the surgeon moves the guide, its outline (and its virtual extensions) appears immediately on the VF images (Fig. 3). The virtual extensions make it easier to align the guide with the more distant anatomical features such as the centre of the femoral head. To satisfy the guide's alignment criteria (see 2.4) the surgeon uses the VF images as follows.

1. *Guide in middle of condyle* – checked both visually and on the various VF views.
2. *Handle of guide parallel with long axis of the tibia* – checked by viewing the guide's handle on the AP and lateral virtual views of the tibia.
3. *Upper surface of the guide parallel with anatomical femur axis* – checked in the lateral virtual view of the femur.
4. *Femoral guide aligned with anatomical axis of femur* – checked in the AP virtual view of the femur where the fin should be parallel to the anatomical axis and the centre line of the guide should pass through the centre of the femoral head.

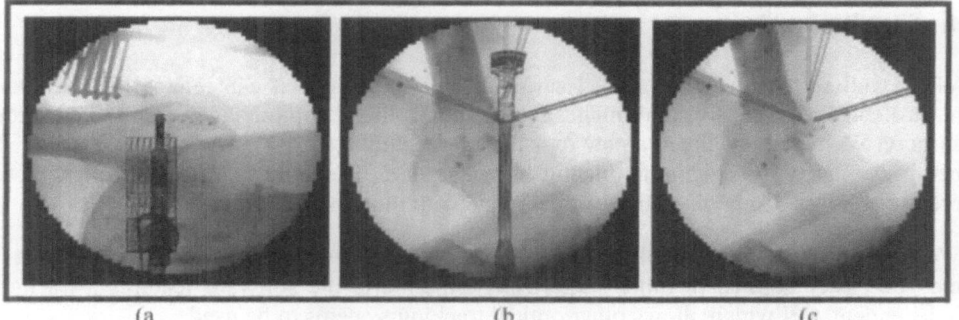

(a (b (c

Figure 3. Virtual fluoroscopy images with overlay of a) instrument, b) instrument with virtual extensions to aid positioning, c) virtual extensions but without instrument.

Once these criteria are met, then the two locating holes for the femoral saw block are drilled. After drilling the first hole, the position of the guide is checked and adjusted using the VF views. The main drill hole is then made and the rest of the procedure then continues as described in 2.4.

3. Results and discussion

A laboratory version of the described VF system is currently being evaluated for effectiveness and efficacy for unicompartmental knee surgery. This evaluation is using plastic bones.

The small H-shaped phantom technique for registration and calibration of this VF system has been used clinically for over 24 months as part of our bespoke computer assisted orthopaedic system for hip trauma surgery [2]. Qualitative assessment of the complete system indicates satisfactory clinical performance in terms of accuracy. Laboratory tests of the phantom indicate a maximum calibration error of 0.5 mm of a fluoroscopic image [3].

©CARS/Springer. All rights reserved.

The software for the detection of the phantom from fluoroscopic has been extensively tested and fine-tuned using a database of over 200 fluoroscopic images of patients.

Our VF approach for unicompartmental knee replacement has several advantages. Basically it simplifies the protocol and instrumentation as it removes the need to drill the intramedullary locating hole and to insert into it the intramedullary rod.

Our VF approach also has advantages over existing VF systems, such as Medtronic Sofamor Danek's Fluoronav™ and Medivision's SurgiGATE. These VF systems use an optically tracked grid that is permanently attached to the C-arm's x-ray receptor. Our VF approach reduces very significantly the optically tracked volume during surgery; it interferes less with existing clinical practice; and image obscuration is significantly reduced.

4. Conclusions

VF is well suited to image guided surgical interventions as it can reduce the radiation hazard considerably as virtual images rather actual fluoroscopic images are used to guide surgery. We have developed a new registration technique for VF. The potential for VF is being evaluated for unicompartmental knee surgery. It should lead to a simpler, more precise and less demanding surgical technique with more consistent results.

We have adopted an extensible modular approach to the design of our VF system. Thus it may be easily applied to other surgeries. Furthermore, the software features a tracker-independent API which allows other optical tracking systems to be used.

Acknowledgements

The authors wish to acknowledge the following fir their support of resources and finance for projects contributing to the research reported: Department of Health, Research Councils supporting the MedLINK programme, the British Orthopaedic Association, the University of Hull and the East Yorkshire Hospitals NHS Trust. The authors also wish to acknowledge all the postgraduate research students, research assistants and the academic and surgical staff who have made contributions to projects contributing results to the reported research.

References

1. JM Boone, JA Seibert and W Blood, "Analysis and correction of imperfections in the image intensifier TV-digitiser imaging chain", *Medical Physics*, 18, 236-42, 1991.
2. WJ Viant, R Phillips, MS Bielby, Y Zhu, JG Griffiths, M Hafez, MN Chawda, KP Sherman, AMMA Mohsen, "Computer assisted positioning of cannulated hip screw", proceedings of *Computer Assisted Radiology and Surgery CARS '99*, Eds. HU Lemke, MW Vannier, K Inamura, AG Farman, pp 751-5, Elsevier, Paris, 1999.
3. WJ Viant, R Phillips, MS Bielby, Y Zhu, JG Griffiths, AMMA Mohsen, KP Sherman., "A technique for a very high accuracy image intensifier calibration", proceedings of *Medicine Meets Virtual Reality*, editors JD Westwood, HM Hoffman, RA Robb, D Stredney, pp 379-80, IOS Press, Newport Beach, 1999.

CARS 2002 – H.U. Lemke, M.W. Vannier; K. Inamura, A.G. Farman, K. Doi & J.H.C. Reiber (Editors)
©CARS/Springer. All rights reserved.

Clinical applications of a laser guidance system with dual laser beam rays as augmented reality of surgical navigation

Nobuhiko Sugano[a], Toshihiko Sasama[b], Shunsaku Nishihara[a], Hisanobu Nakase[a], Takashi Nishii[a], Hidenobu Miki[a], Yasuyuki Momoi[c], Ichiro Sakuma[d], Masakatsu Fujie[e], Sato Yoshinobu[b], Yoshikazu Nakajima[b], Shinichi Tamura[b], Kazuo Yonenobu[f], Takahiro Ochi[a]

[a] Department of Orthopaedic Surgery, Osaka University Medical School

[b] Div. of Interdisciplinary Image Analysis, Osaka University Medical School

[c] Mechanical Engineering Research Laboratory, Hitachi Ltd.

[d] Department of Environmental Studies, Graduate School of Frontier Sciences, The University of Tokyo

[e] Department of Mechanical Engineering, Waseda University

[f] Department of Orthopaedic Surgery, Osaka Minami National Hospital

Abstract

We have developed a novel laser guidance system that uses 2 or more laser beam emitters. Two or more fan-shaped beam tracts intersect in a line that can be controlled in any direction by changing the angle and direction of beam oscillation. The laser guidance system draws cross hairs on a target, and the intersection of the cross hairs is the entry point for a drill or wire. After stabilization of this entry point, the system draws 2 or more lines along the guide sleeve. We have used this laser guidance system in 10 total hip arthroplasty (THA) procedures and 1 open-wedge–type high tibial osteotomy (HTO) procedure. In our clinical experience, this laser guidance system has worked well in the operating room. It effectively draws laser cross hairs on the patient to indicate the entry point of straight surgical tools. The direction of the tools was indicated by parallel laser beams projected onto the guide sleeves. The system assisted surgeons with acetabular cup placement and femoral reaming and rasping in THA. It was also useful for screw insertion and drilling of the osteotomy plane in HTO.

Keywords: Laser beam navigation, total hip arthroplasty, osteotomy

1. Introduction

Most commercial surgical navigation systems display images on a computer monitor positioned adjacent to the surgical scene, and operative procedures are performed using a hand-held pointer and instruments with tracking markers. These systems require that the surgeon performs the mental task of combining 2 sources of spatial information, because the surgeon has to look away from the surgical scene to obtain navigational information from the computer monitor. To solve this problem, we have developed a novel laser guidance system that uses 2 or more laser beam emitters fixed to a stand. This system is combined with our own in-house–developed CT-based navigation system using an optical sensor (OPTOTRAK3020, Northern Digital) [1]. Each beam emitter produces a 0.25-mW

©CARS/Springer. All rights reserved.

red (635 nm) laser beam with a spot radius of 1 mm. The emitter oscillates within a range of 30 degrees at 50 Hz, producing a beam tract shaped like a fan. Two or more fan-shaped beam tracts intersect in a line that can be controlled in any direction by changing the angle and direction of the beam oscillation. This laser guidance system draws cross hairs on a target, and the intersection of the cross hairs is the entry point for a drill or wire. After stabilization of the entry point, the system draws 2 or more lines along the guide sleeve (Fig. 1). When the lines drawn on the sleeve are parallel, the direction of the drill or wire coincides with the line formed by the intersection of the laser beam tracts. The purpose of the present paper is to demonstrate the clinical applications of this laser guidance system and describe its efficacy and limitations.

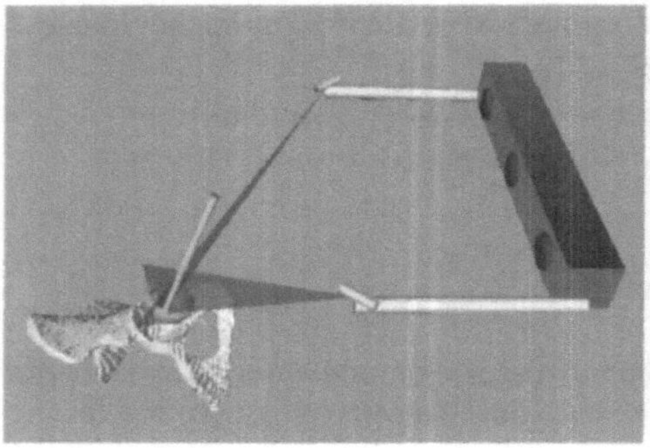

Fig.1: Basic structure of the laser guidance

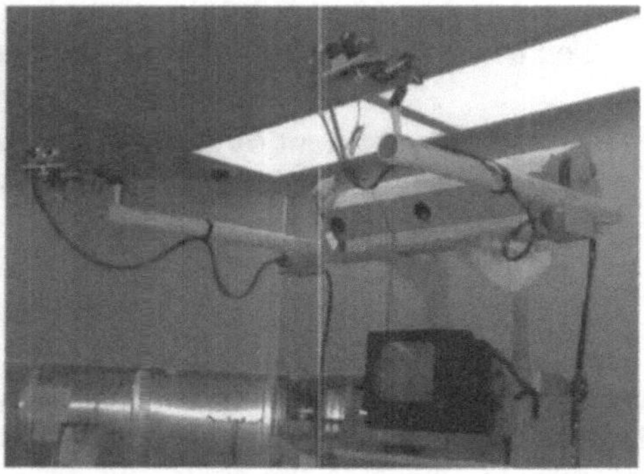

Fig. 2: The laser guidance system in the OR

2. Materials and Methods

We have used this laser guidance system in 10 total hip arthroplasty (THA) procedures and 1 open-wedge–type high tibial osteotomy (HTO) procedure. In the THA procedures, transverse images from the level of the superior anterior iliac spines to the level of the femoral canal isthmus were obtained preoperatively using a helical CT scanner. Several reference images of the femoral condyles were also taken to measure the anteversion. Three-dimensional acetabular and femoral bone surface models were constructed from the CT data. The cup size was determined from the AP diameter of the acetabulum, and the placement of the cup was planned as 40 degrees of abduction and 20 degrees of anteversion. A cementless total hip system with a 28-mm–diameter ceramic-on-ceramic bearing couple (ANCA-FIT, Cremascoli, Milan) was used in the 5 cases with osteoarthritis secondary to hip dysplasia. This system has interchangeable modular neck and head components for adjustment of limb length, offset and femoral anteversion. A cementless total hip system with a physiological femoral head size metal-on-metal bearing couple (Birmingham Hip System and Freeman stem, MMT, Birmingham) was used in the 5 cases with osteonecrosis of the femoral head, and Birmingham hip resurfacing was used in the 1 case with osteonecrosis of the femoral head.

In the operating room, the OPTOTRAK position sensor was positioned on the wall caudal to the patient. The operating table was positioned so that the surgical area was within 2.5

©CARS/Springer. All rights reserved.

m from the position sensor. A rigid bar 120 cm in length was attached to each end of the OPTOTRAK, and a laser beam emitter was mounted at the tip of each bar (Fig. 2). The beam emitters were separated from each other by a distance of 120 cm, and they were 220 cm above the floor. Another laser beam emitter fixed on a stand was positioned cranial to the patient to compensate for any problems with line of sight. Each laser beam was calibrated preoperatively by measuring the position of the beam projected onto a board using a pen probe with LEDs.

In the THA procedures, patients were placed in a lateral decubitus position, and a posterolateral approach was used. A flat plate with 6 LED markers and a rod was fixed to the iliac crest using an extraskeletal fixation system (Hoffmann system, Howmedica). A triangle plate with a socket was fixed to the lateral aspect of the greater trochanter, such that the socket connected to a rod attached to a tracker employing the Hoffmann system. Shape-based surface registration of previously constructed bone models to the real objects was performed [2]. After registration, the laser guidance system was used to guide acetabular cup placement and guide femoral reaming and rasping.

In the HTO procedure, preoperative planning was performed using the 3D models of the femur and tibia. The patient was placed in a supine position on the operating room table. Setup of the OPTOTRAK and the laser guidance system was the same as for THA. A foot brace with a tracker was used for the reference frame of the tibia. Shape-based registration was performed by obtaining surface points of the tibia using a needle with a tracker. After registration, the laser guidance system was used to guide insertion of the first screw, which was fixed with an Orthofix extraskeletal fixation system. The laser guidance system was also used to guide drilling of the osteotomy plane before the final cutting with an osteotome.

3. Results

The 3 laser beam emitters worked well intraoperatively, although shadeless lights had to be turned off so that the laser beams could be seen on the patients or surgical instruments. There were no problems with line of sight. In the THA procedures, acetabular reaming was performed using a guide wire that was inserted under laser guidance (Fig. 3). The guide wire method was especially useful for placement of the cup in the original acetabulum in cases with subluxation of the hip. A guide wire was also inserted into the femoral head and neck in resurfacing hip arthroplasty. Guide wire placement was easy to perform under laser guidance. The entry point of the guide wire was indicated by the laser beam cross hairs. After stabilization of the tip of the wire at the entry point, direction of the wire was controlled using the parallel laser beams projected onto the guide sleeve. Acetabular cup placement was easy and quick, and the difference between the actual and planned orientation of the cup was within 5 degrees. Laser guidance was also useful for the femoral reaming. It was easy to determine the amount of bone to remove from the greater trochanter to avoid varus misalignment. Laser guidance can also be used to adjust femoral anteversion. In the HTO procedure, laser guidance was used to guide percutaneous screw insertion and drilling of the osteotomy plane. The difference between the actual and planned entry point of the screw was 1 mm. The difference between the actual and planned orientation of the screws was within 2 degrees.

©CARS/Springer. All rights reserved.

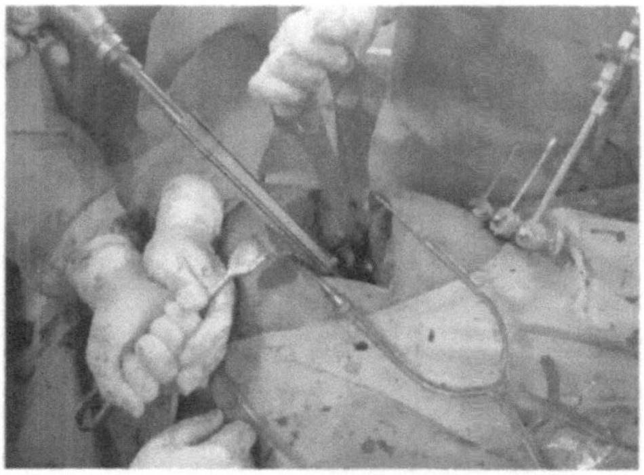

Fig.3: Direction of acetabular reaming was guided by the laser beams, which can be seen by parallel black lines on the hand-hold sleeve in this image.

4. Conclusions

Our clinical experience has shown that the dual-beam laser guidance system works well in the operating room. It was able to draw laser beam cross hairs on patients to indicate the entry point for straight surgical tools. The direction of tools was determined by parallel lasers projected onto the guide sleeves. This system has been successfully used to assist surgeons in acetabular cup placement and femoral reaming and rasping during THA procedures. It has also been successfully used for screw insertion and drilling of the osteotomy plane during an HTO procedure.

Acknowledgements

This study was supported by the future pioneering study promotion project of the Japan science promotion council "The development of the robotic system in the area of the science of surgery".

References

1. Sugano N, et al.: Combined acetabular and femoral surgical navigation in total hip arthroplasty. In: Lemke HU, et al. ed. Computer Assisted Radiology and Surgery. Proceedings of the 13th International Symposium and Exhibition (CARS'99). Amsterdam, Elsevier, 1999. p722-725.
2. Sugano N, et al.: Accuracy evaluation of surface-based registration methods in computer navigation system for hip surgery performed through a posterolateral approach. Computer Aided Surgery 6: 195-203, 2001.

CARS 2002 – H.U. Lemke, M.W. Vannier; K. Inamurc, A.G. Farman, K. Doi & J.H.C. Reiber (Editors)
©CARS/Springer. All rights reserved.

Robust computational osteotomy planning tools for autologous bone grafts in reconstructive surgery

Z. Król[a], M. Chlebiej[b], F. Zerfass[a], H.-F. Zeilhofer[c], R. Sader[c], P. Mikołajczak[b], E. Keeve[a]

[a] Surgical Systems Laboratory, center of advanced european studies and research, Friedensplatz 16, 53111 Bonn, Germany, e-mail: krol@caesar.de
[b] Faculty of Mathematics and Physics, Maria Sklodowska-Curie University Pl. M. Curie-Sklodowskiej 1, 20-031 Lublin, Poland
[c] Department of Oral and Maxillofacial Surgery, Klinikum rechts der Isar, Munich University of Technology, Ismaninger Str. 22, 81675 Munich, Germany

Abstract

This paper presents a method for computer assisted selection of optimal donor sites for autologous osseous grafts in the craniofacial surgery. At the initial graft design stage the surgeon defines in the CT data set the shape of the bone segment to be reconstructed and in the donor region CT data set a set of constraints for the optimization task. This non-automatic step is followed by a fully automatic optimization stage, which delivers a set of sub-optimal and optimal donor sites for a given template. Such approach permits the surgeon to find the best site for harvesting the graft and enables an exact anatomical reconstruction of the osseous section.

Keywords: Computer-aided surgery, autologous grafts, osteotomy planning

1. Introduction

Bone graft surgery is often necessary for reconstruction of craniofacial defects after trauma, tumor, infection or congenital malformation. Since F.H. Albee published in 1915 an influential text on bone graft surgery[1], the bone grafting has became more widespread and attention focused not only on its use, but also on its safety and efficacy. In this operative technique the removed or missing bone segment is filled with bone graft. The mainstay of the craniofacial reconstruction rests with the replacement of the defected bone by autologous bone grafts. There are a number of alternatives to autologous grafts but the autogenous bone is still the best source of bone grafts because it offers the complete histocompatibility and provides the best osteoinductive and osteoconductive stimuli for bone growth. Grafting techniques have markedly changed over the last decades in an attempt to provide better correction of the bone defects, enhance stabilization, and increase the rate of bony consolidation. To achieve sufficient incorporation of the autograft into the host bone, precise planning and simulation of the surgical intervention is required.

This work focuses on the planning of grafting procedures for osseous grafts transplanted from one part to another part of the body in the same individual. The autologous bone

©CARS/Springer. All rights reserved.

transplants can be harvested from different donor sites. Depending on the amount and shape of the bone graft required, it can be harvested from the ilium, rib, cranium, scapula, or tibia bone. For reconstruction of the craniofacial region and particularly for mandibular reconstruction, which is our area of interest, the iliac bone is the most often material of choice because of the anatomical similarity with the recipient region. The major problem in the graft surgery is to determine as accurately as possible the donor site where the graft should be dissected from and to define the shape of the desired transplant. In a number of our previous works [2,3] a novel method and its improvements for selection of optimal donor sites for autologous osseus grafts have been presented. In this work we introduce an improved computer-aided surgery planning system which enables efficient segmentation, visualization and manipulation of the virtual patient model prior to operation. By using a deterministic optimization method the physician can significantly accelerate the selection of the optimal donor site.

2. Methodology

From the medical point of view the osseous graft surgery is an operative technique, where the defected bone is resected, then the designed graft is harvested from the identified donor site and transplanted into the resected section. The reconstructed bone section is then fixed with bone plates and screws, until the healing process is complete. Successful bone graft repair depends on a number of factors. These include (1) close approximation of the shape of the bone section to be reconstructed, (2) supplying of the structural support to the recipient site (3) rigid fixation and (4) minimal lesion of the donor site. To achieve satisfactorily incorporation of the graft into a viable new bony complex, precise planning and simulation of the surgical intervention based on 3D CT studies acquired prior to surgery is required. Inaccurate design and harvesting may lead to loss of the graft. In our continuing work on the computer assisted selection of donor sites for autologous grafts we have developed a method to identify an optimal match between donor region and a given transplant. Let us briefly describe the main idea of the proposed method. More detailed description can be found in our previous publications [2,3].

Considering two pre-operative CT datasets *template* and *donor site* and a rigid transformation $T:\Re^3 \rightarrow \Re^3$, we can pose the problem of matching a desired transplant with the donor region as an optimization problem:

$$v_{opt} = \arg\min\left\{ C(v) \,\middle|\, v \in M \right\}$$

where $C(v)$ is an objective function and $M \subset \Re^6$ is a set of permissible parameter vectors which satisfy some constraints. The goal of the optimization is to find the parameter vector v_{opt} defining a 3D rigid transformation T which minimizes the misregistration measure C between the *template* and the *donor site*. Several similarity criteria have been tested[3] and the most efficient of them have been chosen for our surgery planning system. These include surface matching[4], normalized mutual information[5] and s-distance measure[3]. Each of the matching functions belongs to different similarity measure classes: surface based metrics, voxel based metrics and cross-metrics, accordingly. It enables the surgeon to select the optimal donor site not only in terms of bone surface correlation but also according to the whole morphological information contained in both datasets. Our method consists of two stages. First, the

©CARS/Springer. All rights reserved.

surgeon indicates interactively the osteotomy border lines in the *template* CT dataset and defines a set of constraints for the optimization task in the *donor site* CT dataset. At the second stage a fully automatic optimization procedure delivers a set of sub-optimal and optimal donor sites for a given template. The graft design step and the improved optimization method are discussed in the next two sections.

2.1 Graft design

The goal of the graft design step is to define the shape of the template and the geometrical constraints for the optimization process. At the initial stage the surgeon has to identify the spatial extent of the pathological finding. In our clinical practice the patients with cranio- and maxillofacial disorders have often to undergo different imaging modalities as CT, MRI, PET or SPECT. The registration of these complementary datasets the physician to gain insight into functional and morphological relationships in the region of interest and leads to a better perception of the critical region, particularly when the pathological process involves multiple tissue structures. Thus, the differentiation between pathological

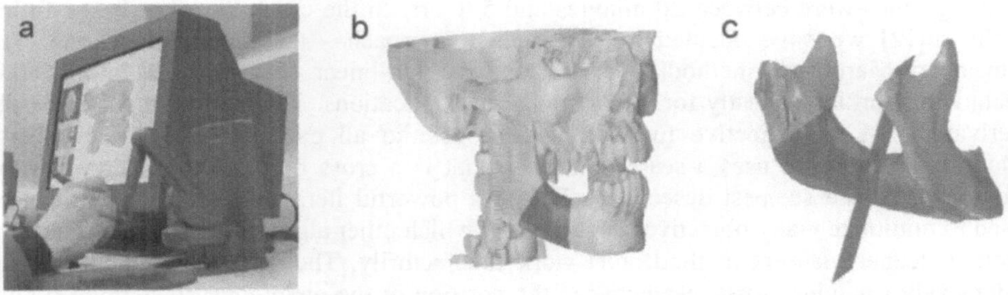

Fig. 1: The graphical user interface of the planning system and the PHANToM haptic interface[6] enabling more intuitive interaction between the user and the virtual objects (a). Designed graft's template and delineated osteotomy lines after the graft design step. (tumor in the alveoral part of the patient's right hemimandible) (b). Mirror technique applied to the large bone defects (reconstruction of the craniofacial area after trauma). The required graft's shape can be defined in the symmetrically mirrored healthy part of the mandible (green) (c).

and healthy structures can be done more successfully, and the likelihood of successful elimination of the lesion is greater with this multimodal approach than with the standard monomodal one. The crucial graft design step is then performed on the segmented CT datasets. For the segmentation of the osseous structures thresholding, region growing, morphological operations, interactive definition of the region of interest and various filters can be applied to the 3D CT datasets. 3D surface models are generated using the marching cubes algorithm. The surgeon can interactive explore and interact with the virtual patient model. The shape of the graft is defined by using simple cutting planes or cutting volumes. Position and inclination of the cutting tool can be controlled using standard computer mouse and keyboard as well as in a more intuitive way by using three-dimensional input devices. Our planning system has been combined with a haptic interface[6] (see Fig. 1a). The cutting plane and manipulation tools are extremely effective given the 6DOF nature of the interaction. For example, the cutting plane can be easily and precisely positioned and oriented within 3D data, which is a particularly difficult problem with the 2D mouse. In the case of large bone defects the graft can be designed using a

©CARS/Springer. All rights reserved.

mirror technique (see Fig. 1c). The healthy side is duplicated, mirrored and aligned with the pathological side. The required graft's shape is then defined in the symmetrically formed template. During this step the surgeon has also to define the donor region in the *donor site* CT dataset (see the bounding boxes in Fig. 2).

2.2 Optimization

Estimation of the optimal transformation vector v_{opt} defining a rigid transformation T_{opt} that minimizes the misregistration measure between the *template* and the *donor site* is the goal of the optimization process. Because the misregistration measures are non-linear functions they can have multiple local minima on the feasible set M[3]. Previously, the simulated annealing[7] - a non-deterministic optimization method - has been applied in our system to solve the optimization problem for all applied misregistration measures. The method is very robust and non-susceptible to local minima. But the drawback is, it is very time consuming approach. Depending on the chosen cooling schedule, on the size of the *template* and the *donor site* datasets and on the applied matching measure the typical running times were between 20 minutes and 5 hours. In the case of surface based fitting technique[2] we have decided to use another approach - the deterministic one. The Levenberg-Marquardt method[8] is a standard non-linear least-squares optimization technique working robustly for a wide range of applications. The method requires partial derivatives of the objective function with respect to all parameters. The Levenberg-Marquardt algorithm uses a search direction that is a cross between the Gauss-Newton direction and the steepest descent[8]. This is a powerful iterative algorithm that can be used to minimize many objective functions, for which other algorithms like Newton or the simple steepest descent method don't work satisfactorily. The surface based fitting uses intensively Euclidean distances between the position of the *template* surface point **p** after being transformed by T_v, and the closest point of the *donor site* surface. By the distance we mean the length of the vector that is defined by that pair of points. To accelerate the distance computation the 3D distance transform method[9] has been applied. We have to keep not only the length but also the three coordinates of the vector, which will be used to estimate derivatives of the objective function in the optimization process. The computation of the distance map is the most time consuming part of the whole process. In some cases we can shorten this time by computing the distance map only for a certain region of interest (see Fig. 2). This new optimisation approach based on the Levenberg-Marquardt algorithm enables, once the pre-processing step has been performed, selection of the optimal donor site in time less than one minute.

3. Results and discussion

A computer aided surgical planning system for selection of optimal donor sites for autologous grafts has been developed. The system provides segmentation and marking tools, which allow the surgeon to delineate precisely the osteotomy border lines in the *template* dataset and to define the geometrical constraints in the *donor site* dataset. By using the haptic interface the graft design step can be performed easier and faster than the standard 2D mouse based approach. It is easy to learn and operate. Different similarity

©CARS/Springer. All rights reserved.

	Case 1	Case 2
Donor region size	81x108x26	181x185x91
# template points	2589	1677
Preprocessing time	26.5 sec	39.7 sec
Optimization time	14.9 sec	10.1 sec

Table 1. Running times for the Levenberg-Marquardt optimization method (surface similarity measure) in the two planning cases showed in Fig. 1 and 2. For the same cases the simulated annealing running times (normalized mutual information) were 51 min 17 sec and 109 min 42 sec accordingly.

criteria and an efficient optimization method have been implemented. The system enables the surgeon to generate a set of sub-optimal and optimal donor sites for a given template. All generated solutions can be explored interactively on the computer display using an efficient graphical interface. Besides various 2D techniques to display matched slices conventional surface rendering techniques have been implemented (see Fig. 2). The two objects can be also rendered as semi-transparent surfaces or combined with volume rendering. Our surgical planning system has been written in C++ with a usage of some external libraries. For creating the graphical user interface and for some 2D graphical operations the Qt library has been used. VTK and OpenGL libraries have been used for 3D visualization and real time interaction as well as Ghost library for the haptics. Because these libraries are fully cross-platform, the system is operating system independent. A reconstructive operation with the 3D planning was performed on 30 patients with osseous defects in different areas of the facial bones. All CT data have been acquired on the Siemens and Philips scanners with high-resolution protocols. The grafts were taken from the area of the iliac crest. Fig. 2a-b show a superposition of the to be reconstructed part of mandible with the pelvis donor site. In the Fig. 2c the graft (designed in the Fig. 1b) harvested from the iliac crest (Fig. 2a) and fixed rigidly to the recipient site by means of metal plates and screws has been shown. Continuous follow-up observations show that there is less loss of transplants, when they are individually designed as well as high improvement of the functional results like chewing ability by exact reconstruction of dental occlusion. Moreover, in most cases the duration of the surgical interventions has been distinctly reduced due to computer-assisted preoperative osteotomy planning.

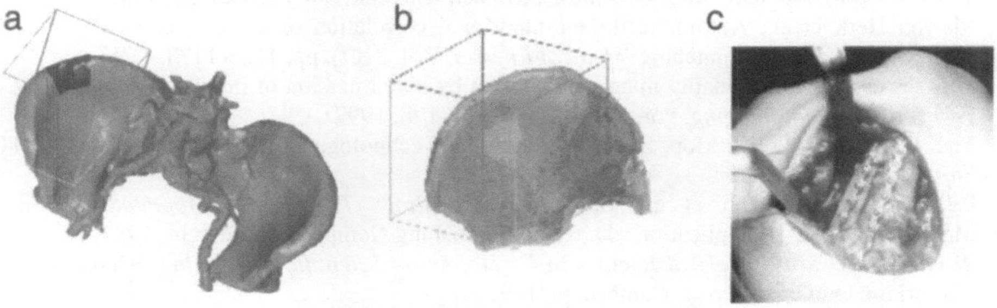

Fig. 2: Pelvis with superposed templates (from the Fig. 2 (b and c accordingly) positioned at the automatically estimated optimal donor sites (a and b). Designed in the Fig. 1b graft harvested from the iliac crest (Fig. 2a) and fixed rigidly to the recipient site by means of metal plates and screws (c).

©CARS/Springer. All rights reserved.

4. Conclusions

In this paper a method to identify an optimal donor site by performing an optimization of appropriate similarity measures between the donor region and a given transplant has been presented. At the initial stage the surgeon has to delineate the osteotomy border lines in the *template* CT dataset and to define a set of constraints for the optimization task in the *donor site* CT dataset. This non-automatic step is followed by a fully automatic optimization stage, which delivers a set of sub-optimal and optimal donor sites for a given template. Such approach permits the surgeon to find the best site for harvesting the graft and enables an exact anatomical reconstruction of the osseous section. The proposed method is generally applicable for various autografts regardless of its shape and the grafting site. The main advantage of this approach is that after determination of the initial conditions and constraints it provides an automatic procedure to find the optimal donor site for the designed template. The new optimization technique based on the Levenberg-Marquardt method enables, once the pre-processing step has been performed, selection of the optimal donor site in time less than one minute (see Tab. 1). Using the haptic device has potential to greatly simplify and improve the interaction with the virtual patient model during the surgery planning. The operation time can be considerably shortened by this approach. In addition, the functional and aesthetical results are optimized. The next steps of this work aim on the graft modeling through parametric surfaces. Future work will also involve combining of our framework with an intraoperative navigation and instrument tracking system to transfer the high precision of the computer-assisted selections of the donor site into the operation situs.

Acknowledgements

This work is supported by BMBF research grant ARSyS-Tricorder #01-IRA08-E.

References

1. F.H. Albee, *Bone-graft surgery,* W.B. Saunders Co., Philadelphia and London, 1915.
2. Z. Krol et al., Computer Aided Osteotomy Design for Harvesting Autologous Bone Grafts in Reconstructive Surgery, Proc. of SPIE Medical Imaging. Vol. 4319, pp .244-251, 2001.
3. Z. Krol, *Computational Methods in the Registration and Visualization of Three-dimensional Multi-modality Medical Data.* PhD thesis, Munich University of Technology, 1998.
4. M. van Herk et al., Automatic three-dimensional correlation of CT-CT, CT-MRI, and CT-SPECT using chamfer matching. *Medical Physics*, Vol. 21(7), pp. 1163-1178, 1994.
5. F. Maes et al., Multimodality image registration by maximization of mutual information, *IEEE Trans. on Medical Imaging*, vol. 16, no. 2, pp. 187-198, 1997.
6. The PHANTOM™ Desktop System, SensAble Technologies, Inc., Woburn, MA 01801, *http://www.sensable.com*
7. P.J.M. van Laarhoven et al.: *Simulated Annealing: Theory and Applications.* Series: Mathematics and its applications. D. Reidel Publishing Company, Dordrecht, 1987.
8. W.H. Press et al., *Numerical Recipes in C: The Art of Scientific Computing,* Second Edition, Cambridge University Press, Cambridge, 1992.
9. G. Borgefors, Distance transformations in arbitrary dimensions, *Computer Vision, Graphics and Image Processing*, 27 (1984): pp. 321-345.

CARS 2002 – H.U. Lemke, M.W. Vannier; K. Inamura, A.G. Farman, K. Doi & J.H.C. Reiber (Editors)
©CARS/Springer. All rights reserved.

3D assessment and simulation of surgical correction of spine deformities by in situ contouring technique

R. Dumas[a], V. Lafage[a], J.P. Steib[b], D. Mitton[a], J.A. de Guise[a,c], W. Skalli[a]
[a] Laboratoire de Biomécanique, ENSAM- CNRS, Paris, France
[b] Hopitaux Universitaires, Strasbourg, France
[c] Laboratoire de recherche en Imagerie et Orthopedie, ETS-CRCHUM, Montreal (Québec), Canada

Abstract

The simulation by finite element of in situ contouring surgical correction is presented for kyphosis and scoliosis reduction. A personalized finite elements model was obtained based on a 3D stereoradiographic reconstruction. This 3D geometric reconstruction was obtained pre and post operatively in order to assess the surgical correction effect as well as validate the simulation. The specific implants and the specific surgical maneuvers were taken into account in the simulation (bringing plastic material and successive loading and release). A reliable correction was measured in 3D for the kyphosis and scoliosis and the simulation render an account of the correction technique (progressive corrections) and of the reduction effects which were consistent with the post operative 3D geometries.

Keywords: scoliosis surgical correction, finite elements simulation, 3D geometrical reconstruction

1. Introduction

The modern surgical treatments of spine deformities are designed to provide a three-dimensional correction. The operative strategy, the specificity of the implants and the correction technique are keypoints for the surgical outcomes. In these terms, 3D measurements and modelling can be reliable help for the understanding of correction phenomena.
The simulation by finite element of scoliosis correction [1][2] and the 3D reconstruction stereoradiographic technique [3] of the patient's spine has been initiated 6 years ago for Cotrel-Dubousset technique [4]. The purpose of this study is to analyse the in situ contouring technique [5] in the cases of kyphosis and scoliosis reduction.

2. Material and methods

2.1 Clinical data

A kyphotic patient (kyphosis angle 50°, 30 years old) and a right thoracic scoliotic patient (Cobb angle 58°, 34 years old) underwent a surgical treatment (by in situ contouring technique) in the *Hopitaux Universitaires de Strasbourg*. Pre operative and immediate post operative standing radiographs were taken on a stereoradiographic device (frontal

©CARS/Springer. All rights reserved.

and lateral calibrated views) in order to obtain the 3D geometrical reconstruction of the spine (T1 to L5) and pelvis.
An extension bending classical X-ray of the kyphotic patient and a left lateral bending classical X-ray of the scoliotic patient were also taken.

2.2 Three-dimensional reconstructions
The 3D reconstruction were obtained by stereoradiography (using NSCP reconstruction [3]) with the calibrated radiographs. The accuracy of the method has been evaluated to 1.1 mm [6]. Then, the reconstructions are analyzed in terms of vertebral 3D orientations (lateral rotation, flexion extension and axial rotation) [7] and spinal lines (in frontal and sagittal plane), expressed in the global reference system [8]. The pre and post operative vertebral 3D orientations were compared.

2.3 Personalized finite elements model and simulation
The model was constructed (Ansys 6.0 software) with the geometry (T1 to pelvis) directly extracted from the 3D stereoradiographic data (Figure1). Bone parts, disc and ligaments were modeled by elastic beams and articular facets were modeled with contact surface elements [1][2].

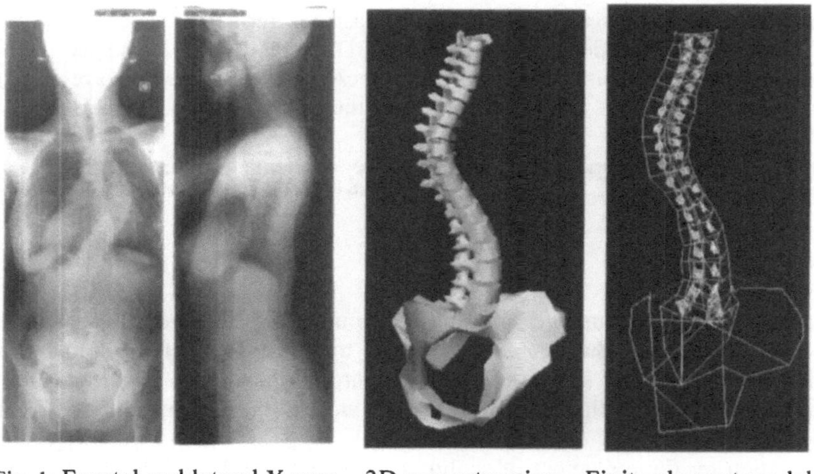

Fig. 1: Frontal and lateral X-rays – 3D reconstruction – Finite element model

The mechanical data were, in a first step, set to standard properties established through experiments in the *Laboratoire de Biomécanique*. Then, they could be personalized by inverse method simulating the bending movements (extension and lateral). The position of T1 and the pelvis measured on the X-rays, were imposed as boundary conditions. The protocol included possible modification of the mechanical properties of the inter-vertebral disc until the error between simulation and radiographic measurements tended to 5° (vertebral 3D orientations) and 5 mm (spinal line).
The surgical correction included two steps, the surgical preparations and the correction maneuvers. Concerning the preparations, the articular facets and the spinous processes were resected (corresponding elements simply deleted in the model) and the patient is lengthened on the table (imposed displacement to the upper vertebrae while the pelvis

©CARS/Springer. All rights reserved.

rests on the Antero Superior Iliac Spines). Then, the implants are constructed at the strategic levels, according to the surgeon choice. Regarding the correction maneuvers, a plastic rod (two bilateral rods in the case of kyphosis) is placed passing through all of the implants (spline computed and meshed with plastic bilinear material). The correction is obtained by bending in situ the rod at successive levels (two opposite moments imposed and released at the end of loading, before going to the next level). In the case of kyphosis, the two rods are bent together in the sagittal plane. In the case of scoliosis, the left side rod is introduced and bent first in both frontal and sagittal planes. Derotation of the screws in lumbar level is also applied with a specific implant holder. The second rod (right side) is further introduced and additional contouring is performed. The last step is compression distraction forces along the rods to put the implants horizontal.
As a validation, the simulated correction was compared with the post operative 3D reconstruction of the spine (expressed in spinal reference system [8] to compare prone and standing position).

3. Results and discussion

The analysis was focused on the sagittal plane of the kyphostic patient and the frontal, sagittal and axial plane of the scoliotic patient.

3.1 Pre and post operative 3D vertebral orientation

Concerning the kyphosis, the upper thoracic vertebrae (T1-T6) were thoroughly in flexion (from 20° to 40°) and that was reduced (60% in average) after surgery. Concerning the scoliosis (Figure 2), all vertebrae were derotated (65 % in average). The axial rotations at the thoracic and lumbar apex (T8 and L1) were 14° and 16° and the post operative values were 4° at both level.

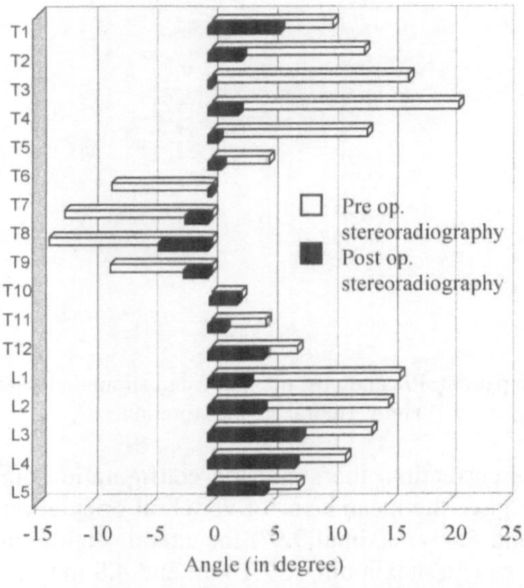

Fig. 2: Scoliotic patient: Pre and post operative vertebral axial rotation

©CARS/Springer. All rights reserved.

These segmental measurements of the 3D orientations are reliable indicators to evaluate the severity of a curve and quantify the surgical effects. The axial derotation is a controversial item of modern surgical correction of scoliosis. For this presented case, the in situ contouring technique demonstrated a whole derotation of the spine.

3.2 Simulation of surgical correction

The mechanical personalization was necessary for the scoliotic patient while the kyphotic one did not presented specific stiffness when simulating the bending movement and comparing with the X-ray measurements.
The simulation of the in situ contouring maneuver yielding the following observations which were confirmed by the surgeons experience:

- The rods present an elastic recoil after each contouring.
- The reduction of the kyphosis/scoliosis is progressive (gradual opening of the curve and elevation of T1).

The simulated configurations were compared with the post operative 3D reconstructions. In the case of kyphosis correction, the mean error of vertebral orientation and spinal line in the sagittal plane were 3.3° (maximal 8.4°) and 2.7 mm (maximal 4.8 mm) (Figure 3).

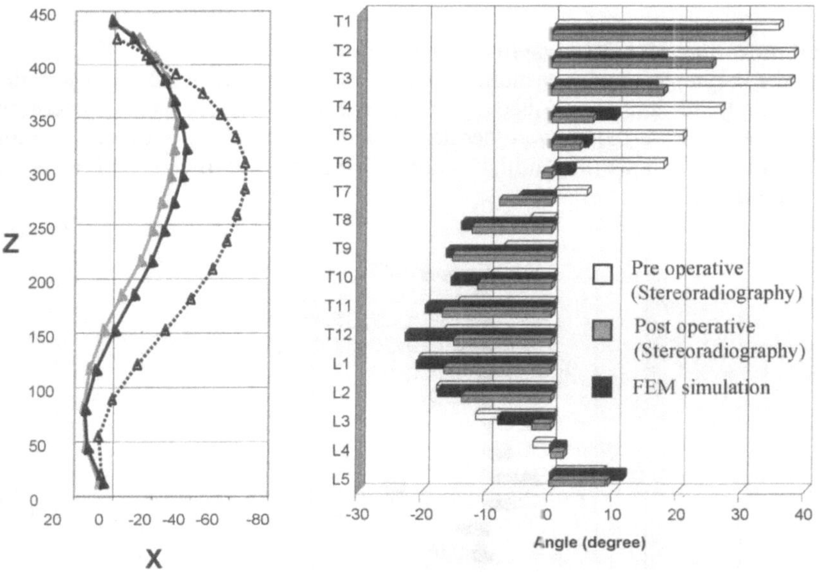

Fig. 3: Kyphotic patient: Pre and post operative and simulated sagittal spinal line and vertebral sagittal rotation

In the case of scoliosis correction, the simulated configuration compared with the post operative 3D geometry gave the mean error of vertebral orientation 3.7° (maximal 7.0°), 3.9° (maximal 12.1°) and 5.0° (maximal 9.9°) for lateral, sagittal and axial rotation. The spinal line comparison gave a maximum of 7.2 mm and 4.8 mm in the frontal (Figure 4) and sagittal plane.

©CARS/Springer. All rights reserved.

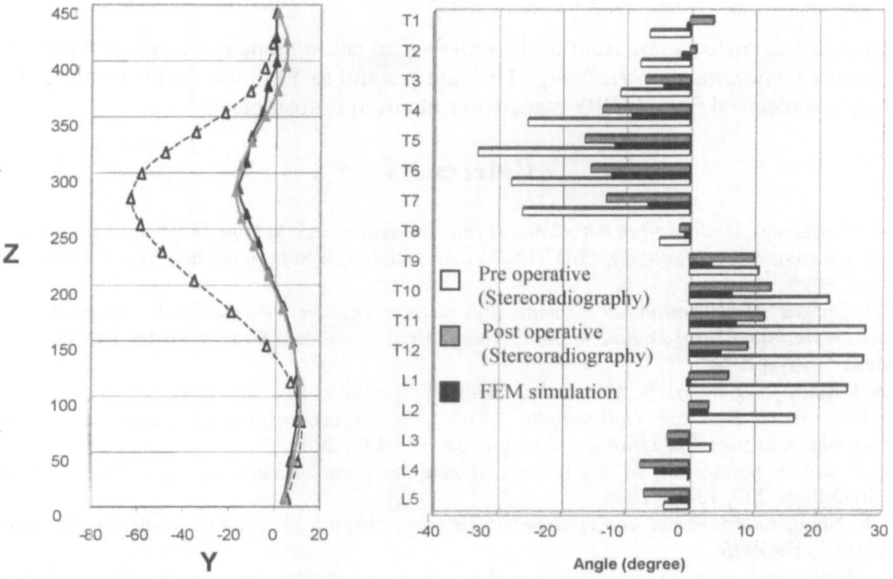

Fig. 4: Scoliotic patient: Pre and post operative and simulated frontal spinal line and vertebral lateral rotation

The simulation allowed to assess the influence of the different steps of the surgery: patient installation, contouring of the first and the second rod, rotation of the screws, compression and distraction forces on the implants.

The maximal error might be due to the modeling of the bending moments. The successive levels to be contoured were selected according to the basic lines of the technique and the load were strictly in frontal/sagittal plane whereas in clinics, the contouring of the rods is *"optimized"* by the surgeons. In the sagitattal plane, the maximal errors might be due to the comparison of prone vs. standing position, especially in the non instrumented (mobile) areas.

4. Conclusion

The 3D stereoradiographic reconstruction of a kyphotic and a scoliotic spine was acquired pre and post operatively in order to assess the surgical effects. Moreover, the personalized finite elements model of both patient was obtained and the simulation of the surgical correction by in situ contouring technique was performed. The simulation includes the specific implants (plastic rods) and the specific surgical technique (successive bending of the rod). The simulation gives reliable results, when compared with post operative 3D reconstruction of the spine. The 3D measurements can be a reliable evaluation of surgical outcomes and the simulation could be a tool, in the future, for the surgical planning.

©CARS/Springer. All rights reserved.

Acknowledgements

The authors acknowledge the team of the radiological and orthopedics surgical departments of *Hôpitaux Universtaires- Strasbourg*. They are grateful to Y. Lafon for his technical help. Funding was received from AGIRS association and from Eurosurgical.

References

1. J-L.Descrimes, *Modélisation par éléments finis du rachis et de la cage thoracique pour l'étude des déformations scoliotiques,* PhD Thesis, Ecole Nationale Superieure des Arts et Métiers, Paris, 1995
2. P. Leborgne, *Modélisation par elements finis de la correction chirurgicale de la scoliose par instrumentation Cotrel-Dubousset,* PhD Thesis, Ecole Nationale Superieure des Arts et Métiers, Paris, 1998
3. D. Mitton, C. Landry, S. Veron, W. Skalli, F. Lavaste, J.A. de Guise, *3D reconstruction method from biplanar radiography using non-stereocorresponding points and elastic deformable meshes.* Med Biol Eng Comput, 38, 133-139, 2000
4. Y. Cotrel, J. Dubousset, M. Guillaumat, *A new universal instrumentation in spinal surgery,* Clin Orthop, 227, 10-23, 1988
5. J. P. Steib, *Lumbosacral and spinopelvic fixation*, chapter 33, Lippincoot-Raven Publishers, Philadelphia, 1996
6. A. Mitulescu, I. Semaan, J.A. de Guise, P. Leborgne, C. Adamsbaum, W. Skalli, *Validation of the Non Stereo Corresponding Points stereoradiographic 3D reconstruction technique.* Med Biol Eng Comput, 39,152-158, 2001
7. W. Skalli, F. Lavaste, *Quantification of three dimensional vertebral rotations in scoliosis: What are the true value ?,* Spine, 20, 5, 546-553, 1995
8. I. A. F. Stokes, *Three dimensional terminology of spinal deformity.* Spine, 19,2, 236-248, 1994

Special Session on Validation of Medical Image Processing in the Context of Image-Guided Therapy

CARS 2002 – H.U. Lemke, M.W. Vannier; K. Inamura, A.G. Farman, K. Doi & J.H.C. Reiber (Editors)
©CARS/Springer. All rights reserved.

White paper: validation of medical image processing in image-guided therapy

P. Jannin [a], J.M. Fitzpatrick [b], D.J. Hawkes [c], X. Pennec [d], R. Shahidi [e], and M.W. Vannier [f]
[a] Université de Rennes France
[b] Vanderbilt University USA
[c] Computational Imaging Science Group, London GB
[d] INRIA Sophia-Antipolis France
[e] Stanford University USA
[f] University of Iowa USA

1. Introduction

Clinical use of image-guided therapy (IGT) systems has grown, creating the need for a common and rigorous validation methodology, as reported in recent workshops and conferences. [1,2,3,4] One key characteristic of IGT systems is that they employ medical image processing methods (e.g. segmentation, registration, visualization, calibration). As a result of this intrinsic structure, validation of IGT systems should include both individual validation of these components, validation of the overall system and a study of how uncertainties propagate through the entire image guided therapy process. Significant progress has been made on IGT system validation recently. Today almost all peer-reviewed publications reporting on the development of new medical image processing methods include a validation section, but this was not always true in the past.

Validation of a medical image processing method allows its intrinsic characteristics to be highlighted, as well as evaluation of its performance and limitations. Moreover, validation clarifies the potential clinical contexts or applications that the method may serve. Validation may also demonstrate a method's clinical added value as well as to estimate social or economic impact. However, standardization of validation processes is required in order to compare various IGT systems. Validation tests can facilitate the user's task of determining whether a particular system meets a given set of clinical requirements.

This short paper identifies the principal requirements of IGT system validation and encourages the medical imaging community to develop a common methodology so we may all share analyses and results in this topic.

2. Validation

IGT system validation is a special case of health care technology assessment (HCTA). Goodman [5] defines the HCTA as the "process of examining and reporting properties of a medical technology" and as the "systematic evaluation of properties, effects and/or impact". Goodman divides this systematic evaluation into the following steps: 1) identify

©CARS/Springer. All rights reserved.

assessment topics, 2) clearly specify assessment problem or question (i.e. assessment objective), 3) determine locus of assessment, 4) retrieve available evidence, 5) collect new primary data, 6) interpret evidence, 7) synthesize evidence, 8) formulate findings and recommendations, 9) disseminate findings and recommendations, 10) monitor impact.

In a transversal approach, the efficacy of diagnostic imaging systems is evaluated at six main levels that span the range from technical performance to societal value. [6] The six levels of efficacy evaluation include: 1) technical capacity, 2) diagnostic accuracy, 3) diagnostic impact (i.e. improvement of diagnosis), 4) therapeutic impact (i.e. influence in the selection and delivery of the treatment), 5) patient outcome (i.e. improvement of the health of the patient), 6) societal impact (e.g. cost effectiveness). An evaluation study must consider only one level at a time but a whole evaluation study should theoretically address all these levels separately.

A key characteristic of IGT systems is that various medical image processing methods are encountered in all stages of an IGT process, in pre-planning, planning, simulation, treatment delivery and post treatment control. These methods have to be validated separately, as well as the overall system. In this paper, we will primarily focus on validation levels 1 to 4. The other levels apply to IGT systems, and should be addressed, but require different skills, and they are beyond the scope of the IGT domain that concerns most engineers and physicists.

3. Criteria of validation

Validation requires the application of defined criteria to a device or process. Common examples of validation criteria which may be applicable to IGT include:

Accuracy: Goodman [5] defines accuracy as the "degree to which a measurement is true or correct". For each sample of experimental data local accuracy is defined as the difference between computed values and theoretical values, i.e., known from a ground truth. This difference is generally referred to as local error. Under specific assumptions, a global accuracy value can be computed for the entire data set from a combination of local accuracy values.

Precision and Reproducibility or Reliability: Precision of a process is the resolution at which its results are repeatable, i.e., the value of the random fluctuation in the measurement made by the process. Precision is intrinsic to this process. This value is generally expressed in the parameter space. Goodman defines reliability as "the extent to which an observation that is repeated in the same, stable population yields the same result".

Robustness: The robustness of a method refers to its performance in the presence of disruptive factors such as intrinsic data variability, pathology, or inter-individual anatomic or physiologic variability.

Consistency: This criterion is mainly studied in image registration validation [7,8,9], by studying the effects of the composition of n transformations that forms a circuit: $T_{n1} \circ \ldots \circ T_{23} \circ T_{12}$. The consistency is a measure of the difference of the composition from the identity.

©CARS/Springer. All rights reserved.

Fault Detection: This is the ability of a method to detect by itself when it succeeds (e.g. result is within a given accuracy) or fails.
Functional complexity and computation time: These are characteristics of method implementation. Functional complexity concerns the steps that are time-consuming or cumbersome for the operator. It deals both with man-computer interaction and integration in the clinical context and has a relationship with physician acceptance of the system or method. The degree of automation of a method is an important aspect of functional complexity (manual, semi automatic or automatic).

Among the most important validation criteria applied in the U.S. market are those required to receive premarket approval for a medical device from the Food and Drug Administration (FDA). Briefly, the criteria are derived from a legal requirement that the device be show to be safe and effective. If a predicate device exists, the FDA may grant approval (510K) based on substantial equivalence in performance. The gold standard for most evaluations is the randomized multicenter (Phase 3) clinical trial, a costly and time-consuming endeavor. For practical reasons, demonstration of feasibility and comparative performance will suffice for journal publication, but not for widespread dissemination and clinical use.

Others factors may have to be studied but are beyond the scope of this paper such as cost/effectiveness ratio, patient acceptance, and outcome factors.

4. Validation requirements

The main categories of requirements concerning validation include: standardization of validation methodology, design of validation data sets and definition of corresponding ground truth, and design of validation metrics. [1,2,3,4,10,11,12]

4.1 Standardization of validation methodology

Actual validation methodologies lack standardization. Without standardization it remains difficult to compare the performance of different methods or systems and even occasionally to really understand the results of a validation process. Standardization is also required to perform meta analysis. Furthermore, the standardization of validation processes may be useful in the context of quality management (e.g. FDA approval). Standardization of validation methodology can be facilitated by common (i.e. standardized) characterisation of image processing methods, of the clinical contexts of validation, and of validation procedures.

4.1.1 Characterization of image processing methods

Common characterization of image processing methods allows describing any method in a generic and standardized fashion from the main characteristics of its process. It begins with a standardized description of the process's components. For instance, an image registration method could be characterized by its component steps [13,14]:

- the class of the computed transformation (e.g. rigid, affine, non linear, if non-linear, type of transformation and number of degrees of freedom),
- the homologous structures (e.g. fiducial markers, lines, surfaces, intensity distributions),

©CARS/Springer. All rights reserved.

- the cost function and optionally the interpolation method,
- the optimisation method,
- the optimisation strategy (e.g. multiscale, multiresolution).

4.1.2 Clinical contexts in validation

The two first stages of an HCTA, as described by Goodman, consist in precisely defining assessment topics (i.e. clinical context of validation) and the assessment objective. Just as the development of new image processing tools in medical imaging requires an accurate study of the clinical context, validation of these new tools has to be performed according to this clinical context. Formalization of the clinical context of validation (also referred as the "necessity of full understanding of problem domain" [11]) is not a trivial task but is essential with regards to clinical relevance. The assessment objective (i.e. goal of the validation study) may be formulated as a hypothesis. The result of the validation process is to confirm or not this hypothesis.

The validation hypothesis can be defined from the specificities of the clinical context of validation. Similarly this hypothesis should be precisely characterized in a standardized fashion. This hypothesis is related to a specific level of evaluation (as defined in paragraph 2.) and is notably defined by the data sets involved in the clinical context and their intrinsic characteristics (e.g. imaging modalities, spatial resolution, dimensions), by the clinical assumptions related to the data sets or to the patient (e.g. regarding anatomy, physiology and pathology), and by the values related to validation metrics representing required or expected results (e.g. accuracy or resolution values). In medical image registration, one example of a level 1 validation hypothesis may be: "In the context of temporal lobe epilepsy, a particular registration method M based on similarity measurements is able to register 3-D T1-weighted MR images (with a spatial resolution around 2 mm and without any pathological signal) to ictal SPECT (with a spatial resolution around 12 mm and with hyper and/or hypo perfusion areas) with a RMS error (evaluated on points within the brain) that is significantly smaller than the SPECT spatial resolution". [15]

4.1.3 Standards for validation procedures

The need for protocols for validation was sometimes outlined as definition of a "unique standardized terminology of validation or evaluation" [11]. The design of models of evaluation processes [10,12] contributes to this standardization.

We can distinguish the main steps of a gold standard based validation procedure as follows. Validation data sets and parameters are used as input by the method to be validated and by the function used to compute the ground truth. Both computations may introduce errors or uncertainties, which have to be taken into account in the comparison. The output of the method is compared to the ground truth for evaluating or validating the method using comparison metrics (i.e. validation metrics)[A]. The result of the comparison function provides a quality index also called "figure of merit" which quantifies distances

---

[A] These validation metrics are chosen according to the validation criterion used in the study.

©CARS/Springer. All rights reserved.

to the ground truth. The results of the comparison are assessed against the hypothesis of the validation process by means of a simple test on threshold or a statistical analysis. This final result provides the result of the validation (i.e. to accept or to reject the hypothesis). Specific statistical approaches have also investigated validation without gold standard (e.g. for studying robustness and internal accuracy of a registration method [16], for comparing quantitative imaging modalities [17]). These approaches may provide an interesting framework for theoretical validation.

4.2 Validation data sets

Some of the most commonly mentioned requirements about validation concern the design of validation data sets, their classification into main families according to the access to the ground truth, and their dissemination through the community [18].

Four main types of validation data sets can be distinguished from absolute ground truth to lack of ground truth: numerical simulations, realistic simulations from clinical data sets, physical phantoms and clinical data sets. The ground truth may be perfectly known, called absolute ground truth (e.g. when using numerical simulations) or may be computed from the data sets (e.g. when using physical phantoms or clinical data sets especially acquired for validation), or finally the ground truth may not be available (e.g. this may be the case when using clinical data sets obtained from clinical routine); in this case the reference for comparison may be given by observers (e.g. manual segmentation vs. automatic segmentation) or by some a priori clinical knowledge or clinical assumptions. In these last two cases the gold standard is called a bronze standard or fuzzy gold standard. Consequently the computation of the ground truth may introduce some uncertainties, which have to be taken into account in the validation process. As it can be noticed, there is a trade-off between clinical realism of the data sets and easy access to ground truth. It is also quite clear that the different types of data sets provide data for different levels of evaluation.

Sharing image databases or patient databases helps validation processes and comparison of performances, and allows robustness studies. These databases must include "hard" and unusual cases (e.g. pathological cases) and be regularly updated with new imaging protocols, new modalities and data from new applications. However, because clinical validation requires clinical image data sets adapted to the local conditions at clinical institutions, the availability of clinical validation data sets will remain difficult until variations among imaging systems will not be quantified and normalized [12].

The experimental conditions defining the validation data sets allow distinguishing effectiveness studies (i.e. benefit of using a technology for a particular problem under general or routine conditions) from efficacy studies (i.e. benefit of using a technology for a particular problem under ideal conditions). [5]

4.3 Validation metrics

The "assessment objective" generally refers to a validation criterion to be studied. Validation metrics and the corresponding mathematical or statistical tools have to be defined according to the validation criterion. Consequently validation metrics have to be chosen or defined according to their suitability to assess the clinical assessment objective.

©CARS/Springer. All rights reserved.

They have to be "clinically useful indicators of outcome". [12] For instance, for accuracy studies in registration, it is now well established that computing or estimating the Target Registration Error (TRE) [19] provides more meaningful information than the Fiducial Registration Error (FRE). The requirement of an overall validation of image guided surgery systems [1,2,4] (i.e. including all its components) should also be taken into account by estimating uncertainty at each stage of the image guided therapy process, and by modelling how uncertainties propagate through the entire image guided therapy process [20]. This allows to study the influence of each medical image processing component within the overall process.

5. Conclusion

Medical image processing sub-systems are key components of image-guided therapy systems, and their intrinsic performances are key factors of the overall IGT system performance. However, their validation still remains driven through a "home made" methodology. As said above, validation of medical image processing methods for IGT should benefit from the definition of common validation data sets and their corresponding ground truth, from the definition of validation metrics adapted to clinical requirements, and finally from the design of common terminology and methodology for validation procedures. Standardized and world wide accepted validation protocols with associated guidelines should also facilitate the comparison of new IGT systems and their acceptance and transfer from research to industry.

References

1. Loew M H, "Medical Imaging Registration Study Project", Report of NASA Image Registration Workshop November 1997. http://www.seas.gwu.edu/~medimage/report97.htm
2. Shtern F, Winfield D et al., "Report of the Joint Working Group on Image-Guided Diagnosis and Treatment", April 12-14, 1999 Washington, D.C. http://www.nci.nih.gov/bip/IGDT_final_report.PDF
3. Cleary K, Anderson J, Brazaitis M, et al., "Final report of the Technical Requirements for Image-Guided Spine Procedures Workshop", April 17-20, 1999, Ellicott City, Maryland, USA. *Comp Aid Surg,* Volume 5, Issue 3180-215, 2000
4. Shahidi R, Clarke L, Bucholz R D, et al., "White paper: Challenges and opportunities in computer-assisted interventions January 2001", *Comp Aid Surg* Volume 6, Issue 3, 176-181, 2001
5. Goodman CS, "Introduction to Health Care Technology Assessment", Nat. Library of Medicine/NICHSR, 1998 http://www.nlm.nih.gov/nichsr/ta101/ta101.pdf
6. Fryback DG and Thornbury JR, "The efficacy of diagnostic imaging", *Med. Decis. Making,* 11, 88-94, 1991
7. Holden M, Hill DLG, Denton ERE, Jarosz JM, Cox TCS, Rohlfing T, Goodey J, Hawkes DJ, "Voxel similarity measures for 3D serial MR brain image registration", *IEEE Trans Med Imag,* 19(2), 94-102, 2000
8. Pennec X, Guttmann CRG, and Thirion JP, "Feature-based Registration of Medical Images: Estimation and Validation of the Pose Accuracy", Proc. of First Int. Conf. on Medical Image Computing and Computer-Assisted Intervention (MICCAI'98), Cambridge, USA, *Lecture Notes in Computer Science,* Springer Verlag, Vol. 1496, 1107-1114, 1998
9. Fitzpatrick JM, "Detecting failure, assessing success", *Medical Image Registration,* Hajnal JV, Hill DLG, and Hawkes DJ ed., CRC Press, June 2001

©CARS/Springer. All rights reserved.

10. Buvat I, Chameroy V, Aubry F, et al., "The need to develop guidelines for evaluations of medical image processing procedures", *SPIE Medical Imaging*, 3661, 1466-1477, 1999
11. Bowyer KW, Loew MH, Stiehl HS and Viergever MA, "Methodology of evaluation in medical image computing", Report of Dagstuhl workshop, March 2001, http://www.dagstuhl.de/DATA/Reports/01111/
12. Yoo TS, Ackerman MJ, Vannier M, "Toward a common validation methodology for segmentation and registration algorithms", Proc. Of Medical Image Computing and Computer-Assisted Intervention (MICCAI 2000), Pittsburgh, USA, *Lecture Notes in Computer Science*, Springer Verlag, Vol. 1935, 422-431, 2000
13. Hill DLG, Batchelor PG, Holden M, Hawkes DJ, "Medical image registration", *Phys Med Biol*, 46(3), R1-R45, 2001
14. Jannin P, Grova C, and Gibaud B, "Medical applications of NDT data fusion", *Applications of NDT data fusion*, 227-267. Kluwer Academic Publishers, Gros X edition, 2001
15. Grova C, Jannin P, Biraben A, et al., "Validation of MRI/SPECT registration methods using realistic simulations of normal and pathological SPECT data", *Proc. of CARS 2002*, Paris, France, 2002
16. Granger S, Pennec X, and Roche A, "Rigid Point-Surface Registration Using an EM variant of ICP for Computer Guided Oral Implantology", Proc. Of Medical Image Computing and Computer-Assisted Intervention (MICCAI 2001), Utrecht, The Netherlands, *Lecture Notes in Computer Science*, Springer Verlag, Vol. 2208, 752-761, 2001
17. Hoppin J, Kupinski M, Kastis G, et al., "Objective Comparison of Quantitative Imaging Modalities Without the Use of a Gold Standard", 17th International Conference Information Processing in Medical Imaging, IPMI 2001, Davis, CA, USA, Insana MF, Leahy RM (Eds.), *Lecture Notes in Computer Science*, Springer Verlag, Vol. 2082, 12-23, 2001
18. West JB, Fitzpatrick JM, Wang MY, et al., "Comparison and Evaluation of Retrospective Intermodality Image Registration Techniques", *Journal of Computer Assisted Tomography*, 21(4):554-566, 1997
19. Fitzpatrick JM, West JB and Maurer CR Jr, "Predicting Error in Rigid-Body, Point-Based Registration", *IEEE Trans Med Imag*, 17(5) 694-702, 1998
20. Viant WJ, "The development of an evaluation framework for the quantitative assessment of computer-assisted surgery and augmented reality accuracy performance", *Stud Health Technol Inform*;81:534-40, 2001

Minimal Invasive Thoracic Abdominal Surgery

CARS 2002 – H.U. Lemke, M.W. Vannier; K. Inamurc, A.G. Farman, K. Doi & J.H.C. Reiber (Editors)
©CARS/Springer. All rights reserved.

What is new in robotic surgery?

Makoto Hashizume[a], Mitsuo Shimada[b], Kohzo Konishi[a], Tomohiko Akahoshi[a], Morimasa Tomikawa[b], Shinichiro Maehara[b], and Keizo Sugimachi[b]
[a]Department of Disaster and Emergency Medicine
[b]Department of Surgery and Science
Graduate School of Medical Sciences, Kyushu University, Fukuoka, Japan

Abstract

This study has demonstrated the feasibility of several endoscopic robotic procedures otherwise the accomplishment was difficult in the conventional endoscopic fashion. The system seems most beneficial in thoraco-abdominal microsurgery or for manipulation in a very small space. Robotic surgery provides the surgeon less stressful, safer and more accurate procedures in the minimally invasive surgery.

Key words: Da Vinci, endoscopic surgery, telesurgery

1. Introduction

Computer-assisted surgical systems are making exceptional progress in the field of minimally invasive cardiac surgery. Two competing systems, Da Vinci by Intuitive Surgical, Inc., and Zeus by Computer Motion, Inc., have targeted cardiac surgery for their introduction to the surgical area. Cadiere (1) reported the use of robotic systems in general surgery cases, however, the feasibility and merits of these procedures have not yet been demonstrated as dramatically in general surgery as in cardiac surgery.

The purpose of this paper is to demonstrate the feasibility and merits of utilizing a robot in thoraco-abdominal surgery (2).

2. Patients and Methods

2.1 Patients

Between July 2000 and February 2002 53 patients underwent robot-assisted endoscopic surgery. They were 22 men and 31 women, and the average age was 57.9 $\pm$ 14.6 years old with a range of 24 to 85. The patients had been admitted to Kyushu University Hospital to undergo treatment utilizing endoscopic procedures. The details of robotic surgery were carefully explained to all patients according to the guidelines of the Institutional Review Board and informed consent was obtained from all of them.

2.2 Methods

The procedures performed in this study were esophagectomy in 1 patients with esophageal cancer, distal two-thirds gastrectomy in 2 patients with early gastric cancer, colectomy in

©CARS/Springer. All rights reserved.

3 patients with early colon cancer (ileocaecal resection, sigmoidectomy and left colectomy), splenectomy in 6 patients (2 idiopathic thrombocytopenic purpura, 1 splenic tumor and 3 hypersplenism), devascularization of the upper stomach in 1 patient with gastric varices, cholecystectomy in 23 patients with cholelithiasis, repair of esophageal hiatus hernia in 2 patients, inguinal herniorrhaphy in 2 patients, giant ovarian cystectomy in 1 patient, tumor resection in 2 patients with esophageal leiomyoma, mediastinal tumor resection in 2 patients (1 thymoma and 1 posterior mediastinal neurogenic cyst), breast tumor resection in 1 patient, esophageal myotomy (Heller) in 1 patient with esophageal achalasia, Nissen fundoplication in 5 patients with reflux esophagitis and thoracosympathectomy in 1 patient with Buerger disease.

The robot (da Vinci surgical system, Intuitive Surgical, Mountain View, CA) consists of a console and a surgical cart with three articulated robot arms. The surgeon sits in front of the console containing a display that presents images obtained by an endoscopic camera inside the patient's body, manipulating joysticklike handles while observing the operative field through binoculars that provide a three-dimensional picture. The surgeon's console provides "Master" manipulators the surgeon uses to control the movements of the corresponding "Surgical " or "Patient Side" manipulators that hold the surgical instruments and the endoscopic manipulator used for the procedure. As the surgeon moves the manipulators on the surgeon's console, the patient side manipulators closely follow the input motions. All of the manipulators are under remote control by the surgeon from the surgeon's console. Electric cables run from the arms to the electronics enclosure in the surgeon's console. The arms have three degrees of freedom (pitch, yaw and insertion) and allow the responsible instrument to move two additional degrees of freedom in the wrist and two additional motions for tool actuation.

A special team was organized to perform robotic surgery. The team consists of three operators (M.H., M.S., K.S.), five assistant doctors, three nurses, and two mechanical engineers.

Operating time, perioperative morbidity, and hospital stay were registered. All data were registered in a computer server at the Kyushu University Hospital.

3. Surgical procedures

After the induction of unconsciousness by the anesthesiologist, the robotic system was set-up by the mechanical engineers and nurses. The surgical cart and the robotic arms were positioned on the same side of the lesion in each case. The whole computer system was set-up and the camera-vision system was prepared. After pneumoperitoneum had been made under a minimal open laparotomy, three trocars were inserted by the assistants: one was for the camera-port and two were for operation arm-port. One or two additional ports measuring 12 mm in diameter were also inserted when necessary on a case by case basis.

©CARS/Springer. All rights reserved.

3.1 Distal gastrectomy

The totally endoscopic procedure of distal gastrectomy was performed with the da Vinci system in the same fashion as that during open surgery. The right gastroepiploic artery, right gastric artery, left gastric artery and each vein with the regional lymph nodes were dissected with a hook type electro-coagulator of the Endo-Wrist™. The vessels were ligated with 2-0 silk by using the forceps type Endo-Wrist™.

The duodenum and the distal stomach were transected, respectively, at the pyloris ring and at the middle of the gastric body, with the autosuture device inserted through the assistant port. Anastomosis of both stumps of the stomach and the duodenum was performed completely in the abdominal cavity with a 3-0 vicryl -atraumatic needle using the needle holder type Endo-Wrist™ in a manual fashion. The surgical specimen was put into a retrieval bag and then was taken out of the abdominal cavity throught the left lower assistant port site with a 3 cm extension. A completely total endoscopic distal gastrectomy with reconstruction using the Bilroth I method was then completed using the da Vinci system.

3.2 Splenectomy

The patient's position and the operative procedures were fundamentally the same as those used in conventional endoscopic surgery. All the surrounding ligaments were transected with a hooked type Endo-Wrist™ electrocoagulator. If necessary, coagulation and hemostasis of the tissues was strengthened by holding the tissue with a conventional endoscopic forceps and by transmitting electric power to the forceps with the Endo-Wrist™ electrocoagulator. The branches of the splenic artery and vein to the upper and lower poles of the spleen were exposed, ligated with 2-0 silk and cut. The trunk of the splenic vessels was finally severed with the autosuture device (Multifire Endo GIA, AutoSuture, United States Surgical, Norwalk, CT, USA) through the assistant port.

3.3 Extraction of the tumor of the esophagus and thorax

The tumor of the lower esophagus was approached laparoscopically and the mediastinal tumor was approached thoracoscopically. All procedures were performed with only the forceps type and the hook type Endo-Wrist™ coagulator. It was easily done with no burning of the surrounding tissues because of the high freedom and few limitations of movement of the Endo-Wrist™ hook type coagulator. The removed tumor was put into a bag and taken out of the cavity.

3.4 Other procedures

The other procedures were all performed according to the above-mentioned robot-assisted procedures and conventional endoscopic procedures.

4. Results

All procedures were successfully performed. No major complication was encountered. There was no mortality. The minor complications were slight stenosis after distal gastrectomy in one patient with early gastric cancer and intraoperative bleeding during splenectomy in one patient with portal hypertension. No surgical treatment was required

©CARS/Springer. All rights reserved.

for the patient with stenosis of the anastomotic site. The intraoperative bleeding was controlled with a conventional electrocoagulator.

The total operative time of average 185 minutes was longer in robot-assisted surgery than that of conventional endoscopic surgery, while actual operation time of the robot was average 117 minutes. There was a learning curve on the operating time of the robot-assisted surgery. The set-up time of the robotic system markedly reduced to half an hour after several cases. The estimated intraoperative blood loss was minimum in patients who had cholecystectomy, while that was less than 200ml in almost all the other operations.

There were no significant differences in number of sedatives administered for postoperative pain, and time period of starting food intake or walking between the robot-assisted surgery and the conventional endoscopic surgery.

However, each procedure such as suturing, ligature, dissection and cutting was significantly easier and faster than that of conventional endoscopic procedures. In distal gastrectomy, for example, all suturing procedures of reconstruction by Billroth I was performed in a manual fashion using the robotic arms. In cholecystectomy no mechanical clips were necessary because both the cystic duct and cystic artery were ligated in a manual fashion. The dissection of the huge dilated vessels in patients with portal hypertension was significantly easier with the robotic assistance than that without the robot because of better three-dimensional vision of the operative field and less limitation of movement of the robotic instruments. Psychological stress was also significantly lower in robot-assisted surgery than in conventional endoscopic surgery, thanks to three-dimensional vision and intraabdominal articulations.

5. Discussion

This study has demonstrated the feasibility of several endoscopic robotic procedures otherwise the accomplishment was difficult in the conventional endoscopic fashion. The system seems most beneficial in thoraco-abdominal microsurgery or for manipulation in a very small space. Robotic surgery provides the surgeon less stressful, safer and more accurate procedures in the minimally invasive surgery. Our study suggests that this system will enable surgeons to perform better procedures due to the increased visualization and enhanced precision, and patients will benefit by being able to return to their normal activities with less pain and trauma associated with traditional operations.

Surgeons have speculated since the introduction of laparoscopic cholecystectomy that computers, three-dimensional imaging, and robotics could overcome the pitfalls of laparoscopy. Only select surgeons are moving beyond these to more technically difficult operations. Robots offer the promise of improvements to laparoscopic surgery that will allow most surgeons to perform more difficult technical operations (3).

The robotics has established a foothold in surgical practice. Commercial systems have been available for a few years, and their value is undergoing stringent scientific evaluation in randomized clinical trials. Although the initial reports are promising, it will be necessary for more long-term, evidence-based outcome studies to prove their efficacy (4).

©CARS/Springer. All rights reserved.

More important, it will be necessary to prove the cost-effectiveness in addition to the other significant non-technical issues such as accommodating the operating rooms, training operating room personnel and surgeons, and gaining acceptance of the technology.

References

1. Cadiere GB, Himpens J, Germay O, Izizaw R, Degueldre M, Vandromme J, et al: Feasibility of robotic laparoscopic surgery: 146 cases. *World J Surg* 25, 1467- 1477, 2001
2. Hashizume M, Shimada M, Tomikawa, et al: Initial experience of endoscopic procedures assisted by a computer enhanced surgical system, *da Vinci. The 6th International Micromachine Symposium*, 49-52, 2001
3. Ballantyne GB: The pitfalls of laparoscopic surgery: challenges for robotics and telerobotic surgery. *Surgical Laparoscopy, Endoscopy & Percutaneous Techniques* 12: 1-5, 2002
4. Satava RM: Surgical robotics: The early chronicles, a personal historical perspective. *Surgical Laparoscopy, Endoscopy & Percutaneous Techniques* 12: 6-16, 2002

CARS 2002 – H.U. Lemke, M.W. Vannier; K. Inamura, A.G. Farman, K. Doi & J.H.C. Reiber (Editors)
©CARS/Springer. All rights reserved.

A new compact robot for manipulating forceps using friction wheel and gimbals mechanism

Takashi Suzuki[a], Etsuko Kobayashi[a], Daeyoung Kim[a],
Hiroshi Inada[b], Takayuki Tsuji[a], Takeyoshi Dohi[c], Ichiro Sakuma[a]
[a] Institute of Environmental Studies, Graduate School of Frontier Sciences,
[b] Department of Precision Engineering, Graduate School of Engineering,
[c] Department of Mechano-Informatics,
Graduate School of Information Science and Technology,
the University of Tokyo. 7-3-1 Hongo, Bunkyo-ku, Tokyo 113-8656 Japan

Abstract

We developed a compact robot for manipulating forceps using a friction wheel and a gimbals mechanism. This robot works as a small slave robot in master-slave robotic system. Rotation and translation (back and forth) of forceps was realized with "friction wheel mechanism". This mechanism does not have limitation in transnational motion of forceps. Determination of forceps insertion direction was realized by a small gimbals mechanism with two degrees of freedom (DOF). Friction wheels had the function of both holding and driving forceps, so we succeeded in making the system compact. The size was 42mm diameter and 89mm long and 250g in weight. Gimbals mechanism realized the two DOF for determining the direction of the forceps. The size was 39mm×54mm ×70mm and 330g in weight. We integrated the two mechanisms into a new compact robot for manipulating forceps. This manipulator is enough small to use three sets without occupying the operating space above the abdomen.

Keywords: Manipulator, friction wheel, Gimbals mechanism

1. Introduction

In abdominal surgery, Minimally Invasive Surgery (MIS) such as laparoscopic cholecystectomy is widely performed. This technique is less invasive than laparotomy, so patients have merits in reduction of postoperative pain, discomfort, medication, and length of hospital stay [1]. However, MIS has some technical difficulties. The forceps have only four Degrees of Freedom (DOF) (three DOF for positioning the tip of forceps and one for the rotation of the forceps shaft). Thus, surgeons need skills to perform required surgical interventions using these tools with less DOF. As an engineering solution, robotic systems for manipulating forceps have been developed [2]. They were effective to extend surgeons' ability and enabled surgeons to perform complicate minimally invasive surgical operations. However, their size was usually large for conventional operating room. Some operation room is too small to install the system. It also caused danger of collision between manipulators and the surgeons. There are difficulties in removing the manipulator system from the operating field when in emergency. Large size of the system limits the number of manipulators used at the same time since the system occupies the

©CARS/Springer. All rights reserved.

space above the abdomen of a patient. Currently commercially available systems have only two manipulators for surgical operations. Some surgical operations require more than three manipulators at the same time. Therefore, we have to develop a compact forceps manipulating robotic system that can manipulate more than three forceps at the same time and does not occupy the operating space above the abdomen. In this paper, we proposed a new compact robot for manipulating forceps using friction wheel and gimbals mechanism. We evaluated the basic performance of the prototype system.

2. Method

2.1. System Requirements

We set the following requirements for the manipulator.
(1) At least, three sets of robotic system can be used simultaneously in the operating field.
(2) The system should be attached to the bedside.
(3) No extra adapter between forceps and manipulator is required.
(4) The manipulator provides the following four DOF:
- Rotation around the forceps
- Translation (back and forth movement) of the forceps
-Two DOF (Pitch and Roll) for determining the direction of forceps
(5) The system has enough power and moving range: The system can bear 0.5kg of weight considering the weight of right lobe of the liver (approximately 0.5kg).

2.2. Construction of Manipulator

We adopted "friction wheel mechanism" [3] and "gimbals mechanism" to realize a manipulating robot satisfying the abovementioned requirements (Fig.1). Friction wheel mechanism realizes the rotation and translation of the forceps. Gimbals mechanism realizes the two DOF for determining the direction of forceps.

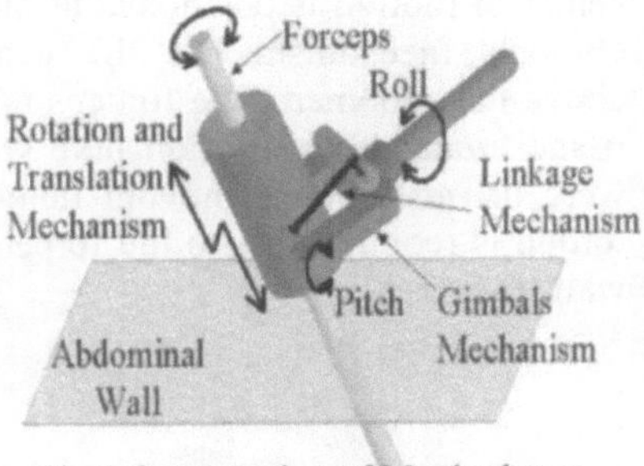

Fig.1 Construction of Manipulator

2.3. Friction wheel mechanism for rotation and translation of forceps

The friction wheel mechanism consisted of three rollers. Those three rollers were placed around the forceps shaft and held the forceps stably. Rollers fit onto the forceps shaft at an angle of 30 degrees inclined. When the forceps rotate, a roller travels spirally on the shaft. Conversely, rollers rotate forceps spirally. As this spiral movement contains rotation and translation, we can rotate and translate the forceps (Fig.2).

We used two friction wheels and two ultrasonic motors. Friction rollers applies two types of friction forces on the forceps shaft: F_1 and F_2 as shown in Fig.3. When we move the forceps in transnational direction, two rollers should be driven as shown in Fig.3 (a) to cancel the radial components of forces F1 and F2. Axis components of the two forces drive the forceps in transnational direction as shown in Fig.3(a). When we drive the friction roller as shown in Fig.3 (b), the rotational motion of the forceps can be realized since the axis components of the two forces are cancelled.

©CARS/Springer. All rights reserved.

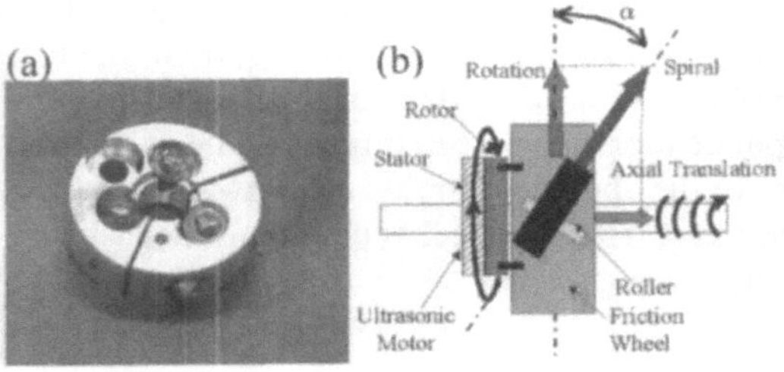

Fig.2 Friction Wheel;
(a) Prototype (b) Mechanism of Motion

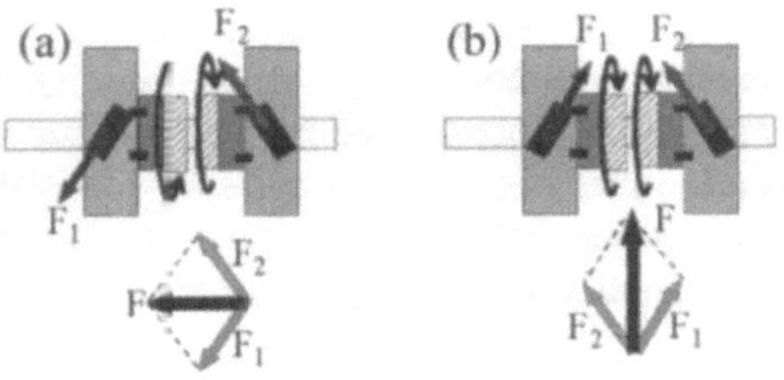

Fig.3 Motion of the Forceps;
(a) Translation (b) Rotation

2.4. Gimbals Mechanism for determination of forceps direction

Gimbals mechanism can simplify the mechanism for determining the direction of forceps. To cover the right lobe of the liver, we set that the length of the forceps inside the abdominal cavity was as long as 200mm, The moving range of pitch and roll movement was set as large as 40 deg respectively. The pitch movement was obtained by a DC motor and the roll movement was obtained by linkage mechanism with a geared DC motor (Fig.1). It is easy to separate sterilized and non-sterilized parts in linkage. On the other hand, the gimbals mechanism has its inherent demerits: In the conventional design of forceps manipulator, the center of motion is positioned at the insertion hole. Gimbals mechanism has the center of rotation above the abdomen. The forceps might damage the tissue around the insertion hole when the forceps were driven in wide moving range. Larger motor torque is required due to the force from abdominal wall (Fig.4).

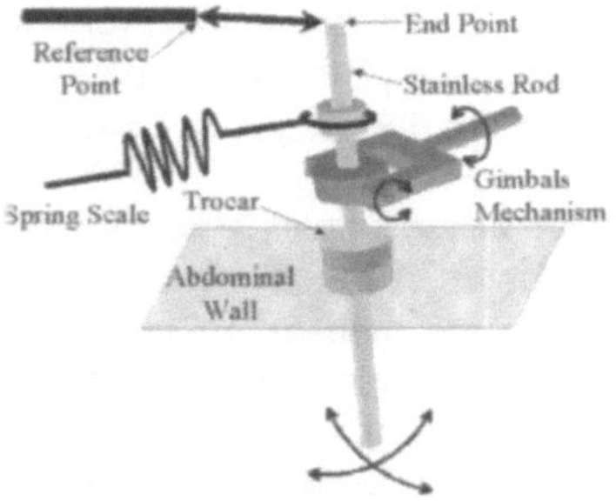

Fig.5 Scheme of the Experiments

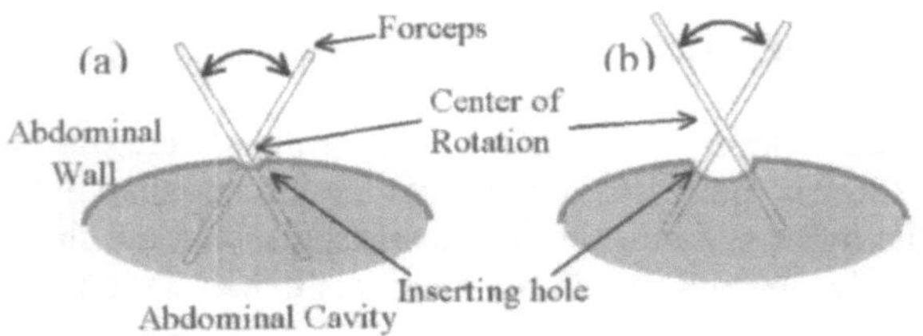

Fig.4 Difference of the Invasion;
(a) Conventional Manipulating (b) Gimbals Mechanism

We conducted animal experiments using a swine to measure required torque to manipulate the forceps when its center of rotation was set above the abdomen. We set the gimbals mechanism above the abdomen and moved the forceps. The angle of the inclined forceps and the force need to incline the forceps were measured (Fig.5). The abdominal wall of the swine was 30 mm thick. The height of the center of rotation was 85mm in Pneumoperitoneum and 65mm in the abdominal wall lifting method. The results are shown in Fig.6.

©CARS/Springer. All rights reserved.

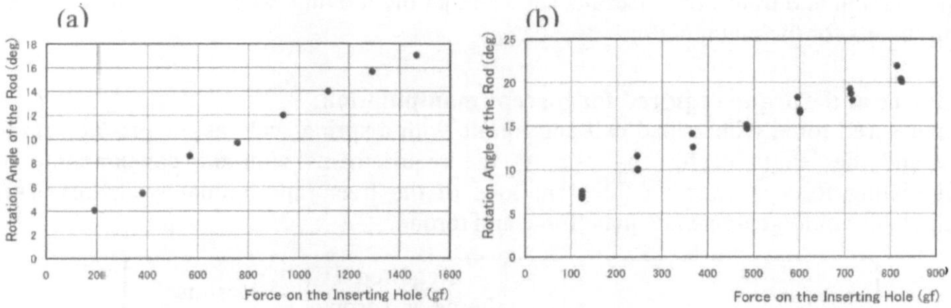

Fig.6 Results; (a) Pneumoperitoneum (b) Abdominal Wall Lifting

We estimated the required torque when the center of gimbals mechanism is set up 45mm above the abdomen. The required torque was 2.6×10^{-1}(Nm) in the case of Pneumoperitoneum and 1.6×10^{-1} (Nm) in the case of abdominal wall lifting. This torque can be obtained using conventional electric motors. During experiments, there were no observable damages at the insertion hole. Thus, it was concluded that the conceivable demerits of gimbals mechanism were not significant.

2.5. Prototype System

The photograph of prototype of the forceps manipulator is shown in Fig.7. Rotation and translation mechanism was 42mm diameter, 89mm long, and 250g in weight. Gimbals mechanism was 39mm$\times$ 54mm$\times$70mm and 330g in weight. Ultrasonic motors and DC motors were controlled in open loop with ON-OFF switches.

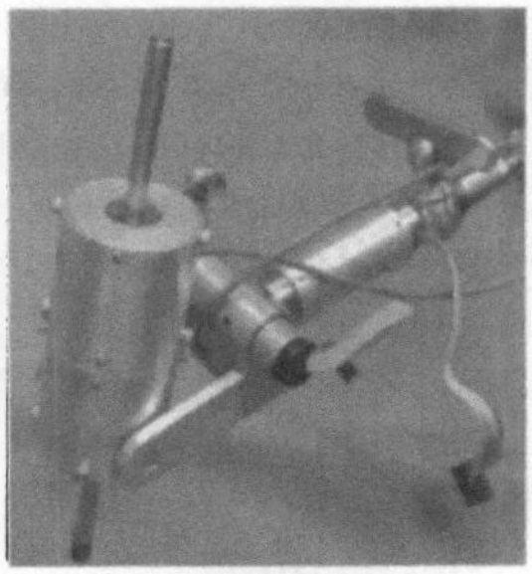

Fig.7 Prototype

3. Evaluation of the prototype manipulator

3.1. Moving Range and Speed

We measured the moving range and speed. We used a digital video camera and measured the moving range on the monitor. The system can provide the required range of motions as shown Table.1.

		Required Moving Range	Moving Range	Max. Speed
Rotation & Translation	Rotation	360(deg)	360(deg)	133(rpm)
	Back & Forth	200(mm)	115(mm)*	23(mm/sec)
Gimbals Mechanism	Pitch	40(deg)	67(deg)	17(deg/sec)
	Roll	40(deg)	360(deg)	45(deg/sec)

Table.1 Specifications of Manipulator (Moving Range and Speed)

The moving range of back and forth movement depends on the length of forceps (indicated with * in the Table.2). The mechanism gives no limitation to the moving range

©CARS/Springer. All rights reserved.

of the rotation and translation. Results showed that the moving range was adequate to the requirements for the manipulator.

3.2. Force and Torque required for forceps manipulation

We measured force with a load cell and torque with a spring scale as the product of the force and the length of forceps. We set the requirements with the consideration of manipulating forceps grasping the right lobe of the liver (approximately 0.5kg). This manipulator could generate adequate force and torque.

		Required Force or Torque	Results
Rotation & Translation	Rotation	1.6×10^{-2}(Nm)	3.9×10^{-1}(Nm)
	Back & Forth	4.9(N)	7.8(N)
Gimbals Mechanism	Pitch	1.2(Nm)	1.5(Nm)
	Roll	1.2(Nm)	1.4(Nm)

Table.2 Specifications of Manipulator (Force and Torque)

3.3. Rotation and Translation of forceps

Friction force between forceps and rollers drove the forceps. However, friction force was difficult to control because friction force was dependent on the condition of the surface. When each force of two friction wheels differs, the movement of the forceps is unstable. We cannot separate the rotation and translation of forceps completely. Forceps move back and forth with rotation, and rotates with translation. We evaluated this unstable movement of forceps. We measured the rotation angle in the 80mm translation and the distance of translation in the 360deg rotation ten times respectively. The average angle was 89.9deg and the average distance was 2.1mm. The results show instability of the movement. This is mainly due to mechanical errors in fabrication and assembly.

4. Discussion

4.1. New Compact Robot for Manipulating Forceps

The mechanism of rotation and translation had no limitation to the moving range. Friction wheels had the function of both holding and driving forceps, so we succeed in making the system compact. The size was 42mm diameter and 89mm long and 250g in weight. Gimbals mechanism realized the two DOF for determining the direction of the forceps. The size was 39mm×54mm×70mm and 330g in weight. We integrated the two mechanisms into a new compact robot for manipulating forceps. We realized all the four DOF required for manipulation of forceps in laparoscopic surgery. This robot is small enough for use of multiple manipulators simultaneously in the abdominal surgery since it does not occupy the operating space above the abdomen.

4.2. Future works

We have to attach rotary encoders to the friction wheels to get positional information of forceps. By calculating the number of revolutions of the friction wheels, we can estimate the position of the forceps. Feedback control contributes to the smooth movement of the forceps, and positional information of the forceps is need for the feedback control.

©CARS/Springer. All rights reserved.

We should consider the Remote Center of Motion (RCM) mechanism. Gimbals mechanism has its center of rotation above the abdominal wall, and this may enlarge the insertion hole and require motors higher torque. The result of experiment on the swine showed that demerits were not so significant. However, enlargement and torque will depend on the thickness of the abdominal wall of patients. RCM mechanism can set the center of rotation at the point remote from actuator, and it has no problem of enlargement of the insertion hole and the high torque of the motor. It is important to add function of Remote Center of Motion to the gimbals mechanism. Robots used in the operation must be washed and sterilized. Gimbals and linkage mechanism simplified the separation of sterilized and non-sterilized parts. Still we have to redesign the robot for easy cleaning and sterilization. We will integrate this compact robot for manipulating forceps with Multi-DOF forceps [4], Wide-angle view endoscope using Wedge Prism [5], and laparoscope manipulator using a five-bar linkage mechanism [6].

5. Conclusion

We developed a new compact robot for manipulation forceps using friction wheels and gimbals mechanism. Rotation and translation mechanism was 42mm diameter, 89mm long, and 250g in weight. Gimbals mechanism for forceps direction determination was 39mm× 54mm×70mm and 330g in weight. This robot had enough power and wide moving range required for forceps manipulation in MIS. Although additional improvement of mechanism is required, the system is promising as miniaturized surgical robot in MIS.

Acknowledgements

This study was supported by the Research for the Future Program JSPS-RFTF 99I00904.

References

1. D.Hashimoto, *Gasless Laparoscopic Surgery*, World Scientific Publishing, 1995
2. Salisbury J. Kenneth Jr., Heart of microsurgery, *Mechanical Engineering* v.120 n.12 Dec 1998, pp46-51, 1998
3. Vollenweider M et al, Surgery Simulator with Force Feedback, *Proceedings of the Fourth International Conference on Motion and Vibration Control (MOVIC98)*, 1998
4. Nakamura R, et al, Multi-DOF Forceps Manipulator System for Laparoscopic Surgery – Mechanism miniaturized & Evaluation of New Interface – *Proceedings of Fourth International Conference on Medical Image Computing and Computer Assisted Interventions (MICCAI2001)*, pp606-613, 2001
5. E.Kobayashi, et al, A Wide-Angle View Endoscope using Wedge Prisms, *Proceedings of Third International Conference on Medical Image Computing and Computer Assisted Interventions (MICCAI2000)*, pp661-668, 2000
6. E.Kobayashi, et al, Development of a laparoscope manipulator using five-bar linkage mechanism, *Proceedings of the 11th International Symposium and Exhibition on Computer Assisted Radiology and Surgery (CAR'97)* pp825-830, 1997

CARS 2002 – H.U. Lemke, M.W. Vannier; K. Inamura, A.G. Farman, K. Doi & J.H.C. Reiber (Editors)
©CARS/Springer. All rights reserved.

Merits of a newly–developed laparoscope manipulator: experiences with 4 cases

Tomikawa M[a], Hashizume M[b], Kobayashi E[c], Yamaguchi S[b], Sakuma I[d], Fujie M[e], Nakamura F[c], Dohi T[c], Shimada M[a] and Sugimachi K[a]

[a]Department of Surgery and Science and [b]Department of Disaster and Emergency Medicine, Graduate School of Medical Sciences, Kyushu University, [c]Department of Precision Machinery Engineering, Graduate School and Faculty of Engineering and [d]Institute of Environmental Studies, Graduate School of Frontier Sciences, the University of Tokyo, and [e]Department of Mechanical Engineering, Waseda University

Abstract

We performed a laparoscopic splenectomy for 4 patients with liver cirrhosis, using a newly-developed laparoscope manipulator that we recently developed. The manipulator was designed for safety and easy control. The manipulator is based on a five-bar linkage mechanism that has two independent motors on the bottom. Also, a zoom-up mechanism of laparoscope was applied to this manipulation system. The moving range was about 25 degrees for both vertical and horizontal directions. The operations were performed using the conventional endoscopic surgical devices or autosuture devices under the laparoscopic view controlled by the manipulator. The laparoscopic view was superimposed by a navigating circle and bar on the videoimage. The integrated image helped the operator manipulating the conventional endoscopic surgical devices throughout the operative procedures. Two thumb-buttons were attached on the holding part of the forceps. By pressing these buttons the operator could control the zoom and the direction of the laparoscopic movement. All patients tolerated these procedures well. All procedures were performed safely and with no problem. No conversion to open surgery occurred. Both mechanical safety and easy control are feasible during laparoscopic surgery using our newly-developed laparoscope manipulator.

Keywords: Laparoscopic splenectomy, laparoscope manipulator, liver cirrhosis

1. Introduction

Laparoscopic surgery has continued to gain in popularity in almost all fields of abdominal surgery. However, the suitability of laparoscopic surgery for patients with liver cirrhosis is still controversial [1]. For example, laparoscopic splenectomy for such patients is still a quite difficult procedure, because the patients often have enlarged spleen, tendency to bleed, portal hypertension and developed visceral venous collaterals. We recently developed a new robotic laparoscope manipulator that can follow a surgeon's wishes without obstructing his manipulation of the laparoscopic instruments [2]. As we expected that the newly-developed laparoscope manipulator would enable us to overcome the

©CARS/Springer. All rights reserved.

various difficulties during laparoscopic splenectomy, we have used the manipulator during a laparoscopic splenectomy for a patient with liver cirrhosis, and reported feasibility of laparoscopic splenectomy assisted by the newly-developed laparoscope manipulator [3]. Since the previous report, we experienced 3 more patients with liver cirrhosis who had laparoscopic splenectomy with the newly-developed laparoscope manipulator. The aim of this study is to evaluate safety and controllability of the newly-developed laparoscope manipulator.

2. Patients and Methods

Four patients were entered in this study. Three of the 4 patients were male and 1 was female. The age was 57±10 (mean±S.D.) years. All patients had liver cirrhosis with hypersplenism. The liver function was Child A in two patients and Child B in two patients. The platelet count and prothrombin time were $62\pm22\times10^3/\mu l$ and 70±16 %, respectively, indicating the tendency to bleed of these patients. The operations were performed as follows. The patients were placed in the right semi-decubitus position. A vertical skin incision was made 2 cm right to the umbilicus about 12 mm in length. A laparoscope was inserted through a trocar applied on the incision and CO_2 gas was infused. Other three vertical incisions were made 12 mm in length at the epigastric region, midclavicular line and midaxillary line along the left subcostal line. The other three trocars 12 mm in diameter were inserted into the peritoneal cavity. Then, the laparoscope was attached to our newly-developed laparoscope manipulator. The manipulator is based on a five-bar linkage mechanism that has two independent motors on the bottom. Also, a zoom-up mechanism of laparoscope was applied to this manipulation system. Electrical devices, such as motors, were set below the operative stand. The moving range was about 25 degrees for both vertical and horizontal directions. The splenic hilum and the retroperitoneum behind the spleen were dissected with electrocautery. The spleen was freed from pancreas tail using 2 or 3 autosuture devices.

These operations were performed using the conventional endoscopic surgical devices or autosuture devices under the laparoscopic view controlled by the manipulator. The laparoscopic view was superimposed by a navigating circle and bar on the videoimage. Two thumb-buttons were attached on the holding part of the forceps. By pressing these buttons the operator could control the zoom and the direction of the laparoscopic movement. When the operating spot was not clear, the operator turned on the zoom-up circle with a thumb-button in his hand. A good zoom-up vision was then obtained. Turning on the navigating circle and bar with the other thumb-button in his hand led the laparoscope toward the indicating direction.

After all procedures using the manipulator, the spleen was packed in a sac, minced with morcellator and took out of the abdominal cavity from the small incision on the midclavicular line. The peritoneal cavity was irrigated with warm saline and adequate hemostasis was confirmed. Fibrin glue was sprayed on the cut edge of the splenic hilum. A Penrose drain was placed at the left subphrenic space through the incision on the midaxillary line. The skin incisions were closed in layers. All patients tolerated these procedures well and returned to the ward in good condition.

©CARS/Springer. All rights reserved.

3. Results

The mean operative time was 292±53 minutes and the estimated blood loss was 290±242g. All procedures were performed safely and with no problem. Neither injury of the body organs nor conversion to open surgery occurred. The mean weight of spleen was 295±208g. The postoperative courses were uneventful with no problems. The mean postoperative hospital stay of the patients was 17±2 days. The integrated image on the video monitor helped the operator manipulating the conventional endoscopic surgical devices throughout the operative procedures. Two thumb-buttons on the holding part of the forceps made the operators' work smooth. The operators could easily control the zoom and the direction of the laparoscopic movement by pressing the thum-buttons. No interference between the instruments and the laparoscope occurred with this manipulation system.

4. Discussion

During laparoscopic surgery, manipulation of the laparoscope is important for smooth work. The assistant holds the laparoscope, and the operator uses both hands to manipulate the long instruments. Holding the laparoscope steady, keeping the view upright and changing the view to the operator's wishes are often difficult for the assistant.

During laparoscopic splenectomy these situations worsen in addition to the difficulties specific to laparoscopic surgery. First, numerous vulnerable visceral vessels are around the spleen. Especially, cirrhotic patients who need to have a splenectomy often have an enlarged spleen, a tendency to bleed, portal hypertension and developed visceral venous collaterals. Second, because the surgical space during laparoscopic splenectomy in the abdominal cavity is away from the port-site area on the skin, interference between the instruments and the laparoscope easily occurs. The longer the distance between the surgical space and the port-site area becomes, the narrower or the closer the positions of the laparoscope and the instruments become.

Our newly-developed laparoscope manipulator overcame these problems during laparoscopic splenectomy in these cases. The laparoscope used in this manipulation system has a zoom-up mechanism to have a close view of the surgical space. Therefore, we did not need to insert the laparoscope closer to the surgical space. Because we experienced no interference with this manipulation system, the operator could perform laparoscopic splenectomy more easily, more safely and more quickly. A minimum blood loss proved the operations were performed safely. Consequently, the recovery of the patients was very quick.

For mechanical safety, the range of movement of the laparoscope was limited mechanically with this kind of manipulator [4]. Therefore, the manipulator did not obstruct the operator's work throughout the operation, with all procedures performed safely and with no problems. Because the manipulator could be placed far from the patient's abdomen, the mechanism offered minimum obstruction to the surgeon's working space. Although the manipulator allowed only limited freedom of the laparoscope, a

©CARS/Springer. All rights reserved.

zoom substituted this movement. Using a zoom is safer than to move the laparoscope mechanically, because of little chance to injure the body organs.

By combining a laparoscopic image with 3D simulation and a planning system using preoperative or intraoperative imaging information such as CT or MRI [5], a surgeon can recognize the more accurate anatomies of the organs and can control the manipulator easily.

We developed a new laparoscopic manipulator. The manipulator was designed for safety and easy control. Using the manipulator, we experienced 4 cirrhotic cases who underwent laparoscopic splenectomy. Both mechanical safety and easy control are feasible during laparoscopic surgery using our newly-developed laparoscope manipulator.

Acknowledgements

This study was partly supported by the Research for the Future Program (JSPS-RFTF 99100902), and the Japan Association for the Advancement of Medical Equipment.

References

1. Hashizume M, Tanoue K, Morita M, Ohta M, Tomikawa M, Sugimachi. "Laparoscopic gastric devascularization and splenectomy for sclerotherapy-resistant esophagogastric varices with hypersplenism." *J Am Coll Surg* 187, 263-270, 1998.
2. Kobayashi E, Masamune K, Sakuma I, Dohi T, Hashimoto D. "A new safe laparoscopic manipulator system with a five-bar linkage mechanism and an optical zoom." *Comp Aid Surg* 4, 182-192, 1999.
3. Tomikawa M, Kobayashi E, Nakamura F, Sakuma I, Hashizume M, Shimada M, Gotoh N, Konishi K, Dohi T, Sugimachi K. "Usefulness of a newly–developed laparoscope manipulator during laparoscopic splenectomy." *CARS2001-Computer Assisted Radiology and Surgery*, Lemke HU, Vannier MW, Inamura K, Farman AG, Doi K (eds.), p1164, Elsevier Science, Amsterdam, 2001.
4. Davis BL, Hibberd RD, Ng WS, Timoney AG, Wickham JEA. "The development of a surgeon robot for prostate. Proceedings of the institution of mechanical Engineers (part H)." *J Engin Med* 205, 35-38, 1991.
5. Iseki H, Masutani Y, Iwahara M, Tanikawa T, Muragaki Y, Taira T, Dohi T, Takakura K. "Volumegraph (overlaid three-dimensional image-guided navigation). Clinical application of augmented reality in neurosurgery". *Stereotact Funct Neurosurg* 68,18-24, 1997.

CARS 2002 – H.U. Lemke, M.W. Vannier; K. Inamura, A.G. Farman, K. Doi & J.H.C. Reiber (Editors)
©CARS/Springer. All rights reserved.

Feasibility of robot-assisted laparoscopic intestinal anastomosis; an experimental study in pigs.

J.P. Ruurda, I.A.M.J. Broeders
Department of Surgery, University Medical Centre Utrecht, the Netherlands
H.P. G04.228, P.O. Box 85500, 3508 GA Utrecht, the Netherlands
jruurda@azu.nl

Abstract

Robotic telemanipulation systems have been introduced recently to enhance the surgeon's dexterity and visualisation in videoscopic surgery, facilitating microscopic suturing and knot tying. The aim of this study was to demonstrate technical feasibility of performing a safe and efficient robot assisted handsewn laparoscopic intestinal anastomosis in a pig model. Thirty intestinal anastomoses were performed. Twenty anastomoses were performed laparoscopically with the da Vinci robotic system, the remaining 10 anastomoses by laparotomy. OR-time, anastomosis-time and complications were recorded. Effectiveness of the laparoscopic anastomoses was evaluated by postoperative observation of 10/20 pigs for 14 days and by testing mechanical integrity in all pigs by measuring passage, circumference, number of stitches and bursting-pressure. These parameters and anastomosis time were compared to the anastomoses performed by laparotomy. In all cases the procedure was completed laparoscopically. The only peroperative complication was an intestinal perforation, caused by an assisting instrument. The median procedure time was 77 minutes. Anastomosis time was longer in the laparoscopic cases than in the controls (25 vs 10 minutes; p<0,001). Postoperatively, one pig developed an ileus, based on a herniation of spiral colon through a trocar-port. For this reason it was terminated on the sixth postoperative day. All anastomoses were mechanical intact and all parameters were comparable to those of the open procedures. Technical feasibility of performing a safe and efficient robot assisted laparoscopic intestinal anastomosis in a pig model was repeatedly demonstrated in this study, with a reasonable time required for the anastomosis.

Keywords: Robotics, anastomosis, intestine

1. Introduction

Recently, robotic telemanipulation systems were introduced with the objective to overcome the problems of laparoscopic surgery [[1, 2, 3, 4, 5]]. These problems exist both in the field of manipulation and visualisation. First, surgeons are limited in manoeuvrability by the need to work through a fixed entry-point, which limits the degrees of freedom of motion to a number of five. Thereby they have to work with an inverted instrument response and variability in scaling of motions. Second, working with an indirect two-dimensional field of view hampers perception of depth. Additionally, the

©CARS/Springer. All rights reserved.

natural eye-hand-target axis is lost by looking at a monitor, compromising normal oculovestibular input[6, 7].
The introduction of robotic systems, such as the da Vinci® system (Intuitive Surgical, Mountain View, Ca) (Fig 1.), aimed at providing a solution towards these problems[8]. This system exists of a console and three-armed robotic cart. Two manipulators and some footpads, integrated in the console, provide the surgeon with direct control over the robotic arms. Two of these arms carry instruments and the third arm carries the camera-system, which is also directly controlled. Manoeuvrability is restored by two additional degrees of freedom at the end-effector of the robotic instruments, mimicking the human wrist. Visualisation is enhanced by the introduction of a double optic system, providing a three-dimensional image of the operative field. This image is projected inside the console, thereby restoring the eye-hand-target axis.
These advantages facilitate the feasibility of complex laparoscopic manoeuvres, such as microscopic suturing and knot tying. Therefore, it should be feasible to perform an intracorporal handsewn anastomosis. The aim of this study is to demonstrate the feasibility of a handsewn laparoscopic anastomosis with the use of a robotic system, by performing intestinal anastomoses in swine.

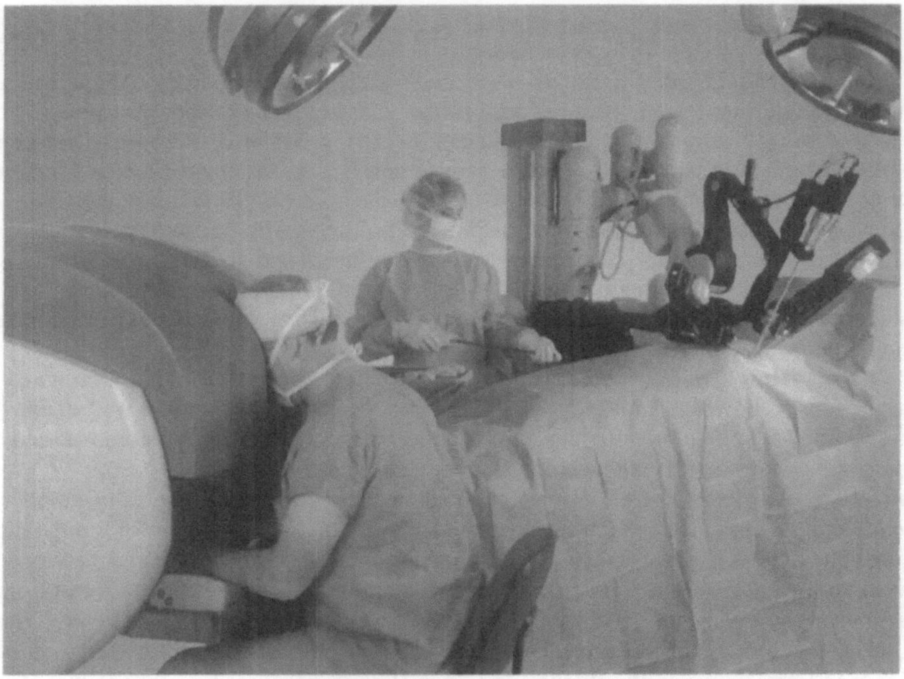

Fig 1. The Intuitive Surgical da Vinci® system

©CARS/Springer. All rights reserved.

2. Methods

After exercise on post-mortem material, 30 female pigs (49-90 kg) were operated. The procedure existed of a division of the rectum at ± 15 cm before the anus followed by a side to side sutured anastomosis. Twenty pigs were operated laparoscopically with the da Vinci® robotic telemanipulation system. Additionally, ten pigs underwent an identical procedure, but through a 20 cm midline laparotomy (control).
The initial ten pigs, operated laparoscopically with the robotic system, were terminated directly following surgery (Group A). Another ten pigs, operated in a similar way, were subsequently observed for 14 days followed by autopsy (Group B).
Conversions and peroperative complications were observed. Total operating time, blood-loss (Group B only, since the other pigs were used in other experiments during the same session) and anastomosis time were recorded. Postoperatively (Group B), first meals, stools and complications were recorded. At autopsy, attention focussed on presence of signs of leakage of the anastomosis and adhesions. The passage, circumference and number of stitches of the anastomosis were evaluated in all groups. Finally, all anastomoses were tested for mechanical accuracy, measuring the bursting-pressure.

3. Results

In Groups A and B, all procedures were completed laparoscopically. There was one complication (Group B), an intestinal perforation, caused by an assisting instrument. Total operative time (skin-to-skin) was 77 minutes (75-120) in Group B. Blood-loss comprised less than 10 ml in 9cases and 100 ml in one (Group B). Anastomosis time was longer in Groups A (33 minutes) and B (25 minutes) than in the controls (10 minutes; $p<0,001$).
All ten pigs (Group B) had their first meal and stool on the first postoperative day. Two postoperative complications occurred; a traumatic arthritis and an ileus. The arthritis was treated with ant-inflammatory analgesics, without further consequences to the postoperative course. The ileus was not expected to improve spontaneously, resulting in termination of the animal on the sixth postoperative day.
At autopsy, there were no signs of leakage in any pig (Group B). The pig terminated for reason of ileus showed a herniation of spiral colon through an abdominal wall defect at a trocar insertion point. In 8/10 pigs, loose adhesions between the anastomosis and the ovarian tube were found, which could easily be detached.
Passage was sufficient in all groups, without anastomotic narrowing. The number of stitches and the circumference of the anastomosis were higher in the control group than in Group A (Table 1, $p<0,001$). There was no difference in these parameters between the control group and Group B. The distance between stitches did not differ between groups.
Bursting pressure was similar in both Group A and the controls (65 respectively 70 mm Hg, NS). In both groups, a burst at a relatively low pressure occurred, due to a large distance (>1 cm) between two stitches. In Group B pressures were higher (145 mm Hg).

©CARS/Springer. All rights reserved.

Table 1

	Group A	Group B	Control	(A-Contr)	(B-Contr)
Anastomosis Time	33 (25-55)	25 (25-35)	10 (9-12)	P<0,001	P<0,001
Circumference	8,5 (8-10)	11,7 (10-15)	13 (11,5-13,5)	P<0,001	NS
Number of Stitches	17 (14-18)	18,5 (17-22)	22,5 (20-26)	P<0,001	NS
Distance between Stitches	0,53 (0,47-0,61)	0,62 (0,48- 0,88)	0,55 (0,50-0,61)	NS	NS
Bursting Pressure (mm Hg)	65 (25-125)	145 (117-178)	70 (37-123)	NS	NS

Table 1: Comparison between robot-assisted laparoscopic handsewn intestinal anastomoses (Groups A and B) and control anastomoses, performed through laparotomy.

4. Conclusions

Robot-assisted laparoscopic handsewn anastomosis was repeatedly proven feasible and safe. No conversions, deniable blood-loss, and only a small number of complications occurred. The complications that were faced, are general problems encountered in laparoscopic surgery, and could not be attributed to the use of a robotic system[9, 10, 11, 12].

Total operating time was acceptable and, although longer than in open surgery, anastomosis time was relatively short in the robot-assisted groups. In conventional laparoscopic surgery, handsewn intestinal anastomosis times of over 90 minutes are common [13, 14, 3, 15]. An explanation for the short anastomosis time in robot-assisted surgery could be found in the increased manipulation and visualisation capacities, allowing surgeons to suture in a smooth and efficient way.

Lack of force feedback is a problem in robot-assisted surgery and resulted in some suture breaks while practising knot tying. This issue could be tackled by exercise and did not result in any problems while suturing anastomoses. All anastomotic parameters were comparable between Group A and the controls, with one failure in both groups. Since it was not compared to a control group, the single conclusion that can be drawn from the bursting pressures in Group B, is the mechanical correctness of the anastomosis.

Now that this technique has proven to be feasible and safe, it will be transported to the clinical setting. In the experimental laboratory advanced anastomotic techniques, such as biliodigestive and vascular anastomosis, in which the capacities offered by the robotic system will be most beneficial, will be assessed in the near future.

©CARS/Springer. All rights reserved.

References

1. Hanisch, E., Markus, B., Gutt, C., Schmandra, T. C., and Encke, A. [Robot-assisted laparoscopic cholecystectomy and fundoplication--initial experiences with the Da Vinci system]. Chirurg: 72; 286-8. 2001.
2. Himpens, J., Leman, G., and Cadiere, G. B. Telesurgical laparoscopic cholecystectomy [letter]. Surg.Endosc.: 12; 1091. 1998.
3. Hollands, C. M., Dixey, L. N., and Torma, M. J. Technical assessment of porcine enteroenterostomy performed with ZEUS robotic technology. J.Pediatr.Surg.: 36; 1231-3. 2001.
4. Lomanto, D., Cheah, W. K., So, J. B., and Goh, P. M. Robotically assisted laparoscopic cholecystectomy: a pilot study. Arch.Surg.: 136; 1106-8. 2001.
5. Meininger, D., Byhahn, C., Markus, B. H., Heller, K., and Westphal, K. [Total endoscopic Nissen fundoplication with the robotic device "da Vinci" in children. Hemodynamics, gas exchange, and anesthetic management]. Anaesthesist: 50; 271-5. 2001.
6. Broeders, I. A. M. J. and Ruurda, J. P. Robotics revolutionizing surgery: the Intuitive Surgical "da Vinci" system. Industrial Robot: 28; 387-91. 1-8-2001.
7. Cadiere, G. B., Himpens, J., Vertruyen, M., Bruyns, J., Germay, O., Leman, G., and Izizaw, R. Evaluation of telesurgical (robotic) NISSEN fundoplication. Surg.Endosc.: 15; 918-23. 2001.
8. Ruurda, J. P. and Broeders, I. A. M. J. Feasibility of robot assisted laparoscopic cholecystectomy. proceedings CARS 2001, ed Lemke, HU ea.; 159-64.
9. Azurin, D. J., Go, L. S., Arroyo, L. R., and Kirkland, M. L. Trocar site herniation following laparoscopic cholecystectomy and the significance of an incidental preexisting umbilical hernia. Am.Surg.: 61; 718-20. 1995.
10. Fritsch, S., Fourquier, P., Gossot, D., Colomer, S., Celerier, M., and Revillon, Y. [Laparoscopic manual intestinal anastomosis: experimental study in a pig model]. Ann.Chir: 52; 574-7. 1998.
11. Kockerling, F., Rose, J., Schneider, C., Scheidbach, H., Scheuerlein, H., Reymond, M. A., Reck, T., Konradt, J., Bruch, H. P., Zornig, C., Barlehner, E., Kuthe, A., Szinicz, G., Richter, H. A., and Hohenberger, W. Laparoscopic colorectal anastomosis: risk of postoperative leakage. Results of a multicenter study. Laparoscopic Colorectal Surgery Study Group (LCSSG). Surg.Endosc.: 13; 639-44. 1999.
12. Nezhat, C., Nezhat, F., Seidman, D. S., and Nezhat, C. Incisional hernias after operative laparoscopy. J.Laparoendosc.Adv.Surg.Tech.A: 7; 111-5. 1997.
13. Msika, S., Iannelli, A., Marano, A., Zeitoun, G., Deroide, G., Kianmanesh, R., Flamant, Y., and Hay, J. M. [Hand-sewn intra-abdominal anastomosis performed via video laparoscopy during colorectal surgery]. Ann.Chir: 125; 439-43. 2000.
14. Bohm, B., Milsom, J. W., Stolfi, V. M., and Kitago, K. Laparoscopic intraperitoneal intestinal anastomosis. Surg.Endosc.: 7; 194-6. 1993.
15. Fingerhut, A., Hay, J. M., Elhadad, A., Lacaine, F., and Flamant, Y. Supraperitoneal colorectal anastomosis: hand-sewn versus circular staples--a controlled clinical trial. French Associations for Surgical Research. Surgery: 118; 479-85. 1995.

CARS 2002 – H.U. Lemke, M.W. Vannier; K. Inamura, A.G. Farman, K. Doi & J.H.C. Reiber (Editors)
©CARS/Springer. All rights reserved.

Evaluation of a magnetic tracking-guided needle placement system featuring respiratory gating in an in vitro liver model

Elliot B. Levy[a], Kevin Cleary[b], Filip Banovac[a], Daigo Tanaka[b], Sheng Xu[c], David Lindisch[b], Neil Glossop[d]
[a]Department of Radiology, Georgetown University Hospital/MedStar Health, 3800 Reservoir Road, Washington, DC, USA
[b]Imaging Science and Information Systems (ISIS) Center, Department of Radiology, Georgetown University Medical Center, Washington, DC, USA
[c]NSF-funded Center for Computer Integrated Surgical Systems and Technologies, Johns Hopkins University, Baltimore, MD, USA
[d]Traxtal Technologies LLC, Bellaire, TX, USA

Abstract

This paper presents our preliminary experience validating a needle guidance algorithm featuring magnetic tracking and respiratory gating for accurate needle placement in the liver using a specially designed phantom. Experimental results suggest that our implementation can facilitate accurate needle placement in this phantom during simulated respiratory-related liver motion.

Keywords: Magnetic tracking, needle placement, liver

1. Introduction

Accurate placement of fine needles within the liver for biopsy or catheterization purposes may be accomplished using CT, MRI, or ultrasound guidance. Respirations commonly must be suspended for accurate CT-or MRI-guided needle placement. In vascular procedures such as TIPS, shunt creation between portal and hepatic veins is most often accomplished without direct real-time guidance, although planar and 3-D ultrasound and MRI guidance has been reported. Recently an interactive image guidance system featuring magnetic tracking coupled to previously acquired 3-D CT images was used to display the real-time position of the intrahepatic puncture needle during TIPS in an animal model [1]. This system featured respiratory gating consisting of a magnetic sensor placed on the animal's abdomen, allowing updating of the needle position only during a designated portion of the respiratory cycle. This algorithm required the placement of 10-20 magnetic markers on the animal's skin to permit image registration. The system accuracy was reported to be 3mm.

In this paper we report our preliminary experience validating a guidance algorithm for accurate needle placement in the liver in a uniquely designed phantom. When coupled with a magnetic tracking system, this prototype features real-time monitoring of respiratory-related target organ motion. For the purpose of phantom design, we assume

©CARS/Springer. All rights reserved.

that hepatic respiratory motion occurs in the craniocaudal direction only and that the liver itself is not deformed by diaphragmatic motion. The respiratory excursion of the liver has been measured as 10mm in previous reports [2, 3]. Furthermore, Davies et.al. [3] initially described upper abdominal respiratory motion by assuming that respiratory motion velocity was either constant or zero. They measured the average dwell time (zero organ velocity) during end-expiration which lasted an average of 1.4 seconds during a mean respiratory cycle time of 4.4 seconds in their group of nine volunteers. The end-expiratory dwell time of the liver was confirmed subsequently by direct measurement of the maximum velocity and peak acceleration values by direct M-mode ultrasound scans obtained at 0.25s intervals.

Our strategy for needle placement and manipulation is patterned after the stepwise conventional "freehand" procedure for static image-guided biopsies. Preoperative images of the target are reviewed for path planning purposes A suitable skin puncture site is chosen from which a needle trajectory unobstructed by interposed viscera can be demonstrated. The angle of trajectory and necessary depth of puncture are determined. Freehand puncture is initiated, guided exclusively by the operator's perception of the desired trajectory. Respirations must be typically suspended during needle movements to prevent undesired organ motion during needle puncture. Needle position is confirmed at the conclusion of the needle drive process by obtaining static images of the target.

For magnetic tracking-guided needle punctures, puncture site and trajectory planning are determined with the assistance of a graphical user interface (GUI) and preoperatively obtained CT dataset. In our model, resting respirations continue throughout the procedure, and needle advancement is performed only when the GUI indicates that respiratory-related organ motion has ceased during the approximately 1.4 sec end-expiratory phase pause. The system tracks the motion of the fixed catheter-based fiducial to determine the timing of the pause in respiratory-related organ motion. Unlike static image-guided procedures, the specifically designed GUI displays 1) the depth of the needle tip relative to the desired depth in graphical fashion, and 2) the position of the needle tip registered with the preoperatively obtained CT dataset. The needle procedure can therefore be terminated by the operator based upon the real-time information and guidance provided by the GUI.

2. Methodology

An abdominal torso phantom (Anatomical Chart Co., Skokie, Il.) was modified by removing the ventral abdominal wall and placing a servomotor-driven platform mount in the "paraspinal" area upon which a foam liver phantom has been secured. The liver phantom contains target thin-walled "vascular structures" created by the removal of barium-coated plastic drinking straws placed within the foam mixture prior to final casting. The resulting air-filled tubes measure approximately 5mm in diameter. The phantom is moderately more firm than the human liver with respect to the tactile sense during needle puncture. The servomotor control system produces linear platform motion which simulates the respiratory motion of the liver. The tracking system consists of a small pyramidal magnetic field generator (Aurora™ Electromagnetic Tracking System, Northern Digital Inc., Toronto, Canada), a system control unit, and one or more sensor interface units. In our implementation we use two magnetically tracked sensors: a catheter

©CARS/Springer. All rights reserved.

and a needle. Both sensors are based on a single embedded 0.9 mm diameter coil. The catheter-based fiducial was placed through the simulated intrahepatic inferior vena cava and into a simulated hepatic vein and fixed in position with a small amount of adhesive. All motion of the liver phantom is therefore tracked by the embedded catheter-based fiducial. The remaining fiducials are calibrated flat skin markers (multi-modality radiographics markers, IZI Medical, Baltimore, MD) which can be readily identified on axial CT images of the torso. The tracked puncture needle is a modified 18 gauge trocar needle with the coil fiducial placed in the stylet (Traxtal Technologies, Bellaire, TX).

For each series of puncture experiments, a total of four skin fiducials were placed on the anterior costal margins. The phantom was placed in a Siemens CT scanner and contiguous 1mm images of the liver obtained. The CT DICOM dataset was transferred to a Windows NT workstation where the axial images were displayed and reviewed in a single window on the GUI. The target vessels were selected and a linear puncture needle trajectory highlighted. The magnetic field generator was placed next to the torso. The registration process was done using the external and catheter-based fiducials. The skin fiducials were identified on the CT images and automatic segmentation was performed to identify the isocenter of each fiducial. The tracked needle was then placed on each fiducial sequentially, thereby recording the position in magnetic space. The catheter-based fiducial was registered in the end-expiratory phase position by identifying the tip of the catheter containing the coil fiducial on the respective CT image. In all experiments, the registration error (root mean square) measured 1-2 millimeters. The skin entry site was determined by placing the tracked needle on the "skin" of the torso, guided in real-time fashion in a third window which displayed the position of the needle tip relative to the previously determined needle trajectory. The correct needle "depth" was compared to the termination target position, and needle advancement ceased when the system graphically indicated the desired needle depth.

3. Results

In initial tests, simultaneous needle puncture of two vessels was performed in the stationary liver phantom to simulate the key step in the specifically modified TIPS procedure [4]. Needle placement was performed by hand by experienced (E.L.) and less experienced (F.B.) operators. Orthogonal biplane fluoroscopic images of the liver phantom were then obtained which confirmed successful puncture of both targets by the single needle pass (Figure 1—note that all figures are on the last page of the paper).

In a second liver phantom, a single vessel served as a target, and guided needle punctures were performed by a single operator (E.L.) on ten occasions during simulated respiratory motion. The respiratory motion ranged from a frequency of 12-40/minute and an excursion distance of 1-2 centimeters. Orthogonal biplane digital images were obtained for each needle pass to confirm successful target puncture (Figure 2). A "guidewire test" was then performed consisting of an attempt to pass a standard angiographic 0.035 inch guidewire through the needle into the targeted "vessel" (Figure 3). The time required to successfully puncture the vessel target after placing the needle tip on the skin was recorded for each needle pass. A picture of the interventional suite and experimental set-up is shown in Figure 4.

©CARS/Springer. All rights reserved.

For needle passes performed during respiratory excursions, success was defined as 1) determination of the needle tip position within the vessel lumen by orthogonal digital images, and 2) successful passage of the guidewire without needle manipulation. For the 10 attempted passes, 8 passes were completely successful. In the remaining two passes, orthogonal biplane images demonstrated the needle tip within the target vessel but in an eccentric position, although withdrawal of the needle tip by 1 millimeter or rotation of the needle was required to allow successful passage of the guidewire. Needle puncture attempts averaged 28.6 sec (standard deviation 34.1 sec), with a prolonged attempt lasting 105 seconds caused by significant needle deflection within the phantom attributed to incorrect insertion of the stylet within the trocar. Needle misalignment was immediately recognized in this case, and needle redirection resulted in a successful puncture.

In all instances, the GUI provided a user-friendly, concise, and stepwise program for needle trajectory planning and needle placement. The rapid needle position update rate provided by the tracking system and interface allows for the real-time display of the position of the needle alignment and depth parameters. The intravascular, fixed catheter-based fiducial permits direct tracking of the respiratory related organ motion for real-time needle placement.

4. Discussion

Potential limitations for widespread implementation of these techniques were revealed in the course of the study. First, the presence of the CT gantry motion and biplane image intensifiers results in distortion of the magnetic field as reflected by increased registration errors. This problem was addressed in the current study by performing the magnetic tracking-guided needle punctures at a distance of at least two feet from the image intensifiers and x-ray sources. Second, in addition to the visual cues guiding needle movement provided by the GUI, the operator can be influenced by the sound of the servomotor initiating a subsequent respiratory cycle. Third, the reported method for respiratory gating would require selective hepatic vein catheterization. The requirement for this minimally invasive procedure may initially limit the implementation of this functionality to other similar, minimally invasive procedures such as TIPS.

Needles can be accurately placed for diagnostic and interventional procedures using static image-guided methods such as conventional CT and real-time guidance including conventional and CT-fluoroscopy and ultrasound. Real-time guidance offers the advantage of concurrent monitoring of the needle position and immediate determination of successful achievement of the intended goal. As a real-time guidance modality, ultrasound is limited by the availability of a satisfactory acoustical window, while CT imaging and particularly CT fluoroscopy is associated with exposure to significant ionizing radiation. Needle placement accuracy is determined by the registration error, stability of the magnetic field, and the operator's dexterity and judgement. Real-time imaging increases the efficacy of the puncture procedure by allowing the operator to distinguish successful and errant attempts and make necessary adjustments.

Magnetic tracking including registration of conventional image space and magnetic space potentially offers the guidance advantages of real-time imaging without the additional radiation exposure. The range of available targets is limited primarily by the resolution of the modality used to acquire the preoperative images. Intravascular or intraductal

©CARS/Springer. All rights reserved.

interventions may be more amenable to magnetic tracking guidance as other real-time imaging modalities may not be applicable or available, and absolute positional accuracy is probably not as significant for successful guidewire introduction into vessels or ducts. Guidance accuracy is usually defined relative to the target *size,* i.e., by the diameter of the vessel or duct, distance from the needle tip to the target, and by the resolution of the imaging modality itself. However, in the case of ducts and vessels, the bevel of the needle and the incident puncture angle may significantly affect the outcome as well.

5. Conclusion

A novel magnetic-based needle guidance system featuring respiratory gating has been successfully tested using a specifically designed phantom. This preliminary effort has highlighted two important obstacles which must be overcome before such a system could be widely implemented in clinical practice. First, observed magnetic field distortion by image intensifiers, C-arms, and the CT gantry in the standard Interventional Radiology or CT suite may significantly degrade the accuracy of the system. Second, the catheter-based fiducial must be retrievable yet fixed within a hepatic vein until successful vessel puncture and introduction of a guidewire has been achieved without causing vessel thrombosis.

The ability to conduct accurate needle placement within targeted hepatic structures during resting respirations offers several advantages. First, patients who are too ill to cooperate with respiratory instructions or who are mechanically ventilated could be successfully approached. Second, the number of needle passes necessary to achieve successful vessel puncture in TIPS could be reduced, thereby reducing the complication rate. The data show that the implemented magnetic tracking system can facilitate accurate needle placement in the phantom during simulated respiratory-related organ motion.

Acknowledgements

The design and construction of the phantom and the software was supported in part by an Academic Transition Award from the Cardiovascular and Interventional Radiology Research and Education Foundation (CIRREF). Portions of this work were also funded by U.S. Army grant DAMD17-99-1-9022. The content of this manuscript does not necessarily reflect the position or policy of the U.S. Government. Thanks are due to Northern Digital Inc. for the loan of the AURORA magnetic tracking system.

References

1. Solomon SB, Magee C, Acker DE, Venbrux AC. "TIPS Placement in Swine, Guided by Electromagnetic Real-Time Needle Tip Localization Displayed on Previously Acquired 3-D CT." *Cardiovasc Intervent Radiol*, **22**: 411-414, 1999.
2. Herline A, Stefansic J, Debelak J, et.al. "Image Guided Surgery: Preliminary Feasibility Studies of Frameless Stereotactic Liver Surgery." *Arch Surg*, **34**: 644-650, 1999.
3. Davies S, Hill A, Holmes R, et.al. "Ultrasound Quantitation of Respiratory Organ Motion in the Upper Abdomen." *Brit J. Radiology*, **67**: 1096-1102, 1994.
4. Banovac, F., Levy, E., Lindisch, D., et al. "Feasibility of Percutaneous Transabdominal Portosystemic Shunt Creation." Accepted for publication in *Surgical and Radiologic Anatomy*, January, 2002.

©CARS/Springer. All rights reserved.

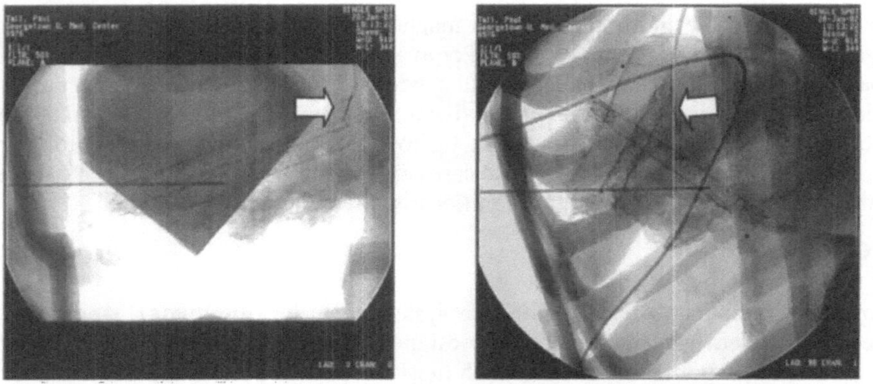

Figure 1: Biplane fluoroscopic images showing a successful magnetic guided puncture of two "vessels" in the liver phantom. The white arrows indicate the tip of the fixed catheter-based fiducial.

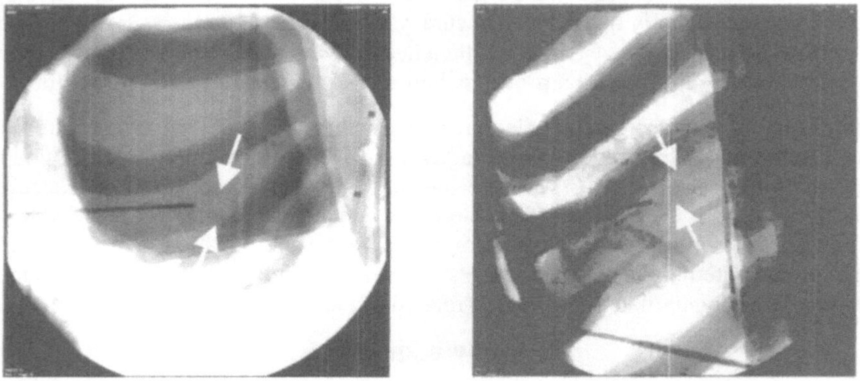

Figure 2: Biplane fluoroscopic images from a successful needle pass to a single vessel during simulated respiratory excursion of 1 cm at a frequency of 24 cycles per minute. The white arrows indicate the "vessel" walls.

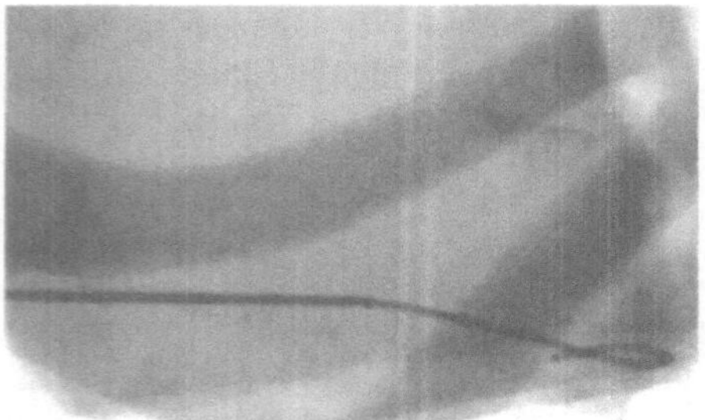

Figure 3: Guidewire test. A/P image showing 0.035 inch diagnostic guidewire inserted through needle into "vessel"

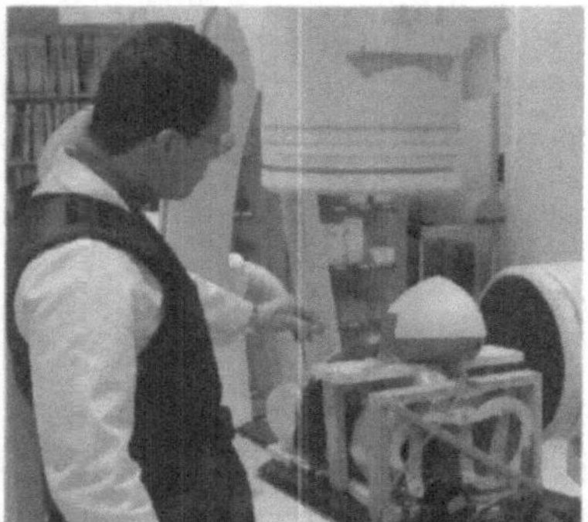

Figure 4: System testing in interventional suite

CARS 2002 – H.U. Lemke, M.W. Vannier; K. Inamura, A.G. Farman, K. Doi & J.H.C. Reiber (Editors)
©CARS/Springer. All rights reserved.

Evaluation of time-loss in robot-assisted surgery

J.P. Ruurda, I.A.M.J. Broeders
Department of Surgery, University Medical Centre Utrecht, the Netherlands
H.P. G04.228, P.O. Box 85500, 3508 GA, Utrecht, the Netherlands
jruurda@azu.nl

Abstract

Robotic surgery systems were introduced recently to deal with the basic disadvantages of laparoscopic surgery. However, working with these systems may lead to time loss due to additional robot-specific tasks, such as set-up of equipment and sterile draping of the system. To evaluate loss of time in robot-assisted surgery, we compared 10 robot-assisted cholecystectomies to 10 laparoscopic procedures by the standard technique. The robot-assisted procedures were performed with the 'da Vinci' robotic telemanipulation system. The total time at the operating theatre was scored and divided in a preoperative, operative and postoperative phase. These phases were further divided in smaller time frames to precisely define moments of time-loss. Although the median total operating theatre time was longer in the robotic procedures, this difference was not significant (144 versus 199 minutes, p=0,131). The preoperative phase was the single phase to cause time-loss due to three significantly longer time frames: set-up of equipment, preparation of materials and sterile draping. In the operative phase, the trocar entry time frame was longer in robot-assisted cases than in standard procedures. Additionally, postoperative theatre clearing was longer in the robot-assisted cases. In conclusion, robot-assisted surgery leads to time-loss during preparation of routine laparoscopic procedures.

Key words: Robotics, laparoscopic cholecystectomy, time analysis

1. Introduction

In recent years, robotic surgery systems have found their way into operating theatres in over a hundred clinics world-wide [1-5]. These systems have been developed with the objective to overcome the traditional problems of laparoscopic surgery. The robotic systems for videoscopic surgery, also named telemanipulation systems, consist of a remote workplace for the surgeon and a tableside robotic manipulator. The remote workplace holds a computer, which exactly translates the motions of the surgeon to the robot-held instruments. These systems offer distinct advantages regarding visualisation and manipulation such as three-dimensional imaging and extra degrees of freedom (DOF) of the instruments[6,7] (Fig. 1.).

Where performing surgery with these systems offers distinct advantages to the surgeon, the use of robotics requires additional steps, mainly during the start of a procedure. The time needed for specific robot related tasks, such as system set-up and sterile draping, adds to the total burden for the operating time schedule, which is disadvantageous in routine surgery [8,9]. Therefore, the aim of this study is to evaluate this time-loss and to

©CARS/Springer. All rights reserved.

define at what point during the procedure it mainly occurs. For this purpose, ten robot-assisted procedures were compared to ten standard laparoscopic cholecystectomies.

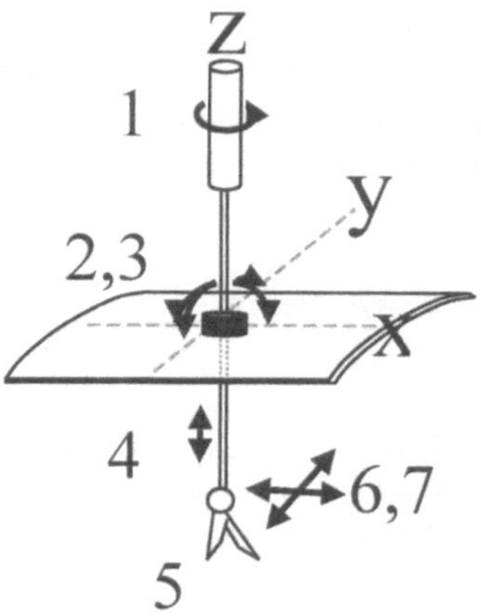

Fig 1: Degrees of freedom in da Vinci robot-assisted laparoscopic surgery: 1: rotation around the longitudinal axis. 2,3,4: Movement in x, y, z directions 5: Movement of the end-effector of the instrument 6,7: Movements of the intraabdominal joints in 2 directions.

2. Methods

Between January and June 2001, 20 laparoscopic cholecystectomies were performed and analysed. Ten of these (Group A) were performed with the da Vinci robotic telemanipulation system (Intuitive Surgical, Mountain View, California)(Fig. 2) [9]. The remaining 10 procedures were standard laparoscopic cholecystectomies (Group B). Selection criteria were identical for both groups. All patients were operated for symptomatic cholelithiasis on an elective basis after cholecystolithiasis was confirmed in all cases with ultrasound. Patients were included in consecutive order, following a visit to our outpatient clinic, and liberally distributed over both groups. All patients gave informed consent for standard and robotic laparoscopic cholecystectomy. In both A and B groups, eight patients were female (80%). The median patient age was 46 years (range 29-72) in Group A, and 54 (24-87) in Group B. During surgery, chronic cholecystitis was found in five patients (Group A: 4, Group B: 1). None of the procedures was converted to open surgery.

All Patients were positioned in the supine position, and standard preparation and draping was performed. Pneumoperitoneum was established at 14 mm mercury by Veress needle technique through a sub-umbilical puncture. A 12 mm (Group A) or a 10 mm (Group B) camera trocar was introduced at this position, followed by the introduction of an 11 mm trocar in the subxiphoid position in both groups. In Group A, a 7 mm robotic trocar was then introduced in the right midclavicular line just above the umbilicus level and another in the left hypochondrium. In Group B, 5 mm instrument trocars were placed in both the lower right abdomen and the right subcostal position. An assistant retracted the gallbladder through the xiphoid (Group A) or the subcostal port (Group B). Both the

©CARS/Springer. All rights reserved.

cystic duct and artery were clipped, and after completion of the gallbladder dissection, it was removed under direct vision through the subxiphoid port. In both midline ports the fascia was closed with Vicryl 2.0 sutures and the skin of all ports with Ethylon 3.0.

Time needed for both the total procedure and the subsequent phases of surgery were compared in both groups. Total time at the operating theatre was defined as time between the entry of the patient at the theatre and departure after surgery. At some occasions instruments or laparoscopy equipment were prepared or dismantled prior to the patient's entry or after the departure. This time was added to the total operating theatre time. The total operating theatre time was divided in three phases: the preoperative phase, the operative phase, and the postoperative phase.

The preoperative phase was defined as the time between the entry of the patient in the operating theatre and the time of the first incision. The preoperative phase was divided into three smaller time frames: the installation of the equipment, preparation of instruments and materials, and the draping of the sterile operative field.. The preoperative time that could not be attributed to any action related to preparation was scored as "undefined time-loss". Total preoperative anaesthesia time was separately scored, and defined as time between the entry of the patient and the moment of release for surgery. The operative phase consisted of a trocar entry period, the period of the actual laparoscopic dissection and the wound-closure. The time between wound-closure and patient departure from the operating theatre was defined as the postoperative phase. Total time needed for theatre clearing after surgery was recorded and started after wound-closure and ended at the time that all materials were dismantled properly and the equipment was stored at the dedicated location. In robot-assisted cases, the theatre clearing time included the de-installation of robotic equipment, which was also scored separately.

All data were analysed using SPSS 7.5 for windows. According the Shapiro-Wilk test, the distribution of all phases and time frames was non-normal. The Mann-Whitney-U test was applied to determine which phases accounted for any significant difference ($p<0,05$). All data are expressed as median time and range.

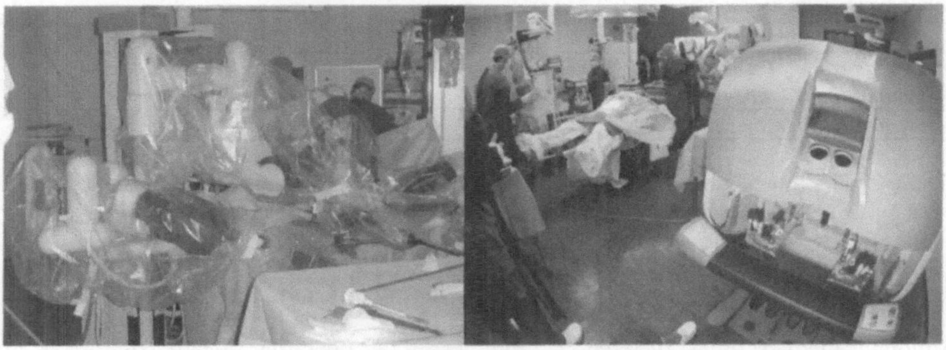

Fig. 2: The da Vinci system in the clinical setting. The three-armed robotic cart on the left, connected to the trocars. The surgeon's console in the right side picture.

©CARS/Springer. All rights reserved.

3. Results

Total operating theatre time in Group A was 144 minutes (111- 234) versus 119 minutes (71-189) in the standard procedures (Table 1). The preoperative phase in Group A was longer than in Group B (p<0.001, Table 1). Also, all individual time frames in the preoperative phase were longer in Group A, except the time frame "undefined time-loss" (Table 2). In the operative phase, the trocar placement, including attachment of the robotic arms, took longer in Group A (p<0,001, Table 2 In the postoperative phase, theatre clearing was shorter in Group B compared to the robot-assisted cases (p=0,041).

Phase	**Robot**	**Conventional**	**P**
Total operating theatre	144 (111-234)	119 (71-189)	0,131
Preoperative	47 (33-69)	27 (21-38)	<0,001
Operative	82 (59-178)	79 (42-150)	0,650
Postoperative	16(8-30)	12(8-22)	0,129

Table 1: Total operating theatre time and the time spent for the different phases of the procedure. Data are expressed as median and (range).

Time-frame	**Robot**	**Conventional**	**p**
Set-up of equipment	7 (6-11)	2 (2-5)	<0,001
Preparation of materials	18 (15-22)	11(8-23)	0,003
Sterile draping *Robot draping*	9 (4-11) 6 (4-8)	3 (2-6)	<0,001
Non-specified time-loss	12 (4-36)	7 (2-18)	0,493
Preoperative anaesthesia	19 (13-40)	18 (14-27)	0,448
Trocar entry *Robotic arm attachment*	20 (13-31) 4 (2-8)	10 (7-16)	<0,001
Dissection	43 (30-149)	64 (23-127)	0,325
Wound-closure *Robotic arm detachment*	11 (8-21) 1 (1-4)	9 (3-15)	0,068
Theatre clearing *De-installation robotic equipment*	14(8-20) 9 (3-10)	9 (3-20)	0,041
Postoperative anaesthesia	11 (3-30)	12 (8-22)	0,568

Table 2: The time spent for the subsequent time frames during the different phases of the surgical procedure. Data are expressed as mean and (range).

4. Discussion

Although median times differed 25 minutes, total operating theatre time was not significantly longer in robot-assisted laparoscopic cholecystectomy than in standard procedures (p=0,131). In both the operative and postoperative phase there was no significant difference between both groups. On the other hand, the preoperative phase of the robotic procedure appeared to be significantly longer than in standard procedures. All

©CARS/Springer. All rights reserved.

separate time frames of the preoperative phase attributed to this difference. The time-loss during installation of equipment can be explained by the need to set-up the robotic cart, console and videocart for each procedure, compared to the set-up of the videocart only in standard procedures. Time-loss during preparation can be explained by the need for additional materials required for the robotic system. Next to the standard laparoscopic set, two sets of robotic instruments, including sterile adapters and trocars, have to be prepared. Obviously, sterile draping took longer, because the three robotic arms of the chart require draping with dedicated covers. Although it was not significant, the excess undefined time-loss may be explained by the novelty of the system, which still tends to create an 'academic' atmosphere and brings spectators that may attribute to time loss by starting procedure related discussions. The preoperative phase exceeded the median time needed for anaesthesia by 19 minutes in robot-assisted cases, compared to only 9 minutes in standard procedures.

In the operative phase, the trocar entry time frame was significantly longer in the robotic group, but this was only partly caused by the time needed to attach the robotic arms to the trocars. An adjuvant reason for the longer introduction phase might be the time needed for the calibration of the 3D-camera system. The median laparoscopic dissection period time was 21 minutes shorter in robotic cases. This could be explained by the improvement of the surgeon's manoeuvrability, offering a smooth dissection. Other explanations can be the difference between operating surgeons (residents compared to experienced surgeons) and the intraoperative findings. Both factors have been discussed extensively [10-12]. For this reason, no conclusions can be drawn to any difference in dissection time in this study. The de-attachment of the robot from the trocars did not cause a difference in wound-closure time.

In the postoperative phase, the median time of robot-assisted cases did not exceed the median time of standard cases significantly. The time needed for clearing of the operating theatre was significantly longer in the robot-assisted cases (14 compared to 9 minutes), and was longer than anaesthesia time in 8/10 cases in Group A. The de-installation of the robotic equipment, comprising the disconnection of the various parts and storage of the system, took in account a major part in this phase, with a median of 9 minutes. In Group B anaesthesia time was longer than theatre clearing in all cases, this explains the comparable outcome of postoperative time in both groups.

These data make clear that the use of a robotic system causes time-loss in the current OR set-up, mainly in the preoperative phase of the surgical procedure. The most potent concept to deal with time-loss during interventions using high-tech equipment is designing technology-dedicated workplaces. One should strive for a spacey videoscopic surgery suite with a permanent robotic equipment setup. The preoperative installation of the apparatus could hereby be eliminated as well as the postoperative time needed for removal and storage of equipment. In our study, this would shorten the preoperative phase by approximately 7 minutes and the theatre clearing phase by approximately 9 minutes, making it shorter than time needed by the anaesthesia team. Another option to limit time-loss is the efficient use of the interval between two surgical procedures. Set-up and sterile draping of the robotic system can be performed during this period and a start can be made with the preparation of instruments. This puts a demand on the team involved, regarding efficiency and dedication, but a serious reduction of operating theatre time will hereby be

©CARS/Springer. All rights reserved.

established. Finally, further development of the robotic systems is required to diminish pre- and postoperative time needed for preparation and clearing of robotic equipment. The time-consuming draping of the robotic arms and the preparation of the materials will be simplified in next generation devices by improving the ergonomics of drape and trocar connectors, offering space for another 11 minutes of time-reduction (Fig 2.).

In conclusion, robot-assisted surgery led to time-loss, mainly during the preoperative phase of routine laparoscopic surgery in a standard operating theatre. This time-loss can be limited by dedicated surgical workplaces, further development of the robotic systems and by creative management of time by the surgical team involved.

References

1. Hanisch E, Markus B, Gutt C, Schmandra TC, and Encke A. Robot-assisted laparoscopic cholecystectomy and fundoplication--initial experiences with the Da Vinci system. Chirurg 72: 286-288, 2001
2. Himpens J, Leman G, and Cadiere GB. Telesurgical laparoscopic cholecystectomy [letter]. Surg Endosc 12: 1091, 1998
3. Hollands CM, Dixey LN, and Torma MJ. Technical assessment of porcine enteroenterostomy performed with ZEUS robotic technology. J Pediatr Surg 36: 1231-1233, 2001
4. Lomanto D, Cheah WK, So JB, and Goh PM. Robotically assisted laparoscopic cholecystectomy: a pilot study. Arch Surg 136: 1106-1108, 2001
5. Meininger D, Byhahn C, Markus BH, Heller K, and Westphal K. Total endoscopic Nissen fundoplication with the robotic device "da Vinci" in children. Hemodynamics, gas exchange, and anesthetic management. Anaesthesist 50: 271-275, 2001
6. Broeders IAMJ and Ruurda JP. Robotics revolutionizing surgery: the Intuitive Surgical "da Vinci" system. Industrial Robot 28: 387-391, 2001
7. Cadiere GB, Himpens J, Vertruyen M, Bruyns J, Germay O, Leman G, and Izizaw R. Evaluation of telesurgical (robotic) NISSEN fundoplication. Surg Endosc 15: 918-923, 2001
8. Marescaux J, Smith MK, Folscher D, Jamali F, Malassagne B, and Leroy J. Telerobotic laparoscopic cholecystectomy: initial clinical experience with 25 patients. Ann Surg 234: 1-7, 2001
9. Ruurda JP and Broeders IAMJ. Feasibility of robot-assisted laparoscopic cholecystectomy. In: Lemke HU, Vannier MW, Inamura K, Farman AG and Doi K (eds). Proceedings CARS 2001, 159-164, Elsevier Science, Amsterdam, 2001
10. Berber E, Engle KL, Garland A, String A, Foroutani A, Pearl JM, and Siperstein AE A critical analysis of intraoperative time utilization in laparoscopic cholecystectomy. Surg Endosc 15: 161-165, 2001
11. Crolla RM, van Ramshorst B, and Jansen A. Complication rate in laparoscopic cholecystectomy not different for residents in training and surgeons. Ned Tijdschr Geneeskd 141: 681-685, 1997
12. Traverso LW, Koo KP, Hargrave K, Unger SW, Roush TS, Swanstrom LL, Woods MS, Donohue JH, Deziel DJ, Simon IB, Froines E, Hunter J, and Soper NJ. Standardizing laparoscopic procedure time and determining the effect of patient age/gender and presence or absence of surgical residents during operation. A prospective multicenter trial. SurgEndosc 11: 226-229, 1997

©CARS/Springer. All rights reserved.

HepaVision2 – a software assistant for preoperative planning in living-related liver transplantation and oncologic liver surgery

H. Bourquain, A. Schenk, F. Link, B. Preim, G. Prause, H.-O. Peitgen
MeVis – Center for Medical Diagnostic Systems and Visualization,
Universitätsallee 29, 28359 Bremen, Germany, Email: bourquain@mevis.de

Abstract

HepaVision2, a user friendly software application for preoperative planning based on CT images in liver surgery is presented. It is intended for both, evaluation of potential donors in living-related liver transplantation and planning of oncologic resections. The planning takes into account the patient's individual anatomy allowing for fully automatic calculation of individual resection proposals including volumetric analysis. The results are visualized in 3D, thus allowing the surgeon to choose the optimal strategy for each patient. The software was tested in over 50 cases by our clinical partners and our institution. Average time needed per case is below one hour, therefore allowing the use of the software application in clinical routine.

Keywords: Living-related liver transplantation, oncologic resections, computer-assisted preoperative planning

1. Introduction

Shortage of cadaveric organs for transplantations leads to an increase in living-related transplantations. For example the number of living-related liver transplantations (LRLT) in the United States of America grew from 86 in 1998 to 219 in 1999 [1]. As the donors are healthy volunteers their eligibility to donate a portion of the liver must be evaluated very carefully before they undergo surgery. It must be assured that both the volume of the transplanted portion and of the remaining liver is sufficient for recipient and donor. Additionally, there are anatomical variants in the vascular or biliary systems that complicate the operation or even interdict it. Examples of these variants are an accessory hepatic vein or an abberant hepatic artery.

New surgical strategies such as anatomical resections of tumors created a demand for more careful preoperative planning of the resection, taking into account the volume of the resected portion of the liver. Preoperative planning is also important in case of multiple liver metastases to decide, whether surgery can be performed in an one-stage approach or if the remaining volume would not be sufficient and therefore the tumors must be resected in several stages with intermittent intervals of organ recovery. To calculate vascular territories and their volumes, it is necessary to segment the liver and the major vessels.

Only a few groups world-wide deal with image analysis for liver surgery planning. A group in France has developed methods for the analysis of clinical data for liver surgery

©CARS/Springer. All rights reserved.

planning [2]. Liver segmentation as well as the segmentation of intrahepatic structures are carried out fully automatically. The underlying idea for the automatic liver segmentation is to start with the segmentation of more prominent surrounding structures (skin, bone, lung, kidney) and thereby restricting the search space for the liver location. The intensities of the parenchyma, the lesions and intrahepatic vessels are estimated by fitting a Gaussian to the image histogram. The methods have been applied to 30 clinical cases and worked reliable in the majority of the cases. The drawback of the automatic approach, however, is a lack of interactive controllability if the assumptions are not fulfilled. A group at German Cancer Research Institute Heidelberg developed a system for liver surgery planning [3] and evaluated its use [4]. Work has been published on preoperative volumetry in the evaluation of liver donors. Most of these papers are based on images from computed tomography (CT) [5,6], while others compare the volumetry results obtained from CT and magnetic resonance imaging (MRI)[7]. Proposals for anatomical resections calculated from clinical CT datasets considering the patient individual anatomy have been described in two publications [4,8]. Different software tools had to be used to obtain these results.

Aim of our work was to develop one comprehensive software assistant that combines all necessary image processing steps needed for both the evaluation of living donors and oncologic resections. The application should be robust, flexible, easy to operate, and sufficiently fast, i.e. time for image analysis should not exceed one hour, thus allowing its use in daily clinical routine.

2. Methodology

Computer-aided preoperative planning in liver surgery is a demanding task that consists of several image processing steps described in detail below. As the first step, the image data normally available in DICOM format are imported Based on these data important anatomical and pathological structures are segmented. These structures are in case of LRLT the liver and the vascular systems. In case of an oncologic resection the tumors must also be segmented.

Liver segmentation is performed with a modified live-wire algorithm, a semi-automatic edge-oriented algorithm as described in [9]. With this semi-automatic algorithm the user has to specify only a few seed points per slice to identify the liver contour. The liver contour is derived by means of a cost function which is used to detect a path with minimal cost (in terms of gray value differences, image gradients and zero crossings of the second derivative). The live-wire contour is interactively determined on a slice about every 10 mm and the contours of the remaining slices are interpolated and subsequently optimized based on the live-wire cost function.

The analysis of the vascular systems is described in [10]. The analysis consists of (1) an image preprocessing step to eliminate inhomogeneities within the liver, (2) segmentation of the vascular structures with a modified region growing algorithm, (3) determination of the centerlines (skletonization) of this segmentation results, and (4) the structural analysis of the vascular trees. From the skeletonized vessels the different vascular systems are separated semi-automatically as shown in Fig.1 and analysis for each of these systems can

©CARS/Springer. All rights reserved.

be performed. This analysis includes, but is not restricted to, identification of the 8 major branches of the portal vein, thus giving a classification similar to Couinaud's scheme.

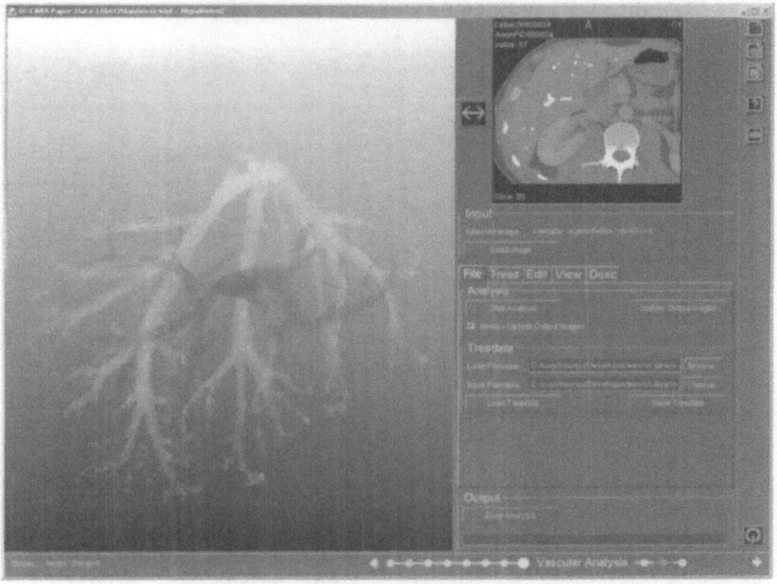

Fig 1: Graphical user interface of HepaVision2. Screenshot for vascular analysis. The different vascular systems are separated by an automatic algorithm and coded with different shades of gray. Visible are the portal vein (dark gray) and the hepatic veins (light gray). These structures are superimposed to the original data in the small display in the upper right corner.

The vascular territories for each of these structures and their volumes are calculated. An example of such a calculation is shown in Fig. 2.
Several methods for tumor segmentation are supported: threshold-based methods restricted to the previously determined liver mask and contour-based algorithms, for example freehand drawing or live-wire. Threshold-based methods which are rather imprecise are more appropriate if the number of metastases is rather large. Volumes of the liver and the tumors are determined by counting the voxels which have been segmented. Partial volume effects, however, are not considered.

In patients with liver tumors a risk analysis, i.e. the calculation of vascular structures and their depending territories affected if the tumor would be resected with a certain safety margin is performed. The safety margins can be adjusted interactively. This procedure is described in detail in [11].

All necessary image processing steps are performed with ILAB4, a R&D platform for image processing and visualization developed at our institution. With ILAB4 modules, each representing an image processing task, are combined graphically to create specialized networks that perform a well defined task. By means of a scripting language a graphical user interface (GUI) can easily be composed. The user interface contains only a subset of the control elements available in the underlying image processing modules.

©CARS/Springer. All rights reserved.

These control elements are carefully chosen to reflect the most frequently needed parameters. Thus, the complexity of the underlying image processing networks are hidden from the user. Also, the user is guided through all necessary processing steps by the GUI.

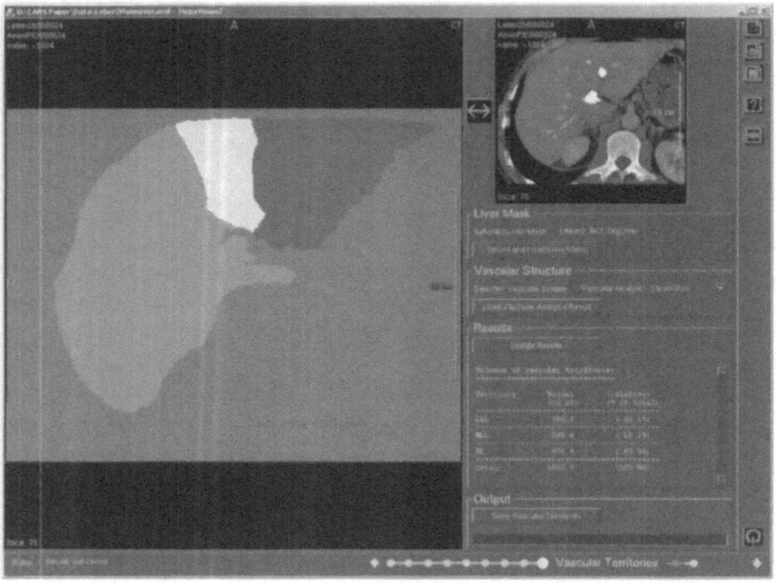

Fig. 2: Vascular territories calculated for the three main branches of the portal vein (right liver lobe – medium gray, medial left lobe –light gray, lateral left lobe – dark gray). Notice also the consistent design of the GUI in comparison with Fig. 1.

All segmentation results are managed by HepaVision2. For this purpose, a data structure has been developed which uses the syntax of the wide-spread XML-format (Extended Markup Language). By choosing XML it is possible to import the results of the planning process into other tools.

In each processing step the GUI consists of two large displays for image data and one region where the control elements are provided. The display regions may be used to display 2d slice data as well a 3d visualization with the usual facilities to control (zoom and rotate) the virtual camera. It is possible to superimpose the segmentation results to the original slice data. HepaVision2 supports the generation of small animations which show interactively rotating 3d visualizations of the relevant structures. These animations are results of image analysis and useful for preoperative discussions.

3. Results

HepaVision2 was tested in our institute on more than 25 clinical datasets, both for living-related liver transplantations and for tumor resections. In the clinical routine it is used on a regular basis for evaluation of donors in living-related liver transplantation at the Hannover Medical School. Preoperative planning of oncologic resections is performed

©CARS/Springer. All rights reserved.

with HepaVision2 at the University Hospitals of Essen and Mainz. Surgery planning with HepaVision2 takes into account the patient individual anatomy of the liver and the vascular structure. Therefore, the volumetry of the vascular territories in evaluation of liver donors is not based on generalized anatomical structures like the main branches of the hepatic veins and the portal vein as in Couinaud's scheme, but is calculated for the individual branching pattern of this patient. In oncological surgery resection proposals are based on the individual branching pattern of major vessels. Tissue at risk from an insufficient blood supply or restricted venous outflow can be calculated for arbitrary safety margins on both the hepatic veins and the portal vein, and the results can be combined.

When comparing our old procedure of preoperative planning with the new software assistant advantages are obvious. First of all, the processing time needed per case is reduced at least by a factor of 2. The speed up is mainly due to the facility to directly import DICOM images, a faster turn-over between image processing steps and the automatic execution of specific actions. The DICOM import also reduces the risk of errors as information like pixel spacing and slice thickness are directly extracted from the DICOM headers. The administration of input data and results is easier as the user does not have to care about filenames. Also, only reasonable entries are shown in selection boxes as possible input images. Image processing is more standardized than with the old networks, thus giving more reproducible results, even if the analysis is carried out by different people.

4. Conclusions

HepaVision2 is a user friendly application, primarily designed to facilitate preoperative planning of liver surgery. It allows the analysis of CT data with calculation of total liver volume, volumes for vascular territories of the main branches of the portal vein and hepatic veins, as well as the tumor volume. Risk analysis provides resection proposals for anatomical resection based on the individual anatomical structure of the vascular systems. Image analysis, without visualization, can be performed in less than 1 hour and is therefore possible in clinical routine for selected cases in oncologic surgery. This effort is always justified for the evaluation of potential living-related liver donors to minimize the risk of healthy volunteers.

Compared to its predecessor which was tied to Silicon Graphics hardware, the new software HepaVision2 is available on Windows-based PCs and it contains better image segmentation methods (in particular those based on live-wire). The functionality has been extended by incorporating a risk analysis module and the workflow was improved considerably.

There are several extensions desirable for the described software assistant. First, the visualization part which is used for the exploration of the final results will be extended to support a more streamlined and standardized approach by means of user preferences. Second, a module for virtual resections, similar to that described in [8] will be integrated. While the underlying algorithms are currently tailored to the analysis of CT data, it is

©CARS/Springer. All rights reserved.

desirable to modify them in a way that they can handle MRI data which are often acquired for LRLT planning, primarily to avoid that the donor is exposed to X-ray radiation.

Acknowledgements

We thank our clinical partners, Prof. Debatin University Hospital Essen, Prof. Galanski, Hannover Medical School, and Prof. Thelen, University Hospital Mainz for providing us with high quality radiological data. The research that lead to the presented results was conducted as part of the cooperation projects VICORA – Virtual Institute for Computer Assisted Radiology (www.vicora.de) and the project Visualization and Interaction Techniques for Oncologic Liver Surgery Planning. We thank all partners who made this publication possible by their continuous support. VICORA is supported by the German Federal Ministry of Education and Research under the grant number 01EZ0010, the latter by the Deutsche Forschungsgemeinschaft (Pe 199/9-1).

References

1. 2000 Annual Report of the U.S. Scientific Registry for Transplant Recipients and the Organ Procurement and Transplantation Network: Transplant Data: 1990-1999. U.S. Department of Health and Human Services, Health Resources and Services Administration, Office of Special Programs, Division of Transplantation, Rockville, MD. United Network for Organ Sharing, Richmond, VA.
2. Soler L, Delingette H, Malandain G, Montagnat J, Ayache N, et al, "Fully automatic anatomical, pathological and functional segmentation from CT scans for hepatic surgery", *Computer Aided Surgery*, Vol. 6(3):131-142, 2001
3. Glombitza G, Lamade W, Demiris AM Göpfert MR, Mayer A, et al, "Virtual planning of liver resections: image processing, visualization and volumetric evaluation", *International Journal of Medical Informatics*, Vol. 53(2-3):225-237, 1999
4. Lamade W, Glombitza G, Fischer L, Chiu P, Cardenas CE Sr, et al, "The impact of 3-dimensional reconstructions on operation planning in liver surgery", *Archives of Surgery*, Vol. 135(11):1256-1261, 2000
5. Higashiyama H, Yamaguchi T, Mori K, Nakano Y, Yokoyama T, et al, "Graft size assessment by preoperative computed tomography in living related partial liver transplantation", *British Journal of Surgery*; Vol. 80(4):489-492, 1993
6. Noda T, Todani T, Watanabe Y, Yamamoto S, "Liver volume in children measured by computed tomography", *Pediatric Radiology*; Vol. 27(3):250-252, 1997
7. Krupski G, Rogiers X, Nicolas V, Maas R, Malago M, et al, "Computed tomography versus magnetic resonance imaging--aided volumetry of the left lateral segment before living related liver donation: a case report", *Liver Transplantation and Surgery*; Vol. 2(5):388-390, 1996
8. Preim B, Selle D, Spindler W, Oldhafer KJ, Peitgen HO, "Interaction Techniques and Vessel Analysis for Liver Surgery Planning", *Proceedings of MICCAI*, Springer, LNCS 1935:608-617, 2000
9. Schenk A, Prause G, Peitgen HO, "Efficient demiautomatic segmentation of 3D objects", *Proceedings of MICCAI*, Springer, LNCS 1935:186-195, 2000
10. Selle D, Peitgen HO, "Analysis of the morphology and structure of vessel systems using skeletonization, *Proceedings of SPIE Medical Imaging*, 4321: 261-271, 2001
11. Preim B, Bourquain H, Selle D, Oldhafer KJ, Peitgen HO, "Resection proposals for oncologic liver surgery based on vascular territories". *CARS 2002*, CARS/Springer, 2002 (in this volume)

CARS 2002 – H.U. Lemke, M.W. Vannier; K. Inamura, A.G. Farman, K. Doi & J.H.C. Reiber (Editors)
©CARS/Springer. All rights reserved.

Preoperatiove prostate cancer volume estimation based on clinically correlated needle biopsy simulation

Jianchao Zeng[a], Roger R. Connelly[b], John J. Bauer[c], Wei Zhang[d]
Isabell A. Sesterhenn[d], Judd W. Moul[e] and Seong K. Mun[a]
[a] ISIS Center, Department of Radiology
Georgetown University Medical Center, Washington, DC, USA
[b] Henry Jackson Foundation, Rockville, MD, USA
[c] Urology Service, Department of Surgery
Walter Reed Army Medical Center, Washinton, DC, USA
[d] Department of Genitourinary Pathology
Armed Forces Institute of Pathology, Washington, DC, USA
[e] Center for Prostate Disease Research, Department of Surgery
Uniformed Services University of Health Sciences, Bethesda, MD, USA

Abstract

This paper presents a new approach to the estimation of preoperative prostate cancer volume using clinically correlated prostate needle core biopsy simulation on a large number of digitized prostatectomy speciemns with clinically localized cancers. The analysis of the 10-pattern and the sextant protocols on cancer volume estimation with age, race PSA, prostate volume, number of positive cores, and 2-way and 3-way interactions of these varaibles in the original regression model as predictors revealed that only three of these variables and two 2-way interactions are needed to estimate prostate cancer volume. The model consists of the main effects of prostate volume, number of positive cores, and PSA plus the 2-way interactions of prostate volume with number of positive cores and prostate volume with PSA, and it explains as much as 40% of the variance of the log cancer volume.

Keywords: Prostate cancer volume, preoperative estimation, needle biopsy

1. Introduction

A number of groups have performed research on estimation of prostate cancer volume based on preoperative factors or variables such as serum PSA, Gleason score at biopsy and clinical stage. D'Amico et al. developed a method to calculate prostate cancer volume based on serum PSA, combined with biopsy Gleason score and ultrasound volume of the prostate [1]. They found that the calculated prostate cancer correlated more closely with the measured prostate cancer volume than that of the Prostate-Specific Antigen (PSA) for all cancer volume groups (0.02 to 9.5 cc), being able to provide a better prediction of extracapsular (ECE) in patients with clinical stage T1 and T2 disease. Chan and Stamey evaluated the formula for cancer volume calculation by D'Amico et al. using a larger data sample of 318 patients who underwent radical prostatectomy after positive systematic

©CARS/Springer. All rights reserved.

sextant biopsy [2]. They, however, did not confirm the usefulness of the equation and it showed that serum PSA correlated with the actual cancer volume even better than the calculated cancer volume. They also indicated that, besides PSA, Gleason score and total prostate volume, more variables need to be taken into account when estimating prostate cancer volume. Kabalin et al. also showed, using 350 consecutive prostate cancer patients, that serum PSA significantly correlated with most morphologic variables that define progression of prostate cancer including cancer volume [3]. They thus suggested that PSA could be used to predict prostate cancer volume and for patient evaluation and treatment decisions. Terris et al. combined the PSA with the TRUS-guided sextant biopsy in order to predict prostate cancer volume [4]. Using 124 patients, they found that the calculated prostate volumes correlated well with the cancer volumes in prostatectomy specimens with the R-square of 0.76. Peller et al. investigated the role of number of positive cores in a sextant biopsy in predicting the stage and volume of prostate cancer [5]. They showed that the number of positive cores might be an important prognostic indicator of pathologic classification and cancer volume, as well as preoperative Gleason score and serum PSA. On the other hand, Egevad et al. suggested that correlation between the core cancer volume in biopsy and the prostate cancer volume could be improved with the increase in number of biopsies [6]. They also indicated that improved biopsy protocols could be used to effectively predict cancers smaller than 1mL in size. Dietrick et al. investigated prostate cancer volume issue in a different way [7]. Instead of formulating an equation to predict specific cancer volume, their study suggested that a core cancer length of 2 mm or more on one or two needle biopsies reliably predicted cancer of 0.5 cc or greater, which was considered a clinically significant volume.

In this paper, we have developed a number of regression models by considering such variables as needle cancer core volumes, number of positive cores, and other predictive variables such as cohort of patient, locations of positive and negative cores, and prostate volume. Biopsy results of two different protocols, a sextant protocol which is widely used clinically and a 10-pattern protocol which was confirmed to be better than the sextant [8], have been initially used in the regression analysis. We have also incorporated the interactions among predictor variables in our regression analyses in order to determine the best possible combination of variables for the estimation of prostate cancer volume.

2. Material and Methods

2.1 Modeling of prostate specimens with clinically localized cancer

Three-dimensional (3-D) prostate surface models were reconstructed from digitized step-sectioned whole-mounted radical prostatectomy specimens with clinically localized cancers using deformable modeling techniques [9,10]. The prostatectomy specimens were first fixed in 10% formalin for 48 hours before being step-sectioned into slices at 2.5-mm intervals in transverse planes, resulting in 10 to 15 slices for each specimen. Each slice was further embedded, sectioned into 4-micron thickness, whole-mounted on a glass slide, and stained with hematoxylin and eosin before being examined by pathologists under a microscope. The pathologists identified key structures from each section and outlined their boundaries. Structures outlined include surgical margin, capsule, seminal vesicles, urethra, ejaculatory ducts as well as all the foci of cancer. The outlined slides were then

©CARS/Springer. All rights reserved.

digitized at a resolution of 1,500 dpi, and slides of a specimen were registered to each other with the help of five fiducial marks on each slide. Prostate surface models were finally reconstructed based on the registered outline information. An example of the reconstructed 3D prostate model is shown in Figure 1.

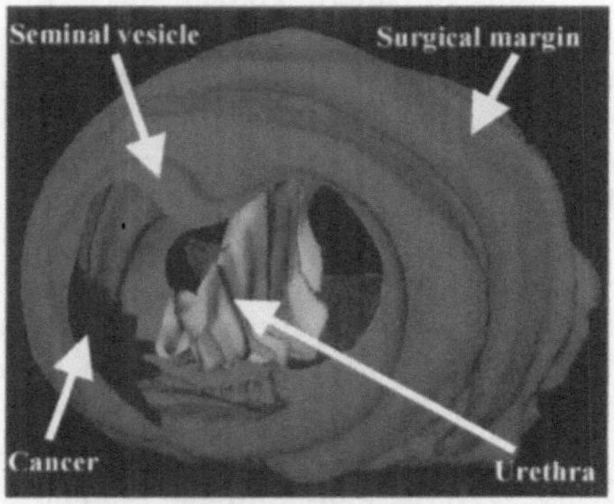

Figure 1. A 3D prostate model reconstructed from prostatectomy specimen

2.2 Prostate needle biopsy simulation and clinical correlation

A 3-D computer simulation system was developed on an SGI Octane workstation using C++ and an object-oriented graphics library OpenInventor [9]. A user can navigate through the reconstructed 3-D prostate model for anatomical inspection. The model can also be geometrically manipulated in 3-D space such as rotation, translation and zooming. The system provides both an automatic and an interactive needle biopsy simulation functions. It was actually used by a number of physicians for prostate needle core biopsy simulation and the user interface proved to be friendly and efficient [11].

We have also preliminarily investigated correlation between our simulation biopsy results and the results of corresponding clinical biopsy, and we have found out that this correlation is statistically significant with paired t-test on 82 patient samples. We randomly selected these 82 patients for whom we gathered clinical biopsy results (such as number of positive sextant biopsies) and compared them with the corresponding simulated sextant biopsy results for the same patients. Among the 82 patients, biopsies of 69 patients (84.1%) were within ±2 positive biopsies of each other. A paired t-test of the null hypothesis of no difference in the number of positive clinical biopsies minus the number of positive simulated biopsies could not be rejected ($p = 0.12$). This result showed a good correlation between the simulated biopsy and the corresponding clinical biopsy.

3. Results

3.1 Multivariable regression model using simulation of the 10-pattern biopsy protocol

We have investigated a regression model using 5 of the 6 available predictor variables to determine which of them correlate significantly with prostate cancer volume. The five variables were number of positive biopsies, prostate volume, age, PSA, and race. Cancer core volume was excluded here since it is highly correlated with number of positive cores.

©CARS/Springer. All rights reserved.

Multivariable regression with backward elimination of insignificant variables showed that the number of positive cores, prostate volume, and PSA value, as well as two of the 2-way interactions, are the only variables that were found significantly correlated with prostate cancer volume. A final regression model involving these variables and interactions for prostate volume estimation for the 10-pattern protocol was as follows:

*Log(cancer volume) = -3.533 - 0.287 * (number positive biopsies) + 1.032 * Log(prostate volume) + 1.748 * Log(PSA) + 0.147 * (number of positive biopsies) * Log(prostate volume) – 0.506 * Log(prostate volume) * Log(PSA)*
This model explained 40% of the variance of the log cancer volume.

Examples of the relationship between the values of the three variables of PSA, number of positive cores and prostate volume with the calculated prostate cancer volume are plotted in Figures 2 through 4 based on the regression model. In Figure 2, it is clear that the prostate cancer volume predicted is getting larger as the number of positive hits increase, and this trend is getting stronger as the PSA value increases. This trend is in line with our expectations. In Figure 3, we observed a proportional relationship between the PSA and the cancer volume predicted: the larger the PSA the larger the cancer volume predicted, which was also noticed by other researchers [3]. What was new in this study is that the proportional increase of PSA and cancer volume was also affected by the size of prostate: the increase of prostate cancer volume with the increase of PSA is degrading as the prostate volume increases. The turning point for prostate volume seems to be around 30cc when the influence of PSA with prostate cancer volume almost vanishes. In other words, for prostates larger than 30cc, the use of PSA in estimating prostate cancer volume becomes less important. In Figure 4, we can see that prostate cancer volume predicted increases with the increase of number of positive cores, and this trend becomes stronger with the increase of prostate volume.

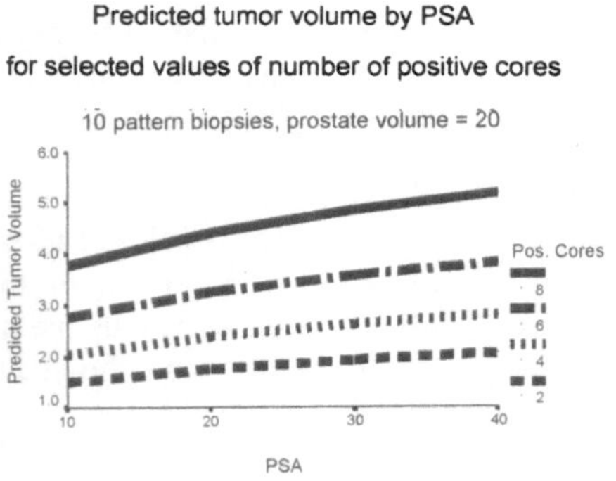

Figure 2. Relationship between prostate cancer volume and PSA values for selected number of positive cores (prostate volume = 20 cc)

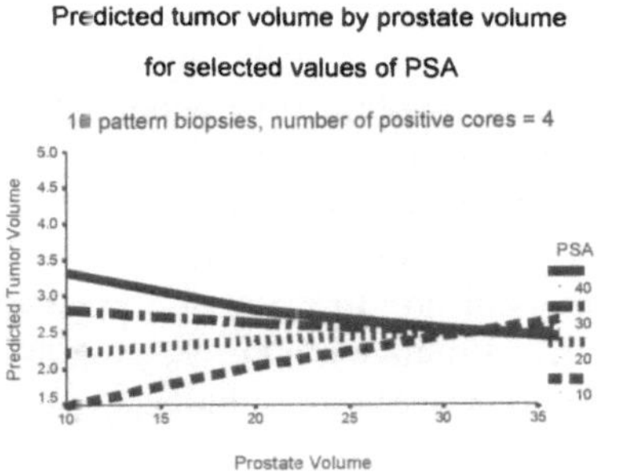

Figure 3. Relationship between prostate cancer volume and prostate volume for selected values of PSA (number of positive cores = 4)

3.2 Multivariable regression model using simulation of the sextant biopsy protocol

The analysis of sextant protocol data followed closely what was done earlier for 10-pattern data. The regression model began with five variables (number of positive biopsies, prostate volume, age, PSA, and race) plus their 2-way and 3-way interactions

©CARS/Springer. All rights reserved.

being used to predict log tumor volume. After backward elimination of insignificant variables showed that the number of positive cores, prostate volume, and PSA value, as well as two of the 2-way interactions, are the only variables that were found significantly

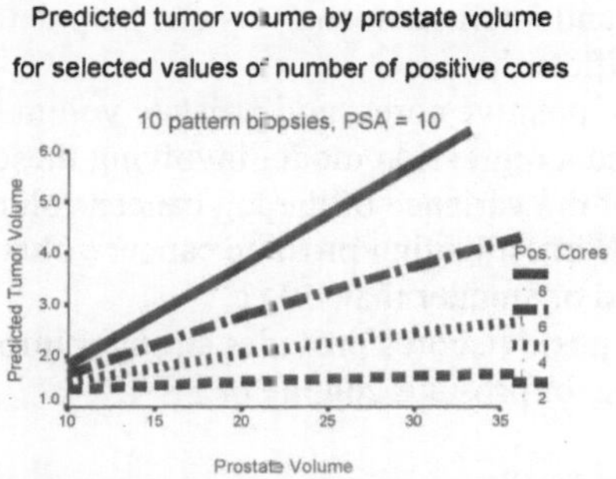

Figure 4. Relationship between prostate cancer volume and prostate volume for selected values of number of positive cores (PSA = 10)

correlated with prostate cancer volume. A final regression model involving these variables and interactions for prostate volume estimation for the 10-pattern protocol was as follows:

*Log(cancer volume) = - 3.867 - 0.518 * (number positive biopsies) + 1.212 * Log(prostate volume) + 1.885 * Log(PSA) + 0.244 * (number of positive biopsies) * Log(prostate volume) – 0.554* Log(prostate volume) * Log(PSA)*

This model is very similar to the one found previously for the 10-pattern data.

4. Discussion

This study is different from most of the existing research on the same issue of preoperative prostate cancer estimation in the following aspects. First, we explored not only the main effect of individual predictor variables as most current research did, but also their interactions in order to find out those group of variables that are significantly correlated with cancer volume. We can thus understand what variables to focus on to best estimate preoperative cancer volume, instead of choosing variables based on assumptions or observations without solid evidance. Secondly, by using clinically correlated simulation, we were able to develop our regression models with biopsy results from multiple biopsy protocols. Initial preliminary results presented in this paper have demonstrated these advantges: similar or better performance with less predictor variables.

5. Conlusions

Being able to accurately and easily estimate prostate cancer volume prior to any treatment has a significant clinical and economical impact on how prostate cancer should be treated for individual patients. It can help avoid unnecessary expensive treatment while maintaining quality of life for the patients, without compromising their potential cures. We have developed a set of statistical regression models to help the physicians estimate

©CARS/Springer. All rights reserved.

preoperative prostate cancer volume based on information from the needle core biopsy. We have come to the following conclusions.

1. Not all variables contribute uniformly to the estimation of preoperative prostate cancer volume and interaction analysis can help determine which variables contribute significantly.
2. PSA, number of positive cores, and prostate volume are found to be significant contributors, and a regression model involving these 3 variables can explain as much as 40% of the variance of the log cancer volume.
3. The role of PSA in estimating prostate cancer volume is more important for prostates around or smaller than 30 cc.
4. The number of positive cores provides stronger information on cancer volume with the increase of prostate volume or PSA.

Acknowledgements

This research is primarily supported by a Biomedical Engineering Research Grant RG-99-0115 of The Whitaker Foundation.

References

1. D'Amico AV, Chang H, Holupka E et al. Calculated prostate cancer volume: The optimal predictor of actual cancer volume and pathologic stage. Urology 49(3): 385-391, 1997.
2. Chan LW, Stamey TA. Calculating prostate cancer volume preoperatively: the D'Amico equation and some other observations. The Journal of Urology, 159(6), 1998.
3. Kabalin JN, McNeal JE, Johnstone IM, Stamey TA. Serum Prostate-Specific Antigen and the biologic progression of prostate cancer. Urology 46(1), 1995.
4. Terris M, Haney DJ, Johnstone IM, McNeal JE, Stamey TA. Prediction of prostate cancer volume using prostate-specific antigen levels, tranrectal ultrasound, and systematic sextant biopsies. Urology 45(1), 1995.
5. Peller PA, Young DC, Marmaduke DP, March WL, Badalament RA. Sextant prostate biopsies: A histopathologic correlation with radical prostatectomy specimens. Cancer 75(2), 1995.
6. Egevad L, Norberg M, Mattson S, Norlen BJ, Busch C. Estimation of prostate cancer volume by multiple core biopsies before radical prostatectomy. Urology 52(4), 1998.
7. Dietrick DD, McNeal JE, Stamey TA. Core cancer length in ultrasound-guided systematic biopsies: A preoperative evaluation of prostate cancer volume. Urology 45(6), 1995.
8. Zeng J, Bauer J, Zhang W et al. Prostate biopsy protocols: 3-D visualization-based evaluation and clinical correlation. Computer Aided Surgery, 6:14-21, 2001.
9. Xuan J, Sesterhenn I, Hayes W et al. Surface reconstruction and visualization of the surgical prostate model. Proc. of SPIE Medical Imaging, Vol 3031, 1997.
10. Zeng J, Kaplan CR, Xuan J et al. Optimizing prostate needle biopsy through 3D simulation. Proc. of SPIE Medical Imaging, Vol. 3335, 1998.
11. Bauer JJ, Zeng J, Weir J et al. 3D Computer simulated prostate models: Lateral prostate biopsies increase the detection rate of prostate cancer. Urology 53(5):961-967, 1999.

CARS 2002 – H.U. Lemke, M.W. Vannier; K. Inamura, A.G. Farman, K. Doi & J.H.C. Reiber (Editors)
©CARS/Springer. All rights reserved.

Resection proposals for oncologic liver surgery based on vascular territories

B. Preim[1], H. Bourquain[1], D. Selle[1], K. J. Oldhafer[2], H.-O.
[1]MeVis – Center for Medical Diagnostic Systems and Visualization, Universitätsallee 29, 28359 Bremen, Germany,
[2]Universitätsklinikum Essen, Klinik für Allgemein- und Transplantationschirurgie, Hufelandstr. 55, 45122 Essen, Germany

Abstract

We describe the generation and visualization of resection proposals for oncologic liver surgery which are based on vascular territories of the portal and hepatic vein. Resection proposals are interactively controlled by one parameter: the desired security margin around a tumor. Resection proposals consider vascular structures inside this margin, dependent vascular structures in the periphery as well as the territories supplied by them. The methods have been applied to artificial data from corrosion casts as well as to 5 datasets obtained in the clinical routine from 3 hospitals.

Keywords: Liver surgery planning, vascular analysis, risk analysis.

1. Introduction

In preoperative planning of liver surgery two major questions have to be answered. Most important is, whether the patient and the liver lesions are suitable for surgery. If this question could be affirmed, the extent of the resection must be determined precisely. If a resection with a sufficient security margin can be performed the probability that all tumor cells were removed increases, leading to a better long-term outcome. On the other hand, for sufficient function of the remnant liver as little as possible liver parenchyma should be resected. Calculation of resection proposals must take both of these contrary objectives into account. The basic idea of generating resection proposals is to consider the patient individual vascular branches in the security margin around a tumor, the dependend branches in the periphery, and the territories supplied by them. Surgery planning is particularly difficult if several liver metastases are present or if a metastasis is located centrally, i.e. near one of the major vessels of the liver. Important factors for the assessment of the resectability are the blood supply of the surrounding tissue and the localization of large intra-hepatic vessels. The term "anatomical resection" comprises all resections that represent vascular territories. These are, for example, segment resections or sector resections, the latter affecting only the vascular territories of smaller branches [1]. In contrast to this, resections that are only based on the extent of the tumor are called "atypical resections". The outcome of these atypical resections seems to be inferior to that of anatomical resections [1].

Intention of this study was to investigate the calculation of resection proposals taking into account both the portal venous and the hepatic venous system. The combination of two or

©CARS/Springer. All rights reserved.

more vascular systems in risk analysis is unique. Especially the importance of the venous drainage was underestimated in the past. A venous congestion can result in restricted outflow, stasis of the blood in the arterial or portal venous system, and consequently thrombosis. Prospects and limits for calculation of anatomical liver resection proposals will be discussed.

2. Related work

Only a few groups world-wide deal with computer support for preoperative planning in oncologic liver surgery. A french group focused their work on automatic segmentation of the relevant structures based on à priori knowledge of typical anatomical variants [2]. Previous work concerning resection proposals focused on the computational methodology for different security margins around the tumor . After graph analysis of the segmented portal vein the branches affected by a resection with a certain security margin were determined and the vascular territories of these branches were approximated. The result of this approximation was displayed as a resection proposal. A shortcoming of the method is that it is based only on one vascular structure, namely the portal vein. This setting does not adequately represent reality where the hepatic artery and portal vein supply blood to the liver and the hepatic veins drain it. Resection proposals should reflect this situation by combining the results for the different vascular structures. Also, in previous work only one clinical example for the successful application was given and the appropriate visualization was not discussed.

3. Image analysis for the determination of resection proposals

The study is based on segmentation methods suitable for parenchymatous organs and tumors [5] and methods for the analysis of intrahepatic vessels [6]. Vascular analysis includes segmentation, skeletonization and separation of different vascular trees and the approximation of vascular territories. For efficient determination of the vascular branches within a certain security margin around the tumor the border voxels are detected by calculating the difference of the tumor and an eroded mask, using a 3×3×3 structuring element for erosion. Distance transformation was applied to all border voxels, thus generating the security margin. The calculation of resection proposals was first applied to two vascular models which result from an analysis of digitized corrosion casts of human livers. One model only contained the portal vein whereas the second model also contained hepatic veins. An artificial sphere (diameter 10 mm) as model for a tumor was placed into these models. The tumor position was translated in 5 mm steps in the x-, y-, and z-direction through the whole vascular model and for each position the affected vascular territories for five security margins were calculated and visualized with different colors. Thus giving about 1500 results for each cast which were summarized in movies for discussion with surgeons. Based on these initial results, selected patient data have been considered. Only cases where it was difficult to define a resection strategy were included. These were patients with tumors close to major vessels or where the decision was difficult due to a central location of the tumor or multiple metastases. Five datasets were chosen, three from a clinical site in Essen (E_1 … E_3), and one from Krefeld (K) and Marburg (M). Each dataset was a contrast enhanced CT scan. The data from E were multislice CT (slice thickness 2.5 and 3 mm), whereas K and M were spiral CT data with 4 mm slice

©CARS/Springer. All rights reserved.

thickness. In E_1 with a central metastasis the goal was to maximize the security margin while keeping the risk of surgery low. Datasets E_2, M and K had multiple metastases (3 or 4, respectively). Resection proposals were generated to support the decision if the metastases should be resected separately or en-bloc. For each security margin the resection proposal is visualized and quantitatively analyzed with respect to the liver volume which has to be resected and the remaining volume. The resection proposals were calculated both for the portal vein and for the hepatic veins. The methods used for the calculation of the security margins were identical. The risk analysis results for different vascular systems are combined. Thus, giving the maximum risk, that either the blood supply or drainage would not be sufficient if the tumor would be resected with this security margin. Fig. 1 illustrates the risk analysis for patient K. The generation of resection proposals is part of our software assistant HEPAVISION which integrates all steps to analyze CT data for preoperative planning in liver surgery [7].

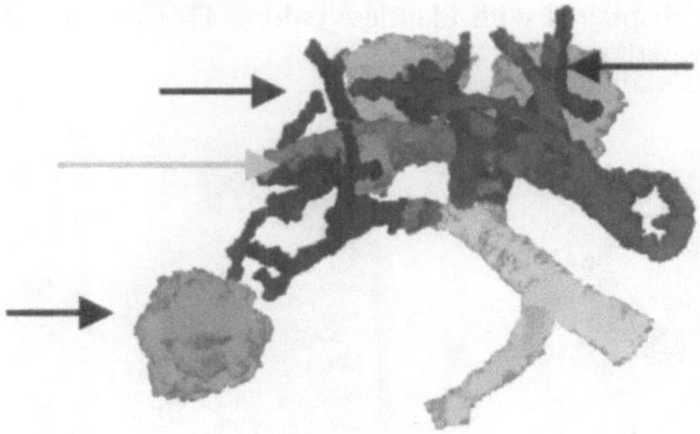

Fig 1: Portal vein and hepatic vein of a patient with four liver metastases (see the arrows). Resection proposals have been calculated for the 5 mm, 10 mm as well as the 15 mm margin. The brightest structure is the portal vein outside the security margin. The darkest structures are branches of either the portal vein or the hepatic vein inside the 5 mm security margin. The portal venous tree is pruned to reveal the major branches affected by a resection with different margins.

4. Visualization and exploration of resection proposals

The visualization of resection proposals can be modified by multiple parameters. Different numbers and sizes of security margins lead to different resection proposals. We provide several ways to modify the visualization of the affected or not affected vascular branches as well as the vascular territories supplied by these branches. Our experience is that it is helpful to use three standard security margins with a distance of 5, 10 and 15 mm around the tumor. As default, we employ the red color for the 5 mm margin which must be definitely resected and orange and yellow for larger margins. Although security margins of more than 10 mm do not improve the outcome it is reasonable to consider these margins. Reasons are that resections can often not be performed exactly as proposed and that the tumor size determined by CT is not perfectly reliable. Often tumors intraoperatively turn out to be larger than expected estimated from the image data. For all security margins the affected vascular branches were color coded and the respective territories were superimposed semi-transparently with the same color. For the liver casts vascular territories were not displayed, as they were identifiable by the corresponding

©CARS/Springer. All rights reserved.

vascular trees. We provide several presentation modes to avoid that too much visual information confuses the viewer. Center lines (the skeleton) of the vascular tree can be displayed instead of a surface rendering of the complete lumen of vasculature. Furthermore, we offer facilities to smooth the segmentation result and to prune the visualization of vascular trees to make the interpretation easier. Another useful option is to use transparency to dilute branches of vasculature which are not in the focus of risk analysis. Vascular territories of the portal vein and drainage territories of the hepatic veins can be visualized separately. For risk analysis the vascular tree affected by a smaller security margin is enhanced by determining the branch with the shortest distance to the tumor. Only branches with a certain diameter are considered. In order to check the validity of the resection proposals and to assess their feasibility it is essential that the results can also be displayed in a 2d slice view. For this purpose, the approximation of vascular territories is transparently overlaid the original radiological data. Corresponding structures in the 2d and 3d view are displayed with identical colors. This is illustrated in Fig. 2 for patient E_2 and in Fig. 3 for patient E_3.

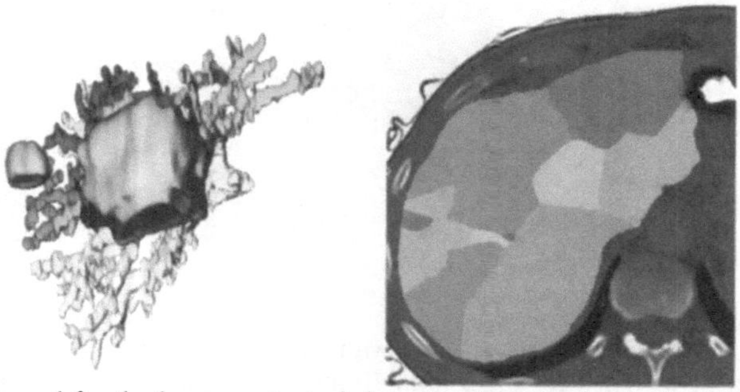

Fig. 2: Resection proposal for the larger metastasis based on the portal vein. Left image: the vascular structures involved for the three standard margins (5, 10, and 15 mm). On the right, the corresponding vascular territories are also displayed.

4.1 Exploration of resection proposals

A typical sequence of interactions is as follows. The user starts the analysis with the metastasis which is probably the most difficult to resect and performs the analysis of security margins for the portal vein. Following this step, the analysis is separately carried out for the hepatic vein and subsequently both results are integrated in one visualization with the vascular trees pruned appropriately. The visualization of the vascular territory should be restricted to one such territory. However, the volumetric analysis is carried out simultaneously for all security margins which have been considered. If other metastases have to be treated, the analysis is carried out for these lesions afterwards and finally an overall visualization and volumetric analysis is carried out.

©CARS/Springer. All rights reserved.

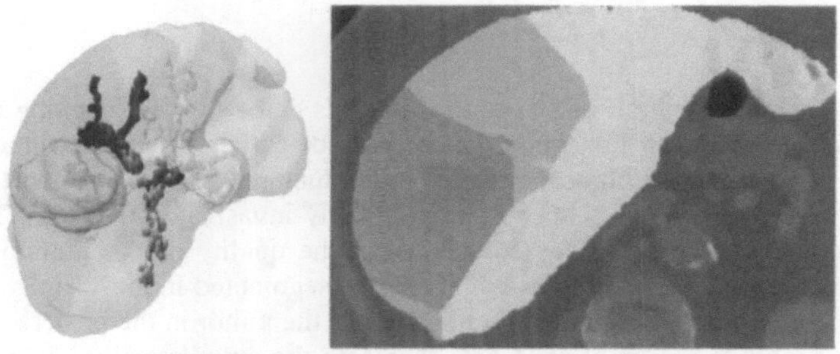

Fig. 3: Risk analysis for the large lesion (see the arrow). It is visualized which branches of the portal vein are inside the standard security margins (5, 10, 15 mm). Dark branches are located in the 5 mm zone, wheras lighter branches are more distant from the lesion. The right image shows the 2d slice view with risk areas transparently overlaid.

5. Results

Resection proposals were first calculated for two vascular models of digitized human liver casts. The resection proposals of selected results for each cast were presented to a surgeon. The shape of the calculated pattern corresponded well to the shape of resection usually applied in clinical practice. Although in clinical data images of less quality is available the approach turned out to be useful for surgeons also in the clinical cases. 4 of 5 cases were regarded suitable for surgery. Patient E_1 could not be resected (even with a small margin of 5 mm the whole portal tree would be affected). Patient E_2 (recall Fig. 2) was regarded not resectable, partly because the remnant parenchyma is rather low, and partly due to an accompanying liver cirrhosis. Patient E_3 (recall Fig. 3) was considered resectable, however, it was decided to treat the patient first with a chemotherapy in order to debulk the lesion. For patient M a hemihepatectomy was carried out. The resection proposal with 15 mm security margin revealed that the remnant parenchyma cannot be increased by resecting the 3 metastasis separately. Volumetric analysis of the resection proposal yielded a volume of 51% of the whole liver parenchyma. Patient K with its 4 metastases had one metastasis too close to the main branch of the portal vein. The other 3 metastases were removed. The remaining metastases was treated by a minimally-invasive therapy which does less damage to surrounding vessels. Results of the quantitative analysis are summarized in Table 1.

Patient	Liver volume	Number and vol. of lesions	Resection proposal 5 mm margin	Resection proposal 10 mm margin	Resection proposal 15 mm margin
E1	1 196 ml	1; 13 ml (1.1%)	1 196 ml (100%)	1 196 ml (100%)	1 196 ml (100%)
E2	1 470 ml	2; 99 ml (6.8%)	201 ml (13.7%)	465 ml (31.6%)	670 ml (45.6%)
E3	2 035 ml	1; 69 ml (3.4%)	327 ml (15.7%)	526 ml (25.8 %)	635 ml (31.2%)
M	1 606 ml	3; 29 ml (1.8%)	101 ml (6.3%)	205 ml (12.8%)	795 ml (49.4%)

Table 1: Quantitative results of risk analysis. All numbers in paranthesis refer to percentage of whole liver volume.

©CARS/Springer. All rights reserved.

6. Conclusion

Generation and visualization of resection proposals can facilitate planning of anatomical resections in patients with liver tumors. The case of patient K revealed that it should be possible to generate resection proposals for individual metastases to support decisions for combined therapies (surgical removal and minimally-invasive destruction). The reliability of the generated resection proposal depends on the quality of the radiological data, in particular on the vascular structures which can be segmented in the vicinity of the lesion. In about 5% of clinical liver tumors the location of the tumor in the posterocentral portion of the liver prohibits a normal approach, therefore the automatically generated resection proposal would surgically be impossible. As the presented resection proposals are not perfectly reliable and sometimes difficult to realize surgically the option to interactively modify these proposals is mandatory. The methods have been applied successfully to clinical data with varying image quality. This clearly indicates that the method is in most cases feasible for preoperative planning. However, the decision whether a patient can tolerate a resection is not fully supported. In particular, primary liver cancer is often inoperable due to the extent of liver cirrhosis which caused the cancer disease. There are several areas open for future work. A larger validation with clinical data could verify the benefit for the clinical routine for centrally located tumors and multiple metastases. The approach can be modified in such a way that also minimally-invasive therapies, such as radiofrequency ablation, are considered. Also for these interventions it is crucial to respect the vascular architecture.

Acknowledgements

We want to thank our colleague Milo Hindennach for generating the visualizations for Fig. 2 and 3. We also thank our clinical partners, Prof. Debatin, University Hospital Essen, PD Dr. Fiedler from Hospital Krefeld as well as Prof. Klose, Philipps University Marburg for providing us with high quality radiological data. We want to acknowledge the support by the Deutsche Forschungsgemeinschaft (Pe 199/9-1).

References

1. Scheele J (2001). "Anatomiegerechte und atypische Leberresektionen" [Anatomical and atypical liver resections], *Chirurg*, Vol. 72: 113-124
2. Soler L, Delingette H, Malandain G et al. "Fully automatic anatomical, pathological and functional segmentation from CT scans for hepatic surgery", *Computer-Aided Surgery*, Vol. 6 (3)
3. Lamade W, Glombitza G, Demiris AM, Cardenas CE, Meinzer HP, Richter G, Lehnert T, Herfarth C (1999). „Virtual surgical planning in liver surgery", *Chirurg*, Vol. 70: 239-245
4. Preim B, Selle D, Spindler W, Oldhafer KJ, Peitgen HO (2000). "Interaction Techniques and Vessel Analysis for Liver Surgery Planning", *Proc. of MICCAI*, Springer, LNCS, Vol. 1935:608-617
5. Schenk A, Prause G, Peitgen HO (2000). "Efficient Semiautomatic Segmentation of 3D Objects", *Proc. of MICCAI*, Springer, LNCS 1935: 186-195
6. Selle D, Peitgen HO (2001). "Analysis of the Morphology and Structure of Vessel Systems using skeletonization", *Proc. of SPIE Medical Imaging*, Vol. 4321: 261-271
7. Bourquain H, Schenk A, Link F, Preim B, Prause G, Peitgen HO. (2002). "HepaVision2 – a software assistant for preoperative planning in LRLT and oncologic liver surgery", *CARS'2002* (in this volume).

16th International Congress and Exhibition on Computer Assisted Radiology

Chairman: **Guy Frija, MD (F)**

Medical Imaging

CARS 2002 – H.U. Lemke, M.W. Vannier; K. Inamura, A.G. Farman, K. Doi & J.H.C. Reiber (Editors)
©CARS/Springer. All rights reserved.

Perfusion weighted MRI: A new tool for epilepsy surgery

J.M. Scarabin [a, b], B. Broche [b], C. Grova [b], C. Argaud [c], M. Schaeffer [d], P. Jannin [b]
[a] Neurosurgery Department, Hopital Universitaire de Rennes
[b] Laboratoire IDM, Faculté de Médecine, Université de Rennes
[c] General Electrics Medical Systems Europe, Buc
[d] Guerbet, Roissy CDG France

Abstract

This paper presents a serie of twenty patients explored with perfusion weighted MRI (pMRI) during interictal state. We applied MR regional cerebral blood volume (rCBV) maps computed from pMRI for studying regional hemodynamic changes compared to interictal stereo-EEG (SEEG) recordings in patients suffering from drug resistant epilepsy. Four original and significant patterns were identified with hypo and hyperperfusion. Perfusion weighted MRI appears a very promising tool for epilepsy surgery.

Keywords: Perfusion weighted MRI, epilepsy

1. Introduction

The initial management of surgical epilepsies routinely requires the use of morphological and functional imagery (e.g. Magnetic Resonance Imaging: MRI, Single Photo Emission Computed Tomography: SPECT, Positron Emission Tomography: PET). This management aims either at performing a tailored cortectomy or at pursuing more invasive presurgical investigations (as depth electrodes or grids) to better delineate the epileptogenic area. Penfield's observations in the thirties provided the first systematic evidence of changes in regional cerebral blood flow (rCBF) associated with focal seizures. The interictal, ictal and post-ictal changes in focal epilepsy have begun to be elucidated in the two last decades with the advent of in vivo imaging techniques such as PET or SPECT. Four types of focal cerebral dysfunction have been reported: during the interictal period, hypoperfusion with SPECT and hypometabolism with PET and during the ictal period, hyperperfusion with SPECT and hypermetabolism with PET. Lot of studies have been performed with functional MRI to localize brain function and/or to evaluate cerebral diseases. Recently functional MRI has been applied to epileptic patients. Two papers reported series of epileptic patients explored with perfusion MRI with endogenous [1] or exogenous [2] contrast showing the same result: an interictal hypoperfusion in temporal lobe epilepsy.

In this paper we present a serie of twenty patients explored with perfusion weighted MRI during interictal state. This technique uses the phenomenon of magnetic susceptibility created by the first passage of concentrated paramagnetic exogenous contrast agents, as for example gadolinium chelates. Thus an evaluation of microcirculation and regional cerebral blood volume (rCBV) is computed. In the present study we applied MR rCBV

©CARS/Springer. All rights reserved.

maps for studying regional hemodynamic changes compared to interictal stereo-EEG (SEEG) recordings in patients suffering from drug resistant epilepsy (14 patients).

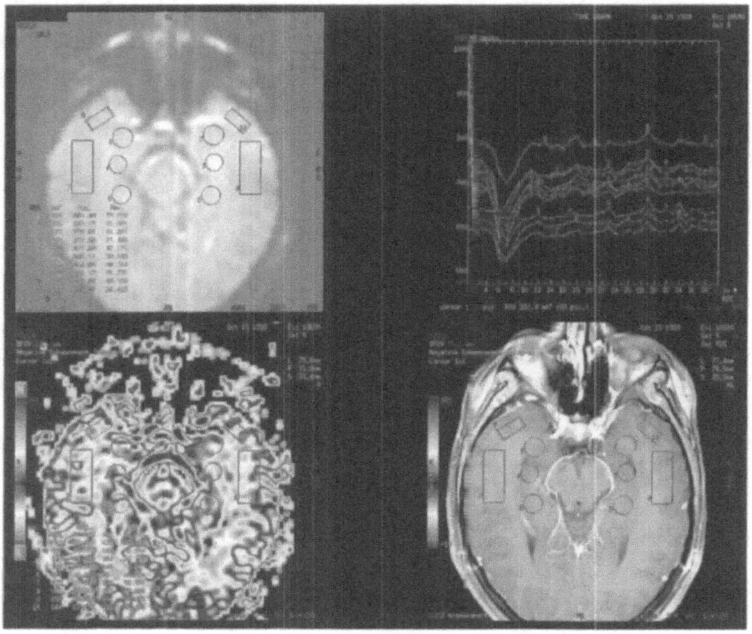

Figure 1: Patient EVA: From left to right and top to bottom: Original pMR EPI image - MR signal curves - rCBV map and ROIs - ROIs mapped on T1 MR images

2. Materials and Methods

We studied 20 patients. All patients had complex partial seizures refractory to maximally tolerated antiepileptic drugs therapy. Eleven patients had unilateral temporal lobe epilepsy and 9 patients had extratemporal epilepsy. The presurgical evaluation included clinical data (video-EEG), neuropsychological evaluation, MRI, interictal and ictal SPECT, and SEEG (for 14 patients). All patients benefited from tailored resections since less than two years. Therefore surgical outcomes were not significant. Informed consent was obtained for all patients.

All MRI studies were performed on a 1.5 T whole-body MR device (Signa Echospeed, GE Medical System, USA). For each patient we acquired conventional T1 weighted spin-echo images for anatomical reference, FLAIR images and perfusion-weighted images. Perfusion weighted MR imaging parameters consisted of 40 acquisitions of 12 slices (FOV: 28*21 cm, matrix: 96*64, thickness: 6 mm). Gradient echo EPI was used (TE: 60 ms, TR: 1800 ms, angle: 60°) to study the extra-temporal regions and spin-echo EPI (TE: 80 ms, TR: 1800 ms, angle: 60°) was performed for temporal regions in order to avoid susceptibility artefacts. After 5 baseline scans a bolus of DOTAREM (gadoterate

©CARS/Springer. All rights reserved.

meglumine) was rapidly injected with a flow rate of 5 ml/sec, followed by a 15 ml saline flush.

Regional cerebral blood volume images were computed using Functool software (GEMSE, Buc-France) according to the method described in [3] (see also [4,5]) (Figure 1). Symmetrical regions of interest (ROIs) were manually defined according to anatomical criteria (Figures 1,2). A Student t-test was performed on each pair of regions of interest (Figures 3,4). Results were finally confronted to anatomical MRI, FLAIR, SPECT and SEEG (for 14 from 20 patients) (Figure 5). SEEG was considered as our Gold Standard as it consists of in situ measurements.

3. Results

Four original patterns were identified with hypo and hyperperfusion.

The first pattern consisted of a hypoperfusion on mesial temporal structures and a hyperperfusion on the lateral cortex observed in a serie of 6 patients (Figure 2). The best significant differences ($p < 0.001$) corresponded to the amygdala and lateral cortex as expected (Figures 3,4). SEEG located the epileptogenic area in mesial temporal structures (Figure 5).

The second pattern is the opposite of the first one. We observed mesial temporal hyperperfusion and lateral temporal hypoperfusion. All 5 patients of this pattern presented characteristic hyper intensities on FLAIR images in the hippocampus and specific SEEG activities. SEEG located the epileptogenic area in mesial and neocortical temporal structures.

The third pattern was observed in a serie of seven extratemporal, more or less complex, focal cortical dysplasia. This pattern consists of a hyperperfusion in the dysplasia, surrounded by a hypoperfusion. All patients presented MR images very suggestive of dysplasia (e.g. hyper intensity in FLAIR images) and a very specific SEEG pattern (i.e. continuous spiking in dysplasia). SEEG located the epileptogenic area in dysplasia only.

The last and fourth pattern was observed in two extratemporal low-grade glioma. This pattern consists of a hypoperfusion in the glioma surrounded by a hyperperfusion and seems very reliable to differentiate the low-grade glioma from the cortical dysplasia. In both cases SEEG shown continuous slow waves and spikes limited to the lesion.

4. Discussion

Although PET, SPECT and XENON-CT may offer similar estimates of time perfusion, perfusion-weighted MRI provides better spatial resolution. It is cost and time efficient when performed as part of a complete MRI examination.

Moreover new original patterns have been introduced in this study that emphasize very exciting theoretical and practical questions. We strongly suspect that hypo and

©CARS/Springer. All rights reserved.

hyperperfusion may coexist during the interictal phases; even if the reference techniques (i.e. interictal SPECT and PET) draw the hypoperfusion and hypometabolism as a rule. However, a meta analysis of SPECT brain imaging in epilepsy [6] performed on forty-six studies found this hypoperfusion in only forty-four percents of temporal epilepsies. A serie of experimental and clinical data clearly exhibits the interictal phase to be so unstable, so heterogeneous in activity and localization that it could have defined as a sub or meta ictal phase [7,8,9]. Thus drug resistant partial epilepsies appear as a ramified system, a complex network consisting of lesional, irritative and epileptogenic areas. We assume that they are made of several interconnected structures, the organization of which depends on the one hand of emerging and spreading events and on the other hand of systems that tend to limit it. Perfusion weighted MRI appears a very promising tool for epilepsy surgery and more than ninety patients have been presently explored.

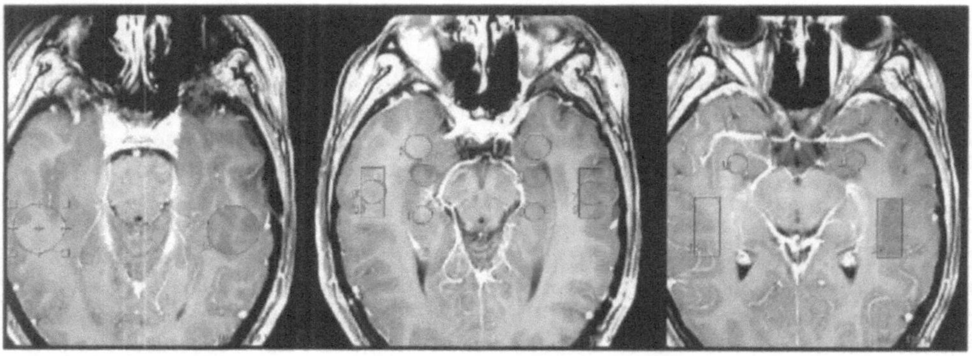

Figure 2: Patient EVA: selected ROIs mapped on T1 MR images – First pattern

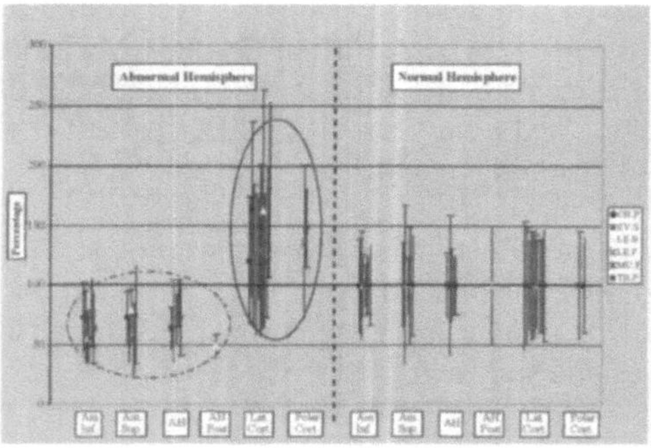

Figure 3: Mean and standard deviation values of relative differences of rCBV measured on symmetrical ROIs and sorted by the selected anatomical areas for the first pattern

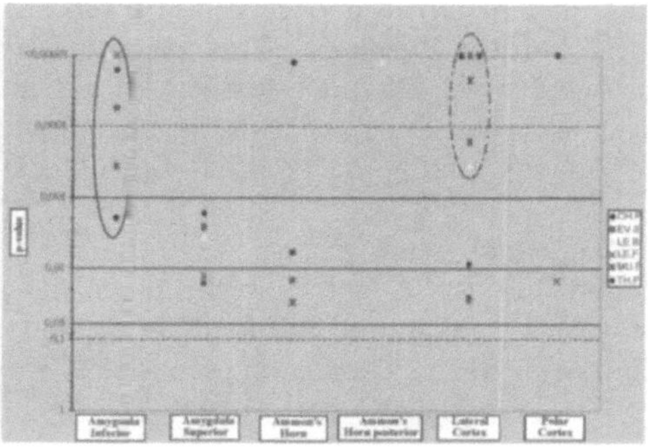

Figure 4: Student t-test p-values computed on each pair of regions of interest for the first pattern

CARS 2002 – H.U. Lemke, M.W. Vannier; K. Inamura, A.G. Farman, K. Doi & J.H.C. Reiber (Editors)
©CARS/Springer. All rights reserved.

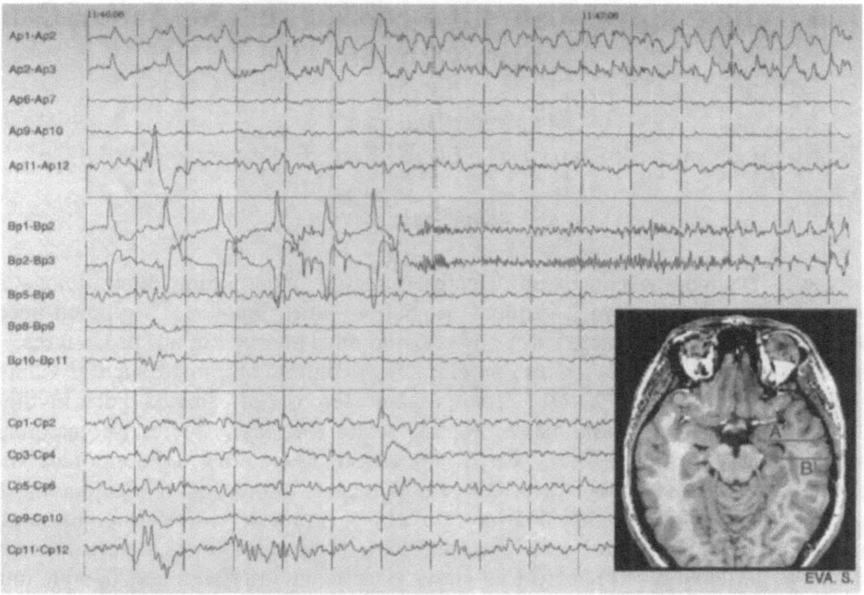

Figure 5: Patient EVA: Characteristic SEEG pattern observed in the first serie corresponding to the first pattern: continuous spiking and frequent infraclinical fast discharges in the amygdala and hippocampus

References

1. Wolf RL, Alsop DC, French JA et al. "Detection of mesial temporal lobe hypoperfusion in patients with temporal lobe epilepsy using multislice arterial spin labeled perfusion MRI", *Epilepsia*, 40:249, 1999 and *AJNR Am J Neuroradiol.*, 22(7), 1334-41, 2001
2. Wu RH, Bruening R, Noachtar S et al. "MR measurement of regional relative cerebral blood volume in epilepsy", *J Magn Reson Imaging*, 9 :435-440, 1999
3. Boxerman J, Rosen B, Weisskoff R. "Signal-to-noise analysis of cerebral blood volume maps from dynamic NMR imaging studies" *J Magn Reson Imaging*, 7:528-537, 1997
4. Ostergaard L, Sorensen AG, Kwong KK, Weisskoff RM, Gyldensted C, Rosen BR. "High resolution measurement of cerebral blood flow using intravascular tracer bolus passages. Part II: Experimental comparison and preliminary results" *Magn Reson Med.*, 36(5), 726-36, 1996
5. Edelman RR, Mattle HP, Atkinson DJ, Hill T, Finn JP, Mayman C, Ronthal M, Hoogewoud HM, Kleefield J. "Cerebral blood flow: assessment with dynamic contrast-enhanced T2*-weighted MR imaging at 1.5 T" *Radiology*, 176(1), 211-20, 1990
6. Devous MD Sr, Thisted RA, Morgan GF, Leroy RF, Rowe CC. "SPECT brain imaging in epilepsy: a meta-analysis" *J Nucl Med.*, 39(2),285-93, 1998
7. Hougaard K, Oikawa T, Sveinsdottir E, Skinoj E, Ingvar DH, Lassen NA. "Regional cerebral blood flow in focal cortical epilepsy" *Arch Neurol.*, 33(8), 527-35, 1976
8. Warach S, Levin JM, Schomer DL, Holman BL, Edelman RR. "Hyperperfusion of ictal seizure focus demonstrated by MR perfusion imaging", *AJNR Am J Neuroradiol.*, 15(5), 965-8, 1994
9. Witte OW, Bruehl C, Schlaug G, Tuxhorn I, Lahl R, Villagran R, Seitz RJ. „Dynamic changes of focal hypometabolism in relation to epileptic activity" *J Neurol Sci.*, 124(2),188-97, 1994

©CARS/Springer. All rights reserved.

Stereo radiography: distortion correction and perception improvement

Alexander Berestov[a]
[a] Canon Development Americas, 3300 N. First St., San Jose, CA, U.S.A.

Abstract

Stereoscopic x-ray imaging can be an effective method for obtaining three-dimensional spatial information from two-dimensional projection x-ray images. This much-needed information is missed in many x-ray diagnostic and interventional procedures, for example in orthopaedic or chest x-ray imaging. New digital equipment such as Canon's Digital Radiography System CXDI-22 can obtain stereoscopic image pairs in digital format, which is ready for fast image processing and display. A stereoscopic image-processing algorithm is proposed in order to improve image quality and depth perception of stereoscopic radiographs taken with conventional or C-arm types of equipment. The steps of the algorithm include illumination correction, geometry conversion and parallax adjustment. Software prototype was developed. Chest phantom images were processed and are shown as examples. The results show significant improvement in both image quality and depth perception.

Keywords: Stereo, radiography, distortion.

1. Introduction

One of the problems with stereoscopic imaging is image distortion in stereoscopic display systems. Various image distortions include depth plane curvature, depth non-linearity, depth and size magnification, shearing distortions and keystone distortions. These problems were addressed in papers [1] and [2]. Another source of distraction in stereo image processing is illumination. When images of the same scene are taken by two different cameras or by one camera shifted horizontally illumination of the scene changes depending on the conditions. This illumination change lead to problems with mathematical analysis, and to difficulties in observing images in stereo. Illumination problem for reflected photography was addressed in [3]. Big problem with stereo imaging is also depth perception. Some people have troubles with observing images in 3D and become tired very fast. It was suggested in [1] that one of the solutions is to minimize the depth range and position the primary area of interest near or behind the surface of the monitor.

Here we propose a three-step stereoscopic image-processing algorithm built to improve image quality and depth perception of stereoscopic radiographs. The first step is illumination correction. We propose adjustment of vertical columns in the images by equalizing the mean and standard deviation of greyscale pixel values. Prior algorithms adjusted histograms for the whole images and neglect illumination changes from left to right due to the rotation. The second step is the conversion of a toed-in stereoscopic

©CARS/Springer. All rights reserved.

geometry into a parallel one. A toed-in configuration has a big disadvantage. The problem lies in the inherent depth plane curvature. This curvature leads to incorrect depth perception and wrong calculations of relative object distances. In order to eliminate this distortion we propose to recalculate projections of the images at the new virtual locations. This transformation should place the images in the plane, which has to be parallel to the base line between two x-ray tube locations used to capture the images. During this procedure the keystone distortion could be eliminated as well. The final step is to adjust the horizontal parallax so that as many people as possible can view the stereoscopic image.

2. Methodology

It would be beneficial if some of the stereo methods used to analyse reflective photography could be applied to the analysis of projected x-ray images. Some of these methods were presented in [4]. Unfortunately, application of binocular stereo methods to x-ray imaging is not easy because there are no visible surfaces on the radiograph, and information about different objects can be located at the same area of the x-ray image. Therefore some new approaches should be developed.

2.1 Illumination adjustment

Very often the difference in contrast and brightness between left and right images of the stereo pair depends on the position of the x-ray source, which illuminates the sensor plate at different angles. In [3] authors proposed the algorithm, which equalized mean and standard deviation of grayscale values in left and right images. The problem with this approach was that equalization was made for the whole image, so the differences in illumination within the images remained unchanged.

In the present paper we suggest to utilize *a priori* known information about the illumination changes within the image and propose the algorithm for brightness and contrast equalization, which eliminates horizontal distinctions between the images. Adjustments proposed in [3] do not change the horizontal variations in contrast and brightness. In order to correct them we take into account the longitudinal trajectory of the x-ray tube.

Let X_1 and X_2 be discrete random variables with values $\{x_i^1\}$ and $\{x_i^2\}$. Then the expected or mean values of $X_{1,2}$ are defined by

$$EX_{1,2} = \mu_{1,2} = \sum_i x_i^{1,2} p(x_i^{1,2}) \; , \qquad (1)$$

where p is the probability function. The quantities

$$EX_{1,2}^2 - \mu_{1,2}^2 = \sigma_{1,2}^2 \qquad (2)$$

©CARS/Springer. All rights reserved.

are the variances of $X_{1,2}$ or the expected values of the square of the deviations of $X_{1,2}$ from their expected values. We would like to adjust variables $X_{1,2}$ so that the expected values $\mu_{1,2}$ and variances $\sigma^2_{1,2}$ would be the same for both variables. In the simplest case we can use the linear transformation:

$$X_2 = aX_1 + b \ , \tag{3}$$

where *a* and *b* are constant parameters. Substitution of (3) into (1) and (2) gives:

$$b = \mu_2 - a\mu_1 \ ,$$
$$a = \sqrt{\frac{\sigma_2^2}{\sigma_1^2}} \ . \tag{4}$$

We propose to adjust the stochastic parameters of the images along the corresponding longitudes of the C-arm path. If the sensor plate rows are parallel to the plane of rotation, the adjustment has to be done for every column of pixels in the images.

Let us consider the pixel brightness level in the column of pixels in one image as X_1 and in another as X_2. This consideration gives as the mechanism of image adjustment. First we calculate expected values and variances for both columns using probability function. In the simplest case of the uniform distribution *p=1/H*, where *H* is the number of rows in the image, but it could be also any other reasonable distribution (exponential, normal, or derived from the data). The second step is pixel brightness recalculation in one or both images using equation (3). We can adjust one image to another, or adjust both images to some values μ and σ^2 (for example, to average values $\mu = (\mu_1 + \mu_2)/2$, $\sigma^2 = (\sigma_1^2 + \sigma_2^2)/2$, or to some other desirable values). Here we adjusted columns with the same number in both images, but it is possible to estimate the average disparity and equalize expected value and variance in the shifted columns.

2.2 Geometry conversion

C-arm configuration of an x-ray system is convenient for fast and accurate stereo pair acquisition. From the geometric point of view it is similar to a toed-in binocular stereo system. The toed-in configuration of the cameras in stereoscopic systems has two significant problems. The first problem is the depth plane curvature, which could lead to incorrect calculations of relative object distances (see [1], [2]). Another well-known effect of the toed-in stereo system is keystone distortion. Keystone distortion causes vertical parallax in the stereoscopic radiograph due to the baseline of the two x-ray sources not being parallel to the surface of the screen. In one of the radiographs, the image of the square appears larger at one side than at the other. In the other radiograph, this effect is reversed. This results in a vertical difference between homologous points, which is called

©CARS/Springer. All rights reserved.

vertical parallax. The amount of vertical parallax is greatest in the corners of the image and it causes difficulties in stereoscopic analysis and image perception. Two approaches were suggested in [5]. The first one also used in [4] was based on the fast correction algorithm, which adjusts the pixels in the images and sets them along the same rows. The method estimates the epipolar geometry in the left and right parts of the images using a correlation matching technique and adjusts the rows of pixel line-by-line. Another approach was to use artificial or natural landmarks to recover epipolar geometry. Those features can be placed or located anywhere around or within the object. Sometimes it is not easy to estimate epipolar geometry or locate fiducial markers in x-ray images due to their projective nature, so here we propose a new approach based on knowledge of system geometry.

The idea is to make the stereo system parallel in 3D space. In order to transform the stereo system, the proposed algorithm projects images onto new virtual planes, which are parallel to each other.

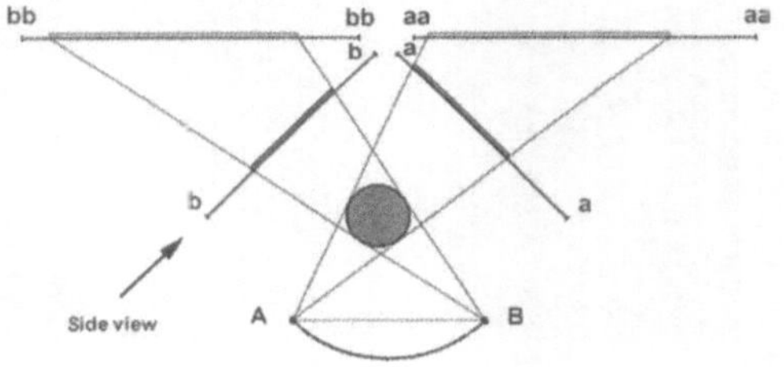

Figure 1a. Conversion of toed-in geometry into parallel geometry for depth curvature correction (top view)

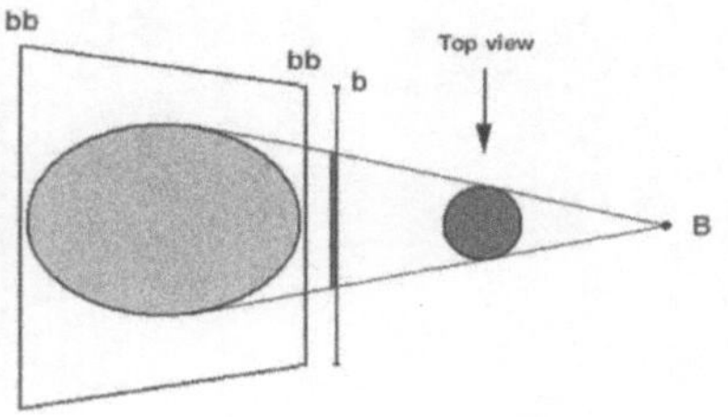

Figure 1b. Conversion of toed-in geometry into parallel geometry for keystone distortion elimination (side view)

In Figure 1a points A and B show the x-ray source location; b-b and a-a are the physical locations of the corresponding digital sensor plates; bb-bb and aa-aa are the new virtual locations of the corrected images. For every pixel of the converted image we locate the corresponding position on the physical sensor plate and assign to it the weighted data from the closest sensors. This transformation places the images in the same plane, which is parallel to the base line between the two locations used to capture the images. When this procedure is done in 3D space vertical parallax caused by keystone distortion is eliminated along with the depth curvature. Figure 1b shows the geometry of the keystone distortion elimination.

2.3 Parallax adjustment

The final step is to change the screen parallax so that as many people as possible may view the stereoscopic image. It was suggested in [1] that the depth range should be minimized and the primary area of interest should be located near the surface of the monitor. This step can be performed manually or automatically. It was suggested in [5] to use physical or artificial pointers during this process. Here we propose another technique based on the knowledge of geometric constraints. The distance from the x-ray source to

©CARS/Springer. All rights reserved.

the surface of the object or to the specific area within it could be used to place the whole object at some specific location.

3. Results

Figures 2 and 3 illustrate the process with side-by-side images. Images can be viewed in stereo with any standard stereoscope.

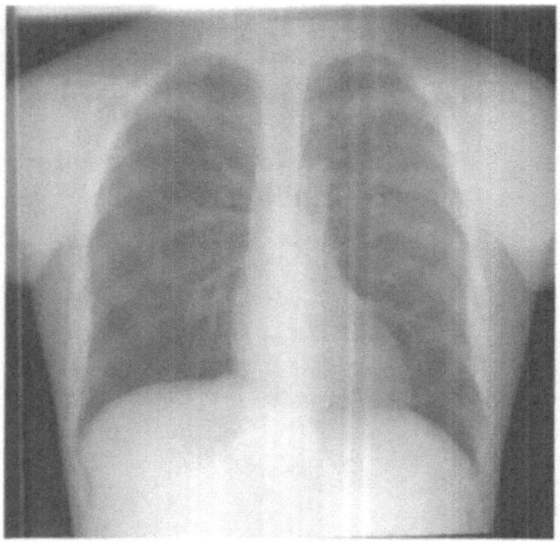

Figure 2a. Chest phantom, original left image

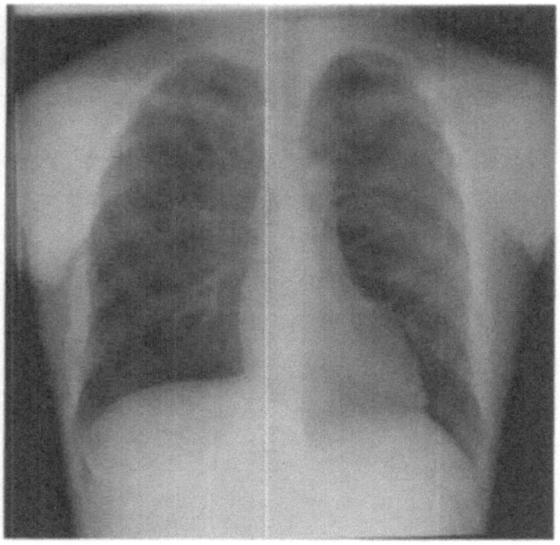

Figure 2b. Chest phantom, original right image

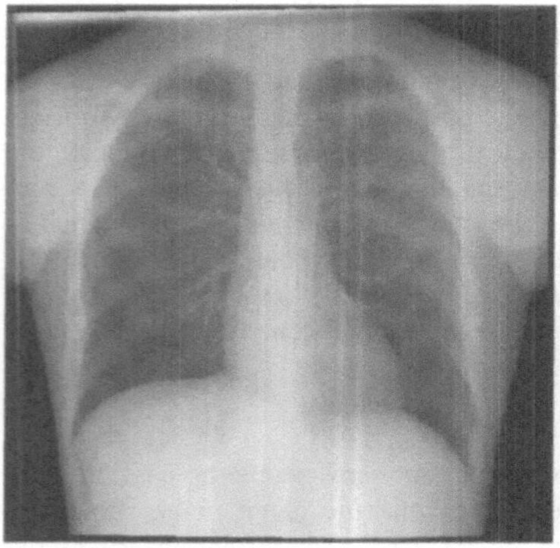

Figure 3a. Chest phantom, processed left image

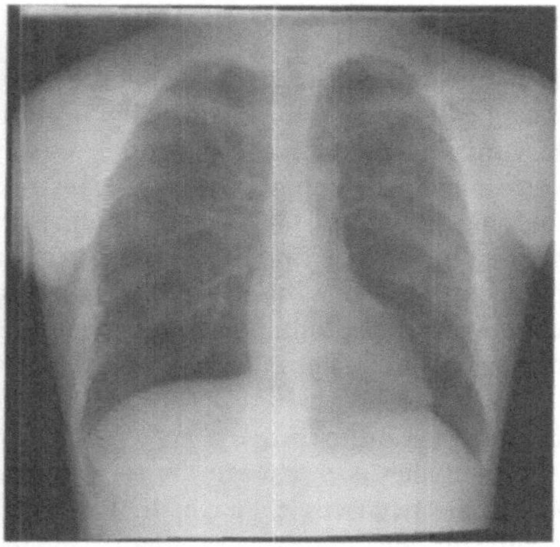

Figure 3b. Chest phantom, processed right image

©CARS/Springer. All rights reserved.

In Figure 2 the original radiograph of the chest phantom is presented. Figure 3 shows processed stereo pair. Images were taken with Canon CXDI-11 by rotation of the phantom for 15° at a focal distance of 72 inches.

There are noticeable illumination differences between the images in Figure 2a and 2b. In images 3a and 3b these effects are completely eliminated. Effects of keystone and depth curvature corrections are the most visible at the edges of the images in Figure 3a and 3b. The most dramatic difference between processed and unprocessed stereo images is when the left and the right images are taken from positions separated by wide angles, when they are differently illuminated, and when the object itself has significant depth. At the same time too wide angle between x-ray shots can lead to losses in depth perception.

A prototype software application was developed. It implements several patented algorithms and has a simple GUI interface with the logic, which allows displaying only the parameters necessary for specific image processing task. It can eliminate keystone and depth curvature distortions, horizontally and entirely equalize histograms in left and right images, position and flip resulting stereo image, create anaglyph and colored versions, save and display the results. In the simplest case of geometric distortion elimination just 3 parameters are required. They are the size of the digital x-ray plate, the focal distance, and the angle between left and right shots.

Parallax adjustment functionality allows positioning of stereo image at any depth in the screen. Required parameters are the distance from x-ray source to the plane of interest or to the surface of the object and, in case of C-arm geometry, the distance from x-ray source to the axis of rotation. If this information is unavailable the object is positioned at some optimum depth, which can be adjusted manually later.

References

1. A. Woods, T Docherty, and R. Koch, "Image Distortions in Stereoscopic Video Systems", *Proceedings of the SPIE,* Vol. 1915, 36-48, 1993.
2. A. Talukdar, and D. Wilson, "Modeling and Optimization of Rotational C-Arm Stereoscopic X-Ray Angiography", *IEEE Transactions on Medical Imaging*, Vol. 18, 604-616, 1999.
3. R. H. Eikelboom *et al.*, "Colour adjustment techniques to improve utility of stereo flicker chronoscopy and chronometry assessment of serial optic disk photographs in glaucoma", *Proceedings of the SPIE* , Vol. 3661, 1336-1344, 1999.
4. A. Berestov, "Stereo Fundus Photography: Automatic Evaluation of Retinal Topography", *Proceedings of the SPIE,* Vol. 3957, 50-59, 2000.
5. A. Berestov, "Stereoscopic X-ray Image Processing", *Studies in Health Technology and Informatics*, Vol. 81, Westwood et al. Editors, 53-59, IOS Press, Amsterdam, 2001.

©CARS/Springer. All rights reserved.

Development and performance evaluation of the first model of 4D CT-scanner

Masahiro Endo[a], Takanori Tsunoo[a], Susumu Kandatsu[a], Shuzi Tanada[a], Hiroshi Aradate[b], Yasuo Saito[b], Masahiro Kusakabe[c], Kazumasa Satho[c], Satoshi Matsusita[c]

[a] National Institute of Radiological Sciences, Chiba, 263-8555 Japan

[b] Toshiba Corp. Medical System Company, Otawara, 324-8550 Japan

[c] Sony Corp. Frontier Science Laboratories, Tokyo, 141-0001 Japan

Abstract

4D CT is a dynamic volume imaging system of moving organs with an image quality comparable to conventional CT. With 4D CT one could carry out not only new diagnoses but also provide new interventional therapy by real-time observation of its procedure. In order to realize 4D CT, we have developed a novel 2D detector on the basis of the present CT technology, and mounted it on the gantry frame of the state of the art CT-scanner. In the present report we describe the design and the results of performance evaluation of the first model of 4D CT-scanner.

Keywords: 4-dimensional computed tomography (4D CT), dynamic volume imaging, 2D discrete detector

1. Introduction

Since the advent of computed tomography (CT) in 1973, dynamic imaging of moving organs in a living person has been one of the biggest dreams in this field [1]. The concept is simply called as 4D CT because it takes 3-dimensional (3D) image with additional dimension of time. With 4D CT one could carry out not only new diagnoses but also provide new interventional therapy by real-time observation of its procedures. Because volume data (3D data) can be acquired by cone-beam CT using a rotation of the cone-beam [2,3], continuous rotation of the cone-beam allows dynamic volume data (4D data) to be acquired. In order to realize 4D CT, we have developed a novel 2D detector on the basis of the present CT technology [4], and mounted it on the gantry frame of the state of the art CT-scanner (Toshiba Corp. Aquillion). In the present report we describe the design and the results of performance evaluation of the first model of 4D CT-scanner.

2. Descriptions of scanner system

2.1 Gantry

The detector and x-ray tube pair is mounted on the gantry frame of the state of the art CT-scanner (Toshiba Corp. Aquillion). Figure 1 shows the geometry of the scanner, and Figure 2 shows a photograph of the gantry. The scanning mechanism can assure a rotation speed of up to 0.5 sec/rotation. However the first model employs 1.0sec/rotation as the

©CARS/Springer. All rights reserved.

maximum speed due to acceleration limit of x-ray tube that covers a wide cone-angle. The x-ray tube is slightly tilted to the rotation axis to cover a wide cone-angle.

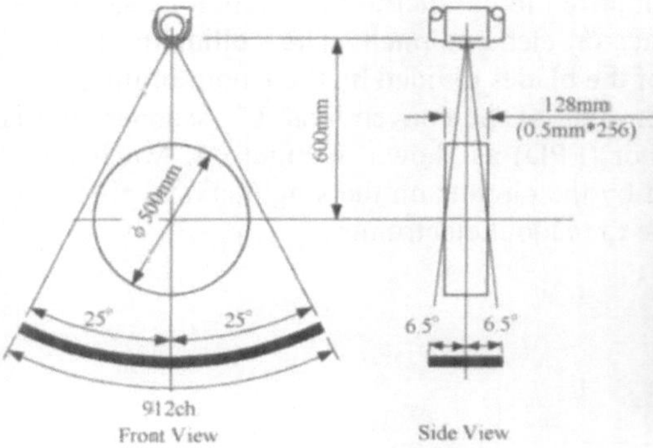

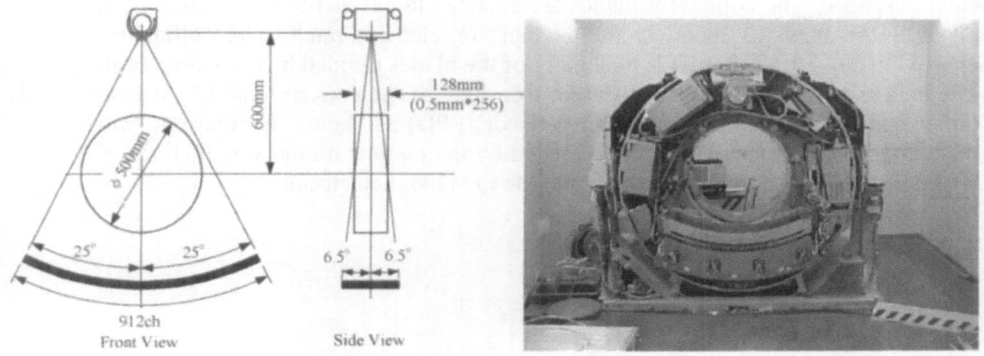

Figure 1. Geometry of the scanner.

Figure 2. Photograph of gantry.

2.2 Detector

The detector is a discrete pixel detector in which pixel data are measured by an independent detector element. The numbers of elements are 912 (channels) x 256 (segments), and the element size is approximately 1mm x 1mm. Data sampling rate is 900views(frames)/sec, and the dynamic range of A/D converter is 16bits. The detector element consists of a scintillator and photodiode. The scintillation material is the same as that for a multi-slice CT detector, and the photodiode is made of a single-crystal silicon, the same as for the multi-slice detector.

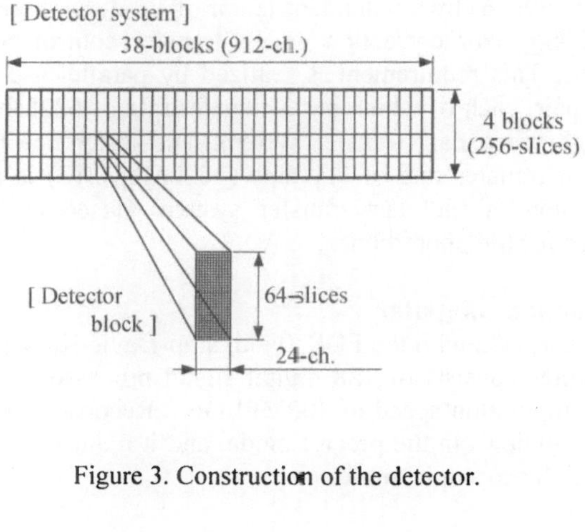

Figure 3. Construction of the detector.

©CARS/Springer. All rights reserved.

Because the size of a single-crystal silicon wafer is limited, the detector system has been realized by tiling detector blocks. One detector block consists of 24 (channels) x 64 (segments) = 1,536elements, while one detector system consists of 38x4=152 blocks. Figure 3 shows the construction of the detector.
The 2D detector has an anti-scatter collimator that is assembly of thin molybdenum blades equally spaced. The collimator blades are adjusted to parallel to the rotation axis, and the pitch of the blade is identical to the detector element pitch. The collimator ratio is approximately 30:1, where it is the height of the blades divided by the length of the gap.
The data acquisition system is different from that of the conventional CT-scanner, and is rather similar to that of a flat panel detector (FPD) as shown in Figure 4. Much faster readout-speed than that of FPD is achieved by the circuits on the single-crystal silicon as well as one-to-one bonding of each data line to readout electronics.

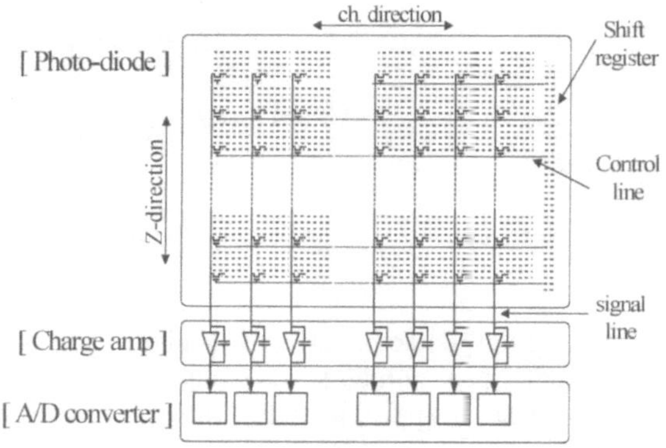

Figure 4. Diagram of data acquisition system.

2.3 High-speed data transfer system

In the present system projection data should be transferred from the rotating part to the stationary part. Since the transfer rate is determined by multiplying the required net rate of 3.4Gbps (=912x256x900x16) by a redundant factor of 1.3-1.4, where the redundant factor is necessary for adding error correction codes, transfer control codes etc, it becomes approximately 5Gbps. This requirement is realized by parallel use of 12 sets of a laser diode – photodiode pair, each of which has a transfer rate of 622Mbps. Figure 5 shows a blockdiagram of high-speed data transfer system. The difference between the required 5Gbps and maximum transfer rate of 7.4Gbps (=622Mbpsx12) is a design margin that accounts for dead time of the data transfer system caused by gaps between light-concentrating devices for the photodiodes.

2.4 Image reconstruction computer

Volume data is reconstructed with the FDK (Feldkamp-Davis-Kress) algorithm [5]. Image reconstruction computer consists of 128 digital signal processors (DSP), each of which has the maximum computation speed of 400MFLOPS. Reconstruction time is 3.5min for 512x512x256 from 900views in the precise mode, and it reduces to 1sec for 128x128x64 from 300views in the fluoroscopic mode.

©CARS/Springer. All rights reserved.

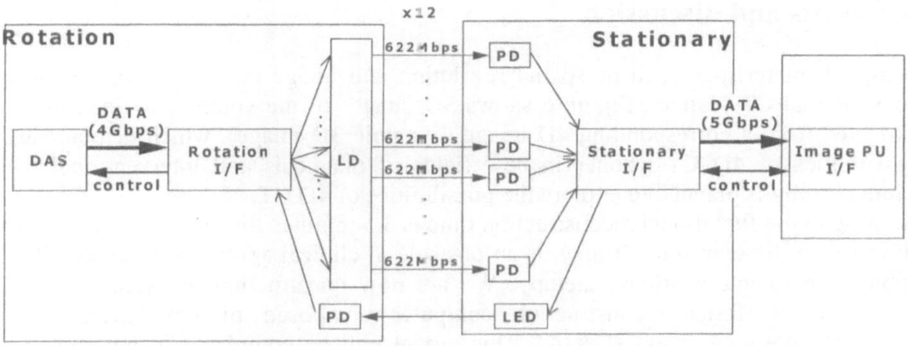

Figure 5. Blockdiagram of high-speed data transfer system. DAS: data acquisition system, PD: photo-diode, LD: laser diode, Image PU: Image processing unit.

3. Experiments

Several phantoms, stationary or moving were scanned with this scanner. Image characteristics were examined with the static phantoms, while the moving phantoms were used to demonstrate the possibilities of 4D images. Dynamic 3D images of moving phantoms were calculated and then displayed. Several volunteers were scanned with this scanner. Their dynamic 3D images are calculated and then displayed. The study protocol was approved by the ethics committee of the National Institute of Radiological Sciences, and each subjects gave written informed consent prior to participating in the study.

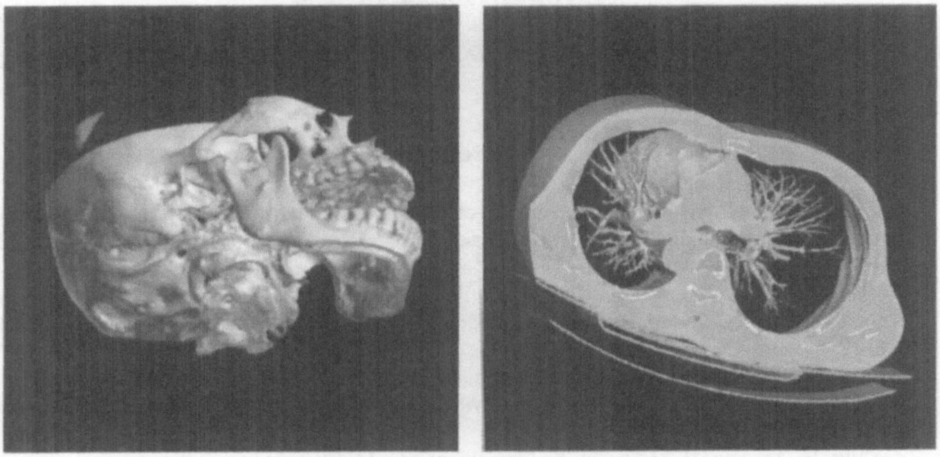

(a) Head image (b) Chest image

Figure 6. 3D images of volunteers extracted from corresponding 4D images.

©CARS/Springer. All rights reserved.

4. Results and discussion

Image characteristics such as spatial resolution and image noise were comparable to a conventional CT-scanner. Figure 6 shows 3D images of the volunteers. Each image was extracted from a corresponding 4D image (dynamic 3D image), which demonstrated the possibilities of 4D CT-scanner in new fields of diagnosis and interventional therapy. Clinical study is planned to explore the possibilities of 4D CT.
Because in the first model reconstruction time is 3.5 minutes for full size matrix and much slower than the scan time, it may be an obstacle in clinical applications, especially in the application to interventional therapy. We are now constructing the second model that installs much faster reconstruction computer composed of next generation field programmable gate arrays (FPGA). This model will be completed in the end of 2003. Table 1 summarizes specifications of the two models.

	First model	Second model
Scan Mode	Cone-beam continuous rotation (4D)	Cone-beam continuous rotation (4D) Helical cone-beam (precise 3D)
Detector	912x256 elements, 1x1mm element size, 16 bits, 900views/sec	The same as the first model
Scan Time	1 sec/rotation (30sec Max)	0.5 sec/rotation (30sec Max)
Reconstruction Matrix	512 x 512 x 256	512 x 512 x 512
Contrast Resolution	Less than 0.5%	The same as the first model
Reconstruction Time	3.5min for 512 x 512 x 256	Less than 1sec for 512 x 512 x 128

Table 1. Specifications of the first and second model of 4D CT-scanner.

Acknowledgement

This work is supported in part by the NEDO (New Energy and Industrial Technology Development Organization), Japan.

References

1. R. A. Robb, "The dynamic spatial reconstructor: An x-ray video-fluoroscopic CT scanner for dynamic volume imaging of moving organs," *IEEE Trans. Med. Imaging*, vol.1, pp.22-33, 1982
2. D. Saint-Felix, Y. Trousset, C. Picard, C. Ponchut, R. Romeas, and A. Rougee, "In vivo evaluation of a new system for computerized angiography," *Phys. Med. Biol.*, vol.39, pp.585-595, 1994
3. M. Endo, K. Yoshida, N. Kamagata, K. Satoh, T. Okazaki, Y. Hattori et al., "Development of a 3D CT-scanner using a cone beam and video-fluoroscopic system," *Radiation Medicine*, vol.16, pp.7-12, 1998
4. Y. Saito, H. Aradate, H. Miyazaki, K. Igarashi, and H. Ide, "Large area 2-dimensional detector for real-time 3-dimensional CT (4D-CT)," *Proc. of SPIE*, vol.4320, pp.775-782, 2001
5. L. A. Feldkamp, L. C. Davis, and J. W. Kress, "Practical cone-beam algorithm," *J. Opt. Soc. Am.*, vol.A1, pp.612-619, 1984

CARS 2002 – H.U. Lemke, M.W. Vannier; K. Inamura, A.G. Farman, K. Doi & J.H.C. Reiber (Editors)
©CARS/Springer. All rights reserved.

Pixels based statistical differences between lung SPECT: experimental approach to help for the diagnosis and the follow-up of pulmonary embolism

S. Bendada, J.M. Rocchisani, J.L Moretti
UPRES2360 & Hôpital Avicenne
74, rue Marcel Cachin
93017 Bobigny, France

Abstract

The statistical parametric mapping method is applied in Neurology for activation studies. We had adapted this powerful method on Lungs SPECT to help for the diagnosis and the follow-up of pulmonary embolism (PE) and other lung diseases. The SPECT slices of pairs of examination were normalized thanks to the total acquired counts, reconstruction background subtracted, smoothed and realigned. Variation in each image was estimated by a filtering approach. A parametric image of statistical differences was finally computed. We had thus obtained a 3D image showing regions of improved or altered region under treatment. We have tested the method on simulated PE images and applied it on various Lung SPECT with good results. A tuning of the various parameters could lead to more a more accurate parametric image. This new approach of lung SPECT processing appears to be a promising useful tool for the physician.

Keywords: Statistical parametric mapping, image matching, lung SPECT

1. Introduction

Pulmonary embolism (PE) is a polymorphous illness, frequent and of difficult diagnosis. The radiological techniques aim to provide direct proof of the existence of a fibrin clot in a pulmonary artery. The gold-standard imaging modality is the pulmonary angiography which is invasive and needs intensive training . During the last decades the ventilation/perfusion lung scintigraphy has been developed as an alternative non invasive imaging modality and used when a clinical suspicion of pulmonary embolism. This technique indirectly reveals PE by showing reduced perfusion in a lung segment downstream from the clot. However the diagnosis of pulmonary embolism based on the sole perfusion lungs with the standard anterior, posterior, both laterals and posterior oblique views is difficult. This is mainly due to false hypoperfusion induced by alveolar pathologies that can be interpreted with a careful comparison of both a ventilation and a perfusion scans. This has led to the development of several sets of controversial interpretation criteria of matched or mis-matched regions. In many cases, this interpretation is inconclusive and some form of medical imaging is required to confirm or to exclude a diagnosis. Therefore, emphasis in the literature has been placed on developing other diagnostic techniques such as spiral CT, Lung SPECT, venous ultrasonography and D-dimer assay. These techniques applied to the diagnosis of

©CARS/Springer. All rights reserved.

pulmonary embolism are still in the early stages of application and their reported sensitivity and specificity varies significantly depending on the size and the location of emboli. Experience using these new technique, training and quality control measures are still maturing in the medical community [1].
We had developed a powerful method on Lungs SPECT to help for the diagnosis and the follow-up of pulmonary embolism and other lung diseases. This new approach is based on parametric image of pixel statistical difference between the ventilation and perfusion images and led to 3D images showing altered regions by the disease or improved ones under treatment.
Difference images are used in other fields on nuclear Medicine for comparing two conditions such as ictal and inter-ictal images of an epileptic patient. However those images take into account neither the local variability of images nor the inter-patient one. Therefore statistical pixel based methods have been developed using two sets of patients in each condition and lead to statistical maps. They gain in importance with PET and fMRI studies and are known as statistical parametric mapping (SPM). Our method derive from these last techniques but differs by the fact that PE sets of patients are not available and that variability has to be estimated.

2. Methodology

2.1 Data

-Patients: A study group of representative cases of normal, PE, PE with airways disease was selected from the clinical data of the department of nuclear medicine of our institution. Patients underwent for a ^{99m}Tc-Technegas-ventilation and ^{99m}Tc-macro-aggregated-albumin lung perfusion SPECT for search of PE. Albumin preparation are injected with the patient in the supine position to insure uniform distribution of flow from the base of lung to the apex. Ventilation SPECT was acquired by a dual-head camera (ADAC Vertex Milpitas, CA, USA, SMVI DST-XL Buc, France) with 64 projections acquired on 360°, in 128x128 matrix, each one during 25 seconds, and contained about 1 million of counts. Perfusion SPECT was then acquired with 10 million of counts. Images were reconstructed using both filtred back projection (FBP) and OSEM.
Images were reviewed and classified by an physician with experience in lung SPECT.
-Synthetic PE lung SPECT: We have simulated defects by inserting holes of different and location on a normal perfusion scan (antérior, posterior, superior and inférior) in order to replicate different real cases of pulmonary embolisms (size and location of the emboli). A rigid body transformation (shift and 3 rotations according to the 3 axis of the 3D space) which simulated mis-registration between ventilation and perfusion was also applied. This image was used for testing our experimental approach.

2.2 Statistical comparison of images

This procedure of comparison of images of Ventilation/Perfusions or Perfusion/Perfusion included the following stages.
- **Transfer and Conversion of format**: Studies were transferred on a station of development SUN Ultra 5 with UNIX (SUN Inc microsystem, Palo Alto, CA, USA) and were converted from the Dicom 3.0 format in Analyze and BRIK formats for treatments.
- **Preprocessing of images** : To minimize the influence of external artefact of reconstruction on the algorithm of registration these were eliminated by applying a 3D

©CARS/Springer. All rights reserved.

mask on the axial scans, thanks to a contour detection for a threshold of about 10% of the maximum pixel. Scans were smoothed then by a gaussian filter of width 10 mm in relation with the FWHM of the system.

- **Normalisation**: The total number of count acquired every exam was calculated to determine which was most elevated The SPECT slices of pairs of examination were normalized. A normalization was done by pondering the most active exam by the ratio of the total number of count weakest by biggest.
- **Coregistration**: Images were warped in the same geometry with the AIR-algorithm [2]
- **Parametric images**: Meaningful voxels by voxel differences were finally calculated with the AFNI software [3] developed for the analysis of fMRI images. This software allows to compute the statistical tests of comparison between two groups of images. A test of comparison in statistical gaussien (t test) was applied then relatively to the null hypothesis. In our case, a group of typical PE perfusion scan is not available since defects are of random distribution and intensity. We assume that the ventilation and the perfusion have in normal cases similar intensities corrupted by noise. We tend to recover disimilarities introduced by PE defects. We estimated SPECT variability by assuming that this image is a good estimate of the mean of its group. Standard deviation was estimated by filtering the SPECT image with gaussian filters of increasing size from 2 to 3 pixels with a step of 0.2 . This procedure allowed to create two groups to be compared by AFNI software. A conventional order of comparison has been chosen: subtraction of ventilation to the perfusion to encourage the positive differences, or of the oldest perfusion to most recent. The described procedure provides a 3D parametric images which the intensity of voxel is the parameter t statistic, and that represent a difference between images. Values of the test are translated in levels of gray. The bottom of the image, the more brigth values and the darker values represent a nul, positive or negative difference respectively. A threshold permits to only preserve the meaningful values that will be displayed by a code of color and superimposed to a image of reference. We chose the image of ventilation or differences in the absence of the anatomical reference such as in neurology.

3. Results

The following figures show some exemples of Lung SPECT processed by our method. They are organized as follow. Row are axial slices (A) and coronal slices (C). Columns represents the Ventilation scan (V), the Perfusion scan (P) and the meaningfull differences V-P superimposed onto the ventilation scan . On figure 6 (D) is the meaningfull differences between the latest perfusion scan and the initial one superimposed onto the raw image of differences. This unique parametric 3D image by pairs of Ventilation/Perfusion exam represents meaningful differences pixel to pixel with a p-value of probability less than 0.05 .

3.1 Synthetic data

Images in figures 1 and 2 show how our method hightlight perfusion defects of various size and location. The process involves the realignement of the perfusion (P) images over the ventilation one (V), the estimation of variability and the statistical voxel by voxel comparison of these images according to our assumptions.

©CARS/Springer. All rights reserved.

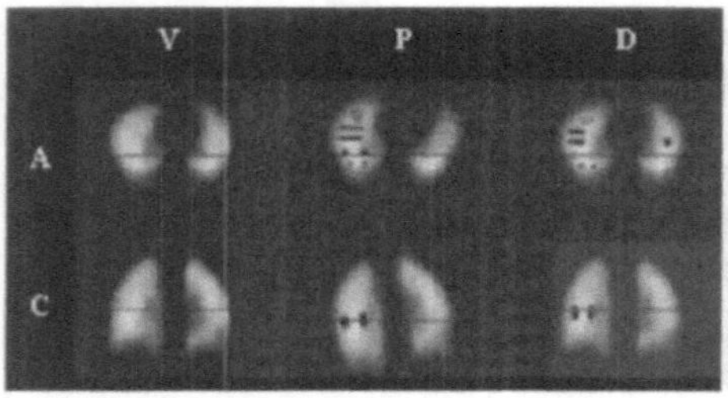

Fig 1. Synthetic PE SPECT with small Perfusion defects.

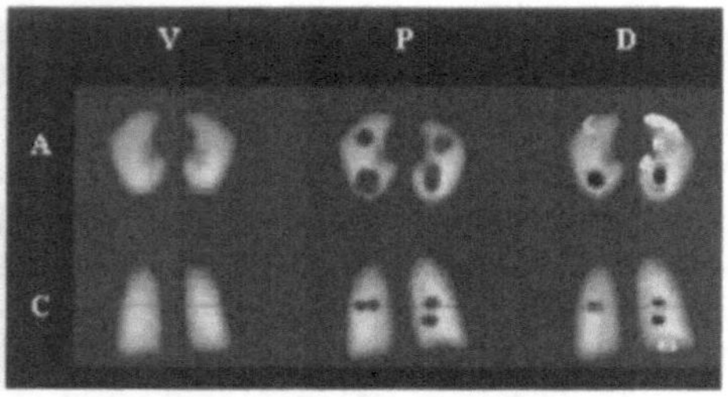

Fig 2. Synthetic PE SPECT with large Perfusion defects.

Defects size were well recovered even for very small defects as well as they location. However some errors may occur on defect edges and on the lung borders. The overall accuracy was estimated by comparing theoretical and measured defect volume. No significant errors were found with a confidence $p < 0.1$.

3.2 Patients data

On normal patients, one can see (Fig 3.) that the ventilation and the perfusion scans are not ideally identical and slight visual differences are well depicted.

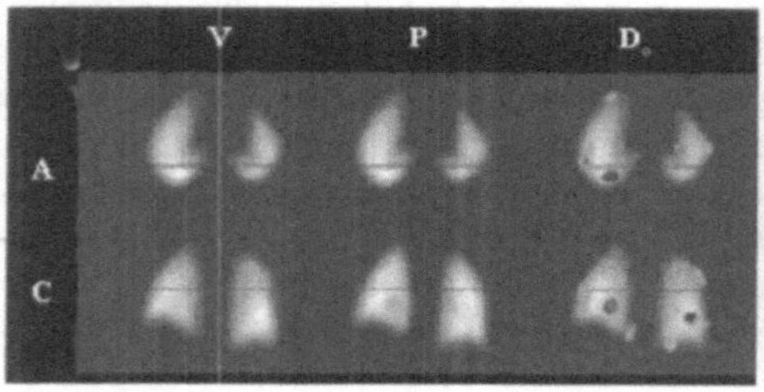

Fig 3. Normal V/P Lung SPECT.

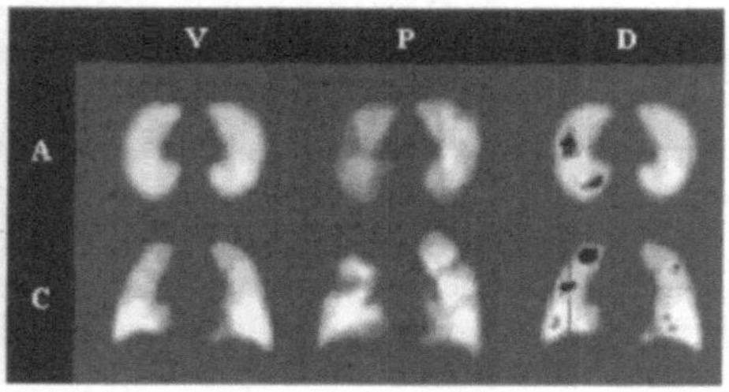

Fig 4. Lung V/P SPECT of Pulmonary Embolism.

On embolic patients, defects of larger sizes are unambiguously found on typical PE scan (Fig 4.) as well as on scan of PE with airways disease. On Fig 5.C, the lower left defect seen on both the ventilation and perfusion was not significant.

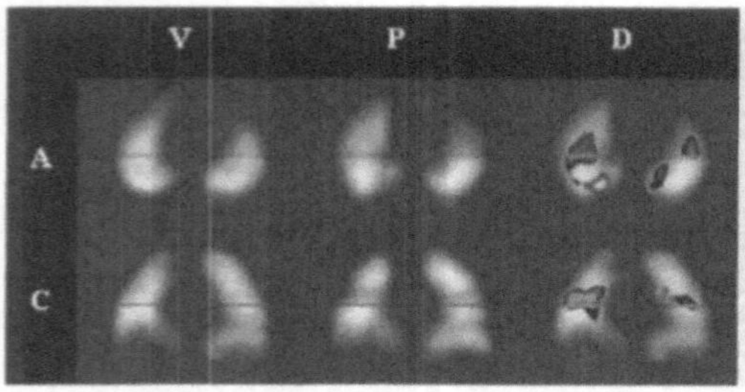

Fig 5. V/P Lung SPECT of Pulmonary Embolism with airway disease.

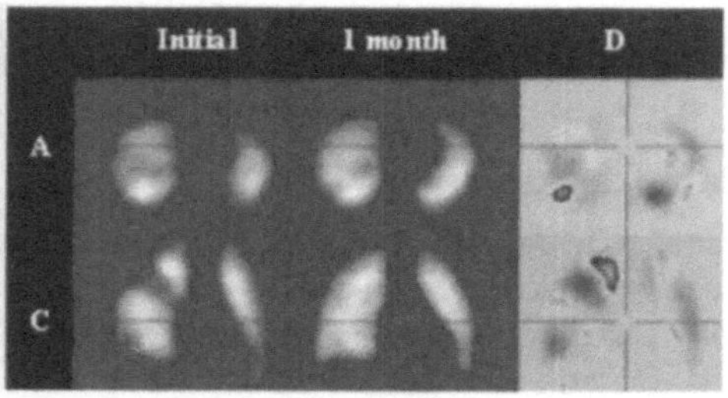

Fig 6. Follow up of Pulmonary Embolism after 1 month of treatment.on Perfusion SPECT

©CARS/Springer. All rights reserved.

The last illustration (Fig 6.) shows how the method can be used on successive perfusion scans for the follow up under treatement of a PE. Remaining unperfused regions are in bright grey while re-perfused appears in dark grey.

4. Discussion

We had thus obtained a 3D image showing altered regions of EP or improved region under treatment. However some artifacts have been seen on the synthetic and real data. This could lead to an altered accuracy mainly for small defects. Several reasons can be invoked. Mis-registration errors may be induced by SPECT an insufficient reconstruction artifacts correction and large defects [4]. Intensity normalization is a known crucial point for SPM method. Estimation of image variability by filtering takes into account some overall physical image properties and is difficult to tune. More relevent and objective techniques [6] could be used. Finally the underlying assumption that intensity in the ventilation and perfusion scans have an intrinsic regular pattern and a strong similarity may not true in pratice [5].

5. Conclusion

We compared in a statistical way differences between images tomoscintigraphic of ventilation and perfusion. The proposed method brings a new synthetic and semi - quantitative approach with the calculation of a parametric images. The interest of this approach is to diagnose a pathology of it is shown on examples and to follow the evolution of pulmonary embolism. However, several improvements could be brought concerning the optimization of treatments and the presentation of results. A tuning of the various parameters and finding a good method of normalisation could lead to more accurate image. This new approach of SPECT lung processing appears to be has promising useful tool for physician.

Acknowledgements

This work was supported by grants of the *Scaler Foundation* and *the Ligue contre le Cancer- Comité de la Seine-Saint Denis*, France.

References

1. Greaves SM, Hart EM, Aberle DR. "CT of pulmonary thrombolism". *Seminars in Ultrasound, CT and MRI*, 18(5):232-237, 1997.
2. Woods RP, Grafton ST, Watson JD, Sicotte NL, Mazziotta JC. "Automated image registration: II. Intersubject validation of linear and nonlinear models". *J Comput Assist Tomogr*. 1998 Jan-Feb;22(1):153-65. http://bishop.loni.ucla.edu/AIR3
3. Cox RW. "AFNI: software for analysis and visualization of functional magnetic resonance neuroimages". *Comput Biomed Res.* 1996 Jun;29(3):162-73. http://afni.nimh.nih.gov/afni
4. J. West, J.M. Fitzpatrick, M.Y. Wang, *et al* . "Comparison and evaluation of retrospective intermodality brain image registration techniques". *Journal of Computer Assisted Tomography*, 1997, volume 21, pages 554--565.
5. Mitomo O, Aoki S, Tsunoda T, Yamaguchi M, Kuwabara H. "Quantitative analysis of nonuniform distributions in lung perfusion scintigraphy". J Nucl Med. 1998 Sep;39(9):1630-5.

Desco M, Hernandez JA, Santos A, Brammer M. "Multiresolution analysis in fMRI: sensitivity and specificity in the detection of brain activation." Hum Brain Mapp. 2001 Sep;14(1):16-27.

CARS 2002 – H.U. Lemke, M.W. Vannier; K. Inamura, A.G. Farman, K. Doi & J.H.C. Reiber (Editors)
©CARS/Springer. All rights reserved.

A fast automatic method for 3D volume segmentation of the human cerebrovascular

M. Sabry M.[a], Charles B. Sites[a], Aly A. Farag[a], Stephen Hushek[b], Thomas Moriarty[b]
[a] Computer Vision and Image Processing Laboratory
University of Louisville, Louisville, KY 40292.
{msabry, syschuck, farag}@cvip.Louisville.edu. http://www.cvip.louisville.edu
[b] Dept. of Neurological Surgery, University of Louisville, KY 40292.

Abstract

We present a new method for 3-D volume segmentation of the human cerebrovascular structures from Magnetic Resonance Angiograms (MRA) and Magnetic Resonance Ventriculargrams (MRV). A slice through the volume containing large vein or artery structures is chosen, which becomes the seed location for the segmentation process. A modified 3-D computer graphics based region-filling algorithm is used to sweep the vascular tree from seed locations in order to track and label the vascular structure. The labelled-segmented images are extracted and a 3-D model is created using VTK toolkit. The 3-D model can then be viewed on a stereo graphics capable workstation or in a Virtual Reality environment. We also present a new maximum intensity projection (MIP) based technique for validating the results. We implemented MIP and used it to project both the segmented and original volume at different angles. Hence, the resultant images from both volumes can be compared side by side, which facilitates validation process.

Keywords: MRA, vascular tree, image segmentation, MIP visualization.

1. Introduction

The human cerebrovascular is a complex three-dimensional anatomical structure. Accurate description of the vascular tree is very important to assist in clinical applications, e.g., surgical planning, quantitative diagnosis, and monitoring disease progress. A variety of methods have been developed for segmenting vessels within MRA. One class of methods is based on statistical model, which classifies voxels within the image volume into either vascular or nonvascular region [1]. Another class of segmentation is based on intensity threshold where points are classified as either greater or less than a given intensity. This is the basis of the iso-intensity surface reconstruction method [2]–[4]. This method suffers from errors due to image inhomogeneities in addition; the choice of the threshold level is subjective. An alternative to segmentation is axis detection known as skeletonization process, where the central line of the tree vessels is extracted based on the tubular shape of vessels [5]. Other approaches for MRA vessel segmentation is the manually defined seed locations for segmentation [6].
Validating the model is very tedious and difficult process since practioners usually rotate the visualized 3-D model by certain angles in order that the views at these angles agrees with the available 2-D images taken by digital subtraction angiography (DSA), X-ray, or

©CARS/Springer. All rights reserved.

MIP. MIP image is the most common way of displaying 3-D MRA. The MIP image is similar in appearance to traditional X-ray but has some characteristics that make it easy to process digitally.
In this paper, we present a new automatic technique for cerebrovascular 3-D volume segmentation based on enhanced intensity threshold image segmentation, and a modified 3-D computer graphics region-filling algorithm. We also present a new fast method for validating results based on MIP algorithm, which will facilitate the validation process done by neurosurgeons.

2. Background

By applying an intensity threshold operator to the MRA data images, we could detect and extract a 3-D model of the major component blood vessels. The 3-D model obtained by this approach usually contains disconnected vascular tree areas and unrelated tissues that get attached to the final output. These are typical problems with threshold-based segmentation. Wilson and Nobel showed that the histogram of the total imaged MRA volume could be classified into three intensity regions [1]. The lowest intensity region corresponds mainly to cerebrospinal fluid (CSF) surrounding the brain tissue, bone and the background air. The middle intensity region corresponds to brain tissue, including both the grey and white matter. The high-intensity region consists of fat, which is found adjacent to the skin, and arteries. Fig. 1 shows a typical histogram of the MRA scan. Since we are interested in the high-intensity region where arteries are found, it is very important to find the grey-scale range for this region [α-255], where α is subjective, vary from one patient to another, and depends on the scan parameters.

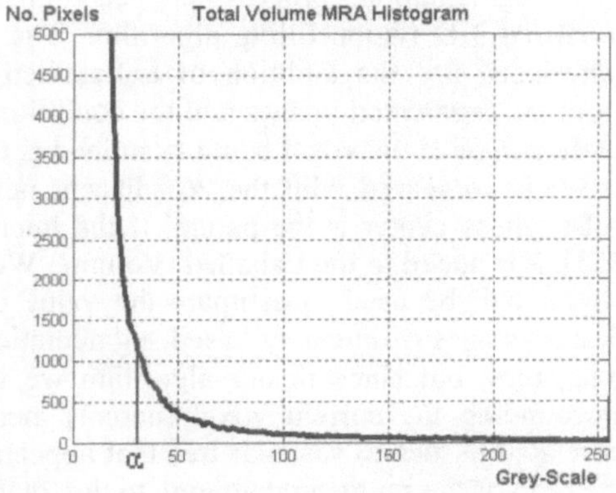

Fig. 1. Histogram of total imaged MRA volume. The intensity range for arteries is [α-255]

3. Methodology

Our vascular tree extraction algorithm consists of three basic steps: vessel segmentation from MRA data, definition of vascular tree, and evaluation/validation of the results.

3.1 Image Seed Selection

The concept we developed for extracting the arteries and veins from MRA and MRV slices is to use "Image Seeded Segmentation". All the MRI images acquired are cross-sectional image slices taken from the lower portion of the nasal cavities and progressing upwards to the top of the skull. Utilizing this acquisition method and recognizing that the vascular system is a tree-like

©CARS/Springer. All rights reserved.

structure with the large coratid arteries located in the neck, it is easy to automatically locate these main blood supply structures. Fig. 2 shows a typical MRA seed image slice. Because of the contrast between the pixel intensities for the coratid artery locations and the surrounding tissues, we isolate these locations by scanning the seed image and tagging all pixels that falls between [α-255] and store them in a stack data structure

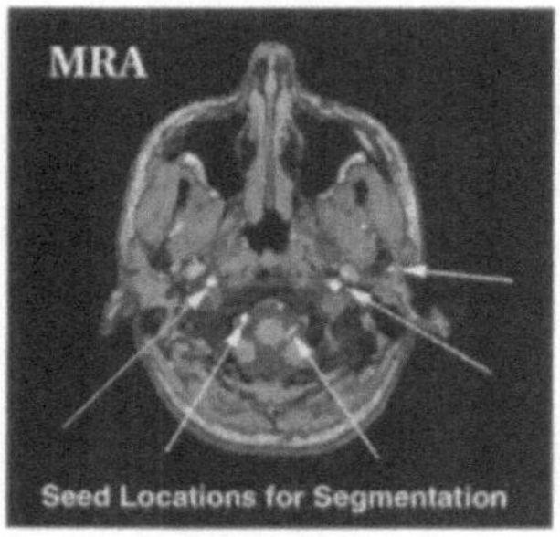

Fig. 2. MRA seed image

3.2 Vascular Tree Definition

The segmentation process is accomplished using a modified 3-D region-filling algorithm. The modifications introduced are the addition of a Labelled-Volume to store the segmented images and the conditions necessary to determine if the voxel being examined is to be included in the labelled set. Each parent voxel is compared with the 26-adjacent neighbour voxels (children) that form a small cube whose center is the parent. If the intensity level of the child falls in the range [α-255], it is added to the Labelled_Volume. We also count the number of segmented voxels, which will be used to estimate the value of α. We mentioned before that one of the disadvantages of intensity-based segmentation technique is having disconnected vascular tree areas, but since in our algorithm we investigate only those neighbours (children) surrounding the current voxel (parent), hence, we eliminate the possibility of having unrelated tissues to vascular tree that appears in the segmented volume. Let's define ζ as the ratio of the segmented volume to the total volume.

$$\zeta = \frac{SegmentedVolume}{TotalVolume} x 100$$

This value can be used to decide if α is too large or too small. From our experience with segmenting large number of MRA data sets validated by the neurosurgeon and neurologist in our research team, we found out that if ζ is larger than [1.5-4.5], there is a high probability that the intensity α is large, and thus can be adjusted automatically downward. Similarly if the percentage is too small, α can be extended upward. Thus, the segmentation process can be done automatically by giving α an initial value. From our experiments, we found that, for images scaled to a grey level between [0-255], initial value for α between [20-40] is a good starting point where it appeared to be the cut-off region between MRA vascular tree and other brain tissues.

3.3 Validation

One of the crucial issues with 3D volumes generated from MRA scans is the validation with respect to the known structures imaged. It is quite difficult to devise validation criteria because of the extent and complexity of the vascular tree. While basic arteries and veins are of known size and significance, the rest of the vascular tree does not have distinct landmarks to recognize. Basic evaluations of these models using phantoms can be employed but there exists no such phantom that mimics the complexity of the vascular tree especially those vessels whose diameters less than 1mm. Practioners usually validate the resulting cerebrovascular volume by rotating the visualized 3-D model by certain

©CARS/Springer. All rights reserved.

angles in order that the views at these angles agree with the available 2-D images taken by DSA, X-ray, or MIP.
We implemented the MIP algorithm such that we can generate any projection of the data volume at any angle. We allowed the rays to rotate around z-axis (slice-axis) by 180° in steps of 5°. We did the same for y-axis and x-axis to cover the virtual sphere that surrounds the MRA volume. We applied the algorithm to both the original and segmented volumes. The generated projected images from all directions at different angles to both volumes can then be compared to each other side by side. This technique will help practioners to evaluate visually the quality of the MRA results fast when compared with traditional methods.

4. Results

The MRA data sets were collected using GE MEDICAL SYSTEMS Genesis Signa MRI system. MRA data set consists of 256x256x117 lateral slices from Nasal Cavity to the top of the skull with 1mm thickness. MRV data set consists of 256x256x84 sagittal slices from ear to ear with 2mm thickness.
The first row of Fig. 4 and 5 show the MRA volume of patient1 and patient2, respectively, projected by the MIP algorithm at angles 0, 25, 45, 90 before segmentation, while the second row of both figures show the resultant images at the same angles after applying our segmentation technique. It is obvious from the results that segmentation technique developed in this paper has successfully segmented most of the MRA structures, even the minor branches down to the limit of the resolution of the used MRI scanner, which is 1mm for a 256x256x128 MRA acquisition. In addition, it also occluded those tissues and noise that form islands in the data volume.
Since stereo viewing is recommended for highly complex 3D vascular structure, we used VTK as a visualization toolkit because of its capability in rendering results in stereo, besides it can be used with virtual reality display environments such as Immersa-Desk system, where our 3-D results are displayed.

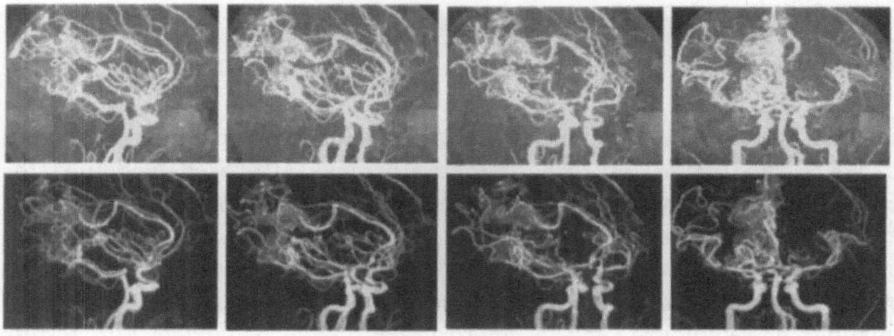

Fig. 4. First row shows the MIP images of the MRA volume of patient1 projected at angles 0, 25, 45, 90 respectively before segmentation. Second row shows the resultant MIP images generated at the same angles after applying our segmentation technique

©CARS/Springer. All rights reserved.

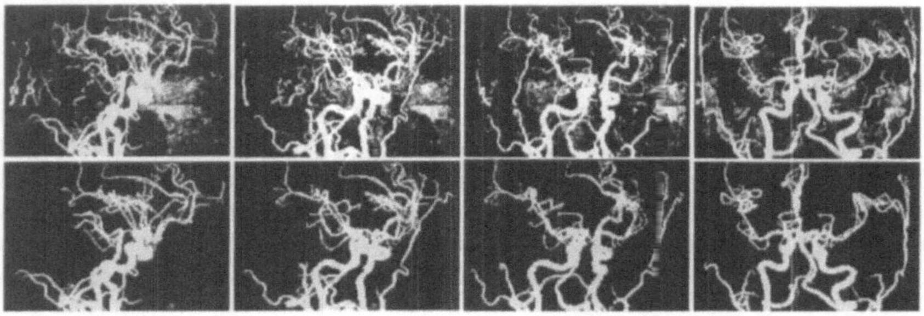

Fig. 5. First row shows the MIP images of the MRA volume of patient2 projected at angles 0, 25, 45, 90 respectively before segmentation. Second row shows the resultant MIP images generated at the same angles after applying our segmentation technique

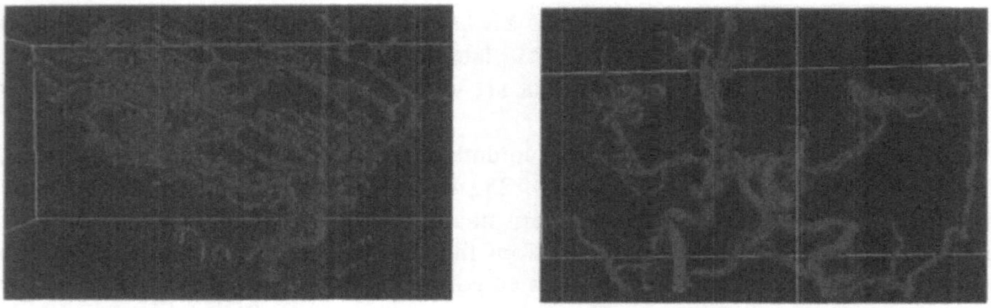

Fig. 6. Left image shows the 3-D visualization of the first column of patient1. Right image shows the 3-D visualization of the last column of patient2

Left image of Fig. 6 shows the 3-D visualization of the MIP images in the first column of patient1, while right image shows the same for the last column of second patient. Speed wise, proposed segmentation algorithm is very fast compared with other algorithms. A typical 256x256x128 MRA are segmented in less than 10 seconds on a single Pentium processor at 300Mhz.

5. Conclusions

We have presented a robust technique for automatic segmentation of the human cerebral vascular from MRA and MRV. We also presented a new MIP-based technique for validating the segmentation algorithm by projecting both the original and segmented volume at different angles and compare the resultant MIP images side by side.
Because we are using simple intensity ranges to determine connectivity, we rely on the consistency of the contrast in intensities from scan to another; otherwise, we have to adjust it manually. A radiologist and a neurosurgeon have validated our results successfully. The accuracy of the results has shown details of the vascular structure down to the limits of the MRI system.
Our final goal is to provide a DICOM network capable stereographic display system, which would accept MRA volumes and render the vascular structures on demand.

©CARS/Springer. All rights reserved.

Acknowledgments

This project has been funded by the Whitaker Foundation Research Grant No. 98-009. The generous support of Norton Healthcare Organization for our medical research through Grants 97-72 and 97-73 is greatly appreciated.

References

1. D. L. Wilson and J. A. Noble, "An adaptive segmentation algorithm for time-of-flight MRA data," *IEEE Trans on Med. Imaging*, vol. 18, no. 10, pp. 938–945, 1999.
2. H. E. Cline, W. E. Lorensen, R. Kikinis, and R. Jolesz, "Three-dimensional segmentation of MR images of the head using probability and connectivity," *Neurosurgery*, vol. 14, pp. 1037–1045, 1990.
3. S. Nakajima, H. Atsumi, and A. H. Bhalerao, *et al.*, "Computer-assisted surgical planning for cerebrovascular neurosurgery," *Neurosurgery*, vol. 41, pp. 403–409, 1997.
4. H. E. Cline, W. E. Lorensen, S. P. Souza, F. A. Jolesz, R. Kikinis, G. Gerig, and T. E. Kennedy, "3D surface rendered MR images of the brain and its vasculature," *JCAT*, vol. 15, pp. 344–351, 1991.
5. Peter J. Yim, Peter L. Choyke, and Ronald M. Summers, "Gray-scale skeletonization of small vessels in magnetic resonance angiography," *IEEE Trans on Med. Imaging*, vol. 19, no. 6, pp. 568–576, 2000.
6. E. Bullitt, el al. "Symbolic description of intracerebral vessels segmented from magnetic resonance angiograms and evaluation by comparison with X-ray angiograms," Medical Imag Analysis, Vol 5; pp. 157-169, 2001.

©CARS/Springer. All rights reserved.

Contrast-enhanced three dimensional MR angiography of pulmonary artery and pulmonary perfusion imaging in pig –a comparison study with DSA

Liu Shiyuan, Dong Weihua, Xiao Xiangsheng
Department of Radiology, Chang Zheng Hospital, the Second Military Medical University, 415# Fengyang Road, Shanghai, China. 200003

Abstract

CEMRA and PPI were performed in 6 healthy pigs and 3 pulmonary embolism models with the gadolinium contrast agents inject rate 3ml/s in different doses (5ml, 10ml, 15ml, 20ml, 25ml) by comparison with DSA, in order to optimize the injection protocol and to evaluate its value in the diagnosis of experimental acute pulmonary embolism. The signal intensities and the signal to noise ratio (SNR) of the pig pulmonary arteries kept increasing with the dosage of agents, but the best angio-pulmonary contrast occurred in 10~15ml(0.25mmol/kg~0.375mmol/kg), while the satisfied dosage for PPI was 15~20ml(0.375mmol/kg~0.5mmol/kg). Although CEMRA demonstrating less obstructed pulmonary arteries than DSA (8/10), but it becomes better (10/10) when combined with PPI. The pulmonary infarction zones showed wedge-shaped perfusion defects in the PPI images, which signal intensity were lower than that of normal areas (137.86±45.32 Vs 330.14±46.52,t=8.40,p<0.001). We concluded that the best dose of contrast agent for CEMRA was 0.25mmol/kg~0.375mmol/kg, and that for lung perfusion was 0. 375mmol/kg~0. 5mmol/kg. It is showed that CEMRA combined with PPI were better than DSA in demonstrating pulmonary embolism.

Keywords: MR enhanced angiography, pulmonary embolism, lung perfusion

1. Introduction

Pulmonary embolism is a common and dangerous clinical entity, with no characteristic clinical symptoms and signs, leaving its diagnosis difficulty [1-4]. It is important to evaluate the pulmonary artery and perfusion states precisely for the pulmonary embolism patients. Nuclear medicine has been long used to evaluate lung perfusion, but the specificity and accuracy are poor because of its low spatial resolution and the overlap with diaphragm and mammary gland. The improvement of MR data acquisition time make it possible to be used in the pulmonary artery imaging and lung perfusion by using contrast medium, but only a few papers were reported [2-8]. The purpose of our study is to optimize the contrast medium injection protocol in thoracic contrast-enhanced MR angiography (CEMRA) and to evaluate its diagnostic value in acute pulmonary embolism.

©CARS/Springer. All rights reserved.

2. Methodology

2.1 Animal cast and experimental procedure

Six Chonghua black pigs (male 4, female 2, average weight 20kg) were provided by Animal Research Constitution of Chinese Academy of Science. Anesthesia: 10 mg ketamine was injected intramuscularly, then the peripheral venous access was established, through which the disoprofol were used to maintain the anaesthesia. Percutaneous right jugular vein was punctured, and 6F pigtail catheter was insert into the main pulmonary artery through 6F sheath in order to perform DSA. MRI enhanced angiography was done using different doses after DSA examination (the examination time between different dose groups must be over 2 Hr), then the optimal injection protocol were chosen by comparison with DSA. Gelfoam particles (3-5mm^3) were injected into the sheath, and the pulmonary artery embolisms were confirmed by DSA examination, then contrast-enhanced MRA and perfusion pulmonary imaging (PPI) were examined using the optimized protocol.

2.2 Contrast-enhanced MRA and pulmonary perfusion imaging (PPI)

Siemens Vision 1.5 T super-conducted imaging system and array head coil were used; Imaging parameters: TR 3.2ms, TE 1.2ms, flip angle 30°, image matrix 128x256, FOV 300mmx300mm, scan slab 64 mm, scan time 7~10s, delay time 0 (contrast medium will reach main pulmonary artery immediately after injected through the sheat). The image matrix, FOV, slice-thick, and the number of partitions could be adjusted according to the different conditions.

Group of auto-control: 5 different dosage of gadolinium (5ml, 10ml, 15ml, 20ml and 25 ml)were injected with 3ml/s flow rate using Meorao Spectris high pressure injector, 15ml saline was injected using same velocity after injection of contrast medium was finished. The signal to noise ratio of the pulmonary artery and parenchyma and the contrast ratio of pulmonary vessels to parenchyma was compared in different groups.

Groups of acute pulmonary embolism: Contrast-enhanced MR angiography and perfusion pulmonary imaging (PPI) were performed using 20 ml contrast medium and 3 ml/s flow rate. The enhancement and signal to noise ratio of pulmonary vessels, normal pulmonary parenchyma and infarct zone were compared.

2.3 Evaluation of images

1) subjective evaluation: The depicted grade of the distal branch of bilateral pulmonary arteries in original and reconstructed MIP images were observed and recorded; meanwhile, the satisfaction of pulmonary perfusion imaging was also analysed at the same time.

2) Quantitative evaluation: the image quality was determined by the signal to noise ratio, while the contrast ratio between vessel and pulmonary parenchyma is the key of contrast resolution of vessels. So, the signal intensity and standard deviation of pulmonary vessels, parenchyma, and background were measured emphatically. Methods of measurement: the signal intensity of three ROIs (region of interested) in bilateral pulmonary arteries and main pulmonary arteries were measured as the enhanced data of pulmonary artery; four ROIs in bilateral upper-lung fields and bilateral infra-lung fields

©CARS/Springer. All rights reserved.

were measured as the parenchyma enhanced data; the four measure points of background were chosen in bi-oxter and both side of neck. The signal intensity and standard deviation of vessels, parenchyma, and background were obtained by the measurement above, the signal to noise ratio (SNR) and contrast ratio of angio-parenchyma were calculated according to the formula behind automatically in Excel.
SNR= mean enhance value of tissue/standard deviation of background
The angio-pulmonary parenchyma contrast ratio = (mean enhance value of vessels-mean enhance value of pulmonary parenchyma) / mean enhance value of pulmonary parenchyma.

2.4 Criteria for identification of pulmonary emboli

1) Criteria of MRA: If the branches of pulmonary arteries in CEMRA images were interrupted and accompanied by perfusion defect in PPI images, then the branch should be defined to be the embolized artery. It will be more definitely if there are not any perfusion defect in the normal pulmonary perfusion images before the gelatine sponged particles were injected into the jugular vein.

2)Criteria of DSA: Normal pulmonary arteries in DSA images appeared smoothly in their natural course, the branches will be cut off if it is embolized; in capillary stage, the filling defect of the embolized pulmonary parenchyma can be depicted.

3)Final decision: After all of the examinations were completed, the pigs were put to death by injecting overdose anaesthetic. Necropsy was done immediately, and the lung specimen was fixed by inject 10% formaldehyde solution through the bronchus. Then the fixed lung specimen was cut open according to the suspected embolized zone provided by CEMRA and DSA. Ordinarily, the infarct area of the specimen is white and hard, serial sections should be done in these portions. If we can find the gelatine sponge in the pulmonary artery and pulmonary infarct under light microscope, and it is the same part as in CEMRA and DSA image, the final diagnosis was made.

2.5 Statistical analysis

The initial data including the mean signal value of pulmonary artery and parenchyma, the standard deviation of background were transferred to Excel table, and the SNR and the contrast ratio of angio-pulmonary parenchyma were calculated automatically. All the data were transmitted to SPSS analysis system. After F test was done between the random groups, Student-Newman-Keuls test was used to analyze the differences among the mean values. A threshold value of P less than 0.05 was statistically significant.

3. Results

3.1 Group of normal auto-control

1) The dose dependent-relationship of signal intensity and SNR of pulmonary arteries (table 1)

©CARS/Springer. All rights reserved.

Table 1 showed, the signal intensity and SNR of pulmonary arteries improved as the dose of contrast medium increased, but the contrast ratio of angio-parenchyma decreased from group 3 (figure 1-4) . The optimized dose for pulmonary MR angiography should be 10-15ml (0.25mmol/kg~0.375mmol/kg) , there is no use to increase the dose continually for depicting of pulmonary artery.

Table 1. The Relationship Between the Effects of CEMRA in Pulmonary Arteries and the Doses of Contrast Medium (x±s) (n=6)

Group of doses (ml)	Signal intensity of pulmonary artery	SNR of the pulmonary artery	Contrast ratio of angio-parenchyma	Depicted branches (Subjective evaluation)
1 (5)	392.83±290.11	53.72±32.41	6.72±4.66	3 (lobar)
2 (10)	848.29±114.15	111.49±29.39*	8.51±3.01	4(segmental)
3 (15)	1022.65±93.05*▲	112.02±40.92*	5.34±3.17▲	4
4 (20)	1163.09±176.67*#▲	123.24±39.42*	3.82±1.55▲	4
5 (25)	1473.92±319.28*▲	135.62±62.68*	5.13±2.93▲	4
F	28.406 (P=0.000)	3.545 (P=0.013)	3.894 (P=0.008)	

* P<0.05 when compared with group 1, ▲ P<0.05 when compared with group 2, # P<0.05 when compared with group 5

2) The dose dependent-relationship of pulmonary perfusion imaging (table 2)

TABLE 2. The dose dependent-relationship of pulmonary perfusion imaging (x±s) (n=6)

Group of doses (ml)	Signal intensity of pulmonary parenchyma	SNR of pulmonary parenchyma	Satisfaction *of PPI (Subjective evaluation)
1 (5)	48.45±13.07	6.88±1.33	0 (no perfusion effect)
2 (10)	99.63±39.84*	12.66±4.91	1 (non-satisfaction)
3 (15)	218.54±129.80*	21.57±14.12*	2(satisfaction)
4 (20)	246.57±172.91*	25.91±16.49*▲	2
5 (25)	351.05±157.54*▲	29.35±12.15*▲	2
F	7.775 (P=0.000)	5.298 (P=0.001)	

* P<0.05 when compared with group 1, ▲ P<0.05 when compared with group 2, # P<0.05 when compared with group 5.

Table 2 showed, the enhancement and SNR of pulmonary parenchyma increased as the dose of contrast medium increased, but the increase of SNR slow down in 15ml-25ml group. We can always acquired satisfactory perfusion images when the dose of contrast medium over 15 ml (0.375mmol/kg) .

©CARS/Springer. All rights reserved.

3) Comparison with DSA: The 5-6 grade of pulmonary artery branches can be depicted on DSA images, CEMRA is not as good as DSA, because only 4 grade of braches can be seen on it. But the quality of DSA perfusion images was not so good as MR PPI.

3.2 The manifestation of acute pulmonary embolism
The MRI and DSA images are satisfactory in 3 pigs of the 6 models, 11 gelatin sponge particles were injected into the 3 pigs and 10 of them were founded in pathological examination. Of the 10 lesions, 3 located in upper lung field, 7 in infra-lung field. All infra lesions were depicted in DSA images, only 1 of the 3 upper lesions can be displayed. In MR enhanced pulmonary angiography and pulmonary perfusion imaging examination, 7 lesions in the infra lung field which corresponding well with the pathological findings; but in the upper lung field, 5 lesions were founded, which means, 2 of them were false-positive, these mainly because of heart beating artifact.

CEMRA (5 lesions) was not as good as DSA (8 lesions) in depicting embolized arteries, but it will improve dramatically when combined with PPI images, in our study, all of the 10 pathological founded lesions were depicted in PPI images. It is usually difficult to define the exact border and extent of the perfusion defect in DSA images, but the images of PPI are serial and there are no overlaps, so the lesions can be easily found. The false-positive lesions mainly come from heart beating artifact. The embolized pulmonary tissues appeared wedge shaped low signal intensity defect (figure 5-9). The mean signal intensity for embolized and normal pulmonary tissue is 137.86±45.32 and 330.14±46.52 respectively, the difference between them is significant (t=8.40,P<0.001).

4. Discussion

Some papers reported that CEMRA and PPI are feasible in the diagnosis of pulmonary embolism[1-4]. Even though, there are still some problems need to be further researched. First of all, no animal experimental reports about the optimal injection protocol for CEMRA and PPI were found up to now. Second, the results were different as the criteria differ. The sensitivity and specificity will be high if the little arteries are not considered, in the other hand, we may get relatively lower sensitivity and specificity when the sub-segmental arteries was regarded. The purpose of our study was to compare the effects of different doses on contrast enhanced MRA and pulmonary perfusion imaging, and to evaluate the diagnostic value of CEMRA and PPI in subsegmental pulmonary artery embolism models.

The best angio-pulmonary contrast is needed in pulmonary CEMRA. As the dose of contrast medium increased, the signal intensity of pulmonary artery and parenchyma increase at the same time. If the signal intensity of pulmonary parenchyma is too high, the angio-pulmonary contrast, which mainly influences the depiction of vessels, will be decreased although the perfusion imaging is satisfied. Therefore, the key point of successful CEMRA examination is to get a balance between vessel and parenchyma enhancement. In our study, table 1 showed that the angio-pulmonary contrast begun went down from group 3, but the signal intensity and SNR of pulmonary artery still went up. The best angio-pulmonary contrast appeared in 10ml(0.25mmol/kg) group when the enhancement of lung tissues was rather low, which suggests it is the optimal doses to

©CARS/Springer. All rights reserved.

perform pulmonary artery MR angiography but not for pulmonary perfusion imaging. Similar results appeared in table 2, where the signal intensity and SNR of parenchyma kept increasing as the dose of contrast medium increased, but the rising speed of SNR was very slow when the dose exceeded 15ml. The subjective evaluation also suggested that similar perfusion effects were found in the last 3 groups that were not necessary to use more contrast medium when the dose reached 0.35 mmol/kg. We concluded that the optimal dose for CEMRA is about 0.25mmol/kg, but above 0.35mmol/kg for PPI.

The embolisms in larger vessels can be depicted easily by any imaging modality, but it remains a challenge to detect embolisms in subsegmental pulmonary arteries. The present experiment was designed mainly to evaluate the value of CEMRA and PPI in the diagnosis of subsegmental pulmonary embolisms. In our results, 11 gelatin sponged particles lead to 10 lesions of pulmonary embolism, one reason that the number of embolized lesions did not corresponded to the injected particles is that the diameter of particles might be too small, another reason might be that two particles entered one vessel. Because the caliber of pulmonary arteries in pig were smaller than those in human being and the breath was not controlled, it was rather difficult to depict subsegmental arteries using CEMRA, these were much a different case in human being. Although CEMRA found less embolized lesions than DSA, but almost all pulmonary infarctions were found after combining with perfusion imaging. The sensitivity of pulmonary perfusion imaging in detecting of embolization is very high, but false-positive results may occur when compared with pathological findings. Both of 2 false-positive lesions in our study located in upper lung field, and mainly because of heart beating artifacts. We believed that, as technique advances in the future, CEMRA would play a very important role in the diagnosis of pulmonary embolism when combined with pulmonary perfusion imaging.

References

1. Yucel EK . Pulmonary MR angiography: is it ready now? Radiology, 210: 301-303,1999.
2. Loubeyre P, Rrevel D, Douek P, et al. Dynamic contrast-enhanced MR angiography of pulmonary embolism: comparison with pulmonary angiography. AJR, 162: 1035-1039,1994.
3. Meaney JF, Prince MR. Pulmonary MR angiography. Magn Reson Imaging Clin N Am, 7: 393-409,1999
4. Gupta A, Frazer CK, Ferguson-JM, et al. Acute pulmonary embolism: diagnosis with MR angiography. Radiology, 210: 353-359, 1999
5. Prince MR, Grist TM, Debatin JF. 3D Contrast MR Angiography. Springer, Germany, P3-52, 1999
6. Steiner P, McKinnon GC, Romanowski B, et al. Contrast-enhanced, ultrafast 3D pulmonary MR angiography in a single breath-hold: initial assessment of imaging performance. J-Magn-Reson-Imaging, 7: 177-182,1997
7. Meaney JF, Prince MR. Pulmonary MR angiography. Magn Reson Imaging Clin N Am, 7: 393-409, 1999
8. Alley MT, Shifrin RY, Pelc NJ, et al. Ultrafast contrast-enhanced three-dimensional MR angiography: state of the art. Radiographics, 18: 273-285, 1998
9. Lentschig MG, Reimer P, Rausch Lentschig UL, et al. Breath-hold gadolinium-enhanced MR angiography of the major vessels at 1.0 T: dose-response findings and angiographic correlation. Radiology, 208: 353-357, 1998
10. Hatabu H. MR pulmonary angiography and perfusion imaging: recent advances. Semin Ultrasound CT MR, 18: 349-361, 1997

CARS 2002 – H.U. Lemke, M.W. Vannier; K. Inamura, A.G. Farman, K. Doi & J.H.C. Reiber (Editors)
©CARS/Springer. All rights reserved.

A virtual training system for linear-type endoscopic ultrasonography

Silke Hacker[a], Ulf Tiede[a], Eike Burmester[b], Thomas Leineweber[b], Karl Heinz Höhne[a]

[a] Institute of Mathematics and Computer Science in Medicine (IMDM), University Hospital Eppendorf, Hamburg, Germany

[b] Department of Hepatology and Gastroenterology, Städtisches Krankenhaus Süd, Lübeck, Germany

Abstract

Endoscopic Ultrasonography (EUS) is used for examinations of the gastrointestinal tract and neighboring organs. With the linear-type EUS highly accurate tumor characterization and staging is possible. However, this most difficult endoscopic procedure is particularly hard to learn. Because of the high flexibility of the endoscope's tip oblique cross-sections can be reached which clinicians are not familiar with. The presented EUS training system that is based on the Visible Human is intended to significantly reduce the training effort of learning this sophisticated technique. EUS examinations in oesophagus, stomach and duodenum can be interactively practiced. Due to the integrated knowledge base it is possible to learn the anatomy as it appears on a sonographic plane. A comprehensive understanding of this special anatomy is necessary for an optimal use of the EUS technique.

Keywords: Endoscopic ultrasonography, virtual reality training system, Visible Human

1. Introduction

Endoscopic ultrasonography (EUS) is a combination of endoscopy and ultrasonography, a small ultrasonic probe being incorporated into the tip of an endoscope. In the past 20 years it has become the most significant advance for imaging the gastrointestinal wall and neighboring organs. The concept behind EUS is to decrease the distance between the ultrasonic source and the organs to be imaged. While endoscopically visualizing the lumen, the probe can be guided and placed adjacent to the area of interest. The short distance between the ultrasonic source and the target permits the use of high frequency, high resolution sound waves which, due to their shorter penetration depth, are not suitable for transcutaneous ultrasonography. High resolution EUS is capable of providing more accurate tumor characterization and staging [1].

Two methods of ultrasound scanning have been applied to intraluminal sonography. The *radial scanner*, that has been the most widely used method, produces a 360° circular scan that is perpendicular to the endoscope shaft. This type of scan facilitates orientation of the probe in the gastrointestinal lumen. The generated images are more or less transverse

©CARS/Springer. All rights reserved.

sections of the human body that clinicians are familiar with due to imaging modalities like computer tomography.
The *linear-type scanner*, that was introduced in the nineties, provides a 120° sector parallel to the shaft axis. This image orientation has allowed the development of biopsy techniques [2]. The biopsy needle can be directed to the target because it is in line with the scanning plane. Unfortunately, this sophisticated diagnostic technique is particularly hard to learn. Because of the high flexibility of the endoscope's tip the scanning plane can be oriented at any oblique angle, making orientation very difficult. Cross-sections can be reached that can not be found in any printed anatomical atlases. Since the position and the orientation of the probe is not visible, anatomical landmark structures have to be identified for navigation. For this purpose a thorough knowledge of oblique cross-sectional anatomy is mandatory for image interpretation. To facilitate the learning of this most difficult endoscopic procedure we have developed an interactive training system that is based on the Visible Human [3]. It simulates a linear-type EUS examination of the gastrointestinal tract while showing the corresponding photographic image sector. With this system orientation and navigation of an echoendoscope in the gastrointestinal tract can be practiced. As well the special anatomical knowledge referring to EUS can be learned.

2. Methods

The EUS training system was developed using the VOXEL-MAN volume visualization environment as an authoring tool [4]. The underlying three-dimensional model is based on the male Visible Human and contains more than 650 three-dimensional anatomical constituents and more than 2000 relations between them [5]. Some structures like the pancreatic and the bile duct that are particularly important for EUS examinations were supplemented for this application.

We calculated virtual EUS scenes for six characteristic positions in oesophagus, stomach and duodenum using an extended QuickTime VR format. The QuickTime VR format provides a two-dimensional matrix of images. The corresponding two degrees of freedom that are controlled by mouse movement were used to simulate the navigation of the ultrasonic probe through the human body. The probe can be rotated in two directions: 360° around the axis of the endoscope and 32° around the roll axis of the ultrasonic fan. For each of the six scenes we calculated 17 x 180 (= 3060) single images.

Each of the scenes consists of a three-dimensional overview image that shows the current position and orientation of the ultrasonic probe in relation to important vessels and organs, and of the corresponding anatomical cross-section (Fig. 1). The cross-sections have been overlaid with a mask, so that only the sector is visible that would be seen in an EUS examination.

We extended the QuickTime format in order to also hold information about the anatomical objects shown (concept of "intelligent movies" [6]). The scenes are connected to a knowledge base containing object descriptions within the structure of a semantic network. Different networks exist for different views, e.g. systematic or topographic anatomy. Within the views the anatomical constituents are linked by relations like "part

©CARS/Springer. All rights reserved.

of" or "branching to". Three different nomenclatures for the anatomical objects are available: English, Latin and German.

3. Results

The precalculated scenes allow an interactive simulation of an EUS examination of a detailed three-dimensional anatomical model in real time. The system runs on a standard PC and does not have any special hardware requirements. The simple user interface makes it easy also for the beginner to navigate the virtual ultrasonic probe through the human body.

The probe can be rotated in two directions by mouse movement. Although the system has only two degrees of freedom to control the probe, instead of six as in a real examination, it has been turned out that all important anatomical landmark structures can be reached. These landmarks that are mostly blood vessels are of particular relevance for the navigation of the probe through the interior of the body because during a real EUS examination position and orientation of the probe is not visible.

Because of the integrated knowledge base visible objects can be interrogated or annotated at any time. This is possible in different languages (see Fig. 1). Likewise, objects can be painted to show their extent. As well it is possible to automatically find a probe orientation for which a selected object is best visible in the associated image sector.
Due to the conjunction of the EUS scenes with a knowledge base it is possible to learn the anatomy as it appears on a sonographic plane. A comprehensive understanding of this special anatomy is necessary for an optimal interpretation of EUS images.

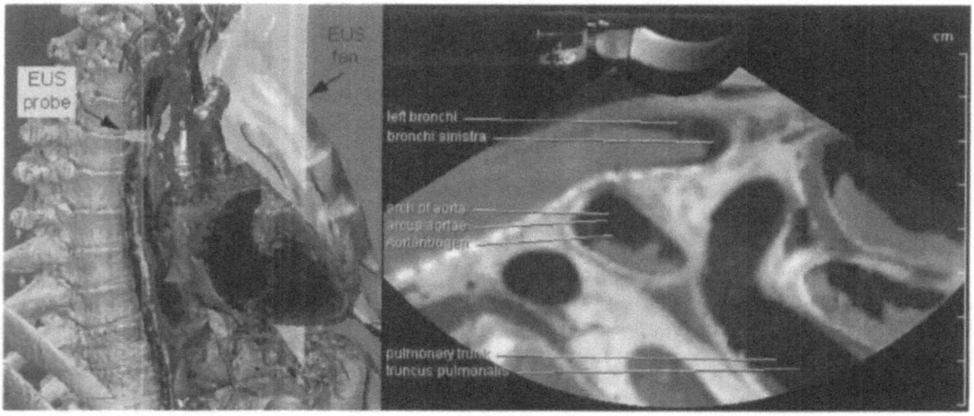

Fig. 1: EUS simulation with the probe located in the middle oesophagus. Left: Overview image that shows position and orientation of the probe. Right: Corresponding anatomical image sector. Here annotations of several anatomical objects in different languages have been made.

To evaluate the suitability of the system for training purposes we tried to generate corresponding anatomical cross-sections to real EUS images. EUS images of individual

©CARS/Springer. All rights reserved.

patients can not be perfectly matched to the Visible Human data due to morphological variations and deformations of organs during an EUS examination. But it still was possible to recreate real EUS images using the presented training system.

Figure 2 shows a endosonographic image of the bile duct and the pancreas with the EUS probe located in the duodenum. The same situation can be seen in the simulated scene in figure 3. Whereas the real EUS image is very hard to interpret not only because of sonographic artifacts, but also due to the unusual angle of vision, the simulated situation is much easier to understand. The photographic representation of the image sector facilitates the identification of the visible objects. At the same time, the three-dimensional model helps to keep track of the current position of the probe and the orientation of its sonographic fan in relation to important landmark structures.

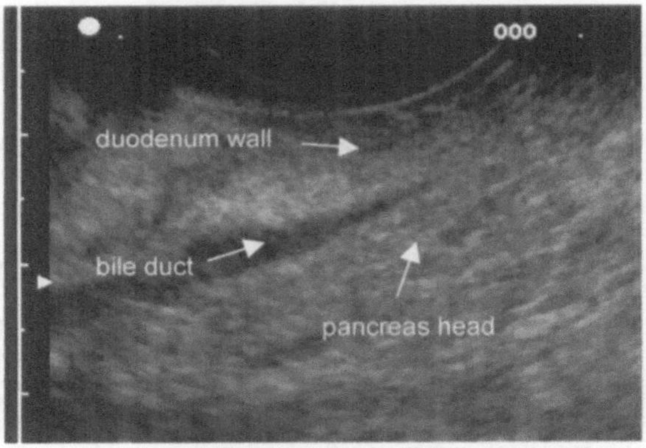

Fig. 2: Endosonographic image of the bile duct and pancreas. The EUS probe is located in the duodenum

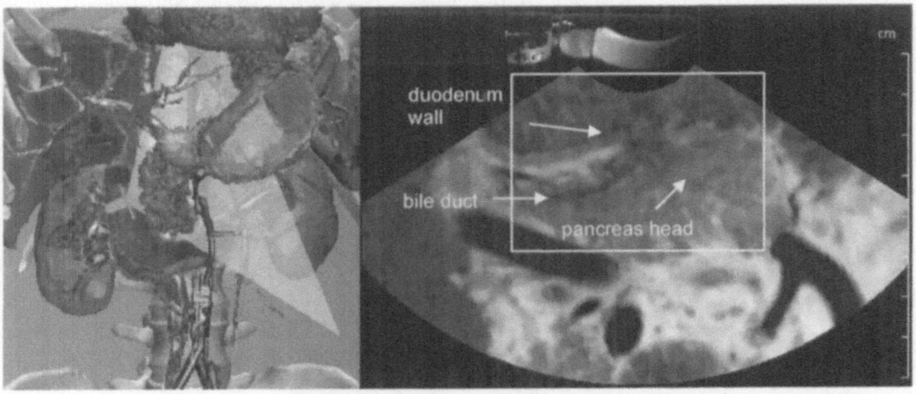

Fig. 3: Simulated EUS examination corresponding to figure 2. Left: Overview image that shows the EUS probe located in the duodenum. Right: EUS image sector based on photographic data. The rectangle marks the area that is visible in the real EUS image in fig. 2.

©CARS/Springer. All rights reserved.

4. Conclusion

The linear-type EUS is a tool for highly accurate tumor characterization and staging, that is often otherwise obtainable only by surgical techriques. However, this method is particularly operator dependent. Its optimal use requires considerable prior experience not only in gastrointestinal endoscopy and abdominal ultrasonography, but also sufficient training with the technique itself. It is expected that with the presented virtual training system the time needed to learn this technique safely could be significantly reduced. It is not only suitable for the beginner but also useful for the expert as a reference system.

A further development of the training system could be the simulation of ultrasonic images calculated from the anatomical cross-sections. However, the calculation of such images has not yet been solved satisfactorily.

References

1. H. Snady, "Role of endoscopic ultrasonography in diagnosis, staging, and outcome of gastrointestinal diseases", *The Gastroenterologist*, pp. 91-110, 1994.
2. T. Rösch, U. Will, and K. Chang, eds., *Longitudincl Endosonography*, Springer, Berlin-Heidelberg, 2001.
3. V. Spitzer, M. J. Ackerman, A. L. Scherzinger, D. Whitlock, "The visible human male: a technical report", *J. Am. Med. Inform. Assoc.*, Vol. 3 (2), pp.118-130, 1996.
4. A. Pommert, K. H. Höhne, B. Pflesser, E. Richter, M. Riemer, T. Schiemann, R. Schubert, U. Schumacher, U. Tiede," Creating a high-resolution spatial/ symbolic model of the inner organs based on the Visible Human", *Medical Image Analysis*, Vol. 5, pp. 221-228, 2001.
5. K. H. Höhne, B. Pflesser, A. Pommert, M. Riemer, R. Schubert, T. Schiemann, U. Tiede, U. Schumacher, "A realistic model of human structure from the Visible Human data", *Meth. Inform. Med.*, Vol. 40, No. 2, pp. 83-89, 2001.
6. R. Schubert, B. Pflesser, A. Pommert, K. Priesmeyer, M. Riemer, T. Schiemann, U. Tiede, P. Steiner, K. H. Höhne, "Interactive volume visualization using 'intelligent movies'", *Medicine meets virtual reality*, J. D. Westwood, H. M. Hoffman, R. A. Robb, D. Stredney (Eds.), Vol. 62 of *Health Technology and Informatics*, pp. 321-327, IOS Press, Amsterdam, 1999.

Image Processing and Display

CARS 2002 – H.U. Lemke, M.W. Vannier; K. Inamura, A.G. Farman, K. Doi & J.H.C. Reiber (Editors)
©CARS/Springer. All rights reserved.

Automated quantification of avascular necrosis of the femoral head (ANFH) from 3D MR images

Reza A. Zoroofi[a, b], Takashi Nishii[c], Yoshinobu Sato[b],
Nobuhiko Sugano[c], Hideki Yoshikawa[c], Takahiro Ochi[d], Shinichi Tamura[b]
[a] Faculty of Engineering, University of Tehran, Tehran 14395/515, Iran
[b] Division of Interdisciplinary Image Analysis
[c] Department of Orthopaedic Surgery
[d] Division of Computer Assisted Orthopaedic Surgery
Osaka University Medical School, Suita, Osaka 565-0871, Japan

Abstract

Avascular necrosis, better known as osteonecrosis, of the femoral head (ANFH), is a disease that causes death of bone. A femoral head with large necrotic lesions may progress to collapse, and ultimately require a total hip arthroplasty (THA). This paper proposes an automatic technique for segmentation and quantitative assessment of necrotic lesions of the femoral head using coronal MRI data. Quantification of ANFH consists of the following steps: (1) Rough segmentation of non-necrotic lesions of the femur by 3D grey morphological operations and 3D region growing techniques. (2) Fitting a 3D ellipse to the femoral head utilizing the anatomical information of the femur, and employing principal component analysis and simulated annealing algorithm. (3) Classification of necrotic and non-necrotic lesions of the femoral head inside the ellipse by a k-means clustering technique. (4) Normalizing the 3-D ellipse to a sphere and extracting features such as size, orientation, centeroid, principal components, etc. of necrotic lesions. Feasibility of the method is demonstrated on 40 sets of in vivo T1-weighted MR images of actual patients.

Keywords: Bone segmentation, femoral head modelling, osteonecrosis quantification

1. Introduction

Avascular necrosis of the femoral head (ANFH) is associated with disruption of the blood flow to the femoral head. Four basic mechanisms are implicated: (I) mechanical disruption, e.g., broken hip; (II) external pressure on or damage to a vessel wall, e.g., vasculitis, radiation therapy; (III) arterial thrombosis or embolism, e.g., sickle cell diseases, prednisone, alcohol; and (IV) venous or blood outflow occlusion, e.g., infection [1]. There are two staging classifications of ANFH, one based on radiographs [2] and the other based on MR signal intensities [3]. The accuracy of radiographic staging may be improved using CT to detect a subchondral lucency indicating advanced stage of the disease. However, that CT does not depict the earliest marrow abnormalities resulting in osteonecrosis. Early diagnosis of ANFH using MRI is important, since the disease occurs in relatively young individuals with an average age of 20 to 50, and since treatment options for more advanced disease are frequently unsuccessful [4]. Hence, finding

©CARS/Springer. All rights reserved.

quantitative criteria to stage the necrotic lesions of the femoral head and assess the susceptibility for collapse or to predict impending collapse for each case before it occurs [11], is an important aspect of the corresponding researches [4], [5], [7]-[11]. In a previous paper [12], we developed a semi-automatic technique for segmentation of ANFH using MRI (T1-weighted) coronal data sets. In this paper, we have improved the performance of the previous technique in terms of accuracy, user interaction, and quantitative assessments. The developed algorithms are integrated in the MEDAL software [18] and available in the Internet.

2. The proposed technique

2.1 Rough segmentation of femur

It is known that MRI data sets are not always in ideal imaging conditions [6]. To reduce the effect of noise and non-uniformity of bone tissues, smoothing of images were applied in the previous work [12]. In some cases, the femur is partly surrounded with fat. In the same manner as of bone tissues, fat tissues are of high density. In the previous work, smoothing was followed by binary thresholding. In this case, surrounding fat tissues of the femoral head may strongly attach bone tissues [See left side image in Fig.1 (a)]. Hence, finding appropriate smoothing parameters, accurate threshold value and number of binary morphological operations will be far from a simple task. Although by selecting higher threshold values and increasing number of binary erosions we may succeed to detach fat and bone tissues from each other, however, due to non-linear nature of thresholding and morphological operations, shape of the extracted femur might be different from the actual shape. In this research, smoothing, thresholding and binary morphological operations were replaced by 3D grey morphological operations and 3D region growing techniques. Three typical slices of a femur with avascular necrosis of the femoral head (ANFH) are shown in Fig.1 (a). Fig. 1(b) depicts the histogram associated with 56 images in the data set. Two separate peaks in the histogram are associated with low and high intensity regions of the image. By employing a bimodal thresholding approach [17], separation of the dark and bright regions of the images was possible. But, as we noted earlier, separation of two bright regions such as fatty and bony tissues were not guaranteed. Fig.1(c) is the result of grey morphological erosions of the images shown in (a). By this operation, nearby bony and fatty regions are well separated. The histogram of the resultant images in Fig. (c) was calculated. The obtained histogram was similar to that of (b). A Gaussian function was fitted to the second peak of the histogram [see arrow in Fig. (b)]. The variance of this Gaussian function was used in the 3D region growing operation. The seed point of the 3D region growing was selected by clicking the mouse button on the femoral head before staring the automatic quantification on the computer. The procedure was followed by a 3D morphological dilation. Fig.1 (d) shows the results of region growing and grey morphological dilation. Next, the procedure followed by filling the holes and binarizing of the images obtained in (d). The results are shown in Fig. 1(e). Overlay of the extracted boundary of femur and original image is shown in Fig.1 (f). The goal of the above operations was to roughly segment the upper part of femur, particularly the femoral head. The segmentation result is used in the next Section to fit a 3D ellipse to the femoral head.

©CARS/Springer. All rights reserved.

2.2 Segmentation of avascular necrosis of the femoral

A femoral head resembles part of a 3D ellipse. In order to develop an automatic method for ellipse fitting [13]-[15], we investigated ten normal femoral heads. Figs. 2(a) to (c) shows three slices of a typical femur. Figs.2 (d) to (f) represent corresponding segmentation results obtained by employing the method proposed in Section 2.1. The overlays of the largest cross-section of a 3D-ellipse and the femoral head are shown in Figs. 2(d) to (f). Point #2 is the centre and the line specified by points #1 and #2 denotes the radius of this circle. The line that are specified by points #3 and #4 separates the femoral head and femoral neck from each other. It was heuristically found that those parts of the femur that are located in the north-west (in the direction of the normal of the line #3-#4), and inside the overlaid circles surround the femoral head tissues. We estimated the above four points by employing the anatomical landmark of the femur. Point #1 is corresponding to the left most point in the data set. Point #2 is the centre of the upper binary component in those coronal slices of the data set that the femur main body and femoral head are separated from each other [see Figs. 2(b) and (e)]. Point #5 is associated with the top most point of the greater trochanter and point #6 is corresponding to the right most point of the lesser trochanter. These points can be automatically obtained from the coronal slices of the data set that only femur body (not femoral head) are available [see Figs. 2(c) and (f)]. The line that separates the femur body and femoral head (line #3-#4) was obtained as follows: from point #2, a perpendicular line with respect to line #5,#6 was drawn. Line #3-#4 was found by drawing a line from the middle of the above perpendicular line in parallel with line #5-#6. By automatically specifying the above circle and line (#3-#4), the search space and initial centre and radiuses of the 3D-ellipse were estimated. Point [c_x, c_y, (0.5 x *depth*)] was used as the initial centre of the ellipses where (c_x, c_y) is the centre of the circle [see Fig. 2] and *depth* is number of slices. Then, in the same manner as of our previous work [12], the principal components, i.e., Eigen values and Eigen vectors of the binary data that were located in the north west of the image (in the direction of the normal of line #3-#4) were calculated. In this case, initial orientations of three major axes of the 3D ellipse were assigned in the direction of three Eigen vectors. By using the above initial values and a simulated annealing technique [16], a 3D ellipse was fitted to the femoral head. Typical results of the proposed technique are depicted in Fig. 3. Fig. 3(a) shows three slices of a data set with ANFH. In Fig. 3(b), the cross section of estimated 3D ellipse are overlaid with these slices. Finally, by using a k-means clustering algorithm [17], bone tissues inside the 3D ellipse were classified into three classes including non-necrotic lesions, low necrotic lesions and high necrotic lesions. These classes of bone tissues are shown as bright, intermediate and low intensity pixels in the overlaid ellipse. Fig. 3(c) shows the result of the surface rendering of the femur with low and high necrotic lesions of the femoral head.

2.3 Quantification of necrotic lesions

After fitting a 3D ellipse to the whole femoral head, the following steps were performed to define a coordinate system for comparisons of femoral heads of different cases: (I) normalizing the 3D ellipse to a sphere; (II) Assigning centre of the sphere as the centre of the world coordinate; (III) Assigning the major axes of the 3D ellipse as the xyz-axes of the world coordinate. In the next step, quantification of avascular necrosis of the femoral head was achieved by calculating the following features: (1) Percentages of the whole

©CARS/Springer. All rights reserved.

femoral head, non necrotic lesions of the femoral head, and necrotic lesions of the femoral head, with respect to the fitted sphere; (2) Percentages of moderate and severe necrotic lesions with respect to the fitted sphere; (3) Distances (mean and standard deviation) of moderate and severe necrotic lesions with respect to both the centre and surface of the femoral head; (4) Angle (mean and standard deviation) of necrotic lesions with respect to the horizontal axis (5) Principal components of necrotic lesions. Statistical evaluation and quantitative assessment of ANFH using the above mentioned features will be reported as a separate article.

3. Results

Data sets of 40 patients were available for evaluations. Among 80 (40x2) femoral heads, 30 femoral heads were either severely destroyed or a total hip surgery were performed for them. In these cases, automated segmentation and quantification were not clinically useful. Hence, the remaining 50 femurs were used in the experiments. In the first part of the experiments the proposed technique for rough segmentation of the upper part of femur was evaluated. That is the ratio of true positive (TP) to wrong segmentation results [wrong segmentation points were obtained by adding false positive and, true negative (TN) pixels.]. Rough segmentation technique was regarded successful if correctly segmented tissues of the femur were above 90%. For results with a performance higher than 80% and lower than 90%, two human operators subjectively made decision about the success or failure of technique. Results with segmentation accuracy of less than 80% were considered as the failure of the algorithm. It was concluded that the technique for segmentation of femur was successful in 47 cases. In three cases, the imaging conditions were very poor and the technique was not effective to deliver acceptable results. In the second part of the experiments, the ellipse fitting technique was applied to the above 47 sets of segmented femurs. The above mentioned evaluation technique was employed to estimate the success rate of 3D ellipse fitting technique. In this case, 43 femoral heads were successfully fitted by 3D ellipses. In four cases anatomical shapes of femurs were abnormal and far from those of typical femurs. For this reason, finding the proposed anatomical landmark shown in Fig. 2 was very difficult and hence the ellipse fitting technique was not successful. In conclusions, 43 femoral heads (out of 50) were automatically estimated. That is, the success rate of the algorithm in the presence of actual clinical data was 86%. For a data set with a size of 256x256x56 pixels, and an IBM compatible personal computer (Pentium IV processor: 1GHZ, Memory: 512 Mbytes) the proposed technique takes around two minutes to quantify non-necrotic and necrotic lesions of the femoral head. All algorithms of this research are implemented in the MEDAL software [18].

4. Conclusion

In this paper, we developed an automatic method for quantification of avascular necrosis of the femoral head (ANFH). The success rate of the algorithm in the presence of actual clinical data was 86%. A 3-D ellipse was automatically fitted to the femoral head. The ellipse was then normalization to a sphere. By this normalization, femoral heads of different patients could be treated in a unique coordinate system and comparative

©CARS/Springer. All rights reserved.

quantification of necrotic lesions of different femoral heads is possible. Developing an automatic technique for assessment of femoral heads with non-elliptic shapes will be considered in our future work. Accumulating enough data sets, extracting corresponding key features, and developing a computer-assisted decision support system for quantification of ANFH are other steps of this research.

Acknowledgements

This work was supported by the Japan Society for the Promotion of Science (JSPS Research for the Future Program).

References

1. http://rothmaninstitute.com/joints/hip/
2. Ficat RP, Arlet J., *Necrosis of the femoral head*, pp.171-182, Williams&Wilkins, Baltimore, 1980.
3. Mitchell DG, Rao VM, Dalinka MK, et al., "Femoral head avascular necrosis: correlation of MR imaging, radiographic staging, radionuclide imaging, and clinical findings", *Radiology*, vol. 162: pp. 709-715, 1987.
4. http://www.mri.jhu.edu.
5. Sugano N, Takaoka K, Ohzono K, Matsui M, Masuhara K, Ono K., "Prognostication of non traumatic avascular necrosis of the femoral head", *Clin Orthop*, vol. 303, pp. 155-164, 1994.
6. Vlaardingerbroek MT, Boer JA, *Magnetic Resonance Imaging, Theory and Practice*, Springer-Verlag, Berlin, 1996.
7. Holman AJ, Gardner GC, Richardson ML, Simkin PA, "Quantitative magnetic resonance imaging predicts clinical outcome of core decompression for osteonecrosis of the femoral head", *J Rheumatol*, vol. 22, pp. 1929-1933, 1995.
8. Ito H, Matsuno T, Kaneda K, "Prognosis of early stage avascular necrosis of the femoral head", *Clin Orthop*, vol. 358, pp. 149-157, 1999.
9. Koo KH, Kim R, "Quantifying the extent of osteonecrosis of the femoral head", *J Bone Joint Surg [Br]*, vol. 77-B(6), pp. 875-880, 1995.
10. Mankin HJ, "Non traumatic necrosis of bone (osteonecrosis) ", *N Engl J Med*, vol. 326, pp. 1473, 1992.
11. Kim YM, Ahn JH, Kang HS, Kim HJ, "Estimation of the extent of osteonecrosis of the femoral head using MRI", *J Bone Joint Surg [Br]*, vol. 80-B (6), pp.954-958, 1998.
12. Zoroofi RA, Nishii T, Sato Y, Sugano N, Yoshikawa H, Tamura S., "Segmentation of avascular necrosis of the femoral head using 3-D MR images", *Computerized Medical Imaging and Graphics* [in press].
13. Wong YY, Yuen PC, Tong CS, "Segmented snake for contour detection", *Pattern Recogn*, vol. 31, pp. 1669-1679, 1998.
14. Ho CT, Chen LH, "A fast ellipse/circle detector using geometric symmetry", *Pattern Recogn*, vol. 28(1), pp. 117-124, 1995.
15. Wu Z, "The robust algorithms for finding the center of an Arc", *Comput Vision Imag Unders*, vol. 62(3), pp. 269-278, 1995.
16. Press WH, Teukolsky SA, Vetterling WT, Flannery BP, *Numerical Recipes in C*, Cambridge Univ. Press, Cambridge, 1992.
17. R. C. Gonzalez and R.E. Woods, *Digital image processing*, Addison-Wesley, New York, 1992.
18. http://www.image.med.osaka-u.ac.jp/reza/medal.html

©CARS/Springer. All rights reserved.

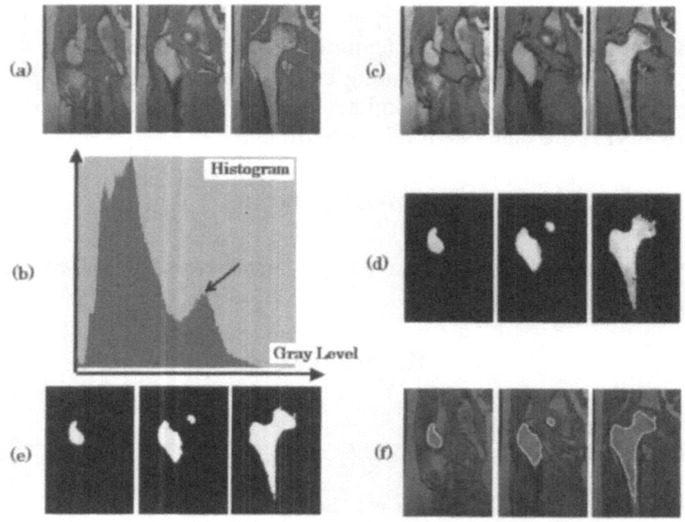

Fig. 1: Rough segmentation of the femur. Details are discussed in Section 2.1.

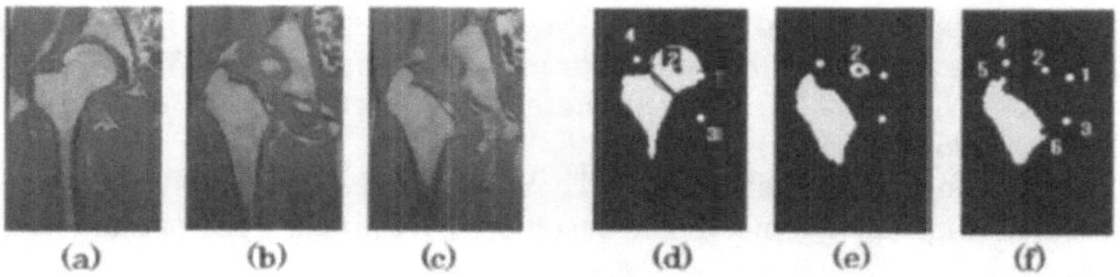

Fig. 2: Procedures for finding the initial values of a 3D ellipse. See Section 2.3 for details.

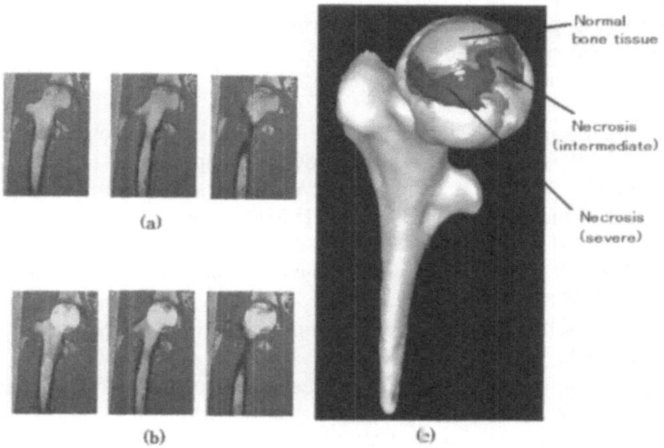

Fig. 3: Classification of non-necrotic and necrotic lesions of the femoral head. (a) Three typical slices of the femoral head. (b) Result of automatic segmentation. (c) Surface rendering of non-necrotic and necrotic lesions of the femoral head.

CARS 2002 – H.U. Lemke, M.W. Vannier; K. Inamura, A.G. Farman, K. Doi & J.H.C. Reiber (Editors)
©CARS/Springer. All rights reserved.

Efficient segmentation of MSCT images by interactive region expansion

Cristian Lorenz, Thorsten Schlathölter, Ingwer Carlsen, Steffen Renisch
Philips Research Laboratories, Röntgenstrasse 24-26,
D-22041 Hamburg, Germany

Abstract

A majority of medical image segmentation problems still refuse completely automatic treatment. These can today only be solved using interactive techniques. Efficient interactive solutions however, require a combination of a fast segmentation technique, an appropriate interaction scheme and the ability of real-time rendering of intermediate 3D segmentation results. This enables the user to instantly intervene and correct the procedure if necessary. Especially challenging is the task of interactive segmentation of large multi-slice CT (MSCT) datasets containing 512^3 or more voxels. In this paper we present an approach for fast interactive prioritised region expansion. A set of user defined seed voxels is expanded according to a given priority criterion. Intermediate segmentation results are frequently displayed to the user. At any time the user may stop or partially undo the procedure. We demonstrate the technique applying it to MSCT data for several problematic areas, such as distinction between bone and vascular structures, bone disarticulation and the segmentation of the bronchial tree.

Keywords: Multi-Slice CT, region expansion, interactive segmentation

1. Introduction

A variety of region expansion algorithms are currently used for image segmentation. They range from simple threshold based region-growing [1] to sophisticated level-set methods [2]. For interactive approaches, it is especially suitable if the region expansion process is steered by a criterion that is related to the probability of a voxel to be part of the desired target object (priority criterion). This means that during the expansion process voxels being more likely to be part of the target object are added before voxels that are less likely. The idea of a "directed" region growing in that sense has been reported in [3]. At a certain point, voxels will be added that the user will no longer consider being part of the target object. Either, this situation is detected automatically by an appropriate stopping criterion (this road is followed in [3]), or as we propose in this paper, the decision is up to user. Given that the intermediate results of the expansion process are frequently displayed to the user, the method proposed in this paper enables the user to stop, continue or even partially undo the expansion process in order to reach the desired degree of expansion. For real-time visualization of intermediate results a special surface shading technique has been developed, similar to the approaches described in [4,5]. The method allows the parallel segmentation of several objects. This can be e.g. used for the virtual disarticulation of

©CARS/Springer. All rights reserved.

joints into its bone components or for the separation of bone and vascular structures in CTA images.

2. The region expansion algorithm

The region expansion algorithm is started with a set of seed-points to which subsequently voxels are added to the following criteria:

- A similarity criterion. During the expansion process this criterion locally determines if a given voxel is added to the object being currently expanded (expansion-object).
- A priority criterion. This criterion determines the order in which the object is being expanded.
- A stopping criterion. If this criterion is met, the expansion process is stopped globally. It can be used to restrict the growing process to a certain number of grow steps, a time interval, a maximal size of the object surface etcetera.

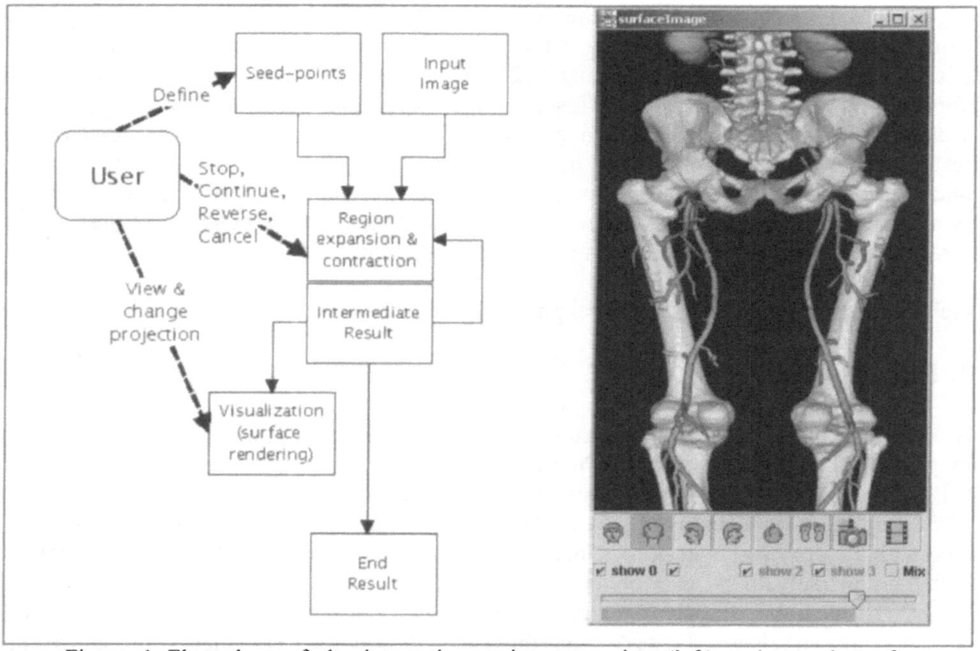

Figure 1 Flow-chart of the interactive region expansion (left) and snapshot of a prototypical realization (right). The user controls the region grower using the slider visible at the lower part of the prototype. The slider position corresponds to a certain number of expansion steps (expansion target) and defines the stopping criterion for the expansion process.

A frequently used similarity criterion for CT data is a lower and upper threshold in terms of a certain Hounsfield (or gray) value range. The priority criterion again may be defined on the basis of Hounsfield values, e.g. "expand first the neighbour with the highest Hounsfield value". Other possibilities are to prefer small gradient magnitudes or a small

©CARS/Springer. All rights reserved.

variance of Hounsfield values in a given neighbourhood. For neighbour voxels of the same Hounsfield value, a first-in first-out strategy applies. Input of the region expansion algorithm is a set of seed voxels being expanded during the process. Different types of seed voxels are allowed to support simultaneous segmentation of several objects. While expanding, an ordered set of voxels to be expanded is maintained (expand-list). The set initially contains the seed voxels. The ordering of the set is defined by the priority criterion. The expansion-process stops if the expand-list becomes empty or if the stopping criterion is met.

The elementary expansion-action consists of the following steps:

- The voxel v with the highest priority is removed from the expand-list.
- The 6-neighbors n_i of v are checked against the similarity criterion. If the criterion is met and the voxel n_i is not already part of the grow-object, n_i is added to the expand-object and to the expand-list.

2.1 Reversible region expansion

In order to give the user complete and immediate control over the expansion process, the algorithm has been designed to allow a reversion of the expansion process. A reversion, i.e. a region contraction, can be achieved in principally two ways: Inversion of the expansion criteria or inversion of the elementary expansion action. Region contraction by inversion of the expansion criteria means basically that the execution of the expansion process is continued, but with a different set of criteria. It turns out that in this case in general it cannot be guaranteed that a given intermediate result of the expansion history can be recovered. In other words, the contraction is in general not an inverted expansion.

In order to guarantee an exact reversion of the expansion process we need to invert the elementary expansion action as shown in Figure 2. The disadvantage of this approach is the additional memory needed to store the history of elements being removed from the expand-list. However, the memory needed to do this scales with the size of the segmented object and not with the size of the 3D image.

Expansion	Contraction
The voxel v with the highest priority is removed from the expand-list.	The voxel v that lastly has been removed from the expand-list is put-back into the expand-list.
The 6-neighbors n_i of v are checked against the similarity criterion. If the criterion is met and the voxel n_i is not already part of the grow-object, n_i is added to the grow-object and to the expand-list.	The 6-neighbors n_i of v that have been added to the expand-list during the associated expansion step are removed from the grow-object and the expand-list.

Figure 2: Elementary action of the expansion and contraction process.

2.2 Performance issues

The target applications of the work reported here deal with large 3D MSCT datasets being processed in a real-time fashion. The requirements with respect to performance and memory consumption are very tight. Appropriate data structures play an essential role for a useful implementation of the described approaches. The basic data structure of a region expansion algorithms is a queue, a dynamic set with a first-in, first-out (FIFO) policy [6]. In case of a priority-criterion based region expansion, the queue has to be re-placed by an

©CARS/Springer. All rights reserved.

ordered set. The optimal realisation of an ordered set depends on the application, especially on the value-range of the order criterion. For an arbitrary value range, a binary tree structure [6] would be a reasonable solution. It delivers the needed operations in $\Theta(\lg n)$ time (given the tree is balanced), n being the size of the binary tree. In case of the integer voxel gray-value being used as order criterion the situation is different. Here, accessing the ordered set in constant time can be achieved. In order to reduce the amount of memory required per queued voxel, information about voxel position and object type is squeezed into a 32 bit integer. Due to the directional expansion process, the information needed to enable an inversion of the expansion process can be efficiently compressed to approx. 3 bits per voxel, leading in total to 35bit / voxel memory consumption during the expansion process.

3. Results

We utilized different combinations of criteria for the region expansion procedure. First, the Hounsfield value of the voxels of a CT image was directly taken as priority criterion. In this case, high-Hounsfield voxels are processed first which is well suited for bone segmentation in CT. Starting from one or more manually placed seed-point, the algorithms expands firstly into the dense parts of the bone (cortex) continuing with bone-marrow and finally reaching the transition zone to soft-tissue. The segmentation of the bone structures in a thorax CT image containing 720 slices of 512x512 pixels took 35s including frequent surface renderings (about 5 renderings/s). Four object types could be separated in parallel: Vertebrae and ribs, sternum, scapulae, and clavicles (Figure 3).

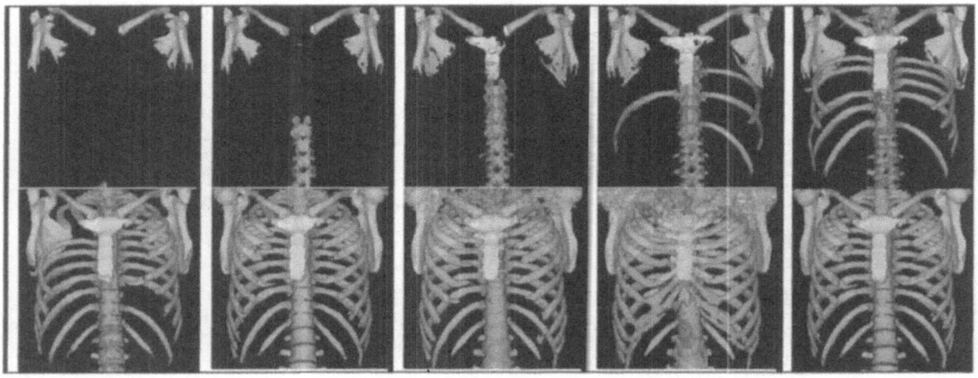

Figure 3: The image series show the segmentation progress of thorax bone structures in a CT image (720 slices, 512x512 pixel matrix). The procedure was initialized with one seed-point for the vertebral column, one seed-point for the sternum two seed-points for the scapulae and two seed-points for the clavicles. The expansion process has been reversed to achieve the end result (right-most image of second row). The procedure took 35 seconds on a 1 GHz Pentium .

©CARS/Springer. All rights reserved.

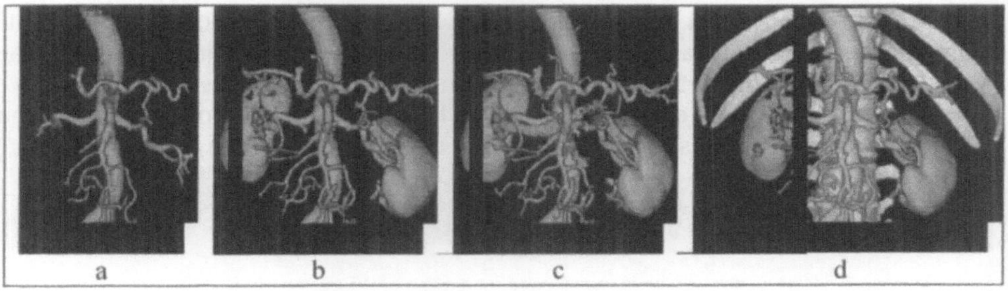

Figure 4: Abdominal angiographic MSCT dataset (323 slices, 512x512 pixel matrix, slice distance 0.70mm, pixel size 0.73mm). Bone and vascularity could be separated using one seed-point for each object type. Images (a-c) show the building up of the contrasted organs: In (a) mainly the larger arterial vessels are visible, (b) shows the arteries and kidneys, in (c) a part of the venous system can be seen. Vessels and bones are displayed in (d), the total segmented volume amounts to about 3 million voxels and was reached after 8 seconds on a 1 GHz PC. Again the priority criterion "grow high Hounsfield voxels first" was used.

The same method is well suited to separate vascular structures from bone structures in CTA images. This is demonstrated in Figure 4 with an angiographic MSCT image of the abdomen. By reversing the priority criterion (expand low Hounsfield voxels first) the method can be applied to the segmentation of the airways. Due to the small difference in Hounsfield values between bronchial lumen and the parenchyma, there is a tendency that

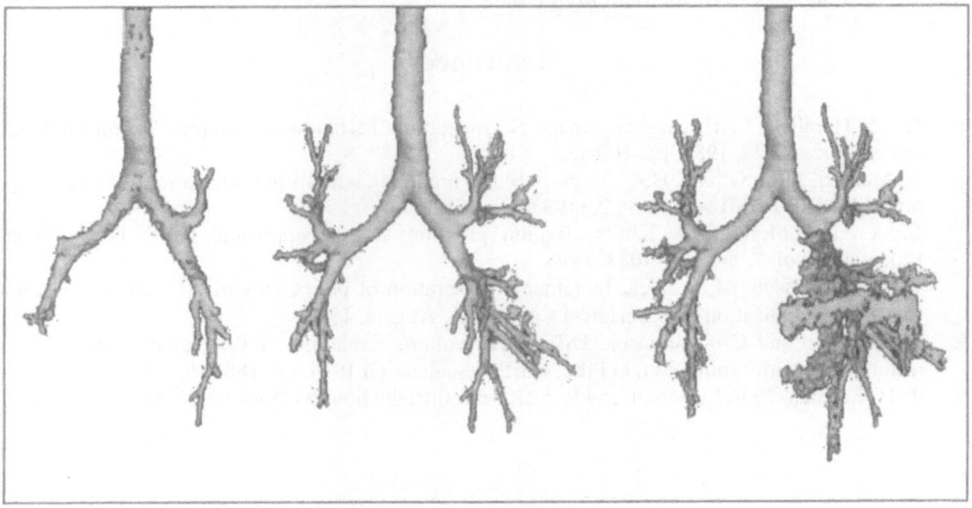

Figure 5: Thorax MSCT dataset (482 slices, 512x512 pixel matrix, slice distance 0.60mm, pixel size 0.63mm). Segmentation of the airways starting from one seed-point placed in the trachea. The priority criterion "grow low-Hounsfield voxels first" was used. Three stages of the region expansion process are shown. Due to the interactive approach, the user could easily select the optimal segmentation result (middle) just before leakage of the segmented volume into the parenchyma.

©CARS/Springer. All rights reserved.

the segmented volume leaks out into the parenchyma. For this reason, threshold or simple region grower based approaches are unable to segment the airways in CT images. The method described in this article has the same problem. However, due to the interactive approach the user is able to detect immediately when the expansion process leaks out and by inverting the grow process he is able to select an optimal result just before the leakage occurs (Figure 5).

4. Conclusions

Today's computer technology in combination with efficient software solutions enables real-time procedures on standard hardware for the segmentation and visualization of large image data sets as produced by multi-slice CT scanners. Combining fast priority steered region expansion algorithms with real-time rendering enables the user to efficiently perform interactive segmentations of medical images. The user can follow the segmentation in progress and may intervene immediately if necessary. The user may stop, continue, cancel or partially undo the segmentation in order to reach the desired result. Based on the described scenario, advanced interaction schemes may be developed, allowing the user further interactions, such as stopping or restricting locally the expansion process, adding further seed-points etc..

Acknowledgements

We like to thank Philips Medical Systems, especially PMS-CT and MIMIT-AD for kind support and the supply of medical image data.

References

1. R. M. Haralick, L. G. Shapiro, Image Segmentation Techniques, Comput. Vision Graphics Image Process., 29, 1985, pp. 100-132
2. R. Malladi, J.-A. Sethian, B.-C. Vemuri, Shape modeling with front propagation: a level set approach!, IEEE PAMI vol.17, no.2, (1995), pp.158-175
3. S. A. Hojjatoleslami, J. Kittler, Region growing: a new approach, IEEE Trans. Imag. Processing, vol. 7, pp.1079-1083, 1998
4. B. Gudmundsson, M. Randen, Incremental generation of projections of CT-volumes, in First Conf. on Visualization in Biomedical Computing, Atlanta, 1990
5. H. W. Shen and C. R. Johnson, Differential volume rendering: A fast volume visualization technique for flow animation, in Proc. IEEE Visualization 1994, pp. 188--195, 1994.
6. T. H. Cormen, C. E. Leiserson and R. L. Rivest, Introduction to algorithms, MIT Press, 1989

CARS 2002 – H.U. Lemke, M.W. Vannier; K. Inamura, A.G. Farman, K. Doi & J.H.C. Reiber (Editors)
©CARS/Springer. All rights reserved.

Automated segmentation of pelvis and femur from 3-D CT images

Reza A. Zoroofi[a, b], Yoshinobu Sato[b], Bahram Borgheai[a], Toshihiko Sasama[b], Takashi Nishii[c], Nobuhiko Sugano[c], Kazuo Yonenobu[c], Hideki Yoshikawa[c], Takahiro Ochi[d], Shinichi Tamura[b]

[a] Faculty of Engineering, University of Tehran, Tehran 14395/515, IRAN.
[b] Division of Interdisciplinary Image Analysis
[c] Department of Orthopaedic Surgery
[d] Division of Computer Assisted Orthopaedic Surgery
Osaka University Medical School, Suita, Osaka 565-0871, JAPAN.

Abstract

This paper presents a method for automatic segmentation of the pelvis and femur from clinical multi-slice computed tomography (CT) data. By defining several features, which represented the difficulty of segmentation, hip joints in the available 60 data sets were divided into four groups. The method consists of the following five steps: (1) Resampling of 3D CT data by a modified Sinc interpolation, to create isotropic volume and avoid Gibbs ringing; (2) Segmentation of bone tissues from other tissues in CT images by a novel adaptive thresholding technique based on a 3D pulses coupled neural networks (PCNN); (3) Estimation of initial boundary of the femoral head and the joint space between the acetabulum and femoral head by a new approach utilizing the constraints of the greater trochanter and femoral head shapes; (4) Enhancement of the hip joint space by a Hessian filter; and (5) Refinement of the rough boundary obtained in step (3) by employing a moving disk technique and the filtered images obtained in step (4). Feasibility of the method is evaluated in the presence of actual clinical data sets.

Keywords: Bone segmentation, pulse coupled neural networks , femoral head estimation

1. Introduction

Automated segmentation of bone is a challenging task. Clinical complications such as osteoarthritis and congenital deformities, technical limitations in CT imaging such as inherent blurring and partial volume effect, as well as narrow inter-bone regions and presence of blood in the bone tissues result in pelvis and femur images with textured regions and weak and diffused boundaries [1]. In the case of hip joint, total hip replacement (THR) is a common orthopaedic procedure performed on over 120000 patients annually in the USA [2]. Automatic segmentation of pelvis and femur from three-dimensional (3D) computed tomography (CT) images is necessary for the purpose of computer assisted surgical planning, intraoperative navigation, and post-operative assessment of the hip joint. Several prominent difficulties of automated segmentation are as follows [3]: (a) the non-uniformity of bone tissue, (b) presence of blood vessels, (c) diffused and weak edges, (d) narrow inter-bone regions, (e) inherent blurring of CT

©CARS/Springer. All rights reserved.

images, and (e) partial volume effect. Segmentation of bone from CT images is traditionally done by thresholding [4] followed by some mending procedure such as connectivity and seeded region growing [5]. This technique fails to work well in the regions such as the hip joint that separated bones are close spatially. In the previous work [6], we developed an interactive method for segmentation of bone from CT images. To create an isotropic data set, we resampled the CT data by a Sinc interpolation technique and smoothed the result. Next, the rough boundary of pelvis and femur was extracted by conventional technique including thresholding, morphological operations, and manual sphere fitting. Finally, the refined boundary of pelvis and femur was found by a moving disk technique [6]. In this research, compared to the previous work, (I) the proposed segmentation technique is automatic; (II) bone tissue is separated from other tissues of CT by an adaptive thresholding technique based on a pulse coupled neural networks [7], [8]; and (III) by imposing several constraints including (a) the elliptical shape of the femoral head, (b) the anatomical information of the greater trochanter, and (c) the geometrical specification of bone tissues, initial boundary of the joint space, i.e. the border between the femoral head and acetabulum is automatically estimated.

2. Materials and methods

2.1 Evaluation of the data sets

The data sets of 60 patients, i.e., 120 hip joints, including 3000 CT slices, were used in the study. Specifications of each group were as follows.

Group #1: in this case, acetabulums and femoral heads in the hip were well separated from each other and distribution of bone intensities throughout the hip were flat and the grey level of bone tissues were considerably higher than those of surrounding tissues.

Group #2: in this group, the joint space was narrow in several slices of each data set. That is, the acetabulum and femoral head were located close to each other. Moreover, the shape of the femoral head was very close to that of a 3D ellipse.

Group #3: the acetabulum and femoral head were close spatially. However, due to pathology and malformation of the pelvis and femur, shape of the femoral head was different from that of a 3D ellipse.

Group #4: in this case, due to the severity of a bone disease and malformation of both the acetabulum and femoral head, lack of the cartilage, the joint spaces in many slices of the hip joints were completely destroyed.

In Fig. 2(a), three axial cross sections of a hip joint with respect to a coronal slice is shown. It is seen that in such a slice, the femoral head and greater trochanter as parts of the femur are detached from each other. We found that the location of a slice with such a property was very close to that of a centre slice. In the data set of a hip joint, one or several slices had the above property. The slice with the largest femoral head bone was chosen as the centre slice. Fig. 2(b) shows two other orthogonal cross-sections with respect to the centre slice of a femoral head.

2.1 Resampling

In the CT data used in this paper, the voxel dimensions were non-cubic: 0.68 x 0.68 x 3 mm^3. Thus, it was necessary to upsample the data in the slice direction. This was done by Sinc interpolation, i.e., zero expansion (zero filling) in the frequency domain. In practice, the modified Sinc interpolation technique mentioned in [10] were employed to reduce the

©CARS/Springer. All rights reserved.

effect of unwanted Gibbs ringing. Using the above technique, the CT data were up sampled by a factor of four which gave the new voxel size 0.68 x 0.68 x 0.75 mm^3 . The voxels are still non-cubic. But compared with original size of 0.68 x 0.68 x 3 mm^3, the new voxel size was found acceptable.

2.3 Segmentation of bone tissues in the hip joint by PCNN

A pulsed coupled neural networks (PCNN) is a single layered, two-dimensional, laterally network of pulse coupled neurons. The network groups the images pixels based on the spatial proximity and brightness similarity. In the previous works, the PCNN was employed for image processing applications including image smoothing, segmentation and feature extraction [7], [8]. As we explained in Section 1, finding an appropriate threshold value for classification of bone from other CT tissues fails in most cases. We have developed a novel PCNN for adaptive thresholding of CT data. Block diagram of one neuron of the PCNN and corresponding explanations are given in Fig. 1.

2.4 Rough estimation of the joint space

After extracting bone tissues of CT images by the PCNN technique, the convex hull of the bone tissues was calculated. The overlay of the convex hull and original CT images for one typical slice of group #2 is shown in Fig. 3(a). It is seen that the bone tissues of the hip joint, including the femoral head, the joint space and the acetabulum were located inside the estimated convex hull. In Fig. 3(a), the centroid of this region was calculated (enumerated as #1). Next, the farthest point in the southwest area of the centre point [enumerated as #2 in Fig. 3(b)] was estimated. From the centre point, normals to the convex hull in the north (up) and east (right) directions were then calculated. The intersections of these normals with the convex hulls were respectively enumerated as points #3 and #4 and are shown in Fig. 3c) and (d). The middle points of lines (#1, #2) and ($\#1,\#4$) were calculated. These points are enumerated as points #5 and #6 and are shown in Fig. 3(e). Points $\#3$, $\#5$ and $\#6$ were employed to draw a circle. This circle is shown in Fig. 3(f) and was used as an initial estimate of the femoral head in the centre slice. By investigating the data sets, it was heuristically concluded that 3D was a good estimate for representing a femoral head. The centre of the circle in Fig. 3(g) was used as initial centre of the 3D ellipse. By experience, average number of slices that contains the femoral head was employed as the diameter of an ellipse in the z direction. Finally, by employing a Hough transform, an initial 3D ellipse with the above parameters, and binary data of bone tissues obtained in Section 2.3, the optimum parameters of a 3D ellipse were estimated. In this case, all one pixels inside the volume were participated to estimate the 3D ellipse. Upper limits of ellipse parameters were obtained from the available sizes of the femoral heads in the data sets. By using the estimated 3D ellipse, boundaries of the femoral head in all slices of a hip joint were calculated. Figs. 3(g) to (i), respectively, show the steps of assigning the initial boundary of the joint space in one typical slice of the hip joint.

2.5 Image enhancement by a Hessian filter

In the previous work, Westin *et al* [9] proposed a tensor-based filter to enhance tube like structure such as vessels, sheet like structure, e.g. the skin, and ball type structures such as tumours from CT images. In another approach, Sato *et al* [10] applied 3D Hessian filter to enhance MRI and CT data. In this work, in a similar manner to previous works [9],

©CARS/Springer. All rights reserved.

[10], we employed a 2D Hessian filter to enhance the joint space between the acetabulum and femoral head in the hip joint. The standard deviation of the Gaussian function in the Hessian matrix [10] was used to control the trade off between the smoothness and preserving of edges.

2.6 Refining rough boundary by a moving disk technique
To cope with a joint space boundary refinement task, the moving disk algorithm [6] was modified as follows: (1) The hip joint images were enhanced by a Hessian filter; (2) the rough boundary of the joint space were smoothed and sorted ; (3) the new value of each boundary point was found by calculating the perpendicular line of each boundary point, adjusting circle around the boundary point, finding the minimum and maximum values of the image [obtained in Step (1)] inside the ROI, binarizing the image inside the ROI for a range of thresholds; (4) the current boundary value was replaced by the closest foreground pixel on the binary ROI. The output of the above algorithm after several iterations gives the refined boundary.

3. Results

The required time for performing automatic segmentation using a IBM compatible PC (Pentium III, 1 GHz, 512 Mbytes memory, ROI: 32x160x160 voxels) was about 6 minutes. Results of automatic segmentation were compared with the manual segmentation results of two experts. We defined three fuzzy terms of *good*, *moderate* and *poor* for evaluations the success rates of the technique, denoted by k as follows. *Good*: (**k**>90%); *moderate*: (65%< **k**<80%); and, *poor*: (**k**<55%). To include the expert decisions in marginal cases, classification of **k** values in the ranges of (80%< **k**<90%) and (55< **k**<65) was made subjectively. It was found that the technique was effective to perform good results with a success rate of 90%, 80%, and 75% for groups #1, #2 and #3, respectively. However, only 30% of the slices in #4 were moderately treated by this technique. This evaluation revealed that fully automatic bone segmentation technique still needs further development for severe clinical cases. A typical result of the proposed segmentation techniques is shown in Fig. 4.

4. Conclusion

In this study, the CT data of 60 actual patients were used for clinical assessments of the proposed techniques. It was concluded that 67% of the slices in the hip joints could be sufficiently segmented by the proposed techniques. Segmentation of the remaining 33% slices was not possible by the proposed techniques. These slices were mostly the hip joints in #4. In this group, bone malformation and pathology seriously affected all proposed techniques. Automatic segmentation of femur and pelvis in severe pathological cases will be considered in our future researches.

Acknowledgements
This work was supported by the Japan Society for the Promotion of Science (JSPS Research for the Future Program).

CARS 2002 – H.U. Lemke, M.W. Vannier; K. Inamura, A.G. Farman, K. Doi & J.H.C. Reiber (Editors)
©CARS/Springer. All rights reserved.

References

1. http://www.hipsandknees.com.
2. Total hip replacement, NIH Consents Statement Online 1994 Sept. 12-14, vol. 12, no. 5, pp. 1-31, 1994.
3. Sebastian TB, Tek H, Cristo JJ, Wolfe SW, Kimia BB,"Segmentation of carpal bones from 3D CT images using skeletally coupled deformable models", *CARS 99*: pp. 1184-1194. 1999.
4. Jain R, Karsuri R, Schunck BG, *Machine Vision*, MacGraw-Hill, New York, 1995.
5. Adams R, Bischof L, "Seeded region growing", *IEEE T Pattern Anal*, vol. 16(9), pp. 641-647, 1994.
6. Zoroofi RA, Sasama T, Sugano N, Nishii T, Sato Y, Yonenobu K, Yoshikawa H, Tamura S., Takahiro Ochi, "Segmentation of Pelvis and Femur from Computer Tomography Images", *Technical Report of the Institute of Elec., Info. and Comm. Eng. (IEICE)*, vol.100, Okinawa, Japan, January 2001.
7. Johnson JL, Padgett ML, "PCNN Models and Applications", *IEEE Trans. Neural Networks*, vol. 10(3), pp. 480-496. 1999.
8. Ranganath HS, Kuntimad G, "Object Detection Using Pulse Coupled Nueral Networks", *IEEE Trans. Nueral Networks*, vol. 10(3), pp. 615-620. 1999.
9. Westin CF, Warfield S, Bhalerao A, Mui L, Richolt J, Kikinis R, "Tensor controlled local structure enhancement of CT images for bone segmentation", *CARS 99*: pp. 1206-1211. 1999.
10. Sato Y, Westin CF, Bhalerao A, Nakajima S, Shiraga N, Tamura S, Kikinis R, "Tissue classification based on 3D local intensity structures for volume rendering", *IEEE T Vis Comput Graph*, vol. 6(2): pp. 160-180, 2000.

(a)

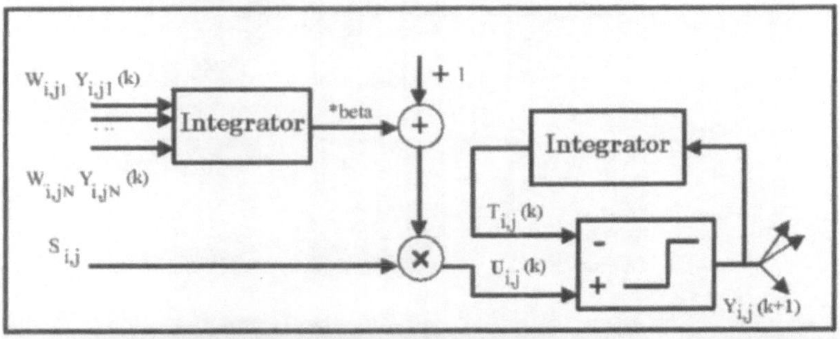

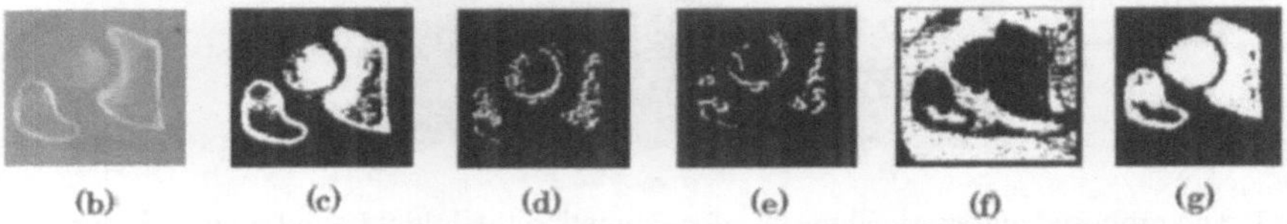

(b) (c) (d) (e) (f) (g)

Fig. 1: (a) Block diagram of one neuron of the pulse coupled neural network (PCNN) for state **k**. There exist a one to one correspondence between the image pixels and network neurons. **S**ij represents an image pixel and is regarded as an independent input of each neuron. The output each neuron, **Y**ij, is used as a dependent input of the neurons which are located in the neighbourhood of pixel **S**ij. **N** represents connectivity. In this research, we selected a value of 26 for **N** to deal with the 3D CT images. As it is seen, PCNN has an iterative nature. **W**ijm denotes contribution of neighbour **m** (**m**=1,2,...,**N**) to the neuron. Cortical bones are located in the boundary of bones are of higher intensities compared to their surrounding tissues. For this reasons, 3D gradient information of the CT data in the neighbourhood of each pixel (here **S**ij) was employed to assign the contribution of neighbourhood pixels. (b) A typical CT image of hip joint. (c) to (f) represent four iterations of the PCNN. Unusual increase in the number of extracted pixels was considered as a sign of background detection. This property was used to terminate iterations. (g) Extracted bone tissues were found by superposition of all results excluding the last result, i.e., by superposition of images extracted in (c), (d) and (e).

©CARS/Springer. All rights reserved.

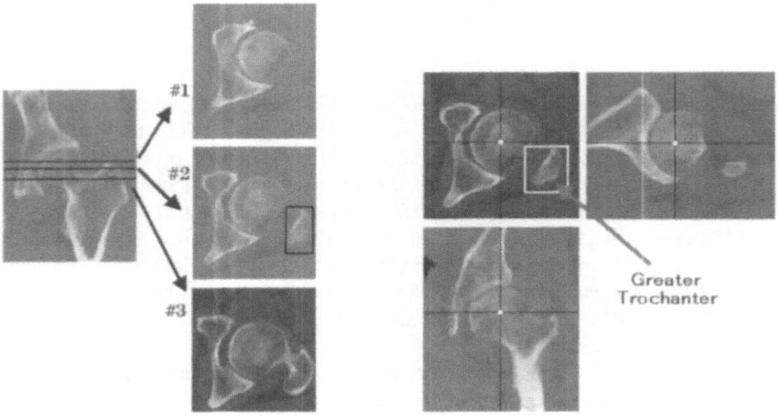

Fig. 2: Finding the centre slice of a femoral head by using the greater trochanter as an anatomical landmark. See Section 2.4 for details.

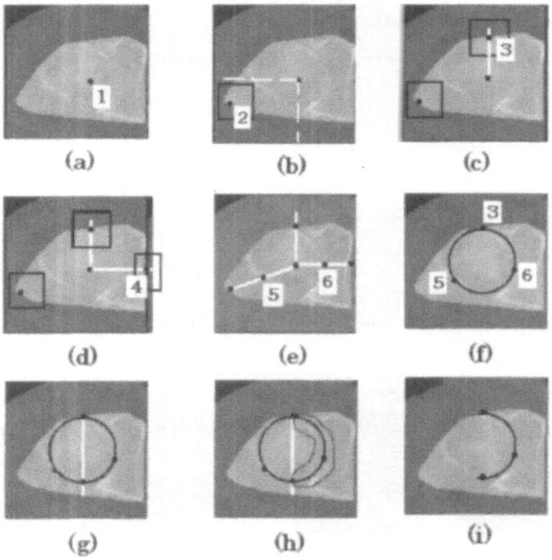

Fig. 3: The proposed automatic algorithm for estimating the initial boundary of a femoral head.

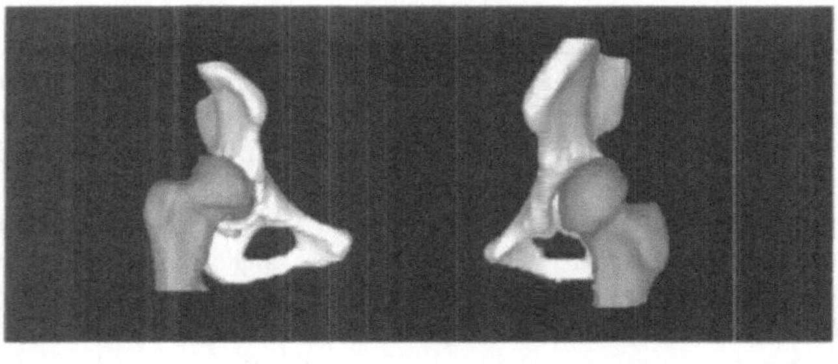

Fig. 4: Surfaces of pelvises and femurs of two typical data sets (in #2) after segmentation are shown.

CARS 2002 – H.U. Lemke, M.W. Vannier; K. Inamura, A.G. Farman, K. Doi & J.H.C. Reiber (Editors)
©CARS/Springer. All rights reserved.

Registration and matching of projection imaging and tomographic imaging. Application to X-rays angiographies and magnetic resonance angiographies.

M. Vermandel[a, b], C. Kulik[b], J.Y. Gauvrit[a], C. Vasseur[b], J. Rousseau[a]
[a]Instistut de technologie Médicale, Pav. Vancostenobel, CHRU de Lille, 2 av. O. Lambret, 59037, Lille cedex.
[b]I [3]D, bat. P2, USTL, 59 655, Villeneuve D'Ascq, France

Abstract

In this paper, we propose a new method for matching vascular imaging modalities without using external frame or external landmarks. First, 3D reconstruction of part of the cerebral vascular tree is performed using Magnetic Resonance Angiography (MRA). Then, this volume is projected on Digital Subtracted Angiography (DSA) image until its best position and orientation are found. Results show satisfactory robustness and accuracy.

Keywords: registration, matching, angiography.

1. Introduction

This study presents a new approach for registration and matching of projection and tomographic imaging. For illustrating the applied method, this paper deals with X-Rays and Magnetic Resonance vascular cerebral images. Several authors [1, 2] describe methods on 2D and 3D registration. Those methods can be classified as two different approaches which are intensity-based registration[1] and feature-based registration[2].

The method described in this paper is based on a 3D modeling of the volume of interest and re-projection algorithm using conic projection properties.

Developments presented have been applied on both phantom and patient images. Pre-operative MRA scans have been used to generate a 3D model of the vascular tree. DSA images were acquired in standard pre-operative conditions.

2. 2D/3D Registration procedure

2.1 Principle

Matching images needs several preliminary steps as registration or researching landmarks changing relations. In order to register MRA and DSA, we propose a method illustrated below (Fig. 1).

©CARS/Springer. All rights reserved.

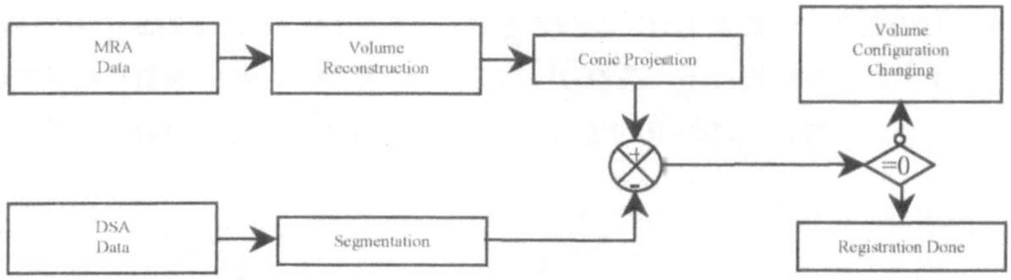

Fig. 1: Block diagram illustrating the methodology applied.

First, MRA and DSA images of considered volume are acquired. Then, a 3D model of the initial volume is reconstructed from MRA. This reconstructed model becomes the anatomic reference linking the two modalities. Then, the model is digitally projected applying conic projection properties. The resulting image is compared to a segmented DSA image through a similarity measure. Finally, the optimal position and orientation of the model in the DSA space is iteratively found. At the end of the process and considering that the structure configuration is known in the MRA referential (thanks to the reconstruction step), the complete matching between the two modalities is immediately obtained.

2.2 Volume reconstruction

The model is reconstructed from the MRA dataset. We first generate a Maximum of Intensity Projection (MIP) [3] as described below (Fig. 2).

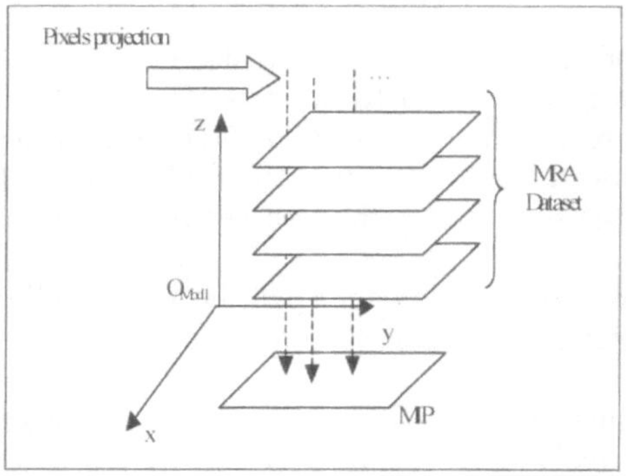

Fig. 2: Maximum of Intensity Projection algorithm.

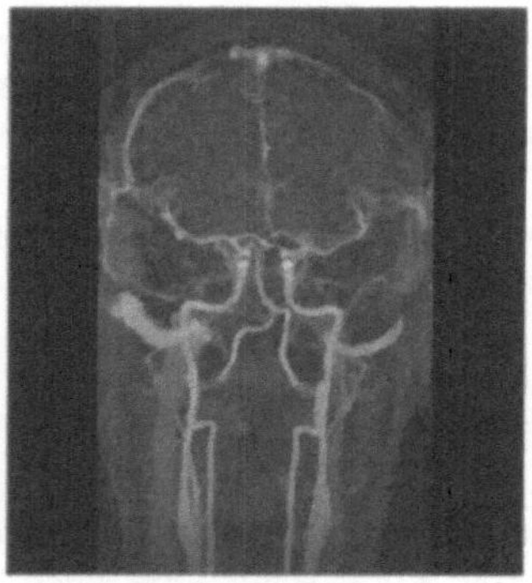

Fig. 3: Resulting image.

The MIP resulting image is used for detecting the vascular structure through the entire MRA dataset, applying fuzzy set theory and data fusion. Fig. 4 shows overlays resulting from an automatic detection performed by the algorithm. Then, the detected surfaces are stacked to reconstruct the model [4] (Fig. 5).

©CARS/Springer. All rights reserved.

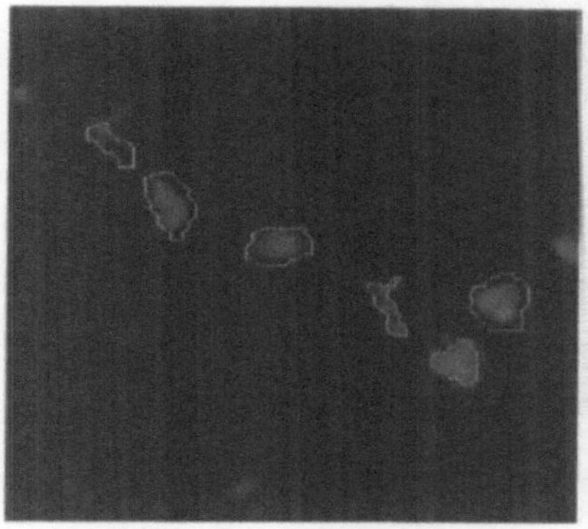

Fig. 4: Detected structure on a MRA image

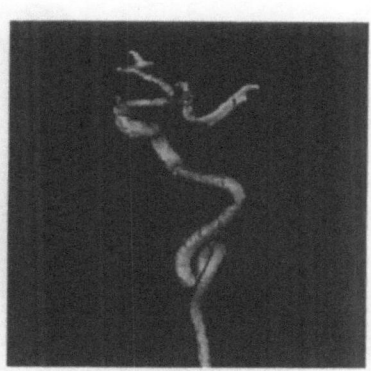

Fig. 5: Model reconstruction from the detected structure

2.3 Initialization

In a such registration problem, six degree rigid parameters describes the 3D volume position in the DSA space.

Research of the best volume configuration in the DSA space can be assimilated as a minimization of energy. The energy applied is computed from the similarity measure described by (1) and known as "quadratic distance between pixels". This kind of similarity measure is already applied in satellite imagery[5].

$$Energy = \sum_{i=1}^{I}\sum_{j=1}^{J}\left(P_{i,j} - P'_{i,j}\right)^2 \tag{1}$$

Where, $P_{i,j}$ and $P'_{i,j}$ are respectively the i and j coordinates pixels of the original image I and the image I' computed from the six rigid-body parameters.

Initially, a multi resolution analysis is done to initialize a first parameters set.

2.4 Finding the optimal registration

To get the optimal configuration we choose to apply an algorithm developed by Salazar[6] and Toral. This method, known as the Hybrid Simulated Annealing (HSA), has the property to change simultaneously the parameters set using a simulated annealing scheme.

As in the standard simulated annealing, the new configuration is accepted using the Metropolis test, with a probability described by (2).

$$P(\Delta H) = e^{\left(\frac{-\Delta H}{T}\right)} \tag{2}$$

The next figure shows an example of optimal registration computed from standard pre-operative image (Fig. 6).

©CARS/Springer. All rights reserved.

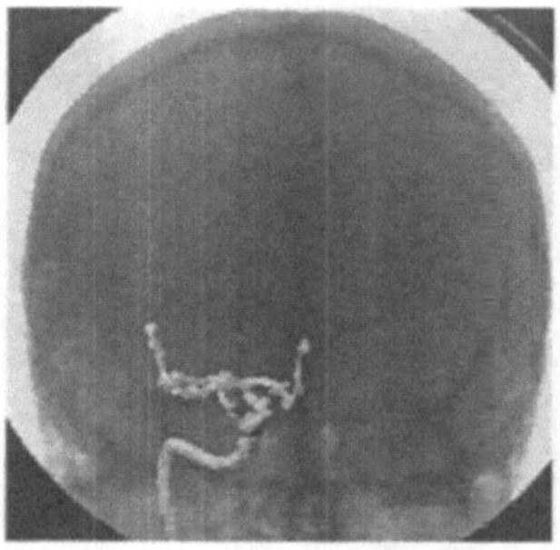

Fig. 6: Optimal registration from standard preoperative image

3. Results

Evaluation criteria are needed for validation of a such registration algorithm. As in standard evaluation experiments, we choose two criterion which are robustness and accuracy. The robustness defines the ability of the method to converge to an unique and optimal solution whatever the starting configuration. To compare with the methods presented in introduction, we have performed experiments as proposed by McLaughlin and al [7] for the robustness. The accuracy is evaluated on the basis of data information obtained from a vascular phantom (Fig. 7 and Fig. 8).

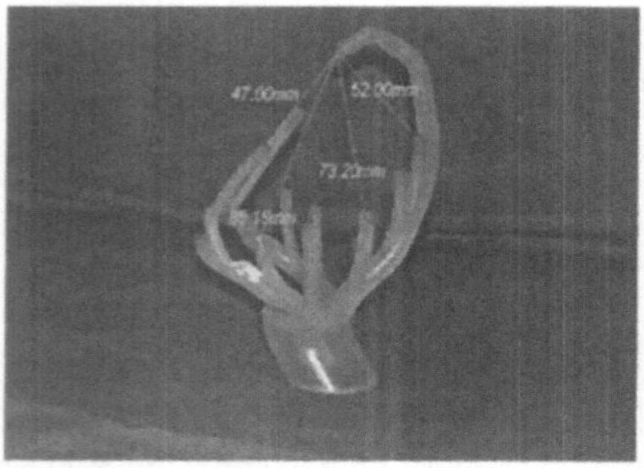

Fig. 7: Phantom used for the test and the validation.

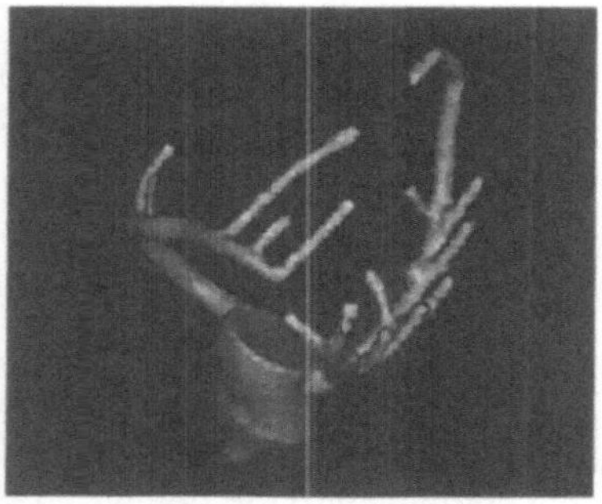

Fig. 8: Model of the phantom reconstructed from MRA.

3.1 Robustness

First of all, an optimal registration is computed Then, starting positions for the registrations were chosen by perturbing this gold standard value. Four experiments were performed with the amount of perturbation increased each time.

Gold standard registration and example of starting perturbed configuration are respectively shown on Fig. 9 and 10.

©CARS/Springer. All rights reserved.

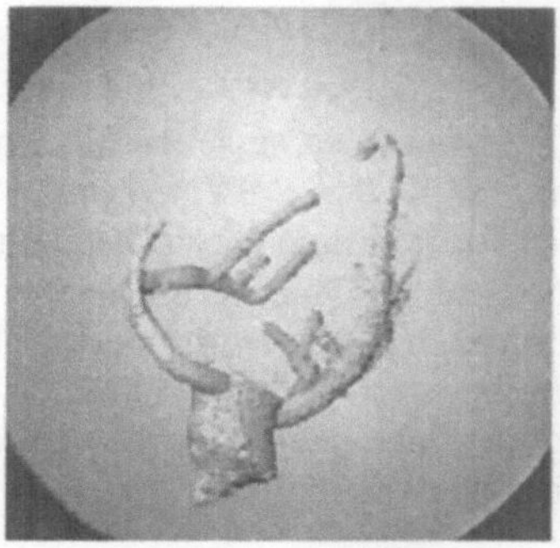

Fig. 9: Optimal registration

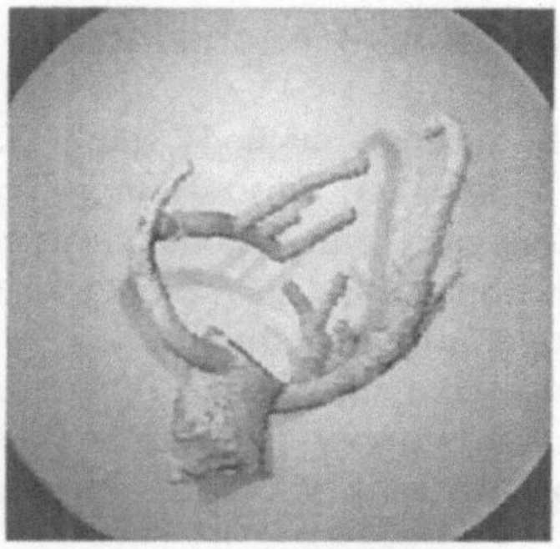

Fig. 10: Example of perturbed starting position

The results of the experiments are illustrated below (Fig. 11), showing simultaneously comparison with the two others introduced methods: intensity-based registration and feature-based registration.

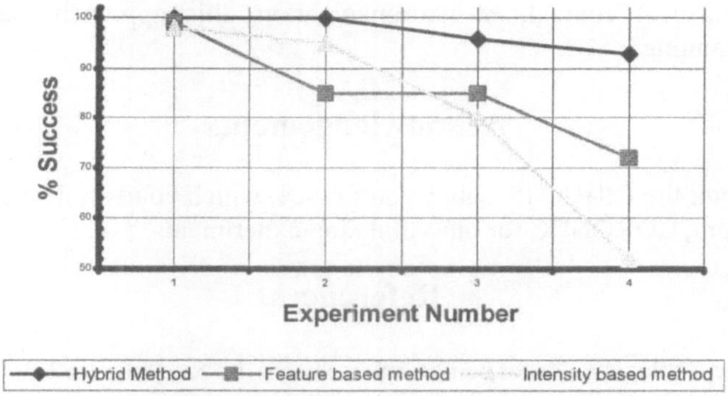

Fig. 11: Results of the robustness experiments

We can observe a good robustness from the hybrid approach. The feature-based and intensity-based method seem to be more sensitive to the perturbing configurations.

3.2 Accuracy

To measure the accuracy of registration, we use Euclidean distance measurements. A number of particular points were chosen on the vascular phantom (Fig. 5). Experiment uses a registration procedure for two different DSA incidences. In this way, measurement is performed using epipolar geometry.

Results of these experiments gives less than 1mm of error between physical and measured distances.

©CARS/Springer. All rights reserved.

4. Discussion - Conclusion

Compare to others methods, the hybrid approach does not need several DSA projection during registration. This advantage enables matching of several DSA projection without calibrating each with the others, which it is required for both intensity and feature based method. Both focal distance and patient table position can be changed at each acquisition without perturbing the registration. A second breakthrough of the hybrid approach is that no manual initialization is required. The registration step is fully automatic. When registration is performed with at least two DSA projection, interactive navigation from DSA to MRA (or MRA to DSA) can be easily performed using epipolar geometry.

Considering the robustness and the accuracy results, the exposed method seems to be efficient for 2D-3D registration. Our registration method is based on several algorithms: a pixel-based approach (as Intensity-based registration), a fast projection algorithm and an effective optimization scheme (HSA)

Applications could be developed from this method. First, the developments of the MRA techniques could be validated using matching and comparison with the DSA as a gold standard. In surgical context, as neuronavigation, this approach may be used for preoperative planning.

Acknowledgements

We wish to thank the CREATIS Lab, Lyon France, which courtesy lets us managed their vascular phantom, CORONIX, for our validation experiments.

References

1. G. P. Penney, “Registration of tomographic images to X-ray Projections for use in image guided interventions”, Phd thesis, University College London.
2. Y. Kita, D. L. Wilson & J. A. Noble, “Real-time registration of 3D cerebral vessels to X-ray angiograms”, *MICCAI’98*, pp. 1125-1133, 1998.
3. Laub G, "*Displays for MR Angiography*", Mag. Res. in Med. vol 14, 222-229, 1990.
4. S. Vial, D. Gibon, C. Vasseur, J. Rousseau,” Volume delineation by fusion of fuzzy sets obtained from multiplanar tomographic images”, *IEEE Trans. on MI*, 20, pp 1362-1372, 2001.
5. M. Svedlow, C. D. McGillem and P. E. Anuta, “Image registration: similarity measure and preprocessing method comparison”, *IEEE Trans. on AES*, 14, pp 141-149,1978.
6. R. Salazar and R. Toral, “Simulated Annealing using Hybrid Monte Carlo”, *Journal of Statistical Physics* 89, p. 1047, 1997.
7. R. A. McLaughlin, J. Hipwell, G. P. Penney, K. Rhode and A. Chung, “Intensity-based registration versus feature-based registration for neurointerventions”, *Medical Image Understanding and Analysis 2001.*

CARS 2002 – H.U. Lemke, M.W. Vannier; K. Inamura, A.G. Farman, K. Doi & J.H.C. Reiber (Editors)
©CARS/Springer. All rights reserved.

Construction of an average CT brain image for brain infarct pattern comparison

Cynthia Jongen, Josien P.W. Pluim, Max A. Viergever, Wiro J. Niessen
Image Sciences Institute, University Medical Center Utrecht, Heidelberglaan 100, room E01.334, 3584 CX Utrecht, The Netherlands

Abstract

An average CT brain image is constructed to serve as a reference frame for intersubject comparison. The use of an average brain image prevents bias resulting from registration to a single patient image. The average CT brain image is constructed from a large number of images by means of rigid registration with scaling, and with normalized mutual information as the registration measure. The construction proceeds in two steps. First a temporary average image is constructed based on a small subset of images. Then this image is used as the reference image for the construction of the average CT brain image. It is shown that registration to the average CT brain image is consistent and effective for the registration of new CT images. Furthermore, registration of new CT images to the average CT brain image outperforms registration to a single patient image.

Keywords: Atlas, average brain, intersubject comparison

1. Introduction

Intersubject comparison of the location of brain pathology requires a common reference frame. The aim of this work is to construct an average CT brain image for comparing brain infarct patterns between groups of stroke patients. Infarct patterns of groups of patients, for example with increasing degrees of internal carotid artery stenosis, can be compared by registering the patient images to the average CT brain image. Once all images are placed in the same reference space location-specific information about infarcts can be obtained, e.g. a probability distribution of size and location of infarcts.

2. Methodology

The average CT brain image is constructed using 96 CT brain images of stroke patients. The construction procedure is fully automatic. The resolution of the CT brain images is typically 0.7 x 0.7 x 4.5 to 5.0 mm for X (left-right), Y (anterior-posterior), and Z (slice) direction. The images are registered using normalized mutual information with rigid transformations and anisotropic scaling [1]. Although the anatomical differences between patients cannot be completely accounted for by the chosen type of transformation, it is preferred to an elastic transformation, which may cause deformation or dislocation of infarcts.

©CARS/Springer. All rights reserved.

The construction of the average CT brain image proceeds in two steps. The first step is the construction of a temporary average image. The second step is the construction of the average CT brain image.

2.1 The construction of the temporary average image

The temporary average image is constructed to prevent bias in the average CT brain image towards a single image. The temporary average image is constructed using a random subset of 32 from the 96 CT brain images. From this subset a starting image is randomly selected and the remaining 31 images are registered to this starting image. To ensure that the temporary average is composed of accurately registered images, we only use the 16 best registered images to create the temporary average. Images with the highest normalized mutual information measure are probably registered most accurately. Therefore we selected the 16 images with the highest normalized mutual information measure. These 16 images are averaged. They are reregistered to the average and then averaged to create the temporary average image.

Step1:

a) randomly select 32 of the 96 CT brain images
b) randomly select 1 of the 32 images
c) register the remaining 31 images to the selected image
d) select the 16 images with highest normalized mutual information measure
e) average the 16 images
f) reregister the 16 image to the average
g) average the reregistered 16 images to create temporary average image

2.2 The construction of the average CT brain image

The average CT brain image is constructed using the temporary average image as registration template. All 96 CT brain images are registered to the temporary average image. Averaging the 96 registered images results in an average CT brain image. The average CT brain image is optimized by iterating the registration step. The iteration is stopped when the average of the normalized mutual information of the 96 images is stable.

Step 2:

a) register 96 images to the temporary average image
b) average 96 registered images
c) register 96 images to average
d) average 96 registered images
e) repeat c and d until the average of the normalized mutual information measure is stable

3. Evaluation

The evaluation of the average brain image construction method focuses on two issues:

a) consistency: how well are the 96 images matched to the average image
b) robustness: is registration to an average brain image more robust than registration to a single brain image

©CARS/Springer. All rights reserved.

a) The consistency of the registrations is evaluated using registrations to a second version of the average CT brain image. This second average image is constructed using the same 96 images, but it is based on a temporary image that was created using a completely different subset from the 96 images. This results in two average CT brain images that are similar except for translation, rotation and scaling. In the ideal case this transformation between the two average CT brain images is the same for each of the 96 individual images that form the two average images.
For each individual image of the 96 images the transformations to both average images are known. Thus for each individual image the transformation between both averages could be calculated. In the ideal situation of perfect registration this transformation is identical for every individual image, since the construction of both average images is based on the same 96 images. Thus the deviation in this transformation is a measure of consistency of the average CT brain image construction.

b) The robustness of registering to the average CT brain image is evaluated by comparing the consistency of registering new CT brain images to the average CT brain images with the consistency of registering these new images to single CT brain images. Hereto, the two starting images that were used for the construction of the temporary average images are used as single images. These two images are chosen since they do not differ in global orientation from the two average CT brain images. So differences in registration consistency are not the result of differences in global orientation. Ten new CT brain images of stroke patients are used. These ten images are registered to both average CT brain images and to both single starting images. The consistency of the registrations is evaluated as was described in the previous paragraph.

4. Results

4.1 Construction

The iteration process of the creation of the average CT brain image converged rapidly. Between iteration two and three of the construction the change in the averaged normalized

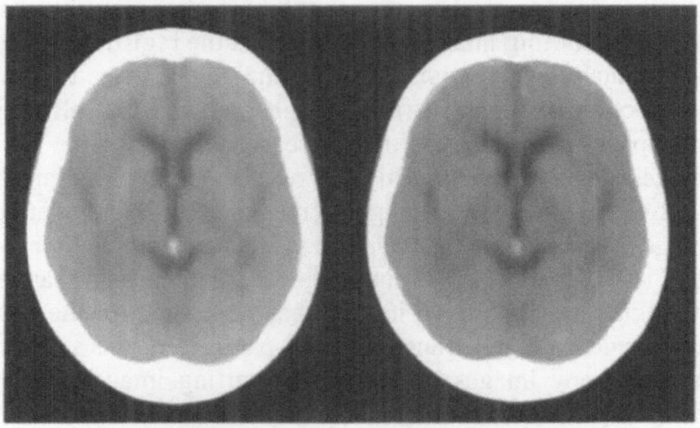

Figure 1: A slice taken at approximately the same position from each of the two average images

©CARS/Springer. All rights reserved.

mutual information was less than 0.5 % for both constructed average CT brain images. Therefore, after three iterations the registration process was stopped. Although only translation, rotation and scaling were allowed during registration, anatomical details were well preserved in both average CT brain images as can be seen in Figure 1.

4.2 Evaluation

The evaluation of the registrations showed that the registrations are consistent. The standard deviations of the calculated transformations between the two average images for all 96 individual images are shown in Table 1. The standard deviations were largest for the transformations involving the slice direction and smallest for the in-plane transformations. This is caused by the large anisotropy in the slice direction.

	Standard Deviations
Rotation around X axis (rad)	0.0351
Rotation around Y axis (rad)	0.0207
Rotation around Z axis (rad)	0.0081
Scaling X direction (factor)	0.0041
Scaling Y direction (factor)	0.0062
Scaling Z direction (factor)	0.0335
Translation X direction (mm)	0.2501
Translation Y direction (mm)	0.7689
Translation Z direction (mm)	1.4657

Table 1: Standard deviations of the transformations between both average images via the 96 individual images

Nearly all standard deviations are of subvoxel magnitudes. This is very small for intersubject registration using rigid transformations with scaling. The consistency of the registration is sufficient for our application of localizing brain infarcts for interpatient comparisons.

The evaluation of the robustness was done by the comparison of the consistency of registration of ten new images to the average CT brain images with the consistency of registration to the single starting images. It showed that the registrations to the average CT brain images were much more consistent than the registration to the single starting images. Visual inspection of the registration results showed that all registrations to the average CT brain images were successful, whereas only half of the registrations to the single starting images were successful. This was reflected in the standard deviations of the transformations between both average images versus the standard deviations between both single starting images, as shown in Table 2. The standard deviations for the registration of the ten new images to the average CT brain images were in the same range as the standard deviations for the registration of the 96 images that were used for the construction of the average CT brain images. For all transformation parameters the standard deviation for registration of the ten new images to the single starting images were larger than for registration to the average CT brain images.

©CARS/Springer. All rights reserved.

	Standard Deviations Registration to Average Images	Standard Deviations Registration to Single Starting Images	Increase (%)
Rotation around X axis (rad)	0.0313	0.0459	146.6
Rotation around Y axis (rad)	0.0156	0.0329	211.2
Rotation around Z axis (rad)	0.0057	0.0443	782.0
Scaling X direction (factor)	0.0034	0.0334	973.7
Scaling Y direction (factor)	0.0044	0.0245	552.4
Scaling Z direction (factor)	0.0242	0.0405	167.1
Translation X direction (mm)	0.2336	4.3266	1852.5
Translation Y direction (mm)	0.8531	1.0922	128.0
Translation Z direction (mm)	0.7393	1.8289	247.4

Table 2: Standard deviations of the transformations between both average images via ten new images compared with the standard deviations of the transformations between the two single starting images via the ten new images

As can be seen in Table 2 the increases in standard deviation ranged from a 1.28 times larger standard deviation for translation in the anterior-posterior direction to an even 18.5 times larger standard deviation for translations in the left-right direction. Thus intersubject registration to an average image is much more consistent than registration to a single image.

5. Conclusions

We have constructed an average CT brain image based on 96 patient CT brain images. The construction of the average CT brain image converged to a stable result in two iterations. The evaluations show that the registration of the images is consistent. This is shown by the small standard deviations of the parameters of the transformation between both average CT brain images. Thus the proposed method provides an automatic and robust way to construct an average CT brain image.
The comparison of registration to the average CT brain images with registration to the single images shows that the use of the average CT brain image as reference frame greatly adds to registration consistency compared to the use of a single image.

References

1. Maes, F., Collignon, A., Vandermeulen, D., Marchal, G., and Suetens, P., "Multimodality image registration by maximization of mutual information", *IEEE Transactions on Medical Imaging*, 16:187-198, 1997

CARS 2002 – H.U. Lemke, M.W. Vannier; K. Inamura, A.G. Farman, K. Doi & J.H.C. Reiber (Editors)
©CARS/Springer. All rights reserved.

Fast Feldkamp-reconstruction for real-time reconstruction using C-arm-systems

K. Kornmesser, B. Schädler, J. Hesser, R. Männer[a], M. Ebert, W. Schlegel[b],
[a] ICM, Universities Mannheim and Heidelberg, B6 23, 68131 Mannheim
[a] Abt. Med. Physik, DKFZ, Im Neuenheimer Feld 280, 69120 Heidelberg, Germany

Abstract

In this paper we present a new technique that allows to reconstruct a series of C-arm x-ray images into a volume within a few seconds instead of minutes. The main innovation is a new architecture that maps this algorithm into FPGA based hardware. This architecture overcomes the typical memory bandwidth limitation in the Feldkamp reconstruction by a sophisticated re-usage of voxel data and projection pixels. It achieves a parallelization speedup that is independent of the available bandwidth; it only depends on the chip-internal amount of resources. We have implemented the architecture into a Xilinx XCV400-4 with one pipeline running and process one projection of size 512×512 within 1 second for a 256^3 volume. A current implementation on a Virtex II XC2V3000 will have 16 parallel pipelines and thus processes 16 projections per second. For assumed 80 projections the system thus requires 5 seconds.

Keywords: Feldkamp reconstruction, real-time x-ray reconstruction, C-arm-systems.

1. Introduction

Three-dimensional information is of great benefit in the investigation of the human morphology. Especially in operation control 3D information about the position of screws in the bone parts is of high relevance. For example, assume that after the operation it should be controlled whether the fixation protrudes within a joint [4]. If this is the case and if the operation wound is still open, a correction is without problems. All other post-operative control (e.g. CT) requires eventually a new operation for the patient. In order to evade these disadvantages, a three-dimensional control in the operation theatre should be a standard in complex cases. CTs in or near the operation room however are beyond the financial possibilities for most clinics. An alternative is the reconstruction based on C-arm systems that are routinely used during operation. The C-arm rotates around the patient within few seconds and registers projection images from a 180° angle area. From these projections a volume is reconstructed using the Feldkamp algorithm [1]. Slicing and 3D rendering then allows to inspect the considered region in detail and allows to proof the correctness of the operation.

Such volume reconstructions can take up to minutes, which stops all activities in the operation theatre in order to see the operation results. Speeding up this processing will allow these three-dimensional investigations to be repeated more often during the operation and thus will decrease the complication rate in critical situations.

©CARS/Springer. All rights reserved.

The question of how to speed up this processing is thus the main topic of this paper.

2. Material and Methods

The reconstruction method used for generating volume data sets from projection images is the Feldkamp algorithm. The Feldkamp reconstruction is not an exact method but gives sufficiently good results and it is very robust [3]. It is assumed that the C-arm rotates about one stable axis and that the projection matrices are known. Based on this information the Feldkamp algorithm proceeds as follows:

First, the C-arm images are distorted and a pre-filtering is performed. This are operations that have the complexity $O(N^3)$ for projection images of size $N \times N$ and for $O(N)$ projections (that are required in order to approximately fulfill Shannons sampling theorem). After this filtering, each pixel value of the projections is reprojected into the direction of the illuminating source. This is an operation that has an overall complexity of $O(N^4)$. Thus, in order to speed up the processing, the reprojection should be optimized.

Optimized implementations of this algorithm on a 500 MHz PC with MMX requires approx. 3-5 minutes for a volume of 256^3 voxels and 256 projections. This reconstruction speed is mainly limited by the memory bandwidth of the PC architecture. As a consequence, faster reconstruction speed requires a higher memory bandwidth; which grows much slower than the CPU performance.

The standard approach is the parallelization of this reconstruction algorithm on massively parallel systems or a cluster of PCs. Due to the algorithmic structure of the Feldkamp method, there is an ideal linear speedup: each processor receives the data from all projections and generates a sub-volume of the final data set. The main disadvantage of this approach is that the cost of that solution increases cubic with the problem size or inverse proportionally with the reconstruction time. This means a high cost for the final reconstruction system.

The issue in this paper is thus: Is there a possibility to keep the cost for reconstruction more or less constant while decreasing the reconstruction time?
If such a solution should be found it can only be based on parallel processing with devices that offer an abundance of resources like FPGAs [2]. For this reason we first implemented our prototype design on a commercial FPGA board and are currently using a board with a more dense FPGA that allows to implement between 16 and 40 parallel processors (depending on the used FPGA model, see fig. 1).

The next question is how to parallelize the algorithm. The naive way for parallelization requires a memory bandwidth that is proportional to the parallelization degree. The main limitation, however, for current FPGA systems is not to have enough internal resources, but to have enough pins to the outside world, to connect enough memory elements (SDRAMs). In addition, scaling the number of memory elements linearly with the parallelization increases the cost accordingly; which should be evaded.

©CARS/Springer. All rights reserved.

The only alternative is thus to find an architecture that can operate with a constant

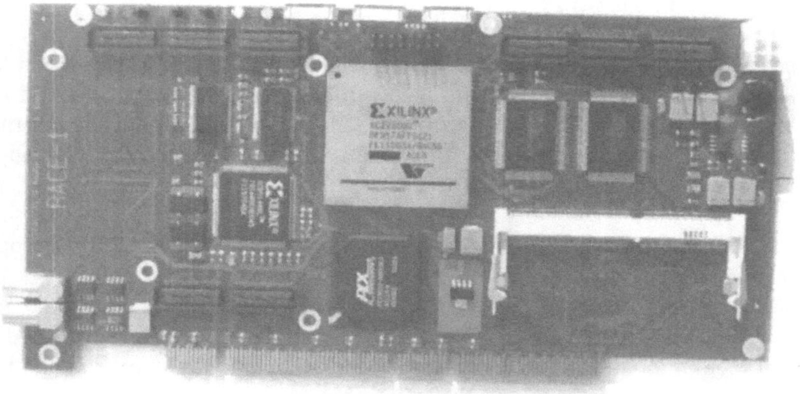

memory bandwidth independent of the internal parallelization degree.

Fig. 1: FPGA-board that will be used for reconstruction (picture from A. Kugel, Informatik V, University of Mannheim)

In order to reduce the memory bandwidth for projection data, one has to select voxels of the volume such that they require access to the same area of the considered projection. These few projection pixels can be loaded into a projection cache so that access to the memory for projection data is not necessary. This approach decreases the demand for projection pixels but does not alleviate the amount of voxels that have to be read from the volume memory. The amount of data to be read is thus still of $O(N^4)$.

If the memory bandwidth for volume data or voxels should be reduced, one has to select projection pixels that contribute to the respective voxels. Here, the amount of projection pixels is not reduced but the amount of read voxels. The bandwidth complexity thus remains the same.

The advantage of caching can only be harnessed if both voxel and projection memory are accessed as seldom as possible. This is achieved by combining both approaches. A sub-cube of size m^3 is loaded onto the processor. This allows to reuse projection pixels. In addition, not only one projection is considered but m^3 projections. This reduces the amount of voxels to be read from memory.

Next, we have to find an architecture that both allows to process m^3 voxels in parallel, i.e. to calculate m^3 contributions to voxels without having a complex communication structure. We found that the following architecture leads to be best results:
During the loading phase each voxel is assigned one slot in a voxel shift register forming a ring. Each clock cycle the voxel shift register is shifted by one, i.e. the voxel of shift register i is shifted to register $i+1 \bmod m^3$ and register i obtains the voxel data from register $i-1 \bmod m^3$. To each of the registers i is assigned a pipeline processor i. This pipeline processor calculates the contribution of projection plane i to the current voxel j in the i-th register. This contribution is added to the respective voxel (being latency L

©CARS/Springer. All rights reserved.

registers ahead). After $L+m^3$ clock cycles each projection contributed to each voxel in the shift register, i.e. $(m^3)^2$ computations have been performed. Finally, the results are stored back into memory. Details can be seen in fig. 2.

To simplify the caching system and to further reduce the memory bandwidth we align projections and volume data. This can either be guaranteed by a stable rotation axis of the C-arm or achieved by rotating the projections during filtering; which is an operation of complexity $O(N^3)$. Further we use the fact that the rays are „relatively" parallel, i.e., we assume that rows in the projection image are reprojected into a slice parallel slab in the volume data with comparable thickness.

If volume and projections are aligned, a slab of the volume data which is perpendicular to the rotation axis is projected onto rows in the projections. Thus to reconstruct such slabs of thickness m consisting of several sub-cubes each pipeline has to load pixels from $(m+1)$ neighboring rows of its respective projection image.

The total amount of data that has to be loaded per slab is $2N^2 \times m$ voxels and $m^2 \times N$ projection pixels. N/m slabs have to be calculated. In addition to consider all projections, this processing has to be repeated N/m^3 times. Thus, the amount of data that has to be transferred is $O(N^2 \times m \times N^2/m^4) = O(N^4/m^3)$. This shows that the overall memory bandwidth is reduced by m^3, i.e., the amount of parallelization. The complexity of this approach is $O(N^4/m^3)$.

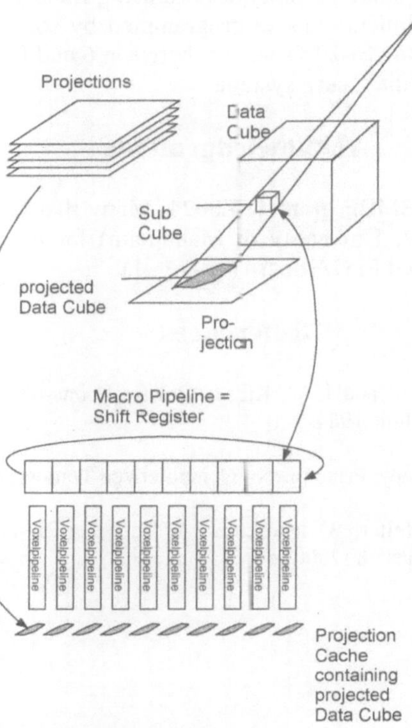

Fig. 2: Architecture of the reconstruction algorithm.

©CARS/Springer. All rights reserved.

3. Results

Each of the pipeline processors performs one voxel update per cycle; i.e. in total the system achieves m^3 voxel updates per clock cycle. However, the required memory bandwidth is independent of this parallelization, so that the performance of the system grows with the amount of resources of the processor; which, for FPGAs, increases roughly by a factor of 2-4 per year. So the overall performance gain using FPGAs increases even faster than for normal processors keeping the interest in the investment in this technology.

We have implemented a prototype system on a PCI-board with one FPGA (Silicon Software microEnable-II with XILINX XCV400-4 [5]). This board that was fabricated 1999 has enough resources to implement one pipeline. This pipeline runs at 30 MHz and reconstructs a volume of 256^3 with 120 projections within 120 seconds. A doubling of the performance would be possible but was considered unnecessary since it serves only as a demonstrator. It should demonstrate the performance of one pipeline processor.

The next implementation that is currently under way uses an Virtex II FPGA [2]. In contrast to the previous FPGA it has fixed-wired hardware multipliers (96 multipliers in a XC2V3000, each 18×18 bit signed data, 5 ns propagation delay). Since hardware multipliers nearly fully consumed the resources of the current FPGA, we calculated that on the new FPGA between 16 and 20 pipelines (16 using fixed-wired multipliers, up to 4 using distributed logic multipliers) can be programmed by software. This will allow to reconstruct the volume a factor 16-20 faster, i.e. between 6 and 8 seconds; which is in the range of the imaging time of the C-arm system.

Acknowledgements

This work is supported by BMBF grant 1EZ0024. Many thanks also to Andreas Kugel and his group (Informatik V, University of Mannheim) for allowing us to try out our architecture on their developed FPGA board (see fig. 1).

References

1. L. A. Feldkamp, L. C. Davis, and J. W. Kress, "Practical cone-beam algorithm," J. Opt. Sot. Amer., vol. 1, pp. 612-619, June 1984.
2. http://www.xilinx.com/
3. A. C. Kak and Malcolm Slaney, Principles of Computerized Tomographic Imaging, IEEE Press, 1988
4. E. Euler, S. Wirth, K. J. Pfeifer, W. Mutschler, A. Hebecker 3D-Imaging with an Isocentric Mobile C- Arm, electromedica 68 (2000) no. 2
5. www.silicon-software.com

CARS 2002 – H.U. Lemke, M.W. Vannier; K. Inamura, A.G. Farman, K. Doi & J.H.C. Reiber (Editors)
©CARS/Springer. All rights reserved.

Trial for making other serially sectioned images (Visible Korean Human)

Min Suk Chung[a], Jin Seo Park[a], Jin Yong Kim[a], Woo Sup Hwang[a], Jae Keun Kim[b], Hyung-Seon Park[c]
[a] Department of Anatomy, Ajou University School of Medicine, Suwon, Korea,
[b] Department of Radiology, Ajou University School of Medicine, Suwon, Korea,
[c] Korea Institute of Science and Technology Information, Daejeon, Korea

Abstract

The Visible Korean Human dataset is being made (Mar 2000 - Aug 2005) as follows. Complete MR and CT images of the Korean cadaver are acquired. The cadaver is serially sectioned (interval 0.2 mm) and inputted into the personal computer (pixel size 0.2 mm) without any missing images. The Visible Korean Human dataset is expected to be more helpful than the Visible Human Project dataset since it will provide Korean images which will help in diagnosing and treating patients belonging to the Oriental race. It also has a complete MR and CT images which will improve the study of MR and CT images. The anatomical images without any missing images will help in reconstructing more complex 3D images. Furthermore, these anatomical images are created with thin interval (0.2 mm) and small pixel size (0.2 mm).

Keywords: Visible Korean Human, serially sectioned images, anatomical images

1. Introduction

The Visible Human Project dataset, which was introduced in 1994 (male) and 1995 (female) by the National Library of Medicine, has been used worldwide in the field of medical imaging. However, there are several problems encountered with the Visible Human Project dataset. First, it is difficult to adapt it to the Oriental race because the shape and size of human organs differ according to the races. Second, it does not include the complete MR and CT images because only MR images of the head were acquired and the lateral parts of upper limbs' CT images were cut off. Third, it has missing anatomical images between the four blocks because the cadavers were divided into four blocks before serial sectioning. Fourth, it does not show the anatomical structures which are smaller than 0.33 mm because the interval of the anatomical images was greater than 0.33 mm and the pixel size of those was 0.33 mm [1-5].

©CARS/Springer. All rights reserved.

The purpose of this study, namely Visible Korean Human, is to make other serially sectioned images which compensate for the problems encountered with the Visible Human Project dataset. Complete MR and CT images of the Korean cadaver are acquired. The cadaver is serially sectioned at 0.2 mm intervals and inputted into the personal computer to make anatomical images (pixel size 0.2 mm) without any missing images. This study is expected to take five years (Mar 2000 - Aug 2005) (Table 1).

Sex	Age	Length	Weight	Cause of death	Period of experiment
Male (first)	65	1,789 mm	53 kg	Brain tumor	Mar 2000 - Feb 2001
Male (second)	60	1,720 mm	65 kg	Traffic accident	Mar 2001 - Aug 2001
Male (third)	33	1,718 mm	55 kg	Leukemia	Sep 2001 - Aug 2003
Female		(to be donated)			Sep 2003 - Aug 2005

Table 1. Cadavers used for the preliminary and main experiments.

2. Methods

To make the Visible Korean Human, three donated Korean male cadavers have been used for the preliminary and main experiments. First and second Korean male cadavers were used for preliminary experiment. Third Korean male cadaver is being used for the main experiment based on his characteristics: he was young, he had average body size of a Korean male, and he had few pathological findings (Table 1).

The MR and CT images of the entire body were acquired at 1 mm intervals. The MR and CT images were transferred to the personal computer via DICOM network, and saved in TIFF format on Piview software (Mediface™).
The cadaver was embedded and frozen. An embedding box was made, and the cadaver was put into the embedding box. The embedding agent (3 % gelatin) was poured into the embedding box and frozen to -70 °C in the freezer.

The embedding box was serially sectioned. A cryomacrotome for serial sectioning of the entire body at 0.2 mm intervals was made (Fig. 1). The cryomacrotome was so large (5 m X 4 m X 3 m) that the laboratory wall had to be removed to transport it into this laboratory. The embedding box was so heavy (1 ton) that a cart was used to transfer it from the freezer to the cryomacrotome and a crane was used to place it on the milling table of the cryomacrotome. The embedding box on the milling table was moved towards the milling disk at 0.2 mm intervals, and then it was moved parallel to the milling disk. At this time, the milling disk was rotated, so that the embedding box was milled at 0.2 mm intervals (Fig. 1).

©CARS/Springer. All rights reserved.

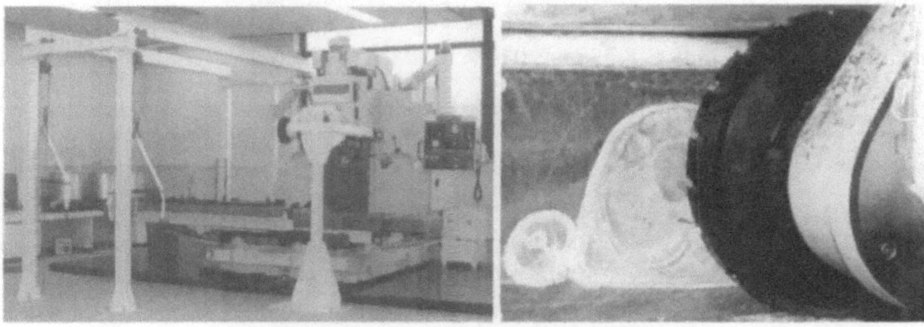

Fig. 1: Cryomacrotome (left) and milling disk and sectioned surface (right).

The sectioned surfaces were photographed and saved on the personal computer. The black curtains were hanged on the laboratory windows, and the fluorescent lights of the laboratory were turned off to make a dark room. Then, strobe lights were flashed on the sectioned surface. Consistent brightness of the sectioned surface was verified using an incident exposure meter. After serial sectioning, the sectioned surfaces (600 mm X 400 mm) were photographed using the digital camera (DSC 560 Kodak™, resolution 3,040 X 2,008) (Fig. 2) while two strobe lights were flashed. The quality (brightness, color, focus, etc.) of the anatomical image (pixel size 0.2 mm X 0.2 mm) made by photographing the sectioned surface was verified on the computer monitor before the next serial sectioning. The anatomical image was saved in TIFF format on two personal computers (Fig. 2).

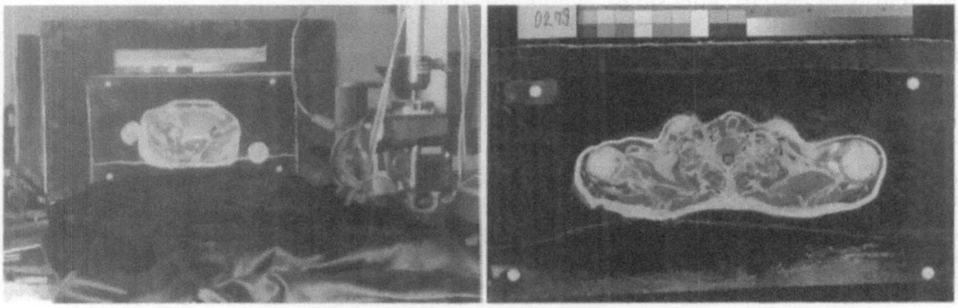

Fig. 2: Digital camera photographing sectioned surface (left). Anatomical image (right).

3. Results

In the main experiment, MR, CT, and anatomical images were acquired. Length of the cadaver was 1,718 mm and interval of the MR and CT images was 1 mm, so that 1,718 sets of MR and CT images were acquired. Each cropped image had 505 X 276 resolution, 8 bit gray color, and 769 KB file size. Length of the cadaver was 1,718 mm and the interval of anatomical images was 0.2 mm, so that 8,590 anatomical images were acquired. Each anatomical image had 3,040 X 2,008 resolution, 24 bit color, and 17,890 KB file size (Table 2).

CARS 2002 – H.U. Lemke, M.W. Vannier; K. Inamura, A.G. Farman, K. Doi & J.H.C. Reiber (Editors)
©CARS/Springer. All rights reserved.

	Interval	Number	Resolution	Color	One File size	Total File size
MR images	1.0 mm	1,718	505 X 276	8 bit gray	769 KB	1.3 GB
CT images	1.0 mm	1,718	505 X 276	8 bit gray	769 KB	1.3 GB
Anatomical images	0.2 mm	8,590	3,040 X 2,008	24 bit color	17,890 KB	153.7 GB
Total						207.0 GB

Table 2. Features of the MR, CT, and anatomical images in the main experiment.

4. Discussion

A voxel, a unit of the 3D images made by volume rendering method, should be a regular hexahedron. First, in the Visible Korean Human, 1 mm sized voxel can be made of the MR and CT images because both interval and pixel size of the MR and CT images were 1 mm (Table 2). The approximate pixel size (1 mm) was decided by the field of view (480 mm X 480 mm) and resolution (512 X 512) of MR and CT images. Second, 0.2 mm sized voxel can be made of the anatomical images because both interval and pixel size of the anatomical images were 0.2 mm (Table 2). The approximate pixel size (0.2 mm) was decided by the size (600 mm X 400 mm) of the sectioned surfaces and resolution (3,040 X 2,008) of the digital camera.

The Visible Korean Human dataset is expected to be more helpful than the Visible Human Project dataset as follows. First, the Korean images will help in diagnosing and treating the patients belonging to the Oriental race. Second, the complete MR and CT images of the entire body at 1 mm intervals will improve the study of MR and CT images. Third, the anatomical images without any missing images will help in reconstructing more complete 3D images. Fourth, the anatomical images with thin interval (0.2 mm) and small pixel size (0.2 mm) will help to show small anatomical structures

5. Conclusions

In this ongoing study, we are trying to make the Visible Korean Human dataset which can compensate for the problems encountered with the Visible Human Project dataset. The Visible Korean Human dataset will be the basis for making better 3D images and virtual dissection software which will be more helpful in medical education. Like the Visible Human Project dataset, the Visible Korean Human dataset will be distributed worldwide free of charge.

References

1. Ackerman MJ, "The Visible Human Project. A resource for education", *Acad Med*, 74, 667-670, 1999.
2. Chung MS, Kim SY, "Three-dimensional image and virtual dissection program of the brain made of Korean cadaver", *Yonsei Med J*, 41, 299-303, 2000.
3. Pommert A, Hoehne KH, Pflesser B, Richter E, Riemer M, Schiemann T, Schubert R, Schumacher U, Tiede U, "Creating a high-resolution spatial / symbolic model of the inner organs based on the Visible Human", *Med Image Anal*, 5, 221-228, 2001.
4. Spitzer VM, Ackerman MJ, Scherizinger AL, Whitlock DG, "The Visible Human male. Technical report", *J Am Med Inform Assoc*, 3, 118-130, 1996.
5. Spitzer VM, Whitlock DG, "The Visible Human dataset. The anatomical platform for human simulation", *Anat Rec*, 253, 49-57, 1998.

CARS 2002 – H.U. Lemke, M.W. Vannier; K. Inamura, A.G. Farman, K. Doi & J.H.C. Reiber (Editors)
©CARS/Springer. All rights reserved.

An alternating-constraints optimization method for volume-preserving non-rigid registration of MR breast images

T. Rohlfing[a], C. R. Maurer, Jr.[a], M. A. Jacobs[b], D. A. Bluemke[b], R. Shahidi[a]
[a]Image Guidance Laboratories, Department of Neurosurgery, Stanford University, 300 Pasteur Drive, Room S-012, MC 5327, Stanford, CA 94305-5327, USA
[b]Department of Radiology and Radiological Science, The Johns Hopkins University School of Medicine, Baltimore, MD 21205, USA

Abstract

We propose in this work a novel optimization strategy for intensity-based non-rigid image registration of contrast-enhanced images with a volume-preservation constraint. The optimization method alternates between under-constrained registration (allowing the elimination of motion artifacts in the subtraction images) and over-constrained registration (enforcing volume preservation of contrast-enhanced structures). We apply our method to pre- and post-contrast MR breast images from 17 patients and demonstrate its capability to simultaneously achieve volume preservation and artifact reduction.

Keywords: Non-rigid image registration, tissue incompressibility, breast MR imaging

1. Introduction

Non-rigid image registration algorithms based on free-form deformations have recently been shown to be a valuable tool in various biomedical image processing applications. One application of particular clinical interest is their application to pairs of native and contrast-enhanced images with the purpose of reducing motion artifacts in the subtraction image [1, 5]. However, a major problem with existing algorithms is that when they are applied to pre- and post-contrast image pairs, they often produce transformations that substantially shrink the volume of contrast-enhancing structures. Contrast-enhancement is an intensity inconsistency between the two images, which is what intensity-based registration algorithms are designed to minimize. Tanner et al. [8] observed this behaviour for contrast-enhanced breast lesions and we have demonstrated it for contrast-enhanced vessels in CT-DSA [2]. This problem severely affects the usefulness of the resulting transformation for volumetric analysis, image subtraction, multispectral classification, and pharmacokinetic modeling.

To address this problem, an additional penalty term is typically added to the intensity-based similarity measure to constrain the deformation to be smooth. Some authors use a mechanically motivated energy term that constrains the "bending energy" of the deformation [5]. A different approach uses "coupled" control points of the deformation to make the contrast-enhanced lesion locally rigid [8]. This approach requires identification of these structures prior to or during registration. Also, it prevents deformation of these structures even in cases where they have actually deformed.

©CARS/Springer. All rights reserved.

We recently introduced an incompressibility (local volume preservation) constraint based on the Jacobian determinant of the deformation [1]. It is based on the assumption that soft tissue in the human body is generally incompressible for small deformations and short time periods. When computing non-rigid coordinate transformations between pre- and post-contrast images, this knowledge can be incorporated into the registration process by penalizing deviations of the Jacobian determinant of the deformation transformation from unity.

When selecting the appropriate weighting factor for the incompressibility penalty term, there is a trade-off between volume preservation and motion artifact reduction. For small penalty weights, artifacts are reduced well at the cost of volume loss of contrast-enhanced structures. For large penalty weights, volume of such structures is preserved but the ability of the deformation to model actual deformations and eliminate motion artifacts is reduced. In particular, large penalty weights often cause the iterative search to get stuck in local minima that can only be escaped from by allowing volume loss. We therefore propose in this paper a new optimization strategy that alternates between smaller penalty weights that allow deformation and artifact reduction and subsequent larger penalty weights that enforce volume preservation. We evaluate the efficacy and robustness of our alternating-constraints optimization method and validate its potential clinical value by applying it to the non-rigid registration of clinical pre- and post-contrast MR breast images from 17 patients.

2. Materials and methods

2.1 Image registration

An initial alignment of pre- and post-contrast images is achieved using a rigid registration method with 6 degrees of freedom (DOFs). Our algorithm is an independent implementation of a technique for rigid and affine registration described in Ref. [6]. It uses normalized mutual information as the image similarity measure [7]. In the first step, this method is employed directly for finding an initial rigid transformation to capture the global displacement of both images. The rigid transformation is then used as the initial estimate for the non-rigid registration.

The non-rigid algorithm is an independent and modified implementation of a technique introduced by Rueckert et al. [5]. The transformation model we use is a multilevel formulation of B-spline based free-form deformation [3, 4]. In addition to the image similarity measure, our technique incorporates an incompressibility penalty term to constrain the deformation of the coordinate space [1, 2]. A user-defined weighting factor controls the relative influence of the image similarity and incompressibility terms, combining both into an overall cost function. The deformation constraint is motivated by the assumption that soft tissue in the human body is approximately incompressible, at least for small deformations and short time periods. The value of the Jacobian determinant of the transformation at (x,y,z) is equal to 1 if the deformation at (x,y,z) is incompressible, greater than 1 if there is local expansion, and less than 1 if there is compression. The deformation penalty term penalizes deviations of the Jacobian determinant from unity (the

©CARS/Springer. All rights reserved.

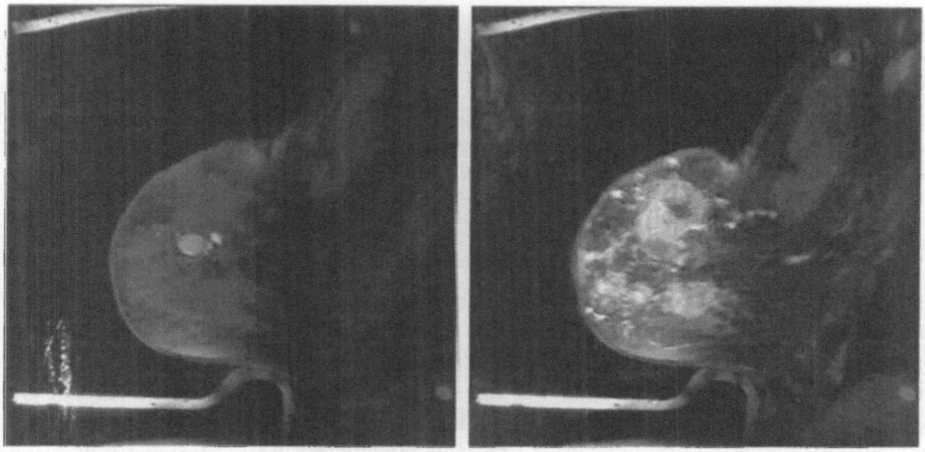

Figure 1. Image data from one of the patients used in this study. Left: Pre-contrast image; right: corresponding post-contrast image.

term we use is the integral of the absolute logarithm of the Jacobian determinant, integrated over the domain of the reference image).

In addition to simply constraining the free-form deformation with a weighted constraint, we also apply a scheme similar to simulated annealing. The idea is to first perform the non-rigid registration with a smaller penalty weight, which allows deformation and motion artifact reduction at the cost of potentially shrinking contrast-enhanced structures. The registration process is then repeated with a higher penalty weight, which enforces incompressibility and volume preservation. The purpose of this alternating-constraints strategy is to help the iterative search process during registration avoid local minima. The deformation penalty term weights used in this study ranged from 0.01 to 1 for the over-constrained steps. The penalty term weights for the under-contrained steps are obtained by multiplying the respective over-constrained weight by 0.01.

2.2 Image data

A total of 17 patients (age range, 18-80 years; median, 45 years) were consecutively referred for MR evaluation of suspicious findings and/or extent of the breast lesion. We applied our non-rigid registration algorithm to MR breast images acquired before and after contrast injection. The MR scans were performed on a 1.5 T MR scanner (General Electric Medical Systems, Milwaukee, WI), using a dedicated phased array breast coil (MRI Devices, Waukesha, WI) with the patient lying prone with the breast in a holder to reduce motion. Fat-suppressed 3-D T_1-weighted FSPGR (T_R/T_E = 20/4 ms, FOV = 18 × 18 cm, matrix = 512 × 160, 60 slices, slice thickness 2 mm) pre- and post-contrast images were obtained after intravenous administration of Gd-DTPA contrast agent (Magnevist, Berlex, 0.2 ml/kg [0.1 mmol/kg]). The contrast agent was hand injected over 10 seconds with MR imaging beginning immediately after completion of the injection. The contrast bolus was then followed by a 20 cc flush. The breast lesion was defined by contrast enhancement and identified by a radiologist. Example images are shown in Fig. 1.

©CARS/Springer. All rights reserved.

2.3 Study design

Constrained free-form deformations were computed, covering a large range of weighting factors for the deformation constraint (0.0001 to 1). All non-rigid registrations started with a 40 mm control point spacing that was successively refined to 20 mm, 10 mm, and finally 5 mm. In parallel, the image data resolution was refined from 4 mm voxel size to 2 mm, 1 mm, until at the final stage the original image data was used.

3. Results

The original volumes of the contrast-enhanced structures in the images from 17 patients ranged from 0.2 to 77.7 ml (mean ± SD, 9.1 ± 19.0 ml). These volumes were determined by semi-automatically segmenting the contrast-enhanced structures in the subtraction image after rigid registration. As other groups have previously reported [8], unconstrained non-rigid registration of pre- and post-contrast images results in volume loss of the contrast-enhanced structures. For the 17 patients considered in the present study, volume loss was between 1.3 and 61.8 percent (23.4 ± 18.3 percent). Our incompressibility constraint preserved the volume of contrast-enhanced structures when weighted with a sufficiently high weighting factor.

Constrained non-rigid registration can still achieve levels of artifact reduction comparable to that produced by unconstrained non-rigid registration. Unfortunately, the more strictly incompressibility or smoothness constraints are enforced (larger relative weight in the optimization function), the more residual artifacts remain. However, this is not a consequence of the constraining of the free-form deformation itself but primarily an effect of the search algorithm used for optimization. Using an alternating-constraint optimization strategy, artifact reduction and volume preservation were both achieved simultaneously.

4. Conclusion

Results on 17 MR mammography data sets suggest that incorporation of an incompressibility penalty term based on the Jacobian determinant improves non-rigid registration of pre- and post-contrast images by substantially reducing the problem of shrinkage of contrast-enhanced structures. Motion artifacts can still be reduced substantially, similar to what can be achieved using unconstrained non-rigid registration. This was especially found to be true when using the proposed two-stage relaxation optimization strategy with alternating under- and over-constraining of the deformation.

Acknowledgements

TR was supported by the National Science Foundation under Grant No. EIA-0104114. MAJ was supported by the National Institutes of Health under Grant No. T32 CA09630. TR, CRM, and RS acknowledge support for this research provided by CBYON, Inc., Mountain View, CA. Computations were performed on an SGI Origin 3800 supercomputer in the Stanford University Bio-X core facility for Biomedical Computation.

©CARS/Springer. All rights reserved.

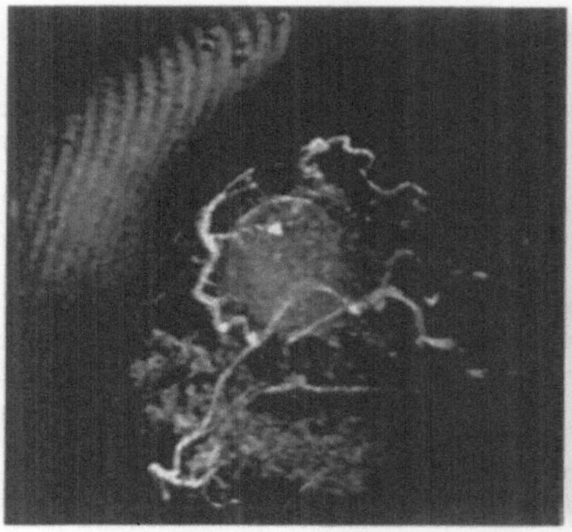

(a) Rigid registration

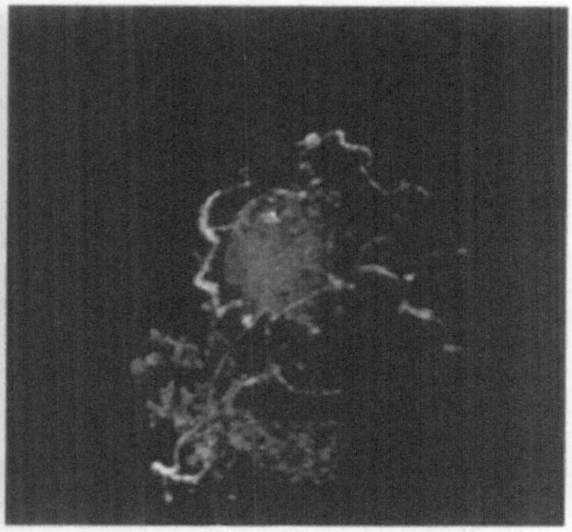

(b) Unconstrained non-rigid registration (25.1% volume loss)

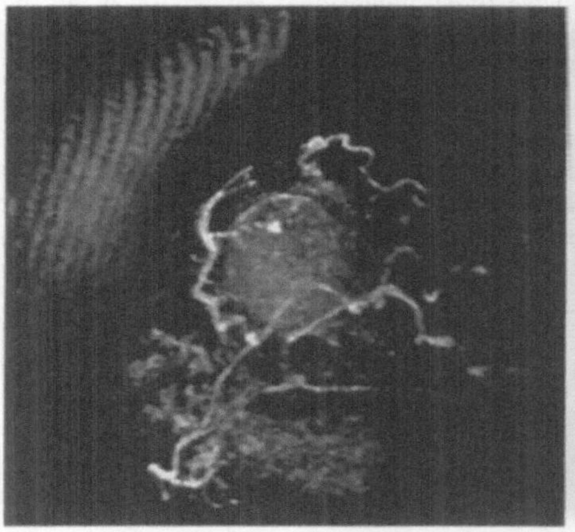

(c) Non-rigid registration with incompressibility constraint (0.1% volume loss)

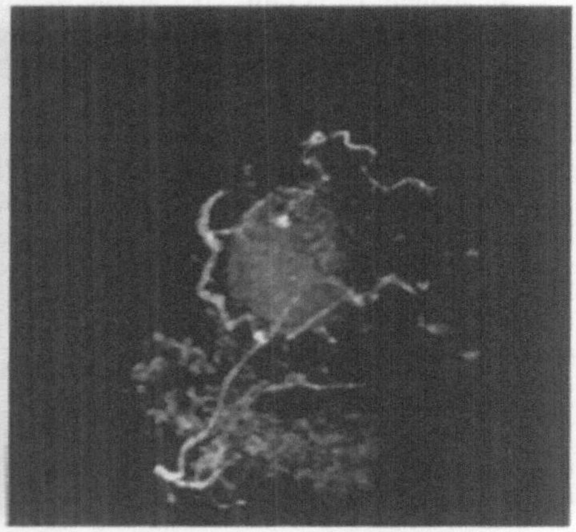

(d) Non-rigid registration with incompressibility constraint and relaxation (1.2% volume loss)

Figure 2. Maximum intensity projections of subtraction images after applying different registration algorithms. Unconstrained non-rigid registration eliminated motion artifacts, but substantially reduced the volume of the contrast-enhanced lesion (*top right*). Using the incompressibility constraint, the lesion volume was preserved but motion artifacts remained almost unchanged (*bottom left*). By alternating between lower and higher constraint weights at each level, virtually all motion artifact is removed with negligible volume loss using the incompressibility constraint (*bottom right*). The images in this figure originate from the same patient as the ones in Fig. 1.

©CARS/Springer. All rights reserved.

References

1. T Rohlfing, CR Maurer Jr. Intensity-based non-rigid registration using adaptive multilevel free-form deformation with an incompressibility constraint. *Medical Image Computing and Computer-Assisted Intervention*, pp 111-119, 2001.
2. T Rohlfing, CR Maurer Jr, J Beier. Correction of motion artifacts in three-dimensional CT-DSA using constrained adaptive multi-level free-form registration. *Computer Assisted Radiology and Surgery*, pp 350-355, 2001.
3. T Rohlfing, CR Maurer Jr, DLG Hill, T Hartkens, WA Hall, CL Truwit, H Liu, AJ Martin, R Shahidi. Intra-operative brain deformation using non-rigid image registration on a shared-memory multiprocessor computer. *Computer Assisted Radiology and Surgery*, 2002 (in these proceedings).
4. T Rohlfing, CR Maurer Jr, WG O'Dell, J Zhong. Modeling liver motion and deformation during the respiratory cycle using intensity-based free-form registration of gated MR images. *Medical Imaging: Visualization, Display, and Image-Guided Procedures* Proc SPIE 4319: 337-348, 2001.
5. D Rueckert, LI Sonoda, C Hayes, DLG Hill, MO Leach, DJ Hawkes. Nonrigid registration using free-form deformations: Application to breast MR images. *IEEE Trans Med Imaging* 18: 712-721, 1999.
6. C Studholme, DLG Hill, DJ Hawkes. Automated three-dimensional registration of magnetic resonance and positron emission tomography brain images by multiresolution optimization of voxel similarity measures. *Med Phys* 24: 25-35, 1997.
7. C Studholme, DLG Hill, DJ Hawkes. An overlap invariant entropy measure of 3D medical image alignment. *Pattern Recognit* 33: 71-86, 1999.
8. C Tanner, JA Schnabel, D Chung, MJ Clarkson, D Rueckert, DLG Hill, DJ Hawkes. Volume and shape preservation of enhancing lesions when applying non-rigid registration to a time series of contrast enhancing MR breast images. *Medical Image Computing and Computer-Assisted Intervention*, pp 327-337, 2000.

CARS 2002 – H.U. Lemke, M.W. Vannier; K. Inamurc, A.G. Farman, K. Doi & J.H.C. Reiber (Editors)
©CARS/Springer. All rights reserved.

Integrating the Insight Toolkit *itk* into a medical software framework

Nils Hanssen, Bartcsz von Rymon-Lipinski,
Thomas Jansen, Marc Liévin, Erwin Keeve
Surgical Systems Laboratory, research center c a e s a r,
Friedensplatz 16, 53111 Bonn, Germany

Abstract

In this paper, we present the integration of an image processing toolkit into our platform-independent medical software framework *Julius*. The *Insight Toolkit* (itk) consists of state-of-the-art segmentation and registration methods, focused on medical applications. In this paper, the focus lies on the integration of the segmentation methods.Each processing filter of the segmentation toolkit is represented as an individual element in the user interface. The central part of every segmentation routine is the anatomical list, which is fully customizable. By clicking on an anatomical entity in this list, the user is guided during the segmentation of the corresponding structure. This guidance is directly dependent on the underlying modality as well as the selected anatomical structure itself.

Keywords: Software framework, segmentation, insight toolkit

1. Introduction

Segmentation of anatomical structures from medical images of different modalities is a central part of the processing pipeline in image-guided surgery. By identifying structures and defining boundaries, parts of the images or volumes can be assigned to anatomical structures, which is important for successional processing or simulation steps. Non-automatic segmentation methods have to be parameterized with a-priori knowledge by the user. This knowledge includes typical voxel values of tissue types in the considered modalities (thresholds) as well as spatial and geometrical properties (seed-points or initial contours).

In this paper, we present the basic concept of anatomy-based segmentation. A customizable knowledge base contains a-priori information about anatomical structures and tissue types for different modalities. By means of this knowledge base, sequences of processing operations from the Insight Toolkit (itk) [1] and their parameters are automatically driven by the medical software framework [2]. The sequences and derived parameter values are displayed in the user-interface. Missing parameters that are mandatory for the operation and cannot be automatically determined have to be supplied by the user.

2. Methods

Our medical software framework serves as a scaffold for any medical image processing application. It is prepared for various use cases that include data-I/O, segmentation, registration, navigation and visualization procedures. All elements of the user-interface

©CARS/Springer. All rights reserved.

are based on the Qt library [3], which is platform independent. The internal representation as well as the visualization of volumetric and polygonal data is based on the Visual Toolkit (vtk) [4].

The open-source toolkit itk provides a collection of C++ classes for medical data representation and processing. It follows a data-flow approach that is based on data objects (representation) that are manipulated by filter objects (processing). Supported generic data structures are n-dimensional images as well as unstructured meshes that are templated over the voxel or vertex type and the dimension. The images are used for holding the acquired medical image data, whereas meshes are mainly utilized as base or helper classes for active contour models or surface-based segmentation algorithms. The toolkit makes intense use of C++ templates, also referred to as *generic programming* [5].

In the following sections, we describe the concept of anatomy-based segmentation as well as the integration of itk in the framework. The presented concepts can be directly transferred to the integration of other third-party C++ processing libraries.

2.1 Anatomy-based segmentation
A central concept within Julius is the anatomical list, which is the starting point for each segmentation procedure (see figure 1, left). It incorporates a comprehensive list of anatomical structures indexed by their Latin and English term. Individual anatomical entities can be grouped by various predefined categories including topographic or functional relationship as well as by tissue type like bone or fat. Custom groups suitable for the current case can be defined. For example, all significant structures for the planning of a knee-intervention can be assembled and handled in a convenient way.

One significant advantage of the anatomical list is that a-priori information can be automatically included in the segmentation, since typical properties of individual structures or tissue types can be stored in an internal knowledge base. This knowledge base, which can be customized via a XML [6] file, contains for example information about typical value ranges of tissue types in the respective modality. Arbitrary custom properties of anatomical entities can be added to the XML file and can be evaluated by the processing filters in the system.

Based on this a-priori information in the knowledge base, the framework can recommend a suitable sequence of segmentation methods and parameters. The typical workflow for a segmentation procedure is as follows:

1) An anatomical entity is selected from the list.
2) The framework suggests a suitable sequence of processing methods and parameters.
3) The recommended sequence of processing methods and derived parameters is shown in the user-interface.

Next, the actual execution of every single segmentation step can be customized and supervised by the user. Missing parameters that cannot be derived from the knowledge-base have to be specified by hand. Intermediate processing results can be inspected in the slice- and volume-views that are part of the framework (see figure 2, right).

©CARS/Springer. All rights reserved.

2.2 Stepcards for processing sequences

The execution of the recommended processing sequences is controlled by user interface elements called stepcards. A stepcard represents one single step of execution that is performed on the data and can be dynamically inserted during program execution. Automatically derived parameters for the processing step are displayed in the stepcard. It is displayed as a Qt-Widget, where the user is able to edit the parameters for the processing step. If interaction with the data, like setting of seed-points or drawing of initial contours is required, the user can click and draw on three orthogonal slice-views. By providing a sequence of stepcards (see figure 2, center), the recommended processing from the pipeline can be monitored. When executing, each stepcard passes its parameters to the corresponding processing filter. The execution of each stepcard can be repeated several times with different parameters until the desired result is achieved. After that, the result is frozen and the next stepcard is displayed.

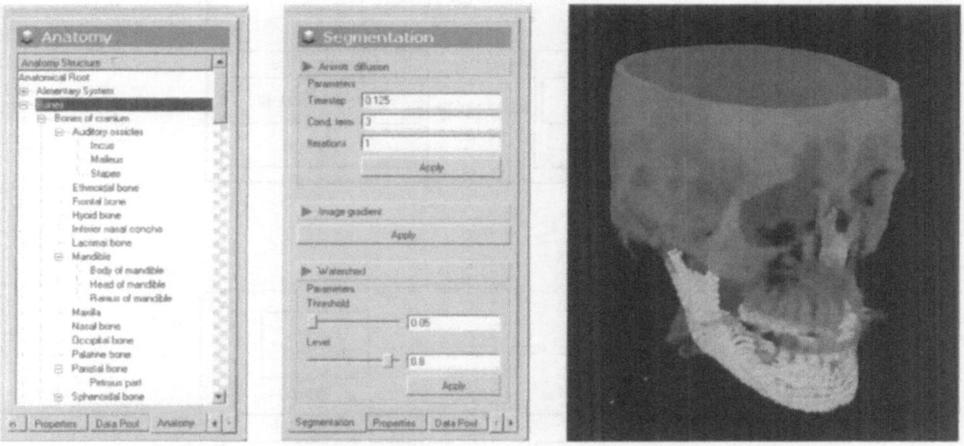

Figure 1. Julius GUI-elements. *Left*: Anatomical list organized by tissue types. *Center*: Stepcard sequence for watershed segmentation. Each step can be applied multiple times until the desired result is achieved. *Right*: Volume view of mandible extracted from CT images with a connectivity filter visualized via hardware-accelerated 3D texture mapping. The seed-points have been specified by the user.

2.3 Integration of ITK in the data pool

The data pool is a collection of data modules, which implement the same consistent interface and encapsulate different data structures with different internal formats. In contrast to a linear processing pipeline, this pool has no prescribed inherent data-flow structure but is first of all a place where data can be stored for processing. The actual data-flow structure from one data module to the other is defined by the methods that operate on the data. The two generic types of data that can reside in the data pool and can be directly visualized are volumetric images and polygonal meshes in 3D. By means of the registry, a globally unique object, the pool can be accessed and data modules can be distinguished by various properties like the type of data, a description string or a modification timestamp. All actions on the pool that result in manipulation of data are encapsulated by controller modules. The input and output types for a controller are specified in the implementation

©CARS/Springer. All rights reserved.

of the module. The controller can automatically take the latest modified data module with the adequate type as input. Depending on the implementation of the controller, the input data is either kept in the pool or is replaced by the output module. While the in-place mode saves memory since it does not keep provisional results, undo-mechanisms are of course only possible, if the data is duplicated. All modules in the framework can reside in an own runtime-library. Thereby, no recompilation of the framework is necessary if new modules are added.

In the current version of Julius, 3D volume objects of itk can be accessed via a data module. With the integrated DICOM-interface itk volume data is added to the data pool and can be displayed with the supported 3D visualization techniques.

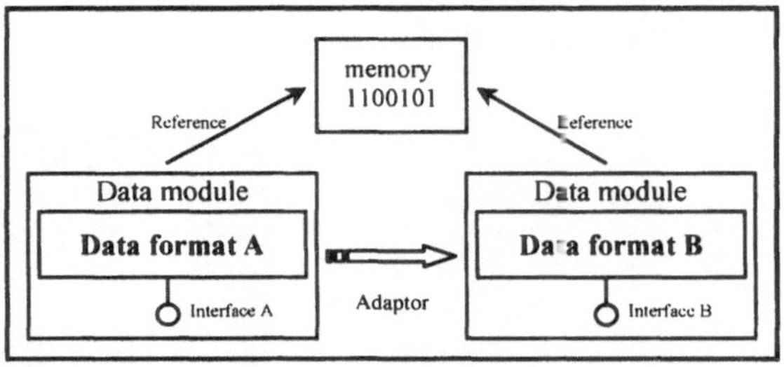

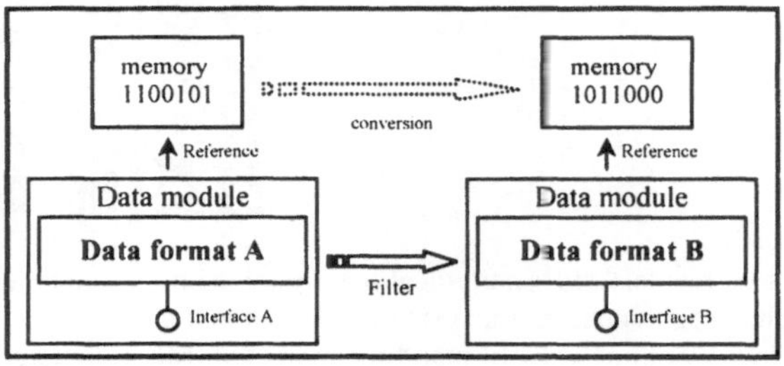

Figure 2. Data format adaptor (top) and data format filter (bottom). Depending on the memory structure, the data from different internal formats can be converted by an adaptor without duplication of memory.

2.4 Data exchange with ITK

At any time, data modules, which encapsulate different internal representations of data, can reside in the pool. In order to perform filter operations from all libraries that are encapsulated in controller modules, the data has to be converted to the appropriate internal format on demand. If the internal representations (in terms of memory usage) of the source and destination format matches, an adaptor for format conversion can be used. This is often true for volume datasets. Thereby, data in the pool is not replicated, but merely gets a new interface that is consistent with the corresponding filter of the library. If the memory format of the source and destination formats do not match, a format conversion

©CARS/Springer. All rights reserved.

filter has to be executed. Thereby, the data has to be replicated and reorganized in memory in order to get the appropriate data type (see figure 2). By means of a data format adaptor, itk volume datasets are connected to the internal volume format of Julius.

First image processing and segmentation filters like anisotropic diffusion, image gradient and watershed segmentation of itk have been integrated. The actual execution is performed by the itk filter object that is encapsulated in the controller module. After the execution, the result of the filter operation is itself encapsulated in a data module and placed in the data pool.

3. Discussion

We presented an anatomy-based segmentation concept in our software-framework Julius, which uses basic a-priori knowledge of structures and tissue types to guide the segmentation. For a selected anatomical structure, image processing and segmentation steps from the Insight Toolkit are recommended and initial parameterizations are suggested. By means of stepcards, the user is able to tune the recommended values and can specify additional parameters that cannot be automatically derived by the system. Data adaptors for volumes have been implemented, which handle the data-exchange between itk volumes and the internal volumetric data format of the framework. Due to the data encapsulation paradigm, further image processing packages can be integrated with minimum effort. By using the standardized XML syntax, custom a-priori information can be added to the knowledge base and can be evaluated by the processing algorithms.

We see this association of anatomical structures and segmentation methods with respect to the underlying modality as a first step towards an expert system for segmentation. For the future, we plan to include region of interests as well as seed-points in the knowledge base.

Acknowledgements

Thanks to Lutz Ritter for providing the anatomical list and its concepts. This work is funded by the German Federal Ministry of Education and Research (BMBF) research grant 01IRA08E – ARSyS-Tricorder. For further information on this research project please refer to http://www.arsys-tricorder.de. The content of this manuscript does not necessarily reflect the position of the BMBF.

References

1. NLM Insight Segmentation and Registration Toolkit, http://www.itk.org, 2001.
2. von Rymon-Lipinski B., Jansen T., "An Extendable Application Framework for Medical Visualization and Surgical Planning," Proceedings Computer Assisted Radiology and Surgery CARS'01, pp. 181-186, Berlin, Germany.
3. Qt library, Trolltech; http://www.trolltech.com/products/index.html.
4. Schröder W., Martin K., Lorensen B., "The Visualization Toolkit – 2nd Edition", Prentice Hall PTR, New Jersey, 1998.
5. Austern M.H., "Generic Programming and the STL: Using and Extending the C++ Standard Template Library", Addison Wesley Professional Computing Series, 1999.
6. Extensible Markup Language (XML), http://www.xml.org..

©CARS/Springer. All rights reserved.

Validation of MRI/SPECT similarity-based registration methods using realistic simulations of normal and pathological SPECT data

C. Grova [a], P. Jannin [a], A. Biraben [a,b], I. Buvat [d], H. Benali [d], A.M. Bernard [e], B. Gibaud [a], J.M. Scarabin [a,c]

[a] Laboratoire IDM, Faculté de Médecine, Université de Rennes

[b] Service de Neurologie, Hôpital Universitaire de Rennes

[c] Service de Neurochirurgie, Hôpital Universitaire de Rennes

[d] Unité INSERM U494, Hôpital Universitaire Pitié Salpétrière, Paris

[e] Service de Médecine Nucléaire, Centre Eugène Marquis, Rennes

Abstract

We propose a validation methodology to study the behaviour of SPECT/MRI similarity-based registration methods in normal and pathological conditions. Validation data sets were computed by simulating realistic SPECT data from 3D T1-weighted MRI data, through Monte Carlo simulations, using a perfusion model built from measurements made on real SPECT data (normal or pathological). Validation of four similarity-based registration methods performed on these simulated data showed a registration mean accuracy significantly lower than simulated SPECT spatial resolution.

Keywords: Registration, validation, SPECT simulations

1. Introduction

The purpose of this study is validation of similarity-based registration methods between Single Photon Emission Computed Tomography (SPECT) and Magnetic Resonance Imaging (MRI). Only few references are focused on validating SPECT/MRI registration methods [1,2]. Registration methods are mainly designed and validated for Positron Emission Tomography (PET)/MRI registration and applied to register SPECT data [3,4]. Traditionally, precision and accuracy of a registration technique are assessed by means of a gold standard. The latter consists of a reference geometric transformation with which registration methods can be assessed. Gold standards are often provided by extrinsic information (e.g. fiducial markers [1], stereotactic frames [3,4]). These evaluations remain limited by the intrinsic accuracy and precision of the registration method used to compute the gold standard. Indeed, the registration method to be validated cannot yield better performances than the gold standard registration method itself. Such evaluations may also require invasive data acquisition and are thus difficult to apply in routine clinical contexts.

We present a validation methodology to study the behaviour of SPECT/MRI similarity-based registration methods in normal and pathological conditions. Our validation hypothesis is to assess whether a similarity-based registration method is able to match 3D T1-weighted MRI data set (showing no pathological signal) with normal or pathological SPECT data sets (showing hyper- or hypo-perfusion areas) with a mean accuracy

©CARS/Springer. All rights reserved.

significantly lower than SPECT spatial resolution. For this purpose, our validation method is based on realistic SPECT simulations from a normal MRI data set. Since simulated SPECT data sets are perfectly aligned with this MRI data set, our method provides a perfect gold standard for registration validation. The use of Monte Carlo techniques to perform simulations, as well as the construction of a theoretical perfusion model deduced from measurements on real SPECT data, allow realistic simulations to be produced. In this paper, our method is applied to simulate normal SPECT and ictal SPECT in the clinical context of temporal lobe epilepsy. Ictal SPECT reflects brain perfusion during an epileptic seizure, as the radioactive tracer is injected just at the beginning of a seizure. These simulated data were then used to estimate and to compare the accuracy of four MRI/SPECT registration methods based on similarity measurements: Mutual Information (MI) [5,6], Normalized Mutual Information (NMI) [7], Correlation Ratio (CR) [8] and Woods Criterion (WC) [4].

2. Material and Methods

2.1 Generation of validation data sets: realistic simulation of SPECT data

The method we present is designed to be able to control both registration geometry and dissimilarities between our data by simulating realistic SPECT data from a normal MRI. First of all, we defined an anatomical model that is an high resolution 3D T1-weighted MRI, and a theoretical perfusion model defined at the MRI resolution. These theoretical models were then used to perform realistic SPECT simulations.

The anatomical model was based on Zubal's head phantom [9], which consists of sixty-three anatomical entities manually segmented and labelled on a normal T1-weighted MRI data set (matrix = 256x256x124, pixel size = 1.1x1.1x1.4 mm). These anatomical entities were classified into seven different types of tissue (i.e. conjunctive tissue, water, brain, bone, muscle, fat and blood), from which the photon attenuation map was derived.

The theoretical perfusion model was computed using Regions of Interest (ROIs)-based measurements performed on real SPECT data. These ROIs were deduced from Zubal's head phantom anatomical entities. To identify functional information in our model, we selected SPECT and MRI data sets from an homogeneous population of normal or pathological subjects, depending on what kind of SPECT we wanted to simulate. Before performing measurements, SPECT data sets and ROIs were localized in a common coordinate system. Rigid registration was firstly realized using Mutual Information [6] between each SPECT/MRI pair of data sets. We then spatially normalized our MRI data sets with the SPM T1 template as described by Friston et al. [10], using the Statistical Parametric Mapping (SPM) software package. We were then able to perform perfusion measurements on these spatially normalized SPECT data sets using spatially normalized ROIs. These measurements provided relative values of brain perfusion for each anatomical entity. The mean perfusion measured for each anatomical entity was used to define the theoretical perfusion model, i.e., the radioactive tracer activity map.

These attenuation and activity maps were used to simulate SPECT data. Using Monte Carlo simulations, we simulated physical processes involved in SPECT acquisition,

©CARS/Springer. All rights reserved.

namely single photon propagation (e.g. Compton scatter, tissue attenuation) and acquisition procedures (e.g. collimator and detector response). Monte Carlo simulations were performed using the Photon History Generator (PHG) software package [11]. 10^9 photons were simulated. A SPECT acquisition with a parallel hole collimator was simulated (64 projections 128 x 128 over 360°, pixel size = 2.2 mm). Tomographic reconstruction used Filtered Back Projection with a ramp filter and the reconstructed data were post filtered using a 3D Gaussian filter with full width at half maximum of 8.8 mm. We finally resampled our simulated SPECT data to obtain voxel dimensions of 4.51 mm that exactly corresponds to the sampling rate used in our clinical acquisitions. Spatial resolution of our simulated data was thus estimated at 10.15 mm, whereas it was measured at 12.4 mm in our clinical acquisitions.

2.2 Registration validation method

These validation data sets (i.e. our simulated SPECT and Zubals'head phantom T1-weighted MRI) were used to compare and validate MRI/SPECT registration methods based on statistical similarity measurements that are widely used in the context of automatic multimodality registration. As our simulated SPECT data are perfectly aligned with MRI by construction, we have a perfect gold standard for registration validation.

The purpose of SPECT/MRI registration methods is to assess a rigid geometric T transformation defined by six parameters (three translations and three rotations). Let the reference image R be our SPECT data set and the floating image F our MRI data set. Similarity-based registration relies on the fact that a similarity measurement S(R, T(F)) is optimal when the data sets are perfectly registered. We studied four statistical similarity measurements: Mutual Information (MI) [5,6], Normalized Mutual Information (NMI) [7], Correlation Ratio (CR) [8] and Woods Criterion (WC) [4]. As recommended by the author, we segmented brain from the MRI data set before registration using the Woods Criterion. The optimisation of these cost functions was achieved using Powell's multidimensional direction set method and Brent's one-dimensional optimisation algorithm for line optimisations. A two-level multiresolution strategy as described by [6] was applied to avoid the pitfall of local optima.

Our validation parameters consisted of N = 50 T* theoretical transformations randomly generated by sampling a 6 parameters vector using a Gaussian distribution (Mean = 0, Standard Deviation = 10 mm or 10° respectively). T* was then applied to the MRI data set and a new unregistered MRI was thus created using trilinear interpolation. We then sequentially launched registration with the simulated SPECT using the four registration methods described above. Let T be the computed geometric transformation. For each registration method, we estimated registration accuracy. The quality index used to assess accuracy was a Root Mean Square (RMS) error measured on a set of n Pi points (n=1600) uniformly distributed within the brain and n Pi points (n=1400) uniformly distributed on the skin, computed as following:

$$RMS = \sqrt{\frac{1}{n}\sum_{i=1}^{n} \|P_i - T^{-1}(T^*(P_i))\|^2}$$

©CARS/Springer. All rights reserved.

3. Results

3.1 Validation data sets: normal and ictal SPECT simulations

The previous method was applied to simulate normal and ictal SPECT data. A population of 22 normal SPECT exams provided by L. Barnden [1] was used to create a normal perfusion model. A pathological model was computed using 15 ictal SPECT of epileptic patients investigated at the Rennes' hospital and who were proved to show temporo-mesial epilepsy (using depth electrodes recordings and surgical outcome). Figure 1 shows the theoretical normal perfusion model and the resulting normal SPECT simulation. Figure 2 shows the theoretical ictal perfusion model and the resulting ictal SPECT simulation. ROIs-based perfusion measurements showed, as expected for ictal SPECT, a hyper perfusion in the right hemisphere, located in the internal structures and the temporal lobe (Figure 2).

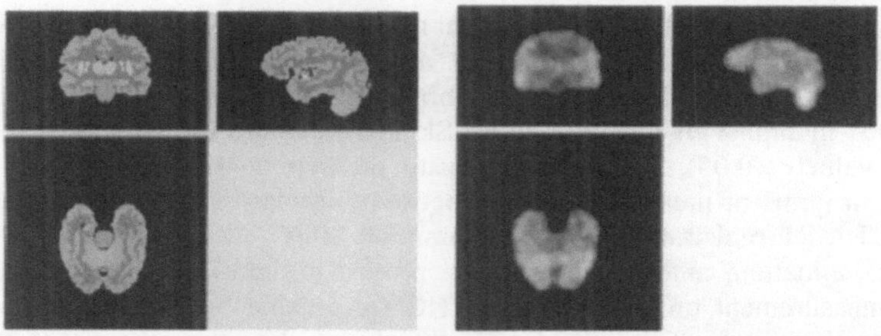

Figure 1: Theoretical normal perfusion model (left) and resulting normal SPECT simulation (right)

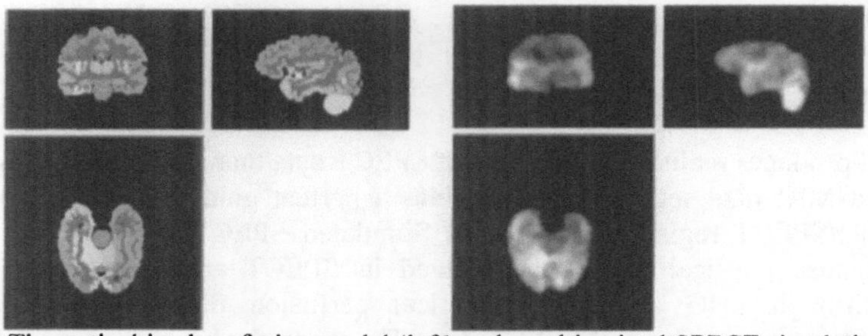

Figure 2: Theoretical ictal perfusion model (left) and resulting ictal SPECT simulation (right)

3.2 Registration validation results

These normal and ictal SPECT simulations were used to perform registration validation. To assess the performances of ictal and normal SPECT/MRI registration respectively, two independent sets of N=50 randomly generated T* theoretical transformations were used. No registration solution was excluded from the results. Figure 3 (resp. Figure 4) shows the distribution of RMS errors for normal (resp. ictal) SPECT/MRI registration, measured within the brain or on the skin for each registration method, using boxplot representation.

©CARS/Springer. All rights reserved.

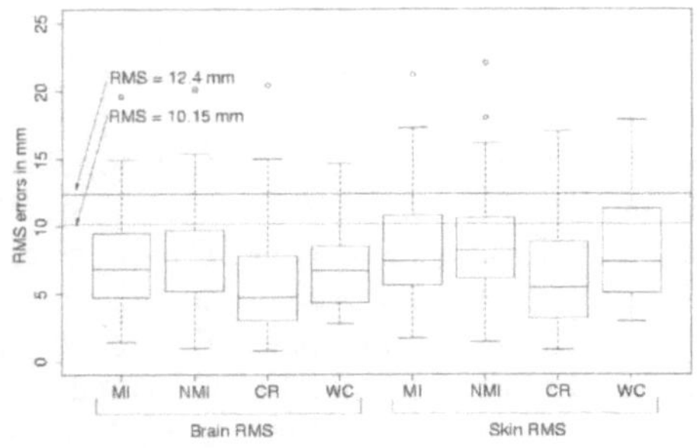

Figure 3: RMS errors distribution for normal SPECT/MRI registration (N=50)

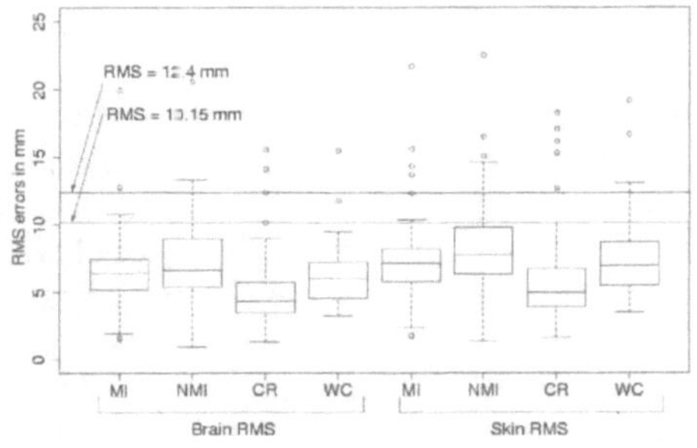

Figure 4: RMS errors distribution for ictal SPECT/MRI registration (N=50)

For each registration method, mean RMS values computed within the brain or on the skin were lower than our simulated SPECT spatial resolution (10.15 mm). Using Student t-test, we rejected the H0 hypothesis (H0: mean RMS > 10.15 mm) at highly significant levels for all registration methods, and for both normal and ictal SPECT/MRI registrations (p-value < 0.001 in almost all cases except for Skin RMS values for MI and NMI for normal SPECT: p-value < 0.05). For each similarity measurement, we found no significant differences in terms of mean RMS values between normal SPECT/MRI registration and ictal SPECT/MRI registration. For both normal SPECT/MRI and ictal SPECT/MRI registration validation, analysis of variance proved a significant effect of the type of similarity measurement on RMS errors (ANOVA p-value < 0.05). However, only the coefficient estimated for CR was significantly lower than the others (t-test p-value < 0.05). Thus CR proved to be slightly more accurate than the other criteria with our simulated data.

4. Discussion

Our method produces realistic simulations of SPECT data that are perfectly aligned with a T1-weighted MRI data set, and thus provides a perfect gold standard to compare and validate MRI/SPECT registration methods. Simulated SPECT data sets are considered realistic because physical processes involved in SPECT acquisition were accurately modelled through PHG and our theoretical perfusion models are deduced from measurements performed on real SPECT data. The theoretical perfusion model defined at the MRI resolution allows the control of the functional information in SPECT data and thus the degree of statistical similarity between simulated SPECT and MRI (e.g. ictal SPECT temporal hyper-perfusion).

We confirmed our validation hypothesis by proving that for the four registration methods, mean accuracy estimated through mean RMS error was significantly lower than our simulated SPECT spatial resolution (10.15 mm). Moreover, we found no significant mean accuracy differences between normal SPECT/MRI registration and ictal SPECT/MRI registration. We hypothesize that it remains enough spatial information in the histograms of our simulated data, especially for ictal SPECT, to achieve accurate registration. However, our simulations may still remain too "perfect" compared to real ictal SPECT. For instance, no radioactive tracer activity was assigned outside the brain, whereas radioactive tracer uptakes were observed within the skin, the muscles or in the parotid

©CARS/Springer. All rights reserved.

glands on some of our clinical ictal data. Nevertheless, our simulation environment allows us to control these different parameters (e.g. by applying different types and amount of noise to our data) in order to further study the behaviour of these similarity-based registration methods in the case of ictal SPECT.

We emphasize the generic aspect of our approach. Actually, this study may be extended to other registration methods or investigate other aspects such as sensitivity to SPECT reconstruction and correction features (e.g. reconstruction filters, attenuation or scatter correction). Our method may also be applied to study other clinical contexts, in particular by simulating other pathological SPECT patterns. Our simulation methodology may finally be useful to validate any other detection or quantification method that involves SPECT, or both SPECT and MRI data.

Acknowledgements

This work was partly supported by grants from the "Ligue Française Contre l'Epilepsie" and from the "Conseil Régional de Bretagne". We also would like to thank Dr. Leighton Barnden (Woodville Hospital Nuclear Medicine Department, Australia) for providing normal SPECT data sets.

References

1. Barnden L., Kwiatek R., Lau Y. et al., "Validation of fully automatic brain SPET to MR co-registration", *European Journal of Nuclear Medicine*, 27(2), 147-154, 2000.
2. Pfluger T., Vollmar C., Wismüller A. et al., "Quantitative comparison of automatic and interactive methods for MRI-SPECT image registration of the brain based on 3-dimensional calculation of error", *Journal of Nuclear Medicine*, 41(11), 1823-1829, 2000.
3. West J., Fitzpatrick J. M., Wang M. Y. et al., "Comparison and evaluation of retrospective intermodality brain image registration techniques", *Journal of Computer Assisted Tomography*, 21(4), 554-566, 1997.
4. Woods R. P., Mazziotta J. C., and Cherry S. R., "MRI-PET registration with automated algorithm", *Journal of Computed Assisted Tomography*, 17(4), 536-546, 1993.
5. Wells III W.M., Viola P., Atsumi H. et al., "Multi-modal volume registration by maximization of Mutual Information", *Medical Image Analysis*, 1(1), 35-51, 1996.
6. Maes F., Collignon A., Vandermeulen D. et al., "Multimodality image registration by maximization of mutual information", *IEEE Trans. on Medical Imaging*,16(2),187-198, 1997.
7. Studholme C., Hill D.L.G., and Hawkes D.J., "An overlap invariant entropy measure of 3D medical image alignment", *Pattern Recognition*, 32, 71-86, 1999.
8. Roche A., Malandain G., Pennec X. et al., "The correlation ratio as a new similarity measure for multimodal image registration", *MICCAI'98: Lecture Notes in Computer Science*, Wells W.M., Colchester A. and Delp S., 1496, 1115-1124, Springer-Verlag, Berlin Heidelberg, 1998.
9. Zubal I.G., Harrell C.R., Smith E.O. et al., "Computerized three-dimensional segmented human anatomy", *Medical Physics*, 21(2), 299-302, 1994.
10. Friston K.J., Ashburner J., Poline J.B. et al., "Spatial registration and normalization of images", *Human Brain Mapping*, 2, 165-189, 1995.
11. Harrison R.L., Vannoy S.D., Haynor D.R. et al., "Preliminary experience with the photon history generator module of a public-domain simulation system for emission tomography". *Conf. Rec. Nucl. Sci. Symp.*, 2, 115 4-1158, 1993.

©CARS/Springer. All rights reserved.

Automatic 3D-reconstruction of the ocular fundus from stereo images

Michael Wünstel und Hagen Schumann
Fraunhofer Institut für Graphische Datenverarbeitung
Fraunhoferstr. 5, D-64283 Darmstadt
Email: michael.wuenstel@igd.fhg.de, schumann@igd.fhg.de

Abstract

The methods of computer vision allow the 3D-reconstruction of an object from 2D stereo image pairs. The EU-Project Glaucad studies the glaucoma disease regarding appropriate geometric characterizations. Our task within this project is to develop a module for automatic 3D-reconstruction of the ocular fundus out of the uncalibrated stereo images. These reconstructions will be used to analyze the changes of the ocular fundus of glaucoma patients. Using methods of computer vision two main demands turned out to produce precise results: A good image preprocessing to compensate the partly changing and difficult recording conditions and a precise registration as prerequisite for the later calculation steps.

Keywords: Computer vision, 3D-reconstruction, glaucoma

1. Introduction

In Germany more than 500,000 people suffer from the glaucoma disease. There exist several types of this illness. In most cases the disease is accompanied with a constantly increased intraocular pressure. This situation might finally lead to the destruction of the blood vessels and nerves in the eye [1]. Newer approaches for diagnosis try to draw conclusions directly out of the 3D-geometry of the ocular fundus. The goal of the EU-Project Glaucad is to find significant geometric characteristics which refer to the disease [2]. Precondition for this attempt is therefore the ability to reconstruct the 3D geometry of the ocular fundus.

The database in this project consists of more than 15.000 stereo slides. Besides the basic requirements needed to apply methods from computer vision this fact leads to stronger demands concerning the reconstruction module:

- Firstly the whole process has to be fully automatic. Only then such a huge number of pictures can be handled.
- Secondly each process step must include an evaluation of its correctness. Due to algorithmical and numerical restrictions the calculation can lack accuracy in most process steps. If the system recognizes algorithmical problems (e.g. based on poor geometric conditions) or numerical problems an estimation of the usability of the result has to be done.
- Thirdly the algorithms have to be optimized concerning their performance.

©CARS/Springer. All rights reserved.

2. Method

The basis of the reconstruction are stereoscopic image pairs of the ocular fundus. They were obtained by taking images from two different positions. There is no further information about the camera, neither about its exact positions nor its orientations given. Also the internal camera parameters like the foci are unknown.
The reconstruction process is done in several steps (see Fig. 1). The first main step is the image preprocessing (Masking, Luminosity Compensation). Here the relevant part of the image is detected and the image is processed to compensate varieties in luminosity. The second step registers the images. These two steps have strong influence on the success of the later calculation steps. The third step consists of the dense matching module where the depth information is calculated in form of a disparity map. The fourth step is the calibration step. The goal there is to calculate the camera position out of the image pair. Here we calculate a certain amount of precise point correspondencies (Sparse Matching). Out of this information the camera parameters can be obtained. Due to the difficult geometric situation this calculation lacks reliability and only can be regarded as an approximation. Therefore the output is currently done using standard camera parameters, but the potential procedure is presented. For the future it is planned to optimize these values using bundle block adjustment.

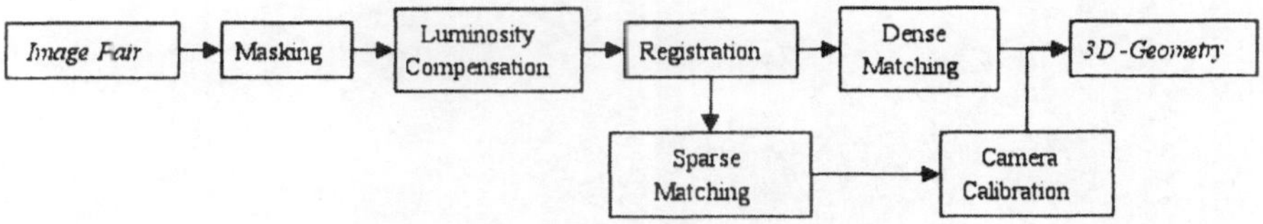

Figure 1: Reconstruction Pipe

2.1 Masking of the Single Images

In the masking step irrelevant parts of the image that would disturb the computation (e.g. patient information, legend) are masked out: To detect the dark background the input images are biniarised. The threshold used for this task is calculated out of the gray value histogram from the originally images using discriminant analysis. Then the pictures are splitted into several coherent regions using a segmentation algorithm [3],[4]. After the detection of the background region the biggest remaining region is identified as the ocular fundus. Thus an image that only contains the interesting part, the ocular fundus, is obtained. Afterwards the results undergo a plausibility check (minimum size, relative size).

2.2 Luminosity Compensation

The process of taking photographies in the eye underlies difficult conditions. This may lead to images with a bad luminositybalance which can have negative effects on the later calculation. The compensation of luminosity results in much more contrast in weak regions.

©CARS/Springer. All rights reserved.

2.3 Registration of the Image Pair

An automatic and precise registration of the images is a fundamental condition for the success of the following steps. To achieve this aim the process is splitted into two tasks: In a first step the received masks are registrated. Thus the displacement resulting from the slide framing or scanning process can be eliminated. In a second step the image contents themselves are registrated using contour based registration (see Fig. 2). The significant contours of the images (predominantly blood vessels) are extracted and biniarised. Using a Chamfer-Matching algorithm [5] the images are registrated by minimizing the distance between the two contours. To improve the robustness of this step the small and less distinct contours are eliminated.

One result is an affine transformation that describes the mentioned displacement. This is used to compensate the error of the scanning process and is necessary for a camera calibration. The second result is a transformation that gives the registration of the blood vessels and is used to make the following calculation steps more robust. After the Sparse Matching and the Dense Matching the results have to be transformed back. The assumption of an affine transformation between the image content can be seen as acceptable approximation due to the given special geometric situation (viewing direction near vertical to the ocular fundus, small depth range).

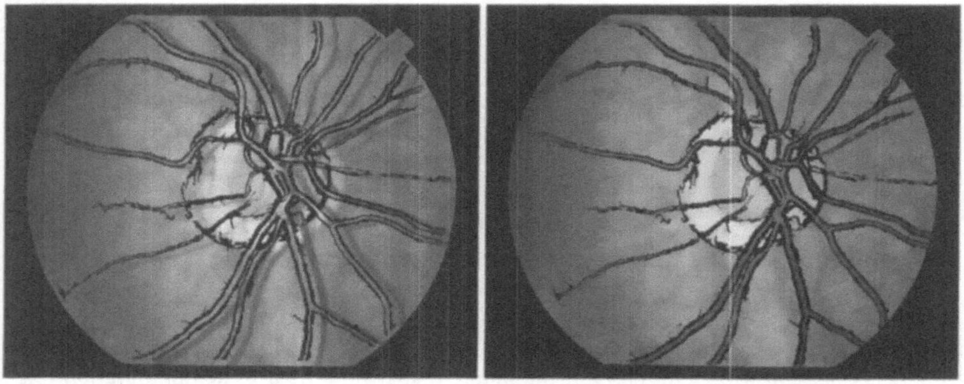

Figure 2: Projection of the contours of the second image before and after the registration

2.4 Dense Matching

The intention here is to find as many point correspondencies of the two images as possible and to detect the relative position in both images. Therefore starting from an image point in one image a template window is guided along a part of the corresponding line in the other image [6],[7]. The image parts are compared using the Normalized-Cross-Correlation (NCC) as measurement. The input are the contour registrated images. Therefore the resulting disparity values have to be transformed to their disparity values in the mask registrated images. The result is a disparity map that encodes the distance of corresponding points in gray values (see Fig. 3).

©CARS/Springer. All rights reserved.

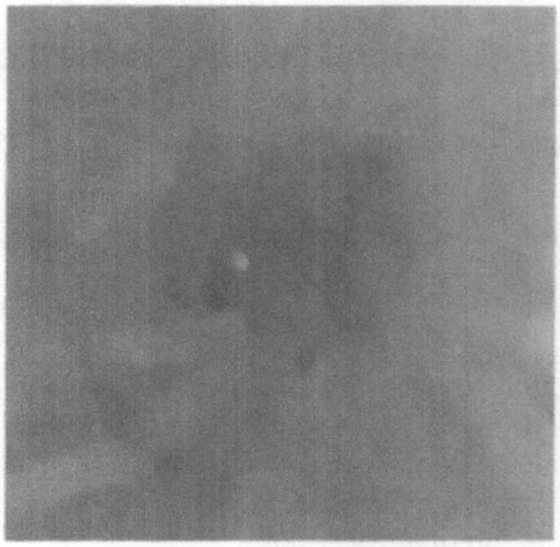

Figure 3: Disparity Map

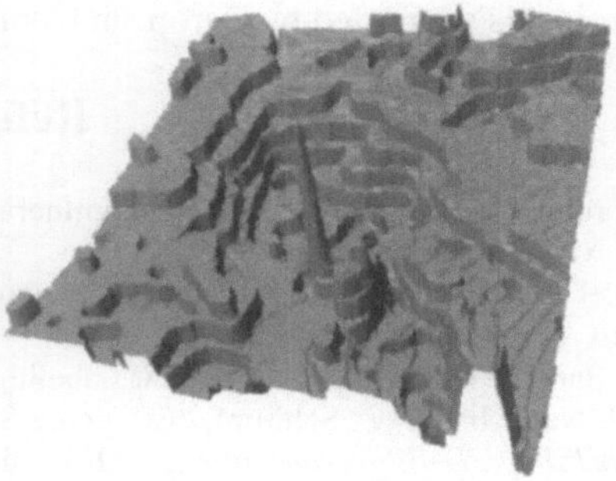

Figure 4: 3D-Reconstruction

2.5 Sparse Matching

At this point some initial point correspondencies are calculated and matched. The algorithm is based on the tracking/matching algorithm by Kanabe et.al. [8]. In a first step a certain number of special feature points in one of the images is detected. Then the corresponding points in the second image are obtained by minimizing the difference of the gray values of a correlation. To improve the robustness for the further calculation the corresponding points are forced to be equally distributed over the image. Here the input are again the contour registrated images. After the sparse matching the positions of the matched points in the mask registrated images have to be calculated.

2.6 Camera Calibration

Using the point correspondencies obtained in the previous step the Fundamental-Matrix can be calculated [9]. To improve the result an iterative process has been implemented that detects weak point correspondencies and excludes them from the calculation. Furthermore special geometric cases are taken into consideration [10].
Generally using this matrix the internal and afterwards the external camera parameters can be calculated. Due to the special geometric situation this problem is ill conditioned [11] and only can be seen as an approximate solution.

2.7 Calculation of the 3D-Geometry

Using the disparity map and the camera parameters a depth map can be obtained. For visualization of the depth information it has to be triangulated (see Fig. 4).

3. Results/Conclusion

We presented a way to reconstruct the 3D-geometry of an object only out of two standard images. In contrast to active systems like laser scanners this technique has the advantage that there is no additional hardware needed to get 3D-reconstructions. Future emphasis of our work will be the increase of the robustness and the calculating speed.

©CARS/Springer. All rights reserved.

Acknowledgements

This project is supported by European Commission from the project QLG1-2000-00651.

References

1. Norbert Pfeiffer, "Eine neue Glaukomtherapie", *Forschungsmagazin der Johannes Gutenberg-Universität Mainz*, 108-117, 2/95.
2. Axel von Freyberg, Jörg Peters, "Glaucoma Prevention by Computer Aided Diagnostics", *http://www.glaucad.com*, 11. Oct. 2001.
3. H. Samet, "Connected Component Labeling Using Quadtrees", *ACM Journal*, 1981.
4. P.J. Neugebauer, C. Schimpf, "Effiziente Skulpturierung von 3D-Modellen aus Tiefenbildern", *Workshop 3D-Bildverarbeitung*, TAE Esslingen, June 1996.
5. Gunilla Borgefors, "Hierarchical Chamfer Matching: Parametric Edge Matching Algorithm", *IEEE Transactions on Pattern Analysis and Machine Intelligence*, 1988.
6. Lutz Falkenhagen, "Depth Estimation from Stereescopic Image Pairs Assuming Piecewise Continous Surfaces", *Proc. of European Workshop on combined Real and Synthetic Image Processing for Broadcast and Video Production*, Hamburg, 1994.
7. Lutz Falkenhagen, "Hierarchical Block-Based Disparity Estimation Considering Neighbourhood Constraints", *International workshop on SNHC and 3D Imaging*, Rhodes, Greece, 1997.
8. Jianbo Shi, Carlo Tomasi, "Good Features to Track", *Conference on Computer Vision and Pattern Recognition*, 1994.
9. R. Hartley, A. Zisserman, *Multiple view geometry in computer vision*, Cambridge University Press, 2000.
10. Philip Hilaire Sean Torr, "Motion Segmentation and Outlier Detection", PhD Thesis, Department of Engineering Science, University of Oxford, Hilary Term, 1995.
11. M. Pollefeys, R. Koch, L. Van Gool, "Self-calibration and metric reconstruction in spite of varying and unknown internal camera parameters", Katholieke Universiteit Leuven, 1997.

CARS 2002 – H.U. Lemke, M.W. Vannier; K. Inamura A.G. Farman, K. Doi & J.H.C. Reiber (Editors)
©CARS/Springer. All rights reserved.

Performance evaluation of LCD displays

H. Roehrig[1], J. Fan[2], T. Furukawa[3], M. Ohashi[4], A. Chawla[2], K. Gandhi[2]
[1] The University of Arizona, Department of Radiology, Tucson AZ 85724
[2] The University of Arizona, Department of ECE, Tucson AZ 85724
[3] Data-Ray Corporation, Westminster, CO 80234, USA
[4]Spectratech., Inc, Tokyo, Japan

Abstract

This paper presents measurements of display function, spatial resolution (MTF), grayscale precision and spatial noise of three monochrome LCDs. Each of these LCDs features a different method to increase the grayscale precision: Frame Rate Modulation, Sub-Pixel Modulation and Aperture Modulation. A CCD camera was used for the evaluation. It imaged a small portion of the LCD, usually with over-sampling of between 115:1 and 8:1 CCD pixels per LCD pixel. The evaluated systems have image quality that in many respects is superior to CRT displays. Most impressive is the spatial resolution. The MTF of the systems investigated is almost unity. The typically 8 bits grayscale precision can be significantly increased by temporal as well as spatial modulation techniques. It appears that the aperture modulation technique alone can achieve a precision of 10.8 bits or 1800 distinct luminance levels. Spatial noise was evaluated in terms of single pixel signal-to-noise ratio and in terms of the spatial noise power spectrum. Single pixel signal-to-noise ratios for one LCDs were in the order of 100:1, and for another one the spatial noise power density of the normalized NPS at spatial frequencies below the LCD Nyquist frequency of 2.4 lp/mm was about 3.1E-5 mm^2, values which are in the order of those from high performance CRTs.

Keywords: LCD, MTF, spatial noise

1. Introduction

In most radiological imaging workstations today, the monochrome cathode ray tube (CRT) is the electronic display of choice. It offers the best performance, and it is the most highly developed and reliable electronic display in common use. CRT systems with pixel matrices of up to 2048 x 2560 pixels are commonly used for soft copy diagnosis. Despite this status, the CRT is not perfect. It is bulky, has a curved surface and suffers from loss of information due to non-isotropic Modulation Transfer Function (MTF) and Veiling Glare. A space saving display with a flat surface similar to the conventional film/lightbox is still the dream of the radiologists.

A great deal of effort has been devoted to active-matrix liquid crystal displays. Initially it appeared that it would take perhaps as much as a decade, until these LCD systems would replace the CRT in medical applications. Recent developments forced a reevaluation of this prediction. LCD displays are now offered with dynamic range of up to 600:1 (exceeding that of CRTs) and with pixel matrices of 1536 x 2048 and even 2048 x 2560.

©CARS/Springer. All rights reserved.

It is of great importance to evaluate the information transfer characteristic of these LCD displays relative to those of typical high performance CRTs .The MTF of the LCDs of course will describe the information transfer with respect to spatial detail. This is particularly important since the MTF of CRTs is one of their weakest points on account of the limited bandwidth of their video amplifiers.

Spatial noise of the LCD is of interest with respect to display of small contrasts and the desired precision of luminance levels. On CRTs the low contrast performance is affected by the phosphor granularity and known to be different for the phosphors P45 and P104. No information on the magnitude of spatial noise of LCDs was available at the beginning of this project.

This paper presents measurements of display function, spatial resolution (MTF), grayscale precision and spatial noise of three monochrome LCDs. Each of the LCDs investigated features a different method to increase the grayscale precision: (1) Frame Rate Modulation, (2) Sub-Pixel Modulation, and (3) Aperture Modulation. The pixel matrix of the first two types is 1536 x 2048 and a pixel size of 0.207 mm, while the last type features a pixel matrix of 1024 x 1280 and a pixel size of 0.312 mm.

Figure 1 shows the pixel structure of the first two LCD types, while Figure 2 shows the pixel structure of the last LCD type.

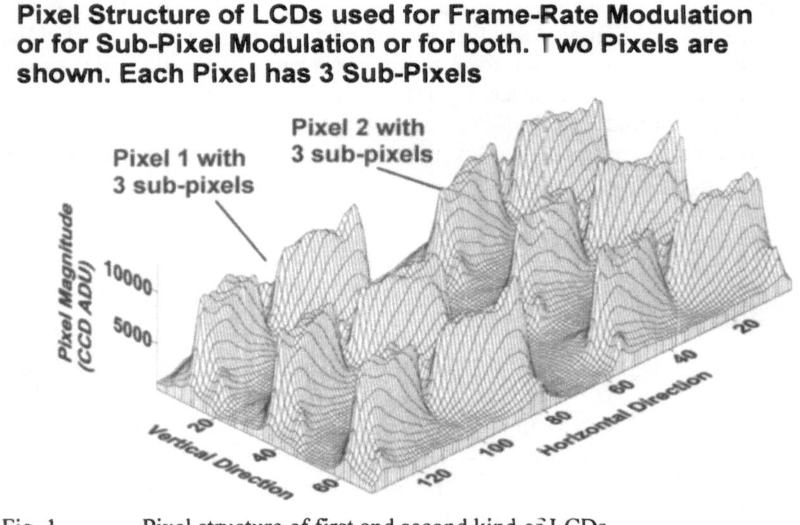

Fig. 1 Pixel structure of first and second kind of LCDs

2. Method and procedures

The evaluation was done similar to the well known method to perform CRT evaluation: Test patterns such as single lines on a uniform background or uniform fields were displayed by the LCD at different luminance values and a high performance CCD camera was used to image a portion of the test images displayed by the LCD. The optical

©CARS/Springer. All rights reserved.

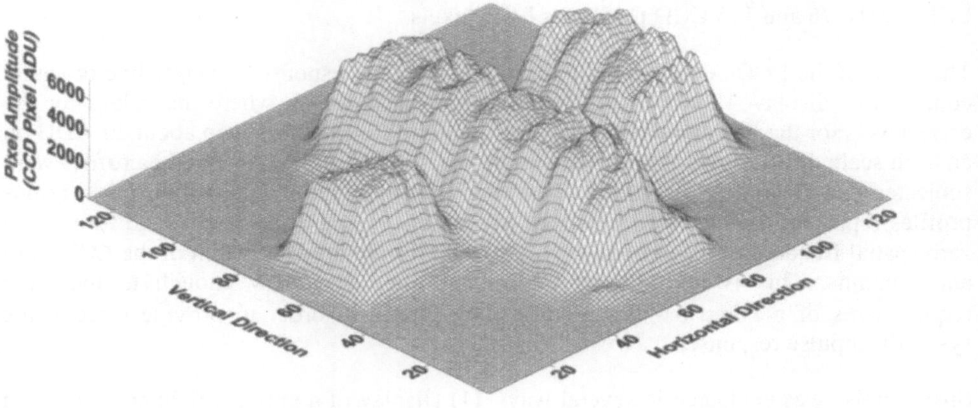

Fig. 2 Pixel structure of Aperture Modulated LCD.

magnification was chosen to achieve a certain amount of over-sampling. Over sampling was necessary for two reasons: First to minimize the influence of the CCD camera's MTF on the measurement of the LCD's MTF and secondly, but most importantly, to permit treating the inherently sampled LCD display as a quasi continuous display permitting use of Fourier Transform Techniques. An additional consideration with respect to the use of Fourier Transform Techniques was the use of small signals as the LCD systems are non-linear.

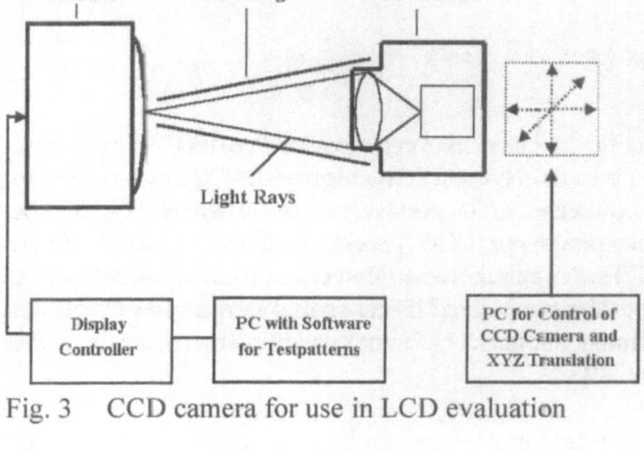

Fig. 3 CCD camera for use in LCD evaluation

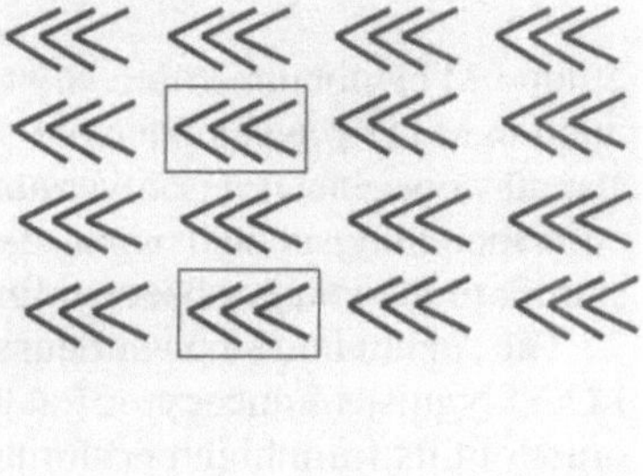

Fig 4. Schematic illustrating image of LCD pixels with high magnification and ROIs to find the mean CCD response per pixel

©CARS/Springer. All rights reserved.

Fig. 3 is a schematic, illustrating the use of the CCD camera for the LCD evaluation. Over sampling was expressed as the ratio of the number of CCD pixels per LCD pixel. The most common values of over sampling for this evaluation were 8 CCD pixels per LCD pixels, 76 and 115 CCD pixels per LCD pixels.

The MTF of the LCDs was derived from the LCD's line response. A single line or single column was displayed on the LCD on a uniform background, where the values for the drive-levels for the line and the background did not differ by more than about 20 ADU on an 8-bit scale. Profiles were generated in the CCD images of the line and the profiles were subjected to 1-D Fourier Transforms. The results of the Fourier Transform of the various profiles represent the raw un-normalized MTFs. They need to be normalized to unity at zero spatial frequency and subsequently corrected for the inherent width of the LCD lines and columns. This is because the LCD lines are not narrow enough to meet the requirements of a Dirac δ - Function as they should in order to provide directly the system's impulse response.

Spatial noise was evaluated in several ways. (1) Display of a uniform field and taking an image with the CCD camera at very high magnification of 76 CCD pixels per LCD Pixel. Then placing ROIs over each pixel as shown schematically by Figure 4 to determine mean and standard deviation of the pixel intensities in the fashion of a pulse-height distribution. (2) Display of a uniform field by addressing all LCD pixels in a relatively small area to the same luminance, taking a picture of the uniform field with the CCD camera (using a magnification of 8:1) and analyzing the CCD camera image with 2-D Fourier Transform Techniques to find the Noise Power Spectrum. (3) Display of a uniform object (a square of about 50x50 pixels) in the center of a uniform background with object and background addressed by a difference of 1 ADU to generate a luminance difference. This difference of 1 ADU is slowly moved over the whole dynamic range of the system . The CCD camera images object and background using a magnification of 8:1 and determines the luminance step.

3. Results

Some MTFs obtained are shown in Fig. 5. They are very close to "perfect" in the sense that the MTFs reach values of 95 % up to the Nyquist frequency of 2.47 lp/mm. A map of spatial noise in terms of variation of mean LCD pixel values is shown in Fig. 6. The corresponding spatial signal-to-noise ratios per LCD pixel are in the order of 100:1, similar to the values observed for CRTs. A spatial Noise Power Spectrum is shown in Fig. 7. The spatial noise power density of the normalized NPS at spatial frequencies below the LCD Nyquist frequency of 2.4 lp/mm is about 3.1E-5 mm^2, values which also is in the order of that from high performance CRTs.

With Frame Rate Modulation 1024 different gray steps can be generated while with Sub-Pixel Modulation only 766 levels can be generated. It appears, that all levels can be detected by a human observers (one at a time). It also appears that the aperture modulation technique alone can achieve a precision of 10.8 bits or 1800 distinct luminance levels. But in the latter case, spatial noise may be preventing detection by the human observer. This is not clear at this time.

©CARS/Springer. All rights reserved.

4. Discussion and conclusions

LCD displays appear to be highly efficient systems with respect to the MTF. With MTF values of close to unity they are almost ideal which seems to be consistent with the reports of clinicians who love to read clinical images on these types of LCD displays. Of great concern are the many spikes with very high power in the Noise Power Spectra, resulting from the fact that an LCD pixel is not simply a continuous Gaussian type Point-Spread-Function rather it consists of at least 3 if not even 6 separate structures. Although these structures are not visible to the human observer when he chooses a sufficiently large viewing distance, the power in those spikes may still affect the detection during soft-copy reading. Therefore more work is necessary in order to get a more complete picture of the information transfer characteristics of these LCD displays.

Acknowledgement

This work was supported by the Data-Ray Corporation

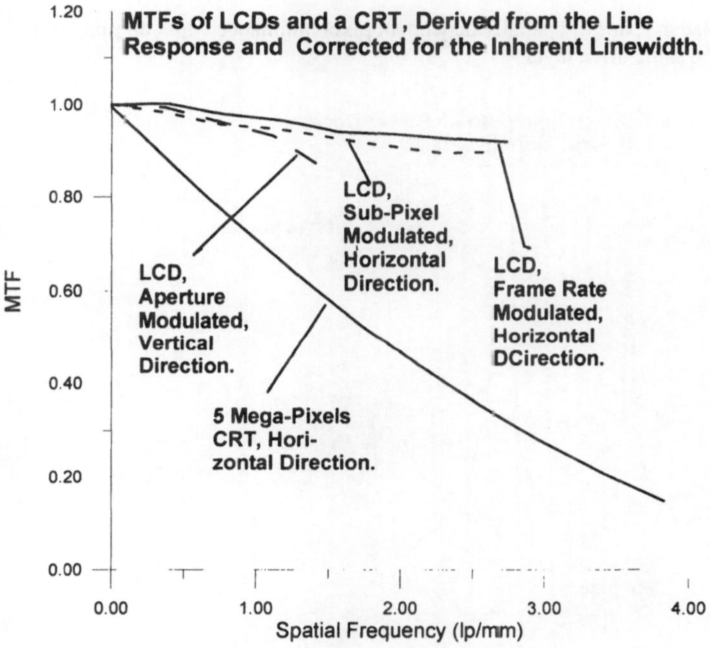

Fig. 5. Some MTFs of LCDs and a CRT

©CARS/Springer. All rights reserved.

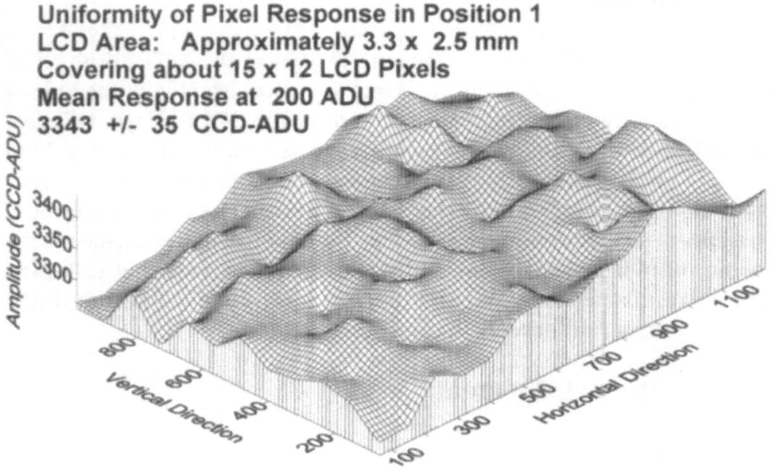

Fig. 6 Map of spatial noise in terms of spatially dependent pixel luminance while all pixels are uniformly addressed with the same drive level

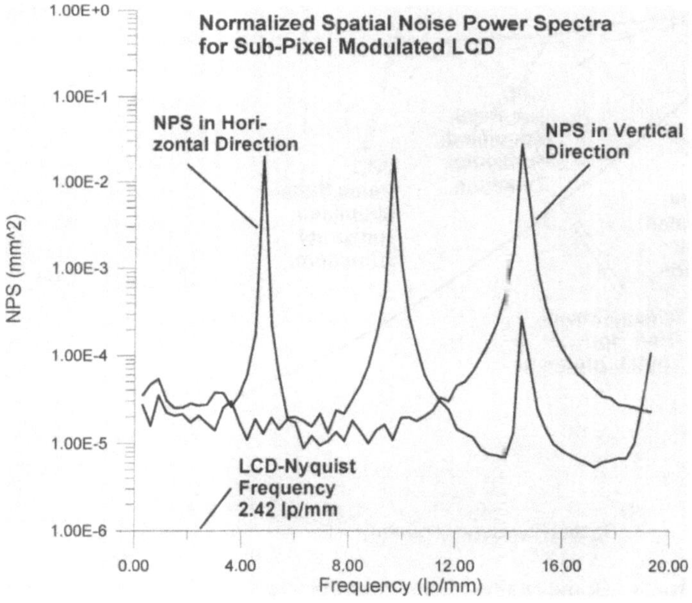

Fig. 7 Normalized Spatial Noise Power Spectrum of an LCD with a pixel Matrix of 1536 x 2048

CARS 2002 – H.U. Lemke, M.W. Vannier; K. Inamura A.G. Farman, K. Doi & J.H.C. Reiber (Editors)
©CARS/Springer. All rights reserved.

Fast volume rendering based on software optimisation using multimedia instructions on PC platforms

Kensaku Mori[a,b], Yasuhito Suenaga[a], and Junichiro Toriwaki[a]
[a] Graduate School of Engineering, Nagoya University,
Furo-cho, Chikusa-ku, Nagoya 464-8603, Aichi, JAPAN
[b] Image Guidance Laboratories, Department of Neurosurgery, Stanford University,
300 Pasteur Drive, Stanford, CA 94305-5327, U.S.A.

Abstract

This paper describes a fast software-based volume rendering method based on software optimization using SIMD instructions equipped in PC processors currently available. This method achieves fast rendering speed by highly optimizing instructions of software rather than optimization of algorithm. The proposed software can render 3-D volume of 512x512x488 voxel size at about six frames per second in maximum with perspective projection, arbitrary light source position, reflection computation of ambient, diffuse and specula reflections, and *on-the-fly* surface normal computation on a conventional Intel Pentium-based PC platform which has single or more CPU(s) without special graphics hardware. We can also change color and opacity tables that define color and opacity transfer functions during the rendering process. The change is reflected on rendered images immediately. This software achieves fast rendering speed without any special hardware including graphics boards. We implemented the proposed software in a virtual endoscopy system (VES). The experimental results show that it can render endoscopic views at six frames per second.

Keywords: Volume rendering, SIMD instruction, fast rendering

1. Introduction

Recent progress of three-dimensional (3-D) scanner, such as multi-detector row computed tomography (CT) or magneto resonance (MR) scanners, enabled us to take precise volumetric images of human bodies. Visualization of these large size 3-D images is becoming much important in clinical field. Volume rendering (VolR) is a well-known and very strong technique to visualize 3-D volumetric images [1, 2]. VolR enables us to render 3-D images by only defining the color and opacity transfer functions. It can visualize not only the surfaces of anatomical structures but also their contents by setting the transfer functions as semi-translucent. Explicit extraction of anatomical structures is not required for rendering. However, VolR usually requires much computation time for generating images. This is because that we need to compute shaded values on many sample points along rays and perform weighted accumulations in the case of a ray casting method. When we use VolR in clinical diagnoses, interactive visualization is very important. Real time or semi real time rendering is required without any degradation of rendered images.

©CARS/Springer. All rights reserved.

Several publications describe fast volume rendering by improvements of algorithms, such as splatting or shear warp methods [4-8]. Some papers try to achieve high rendering speed by using parallel computers or special graphics boards. Although these methods can render images at reasonable speed, they have some limitations, i.e. fixed light source position, only parallel projection, requirements of special hardware, or pre-computations.

In recent years, processing performance of CPUs used in conventional PCs drastically increased. As the increase of demands of multimedia processing, the recent CPU equips some special instructions for multimedia applications such as SIMD (Single Instruction Multiple Data) and cache control instructions. This paper shows the framework to achieve high speed of VolR by using these instructions. The method proposed here uses only CPUs to perform high-speed volume rendering. Since special hardware is not necessary in the rendering, the proposed method is quite useful for clinical use. This method achieves fast rendering speed by highly optimizing instructions of software rather than optimization of algorithm. The proposed software can render a 3-D volume of 512x512x488 voxels at about six frames per second in maximum with perspective projection, arbitrary light source position, reflection computation of ambient, diffuse and specula reflections, and *on-the-fly* surface normal computation on a conventional Intel Pentium-based PC platform which has single or more CPUs. We can also change color and opacity tables that define color and opacity transfer functions during the rendering process. The change is reflected on rendered images immediately. In Section 2, we briefly describe optimization methods of software for volume rendering. Several optimization techniques are shown here. Section 3 shows rendering time achieved by the proposed method with comparison with a non-optimized method. We also add discussion in the same section.

2. Methods

2.1 Volume rendering by ray casting

In our VolR method, we use a ray casting method to generate VolR images. Basically, the ray casting performs VolR by casting a ray that starts at the viewpoint and passes through the pixel on the screen. Prior to a rendering process, we define the color and opacity functions that show relations between voxel values and color and opacity values. In an actual program, these are implemented as look up tables. Weighted accumulation of the shaded color of each voxel is performed along the cast ray. Shaded value at each sample point is calculated from the voxel value, the normal vector at the sample point, the light source direction, and the vector that connects the viewpoint and the sample point. Each pixel value of the rendered image is computed by the weighted accumulation operation. The color and opacity values at the sample point are obtained by interpolating eight voxels on the image grid around the sample point and referring the color and opacity tables with the interpolated value (Requirement I: Fast interpolation). The normal vector is also computed by interpolating eight normal vectors of eight-neighbors points. At each neighbor point, the normal vector is computed by calculating a gradient vector from gray values and normalizing it (Requirement II: Fast vector normalization). Shaded value can be calculated from the normal vector at the sample point, the light source direction and the vector connecting the viewpoint and the sample point (Requirement III: Fast dot-product computation). The casting process is performed for all pixels of the rendered image. Each ray also has a lot of sample points. Huge memory space is accessed in the rendering process (Re-

©CARS/Springer. All rights reserved.

quirement IV: Fast memory access). It also needs to skip translucent parts fast, since these parts provide no effect to the rendered image (Requirement V: Fast ray skip).

2.2 Optimization

(a) Utilization of SIMD instructions for Requirements I, II, and III

The latest CPUs have SIMD instructions to process multimedia-oriented data such as images, videos or audios. SIMD instructions can handle multiple data simultaneously. In Intel Pentium III or 4 processor, we can perform basic numerical operations of four single precision floating-point data only by one instruction (c.f., addition, subtraction, multiplication and division) (Fig. 1). In the rendering process, we use these instructions for interpolation, dot product computation, and vector normalization. In the vector normalization process, we need to compute square root value of the squared length of a vector and to divide the vector with its length. We utilize the instruction that simultaneously computes the square root values and their reciprocal numbers.

(b) Avoiding zero division for Requirement II

The lengths of gradient vectors become zeros in constant-intensity areas. These cause zero division exceptions of CPUs in the vector normalization process. Although we usually use conditional branches that check divisors to avoid the exceptions, this leads performance degradation caused by pipeline stalls of the processor. The proposed method avoids this problem by adding very small ignorable constants to divisors and executes normal division operations.

(c) Fast computation of absolute values for Requirement III

In the calculation process of shaded values, it is required to compute the absolute values of the dot products of the light source and normal vectors. The method executes this process by directly changing the flag-bit of a floating-point value, which shows positive or negative. This operation is also performed for four values simultaneously by using a SIMD instruction.

(d) Optimization of memory allocation for Requirement IV

We divide the whole of an original image into a set of small subimages. This process is called *tiling*. This special memory allocation prevents miss-hits of the cache memory when the method accesses to the neighboring voxels of sample points. The size of tiling is determined based on the size of the cache memory of a CPU.

(e) Fast ray skip in translucent part for Requirement V

Regions of zero opacity values (translucent regions) give no effect to the final image. While the opacity value at a sample point is zero in casting, we perform the casting process with the interval step of double of the voxel size. When the casting process finds the opaque (including semi-translucent) sample point, the casting process goes back for one voxel unit and continues the casting with one or less voxel-size intervals predefined. Skipping is very important to achieve higher speed. In the casting process, we compute the opacity value at a sample point at

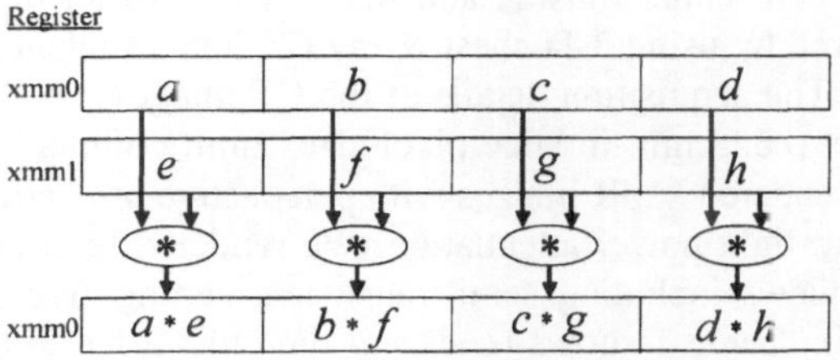

Fig. 1. An example of operations using SIMD instructions equipped in Intel Pentium processors. In this example, four multiplications are executed simultaneously by one instruction.

©CARS/Springer. All rights reserved.

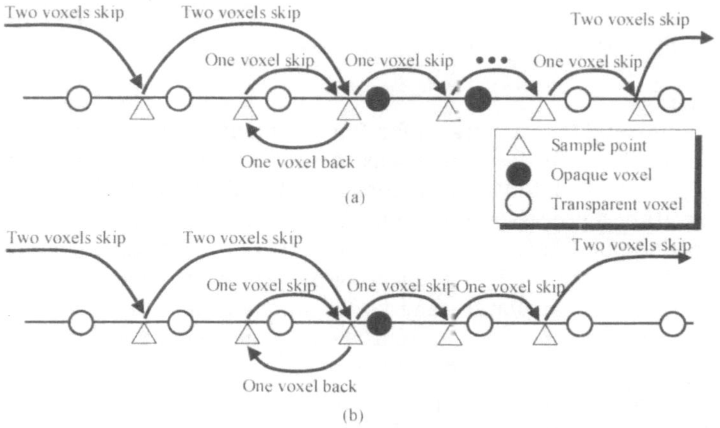

Fig. 2. Illustration of ray skipping. (a) In translucent area, the cast ray runs with the interval of two voxel size. When we find an opaque sample point, the ray goes back and runs with the interval of one voxel size. (b) This method can also find a solitary opaque point effectively.

first. If it is zero, we proceed to the next sample point immediately.

(f) Utilization of cache control instructions for Requirement IV

VolR accesses huge memory space in its rendering process. Usually the access speed of the main memory is much slower than CPU speed. This means that the CPU must wait to load gray values of the input image to registers. The proposed software performs prefetching of the content of the main memory to the cache memory for avoiding this problem by using cache control instructions equipped in the CPU.

(g) Utilization of multi processors

In the ray casting method, each ray can be computed separately. Hence we assign independent rays to processors installed in a PC.

3. Experimental results and discussion

We implemented the fast VolR routine on a conventional PC that has two Intel 2.2 GHz Xeon processors and two giga-bytes main memory. The software was developed by using the Intel C++ compiler. We used the VolR routine as a rendering engine of our virtual endoscopy system (VES). This system can render outside and inside views of an input image. The rendering speed was measured by using 3-D chest X-ray CT images taken by helical and multi-detector CT scanners. The acquisition details of the CT images are: 512 x 512 pixels, 118 or 488 slices, 0.625 x 0.625 mm in slice pixel size, 2mm collimation, and 1mm reconstruction. The software rendered VolR images with perspective projection, specula reflection, spotlight lighting, and light power attenuation. We rendered both outside views and virtual bronchoscopic views including semi-translucent setting. We set 256x256 (pixels) as the rendering matrix. Table 1 shows rendering time measured in the experiments. For comparison, we also measured rendering time of the rendering method not using the above mentioned optimization techniques. The experimental results show that the proposed method is about four times faster than the non-optimized method. The average of rendering speed was about six frames per seconds for bronchoscopic views.

©CARS/Springer. All rights reserved.

This rendering speed is sufficient for clinical use. This VolR software achieves fast rendering by optimizing the software of the ray casting method. It is also possible to modify rendering algorithms with keeping high frame rate. This method does not require any precomputations such as normal vectors or shade values computations. In our preliminary experiment, it was possible to dynamically update the content of a volume with keeping high frame rates. This shows that the proposed method is also useful for visualization of time variant volume data.

4. Conclusion

This paper describes a fast software-based volume rendering method based on software optimization using SIMD instructions equipped in PC processors currently available. This method achieves fast rendering speed by highly optimizing instructions of VolR software rather than optimizing rendering algorithms. The proposed software can render a 3-D volume of 512x512x488 voxels at about six frames per second with perspective projection, specula reflection, spotlight lighting, and light power attenuation on a conventional Intel Pentium-based PC machine that has dual CPUs. This software achieved fast rendering speed without any special hardware including graphics boards. Also it demonstrated the potential of real-time interaction of clinical 3-D data on the conventional PC without special hardware

Acknowledgements

Authors thank our colleagues for their useful suggestions and discussion. K.Mori thanks Dr. Ramin Shahidi and Dr. Calvin Maurer, Jr., of Stanford University for providing him an opportunity to write this paper. Parts of this research were supported by the Grant-In-Aid for Scientific Research from the Ministry of Education, the Grant-In-Aid for Scientific Research from Japan Society for Promotion of Science, and the Grant-In-Aid for Cancer Research from the Ministry of Health and Welfare of Japanese Government.

Table 1. Comparison of rendering time. *VE* means a virtual endoscopic view.

Scene No.	Rendering time		Accel. ratio	Volume size	Remarks
	With optimization.	Without optimization			
Scene 1	0.25	0.88	3.52	512x512x118	Pulmonary Vessels
Scene 2	0.16	0.63	3.94	512x512x118	VE (bronchi)
Scene 3	0.20	0.89	4.45	512x512x118	Pulmonary Vessels
Scene 4	0.27	1.44	5.33	512x512x489	Whole body
Scene 5	0.14	0.58	4.14	512x512x489	Whole body
Scene 6	0.16	0.56	3.50	512x512x489	VE (bronchi)
Scene 7	0.39	1.64	4.21	512x512x489	Pulmonary Vessels
Scene 8	0.31	1.47	4.74	512x512x489	VE (stomach)
Scene 9	0.80	2.88	3.60	512x512x489	Semi-translucent
Scene 10	0.28	1.22	4.36	512x512x489	Pulmonary Vessels

©CARS/Springer. All rights reserved.

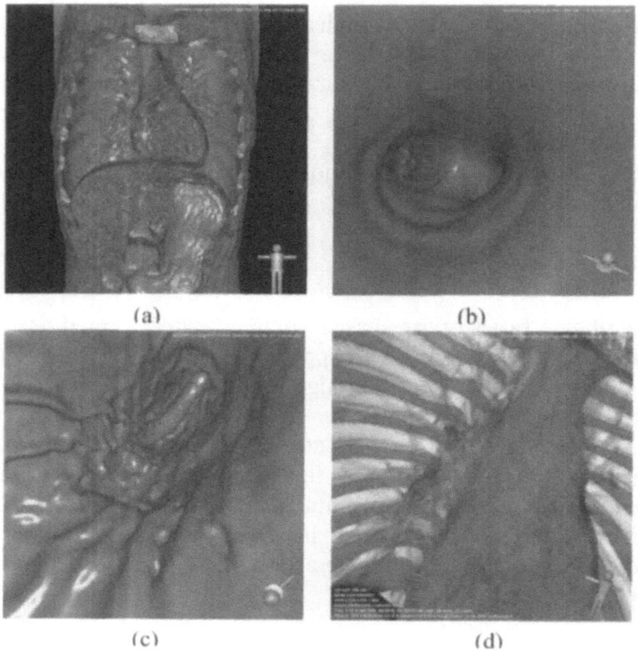

Fig. 3. Examples of rendered images for measuring rendering time. (a) Whole body view with a cutting (Scene 5), (b) virtual bronchoscopic view (Scene 6), (c) virtual gastroscopic images (Scene 8), and (d) pulmonary vessels with semi-translucent setting (Scene 9)

References

1. Marc Levoy, "Display of surfaces from volume data", *IEEE Computer Graphics & Applications*, Vol. 8, No. 3, pp. 29-37, 1988
2. Rovert A. Drebin, Loren Carpenter, Pat Hanrahan, "Volume rendering. Computer Graphics", *Proc. ACM SIGGRAPH '88*, Vol. 22, No. 3, pp.65-74, 1988
3. Lee Westover, "Footprint evaluation for volume rendering", Computer Graphics, *Proc. ACM SIGGRAPH '90*, Vol. 24, No. 4, pp. 367-376, 1990
4. Philippe Lacroute, Marc Levoy, "Fast volume rendering using a shear-warp factorization of the viewing transformation", Computer Graphics, Proc. ACM SIGGRAPH '94, Annual Conference Series : 451-458, 1994
5. Kwan-Liu Ma, James S. Painter, Charles D. Hansen, et al., "Parallel volume rendering using binary-swap compositing", IEEE Computer Graphics & Applications, Vol. 14, No. 4, pp. 59-67, 1994
6. Harvey Ray, Hanspeter Pfister, Deborah Silver et al., "Ray Casting Architectures for Volume Visualization", IEEE Trans on Visualization and Computer Graphics, Vol. 5, No. 3, pp. 210-223, 1999
7. Milos Sramek, Arie Kaufman, "Fast Ray-Tracing of Rectilinear Volume Data Using Distance Transforms", IEEE Trans. on Visualization and Computer Graphics, Vol. 6, No.3, pp. 236-252, 2000
8. Steven Parker, Michael Parker, Yarden Livnat et al , "Interactive Ray Tracing for Volume Visualization", IEEE Trans on Visualization and Computer Graphics, Vol. 5, No. 3, pp. 238-250, 1999

CARS 2002 – H.U. Lemke, M.W. Vannier; K. Inamura, A.G. Farman, K. Doi & J.H.C. Reiber (Editors)
©CARS/Springer. All rights reserved.

Interactive tutorials: development of a large scale 3D database of pathological cases using interactive volume rendering technique

H. Shin[a], U. v. Jan[b], M. Galanski[a], H.K. Matthies[b],
[a] Diagnostic Radiology
[b] Institute of Medical Informatics
Hannover Medical School
30623 Hannover, Germany

Abstract

3D rendering is recognized as an efficient educational tool to present human anatomy and included pathologies. In The Visible Human Project it is in use as an interactive 3D atlas. For 3D visualization all anatomic structures of the body was precisely segmented, which is a very time and cost consuming task. Thus, it is not feasible for larger databases as detailed segmentation of each individual case is unreasonable. Therefore we started a project focusing on direct volume rendering techniques to build a large scale 3D database of pathological cases intended as an interactive learning tool for medical students.

Keywords: 3D Rendering, volume Rendering, web based learning

1. Methods

As a starting point we focused on computed tomography data of 30 patients covering following areas: trauma, pathologies of the thorax / abdomen and CT Angiography. All examinations were performed on a Multislice CT scanner (GE Lightspeed QX/i, Siemens VolumeZoom) using a slice collimation of 1 – 2.5 mm resulting in volume data sets of high resolution in all three dimensions. Following data conversion, a program utilizing the image processing library of the Visualization Toolkit (vtk 4.0, Kitware inc., USA) with integrated functionality for the VolumePro VP1000 card (Terarecon inc., USA), was used to interactively visualize all data sets. The VP1000 allowed for hardware accelerated volume rendering [1]. It was also possible to embed opaque and translucent polygon surfaces within the volume data generated by the Marching Cubes algorithm implemented in VTK (fig. 1). The segmented results can be shown either separately or overlaid with the original volume data to allow a more precise insight in these cases. All investigations were performed on a standard PC (dual Pentium 1GHz, 1GB memory) equipped with the VP1000 card. A graphical user interface was designed to allow for interactive variation of transfer functions (opacity, color and gradient) and to use cutting planes to crop the volume. To facilitate the adjustment of the transfer functions [2-4], presets of each individual data set optimizing the visibility of important anatomic structures and the underlying pathology were provided (fig. 2).

©CARS/Springer. All rights reserved.

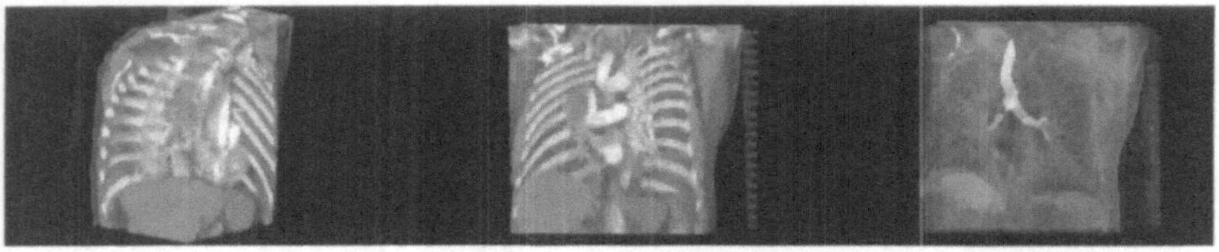

(a) (b) (c)

Figure 1. Patient with centrally located bronchial carcinoma. a. and b. show volume rendered subvolumes of the patient. In c. the same subvolume of b. is visualized with different parameter settings for volume rendering showing both lungs transparently. Additionally, the segmented tracheobronchial tree is embedded in the volume. Note the considerable compression of the right main stem bronchus caused by the tumor.

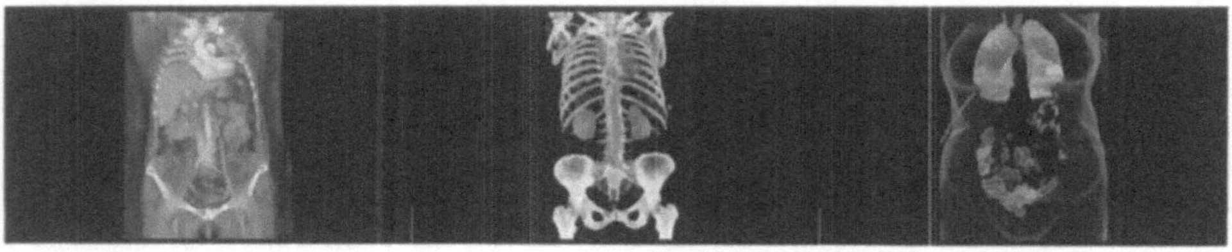

(a) (b) (c)

Figure 2. Examples of supplied presets of transfer functions: In this patient three settings for viewing of soft-tissue (a), bone (b) and air-filled structures (c) were provided.

The datasets and corresponding predefined transfer functions and other parameters (e.g. camera position) were stored in a MySQL database. Access to the database was provided via a web based interface (fig. 3) that was implemented using Apache 1.3 as web server software and PHP 4 with the ADODB library. The ADODB library [5] is an easy to use interface providing access to a variety of databases and would make it possible to switch to other database systems (e.g. for larger scale databases) with minimum effort if necessary.

The camera can be moved to predefined positions for defining a specific view depending on the subject under investigation. This makes it possible to direct the students attention to the most interesting regions of the dataset.

Datasets can be selected by specifying keywords (fig. 3). For each of the resulting datasets, a TCL parameter file will be created that can be loaded into our standard Tcl/TK visualization application. In addition to using the predefined transfer functions, visualization parameters can be changed comfortably in the web interface.

©CARS/Springer. All rights reserved.

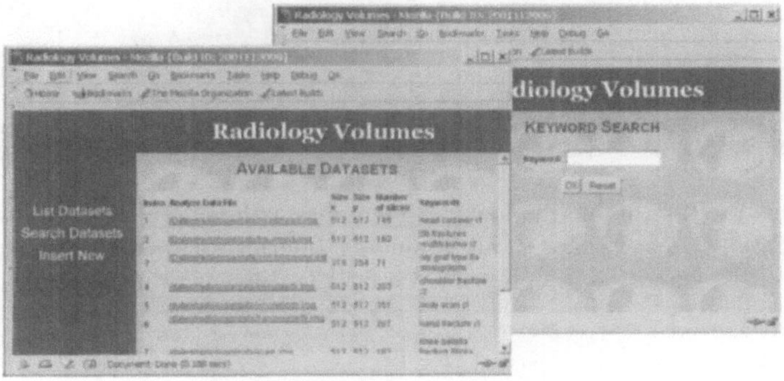

Figure 3: Access to volume datasets via web based interface.

2. Results

Without radiological training medical students were able to work with the case-based 3D-presentations. With basic anatomic knowledge they could interact and work with the different 3D data sets to gain a deeper understanding of the underlying pathology. In comparison to serially-sectioned slices anatomic orientation was greatly facilitated (fig. 4). In the trauma cases complex fractures and accompanying soft tissue injuries were better appreciated as volume rendering allowed for excellent discrimination of soft-tissue and bone injuries (fig. 5). Also parenchymal lesions of the liver were depicted including details (e.g. compression and shifting of the surrounding vessels, dilation of the bile duct: Beispiel Lebergefäße). All pathologies of the CT- angiography cases could be visualized without time consuming segmentation. Using appropriate settings of the transfer functions and cutting planes concurrent visualization of different pathologies (soft- and hard plaques, aneurysm and stenosis) were possible. Even dissection membranes could be visualized.

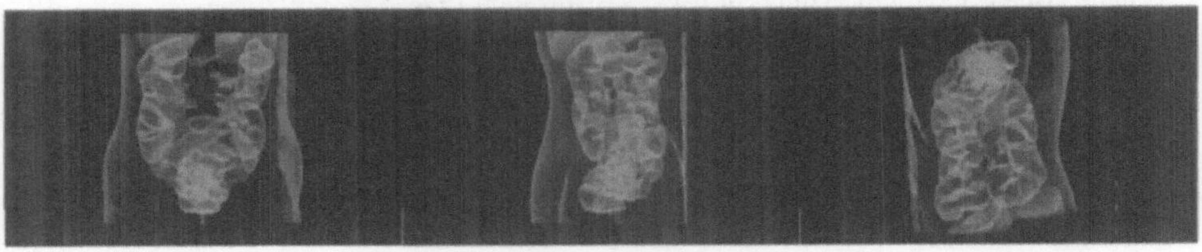

Figure 4. Virtual Colonoscopy: Hardware accelerated volume rendering allowed for 3D interaction at near real time. By changing the viewing angle and / or using cutting planes, overlaying loops impeding the visibility of concealed areas of the colon could be resolved. This facilitated the recognition of the anatomy and potential pathologies of the data.

©CARS/Springer. All rights reserved.

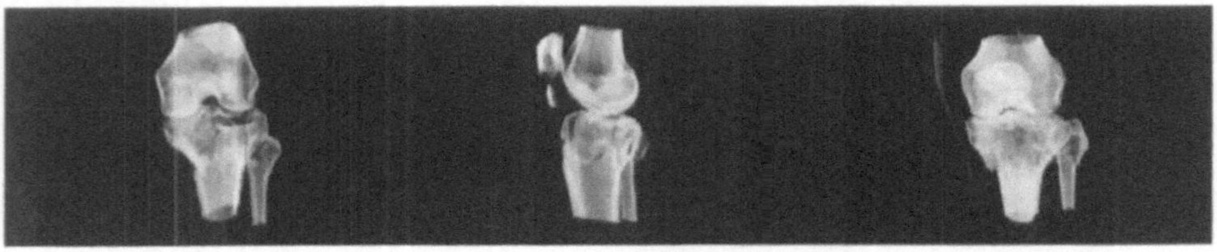

Figure 5. Complex fracture of the tibial head. Interactive volume rendering allowed for precise assessment of size and shape of all fragments. Interior fragments could be identified and also the extension of defects. Even fracture lines within spongious bone could be delineated.

3. Conclusion

Volume Rendering allows the development of large scale 3D-databases of pathological cases in a time and cost effective way. Near interactive rates can be achieved even with Multislice-CT data (CT volumes up to 512 x 512 x 1000 voxels) using hardware accelerated volume rendering.

Acknowledgements

This work is a partner project of the BMBF-granted project "Teaching and Training Network in Neurosurgery" (TT-Net).

References

1. Pfistner H, Hardenbergh H, Knittel J, Lauer H, Seiler L. The VolumePro real time ray-casting system. Proceedings of ACM SIGGRAPH 1999; 251-260.
2. Calhoun PS, Kuszyk BS, Heath DG, Carley JC, Fishman EK. Three-dimensional Volume Rendering of Spiral CT Data: Theory and Method. Radiographics 1999; 19,3: 745-764.
3. Fang S, Biddlecom T, Tuceryan M. Image based transfer function design for data exploration in volume visualization. Proceedings of IEEE Visualization 1998; 319-326
4. König AH, Gröller EM. Mastering Transfer Function Specification by using VolumePro Technology. http://www.cg.tuwien.ac.at/research/vis/vismed/ATFSpec/
5. Lim J: ADOdb Database Library for PHP: Create Portable DB Apps. http://php.weblogs.com/ADOdb/

Image Management and Communication

CARS 2002 – H.U. Lemke, M.W. Vannier; K. Inamura, A.G. Farman, K. Doi & J.H.C. Reiber (Editors)
©CARS/Springer. All rights reserved.

RIS/PACS integration in a Web environment

R. Passariello (1), G. Venturi (2), V. Campanella (1), S. Simonetti (2), C. Catalano (1), A. Fiumicelli (2)
1 Department of Radiology, University of Rome "La Sapienza"
2 Ferrania Imaging Technologies –LifeImaging Division - www.ferraniait.com

1. Introduction

Current market research studies and surveys concerning the evolution in Medical Diagnostics for Images and Health Care agree that there will be a definitive increase in the use of digital technology as well as Information and Communication Systems [1] over the next five years. A technological change will take place along with an operative modification that will lead to a change in the customer-supplier relationship. The supplier will be requested not only to provide a product or a solution but a series of professional support and consultation services that can be used for the design, transition and then optimised use of technologically diverse and perfectly integrated platforms. Information system installations for medical applications often have not met the expectations of Health Care professionals for various reasons: complex and fragile construction, high costs, redundancy and mainly local information management, problems in ensuring interoperability between different manufacturers' systems and sometimes even between solutions from the same producer.

Recently, we have experienced and taken part in a technological revolution involving the Internet and the Word Wide Web platform that is changing the information technology world and affecting the entire commercial and social organisation. This technology, defined as Web technology, has proven to be capable of distributing information over a very broad area, thus eliminating geographic distances and significantly increasing the information processing potential of easy-to-use and inexpensive machines, such as Personal Computers. Web technology has already radically changed information management models in the financial world, in trade, in company information systems and in the mass media. It's quite likely that use of this technology in new-generation medical information systems will have revolutionary effects even in the health sector. The new systems can be modular and open, while performances will be able to be adapted to satisfy each customer's functional and economic needs. They will also be easy to integrate with all commercial applications based on such an infrastructure.

All the information involved in the diagnostic process can be managed by a standardised system and can be integrated with the external information world. The information will be distributed inside and outside clinics and can be accessed by anyone who has the right to do so, in compliance with privacy and security requirements. Though physically located in a single point, the information will be "virtually" available throughout the area, with the specific and ambitious objective of creating a virtual hospital located wherever there is a need for information: hospital ward, out-patient's clinic or patient's home.

©CARS/Springer. All rights reserved.

2. The role of the industry in transferring information technology innovation in the health field

2.1 Characteristics of medical information systems

Development, marketing and maintenance of a medical information system is a complex process that requires large investments and an advanced company organisation.
In fact, the problems to be solved are not only technological by nature, but they also involve work organisation models, compliance with legal regulations and economic assessment plans. The customer has four types of requirements when ordering a medical information system:
Technological: "Critical Mission" System that can manage large volumes of data, guaranteeing the diagnostic quality of the image, fast turnaround time and conformity with standards. It's also easy to use, flexible and scalable in relation to the growth dynamics of the structure, robust and reliable.
Organisational: Optimisation of the diagnostic flow, guaranteeing multi-vendor interoperability, providing training and personal instruction courses, while ensuring maintenance with immediate intervention.
Legislative: Compliance with regulations concerning maintenance of medical data. It guarantees privacy and data security.
Economical: It offers a return on investment plan in specific time periods and maintains the investment over time.

2.2 Evolution in medical information systems

Information Systems to manage images and medical data (Image Management System) cropped up around the end of the 1980s when the digital acquisition procedures began being used in the larger hospitals. At that time each procedure was considered an isolated system and simply connected to the display station and a dedicated printer. Penn University was the first to demonstrate how different procedures could be digitally linked to a single central processing unit, thus centralising image management and greatly increasing management efficiency and reducing costs. Thus, the first IMS system was born. In Italy, the first digital image distribution system was developed by our group at the University of L'Aquila in a cooperative effort with 3M. Since the procedures at that time all operated on proprietary platforms, with data coded in the proprietary format of various manufacturers, the first commercial IMS products were developed by those same producers in a closed environment, i.e. that could manage and connect only the equipment built by that same manufacturer. At the same time, some software houses attempted to develop open systems that could connect systems developed by different manufacturers operating on commercial hardware.

The potential of the initial systems, together with the growing distribution of digital procedures, created a need to code (standardise) the format of the medical images so that open systems could be developed with having to adopt the standards utilised by the procedure manufacturers. The American National Association of Electric Machines and the Radiology Society of North America (RSNA) commissioned a number of American companies and universities to develop a standard that could code and manage all operations carried out on digital radiological images. At the 1993 RSNA convention, the DICOM (Digital Imaging and Communication in Medicine) standard was presented for the first time [2]. The standardisation turned out to be a decisive factor for the distribution

©CARS/Springer. All rights reserved.

of IMS products. With the decisive contribution by the medical-scientific sector, the procedure manufacturers quickly adapted to the standard, while a growing number of specialised software houses began to offer open systems. Naturally, competition accelerated the continuous improvements in the system and began the process to reduce costs even further. However, those costs remained high since expensive and specialised equipment was required to deal with the complexity of the systems.

The second key event behind the development of the IMS products took place in the middle of the 1990s, when increased PC calculating power (introduction of Intel's Pentium II microprocessor), lower hardware costs and the advent of Client/Server technology provided the final impetus to develop the IMS products that could operate on less expensive platforms and use standard components, thus significantly reducing costs. Finally, the explosion of the technology relative to the distribution of the Internet and the World Wide Web provided the technological tools needed to develop medical systems that could be integrated with the external information world, efficiently distribute information throughout the area and require even lower investments. In the meantime, DICOM, HL7 [3] and IHE [4], became reference standards whose compatibility is an indispensable requirement for every system used in the medical field, just like HTTP [5] and XML [6] became the reference protocols for distribution and interoperability with management information systems.

3. Web technology characteristics

3.1 Special features of web technology with respect to the Client/Server model

Most of the RIS/PACS systems on the market are based on the Client/Server model. This model, which is typical of the systems developed in the 1990s, utilises a high-performance server machine, on which to implement the complex processing operation, and a set of client machines, for which the user has direct access, to implement the data display software. Communications between server and client and the visual interface with the operator are developed according to proprietary protocols. Only the clients for whom the corresponding software has been installed can access the server. Therefore, Server and Client are strictly related and any change in the server implies that changes must be made with the client. In addition, the configuration is rigid. If one client machine is added, special software must also be installed. In fact, different software versions may be incompatible and, therefore, to add just one client, it might become necessary to update the software on the server as well as all the clients that were previously installed. This operation may also require updates to the hardware. The developer manages the transmission between Server and Client and performances vary significantly according to the implementation. Finally, the Client/Server model is designed to operate in a local network and is difficult to implement on a geographic network or on the Internet.

Because Web technology is based on international standards, it gets around all these problems. With this technology, a server machine also handles the complex processing operations, but the communication to clients is carried out using a standard protocol while the data display interface is standardised and incorporated within the client machine operating system (web browser). Therefore, client management is no longer tied to the server and can be managed independently by the user. Since it is standard, the transmission is managed at the operating

©CARS/Springer. All rights reserved.

system level, thus offering greater guarantees in terms of efficiency and stability. In addition, Web technology dos not make any distinction between local network, geographic network or the Internet, ensuring that the operating model remains the same in all three environments. Another advantage offered by Web technology is that different applications can be integrated as simple web "plug-ins", thus using different applications within the same environment and generating systems that combine a high degree of application customisation while maintaining a very general system structure.

In summary, Web technology has three special features:

It concentrates the entire processing operation, specific to the application, on one server machine and standardises the procedures involving access and transmission from the server to the user connected with the computer.

For the user interface it uses standard browsers that are already integrated into new-generation operating systems or, in any case, are easy to install and free.

It can be used to distribute information on a local or a geographic network, ensuring access to the same information by anyone with access authorisation, no matter where they are located.

This offers significant advantages for both the system client/user and for the vendor company. With Web technology, the customer can use standard machines as the client, without having to install dedicated software and it's also possible to add, replace and change the number of connections as required. In addition, the customer can access his server application locally within the Intranet and from a remote location on the Internet since access is available to the same application and with the same environment.

The company that sells the system has the advantage of acquiring greater control over all its parts, since they are installed on a single machine, thus greatly simplifying the necessary maintenance and updating procedures. Finally, Web technology is used to integrate different applications as "plug-ins" of a system, thus making it possible to use different applications within the same environment and to generate systems that combine a high degree of application customisation while maintaining a very general system structure. For example, it will be possible to introduce voice recognition, electronic signature certification or biometric recognition algorithms, without requiring any dedicated development operations.

3.2 Security issues

When transmitting sensitive information, such as medical data, on a 'public' network, some precautions must be taken to comply with Privacy regulations and to guarantee the efficiency and security of that data transmission [7]. The new-generation medical information systems generally use protection mechanisms similar to those used in electronic trade and in Web financial transactions that, to the present, have proven to be reliable and inaccessible to unauthorised users.

The main transmission protection mechanisms include:

128-bit public and private key information coding.

Transmission based on the SSL protocol.

Private/public network separation using Firewalls.

Possibility of configuring VPN (Virtual Private Network) networks.

©CARS/Springer. All rights reserved.

4. Web-based distribution of diagnostic information

4.1 Web systems for distributing information within image diagnostic departments

There are many economic as well as productive advantages in using web-based systems within diagnostic image departments. Using standard hardware as client access stations greatly reduces investment costs, increases equipment service life and fully optimises and enhances the efficiency of each component. The standardisation inherent to the Web protocol makes the structure independent in managing the system configuration, eliminating all constraints with the software vendor company. The same standardisation makes the system learning phase simpler, easier to use and reduces the information technology skills required within the department. Maintenance costs are reduced since they are basically limited to the server components. In addition, component maintenance and updating can be carried out using a remote connection, and this makes response time as quick as possible while lowering the relative costs.

The Web platform is a remarkable tool for distributing images and information to requesting departments. All authorised departments can obtain immediate access to the information to which they are entitled, without having to acquire particular equipment and simply using the local hospital network and common PCs. Finally, through XML, it is possible to connect different specialised systems and/or different data banks within the same environment. Therefore, it is easy to integrate the medical information system with the hospital information system (HIS), the enterprise information system (ERP), or with the data banks of the Single Appointment Centre (CUP) and the Health Records Office.

4.2 Web systems for distributing information throughout the area

One of the special features of the health care system is certainly the relationship that has been established between the family doctor and his or her patients. In fact, it is this important professional Health Care figure that represents the first and, as we will see, the last link in the chain of the structured and complete national health system. Thus, it is the family doctor, who acts as the interface between the patient and the health world, whom patients instil their trust, often establishing a friendship that goes beyond the mere professional relationship. However, the family doctor often has problems in obtaining access to specialised information and the patient may be forced, on an individual basis, to contact other figures in the health and medical world and must interact, generally in person, at different times and places, with a series of 'windows' to do various tasks, such as making an appointment for a test, paying a fee and picking up results. These administrative operations, that add no value to the diagnostic and/or treatment process, may be further hampered by delays, inconveniences and errors and cause fatigue and generate frustration for the resident/patient.

Distribution of the communication and information through the Internet can play a fundamental role in the process of sharing important images and data. This would help improve the national health service as well as the patient's quality of life. It would get the family doctor involved in the entire diagnostic testing 'health and medical' process, ensuring complete information and providing access to all data relative to the 'Patient's Electronic Health Chart', once again making that doctor the patient's main point of reference. It would increase the family doctor's opportunities to continuously update

©CARS/Springer. All rights reserved.

his/her professional skills through access to data banks containing representative and reference case studies. It would increase the accuracy of the diagnoses, ensuring the active involvement of several specialists and/or colleagues of the family doctor. It would provide better service to the patient, in terms of time and quality, providing him/her with more detailed explanations that are easier to understand. Automation and centralisation of all the 'medical' data together with the non-diagnostic component may lead to additional savings in terms of resources for the Administration as well as for the population.

Thanks to the use of the Internet and the Web platform to be network-linked to the CUP (Single Appointment Centre), the Health Records Office, the Image Diagnostics Departments distributed throughout the area and the family doctors, it would be possible to create a single Virtual Hospital or Heath Care Organisation where information, although being physically located in another site, is "really" available throughout the area, in the hospital, family doctor's clinic or even the patient's home.

5. Use of the Web at the Policlinico Umberto I - Rome

In our department, in cooperation with Ferrania Imaging Technologies, we have developed a system based on Web technology to manage and distribute images and diagnostic information at the Policlinico Umberto I of Rome and throughout the area [8, 9].
The project includes three development phases and the second phase is currently in progress:

- Development of the intradepartmental system
- Distribution of information to hospital departments
- Distribution of information throughout the area

6. Conclusions

Image diagnostics is going through a transition from analog to digital technology. This transition is turning out to be slower and more difficult with respect to the initial expectations. However, we believe it is an inexorable process that can really improve the diagnostic process and help enhance the quality of the Health Care Service and, more generally, the quality of people's lives.
Web technology can make a decisive technological contribution. However, to be successful, the process cannot be based only on technology, and thus must also integrate organisational, cultural and economic aspects.

References

1. Diagnostic Imaging Scan – Market Report, Miller Freeman, 1999
2. Dig. Imaging and Communication in Medicine, Part 1-10, Nema Standard Publ. 1992-2000. ww.rsna.org
3. Health Level Seven, Version 2.3, Health, Level Seven Inc. 1996. www.hl7.org.
4. Integrating The Healthcare Enterprise, Tech. Framework Year 3., HIMSS/RSNA Ed., 2001. www.rsna.org.
5. Hypertext Transfer Protocol Specifications. Word Wide Web Consortium, 1999.
6. Sturm J. Sviluppo di soluzioni XML. Mondadori 2000.
7. Eng J. Computer Network Security for the Radiology Enterprise. Radiology, August 2001.
8. Passariello R. Intranet nella diffusione RIS/PACS. Convegno di Radiologia Informatica, Pisa 2001.
9. Campanella V. Diffusione Web e Stategie Tecnologiche di un Moderno Sistema RIS/PACS. Convegno Nazionale AIFM, Brescia 2001.

CARS 2002 – H.U. Lemke, M.W. Vannier; K. Inamura, A.G. Farman, K. Doi & J.H.C. Reiber (Editors)
©CARS/Springer. All rights reserved.

Implementation of RIS/PACS at Princess Alexandra Hospital Brisbane, Australia

B Crowe
Health Informatics Society of Australia, Canberra Australia
Email: bernie.crowe@acslink.aone.net.au

Abstract

Princess Alexandra Hospital (PAH) let a contract for the provision of a RIS/PACS system with Agfa/Cerner in April 1999. The contract was arranged in conjunction with the Royal Brisbane Hospital/ Royal Women's Hospital and Royal Brisbane Children's Hospital. The purpose of the contract was to enable the distribution of medical images and reports throughout the hospitals in digital form. It was anticipated that the introduction of the new system would lead to greater efficiency in the delivery of radiology services and would provide an improved service to clinicians to facilitate patient management.

An Assessment Study was conducted in parallel with the project implementation into the effect of RIS/PACS on both the Radiology Department and the hospital at PAH. Prior to the signing of a contract with Agfa/Cerner in April 1999, a great deal of effort was directed into project planning activities. The implementation of the Cerner RadNet RIS (April 2000) and installation of Agfa ADC Computed Radiography systems in the Emergency Department (July 2000) and Intensive Care Unit (August 2000) provided experience with digital technology. The Agfa IMPAX PACS and archive were installed in the old hospital (January 2000) prior to the physical move to the new hospital (May 2001). The project resulted in the establishment of a filmless imaging environment at the new PAH hospital with images distributed to clinicians via the Agfa Web 1000 on 143 Clinical Review Workstations in the wards and in 19 theatres.

The installation of a RIS/PACS to create a "filmless" hospital has been a major project. The PAH is a 720 bed hospital providing all services of an acute care teaching hospital, and has moved into a new building during the implementation of the RIS/PACS/CR. The result has been a new hospital with a new radiology reporting and digital image distribution system that has increased radiologists' productivity at a time of increasing volume and complexity of workload.

Keywords: PACS, evaluation, productivity, workflow

1. Introduction

The planned rebuilding of the major tertiary hospitals in Queensland, Australia, under the State Government's AUS $2.4 billion health capital works program, provided the impetus to implement PACS. Queensland Health entered an AUS $25M contract in April 1999 to implement a Picture Archive and Communications System (PACS) at four major public teaching hospitals in Queensland. RIS/ PACS/CR was implemented at the Princess Alexandra Hospital (PAH) and the Herston Hospitals Complex, which includes Royal Brisbane Hospital, Royal Women's Hospital and Royal Brisbane Children's Hospital. The contract was subsequently extended to include the Townsville General Hospital.

©CARS/Springer. All rights reserved.

Agfa-Gevaert Limited (Agfa) was selected as the prime contractor for the PACS implementation. Agfa's subcontractors were Cerner Corporation for the provision of the RadNet Radiology Information System, Sun Microsystems Australia Pty Ltd, Storage Technology of Australia and Compaq Computer Australia. A change management consultancy was arranged with Convergent Technologies Group (CTG) Healthcare Consulting. An Assessment Study was performed by Bernard Crowe & Associates. Initial planning for PACS commenced in 1995 with the establishment of the Medical Imaging Digital Acquisition and Archiving Communications (MIDAACS) Working Party at the Herston Hospitals Complex. The radiological workload at the three Herston Hospitals was 180,000 examinations per year.

The MIDAACS Committee commissioned a PACS feasibility study that was completed in April 1996. Following acceptance of the feasibility study a Request for Information (RFI) was issued in November 1996. Subsequent to the RFI it was decided to include the Princess Alexandra Hospital, also under redevelopment which had a radiological workload of 100,000 examinations per year. In November 1997, a Request For Offer (RFO) was released. In June 1998, following extensive evaluation of the offers, Queensland Health announced Agfa-Gevaert Limited as its preferred supplier for PACS. A period of contract negotiations then occurred, culminating in the signing of a contract between Queensland Health and Agfa-Gevaert Limited in April 1999.

2. Methods and results of assessment study

At PAH it was planned to implement PACS over a number of phases. The first two phases occurred in the existing hospital building with subsequent phases occurring in the new hospital. The first two phases involved establishing PACS for the existing "digital" modalities i.e. Computed Tomography (CT), Magnetic Resonance Imaging (MRI), Digital Subtraction Angiography (DSA), Digital Subtraction Imaging (DSI) and Ultrasound. Following the implementation of the Cerner RadNet RIS (April 2000), Agfa ADC Computed Radiography systems were installed at PAH in the Emergency Department (July 2000) and Intensive Care Unit (August 2000). Hard copy images were produced at PAH during these two phases. Following relocation to a new hospital on the Princess Alexandra Campus, the RIS/PACS became operational in May 2001.

This implementation followed an 18 month schedule where all medical imaging modalities (a total of 16 devices plus 7 Computed Radiography (CR) plate readers) were connected to the PACS and patients' images and reports were stored in digital form in a long term archive. These images and reports are immediately available on 143 dedicated Clinical Review Workstations through the PAH wards, clinics and operating theatres. Radiologists report images on 19 Dual Screen Diagnostic Workstations within the Radiology Department. In addition, a diagnostic review station is located in the Intensive Care and Emergency Department. A phased approach to implementation was adopted so that experience could be gained in implementing PACS across the full range of imaging modalities while minimising the disruption to radiological service delivery. Lessons learned during the first two phases ensured a smooth implementation of PACS in the new hospital. The final outcome for the Radiology Department was a "filmless" environments, i.e. no darkrooms and no dedicated film storage.

©CARS/Springer. All rights reserved.

The Assessment Study of the implementation of PACS, undertaken by Bernard Crowe & Associates, was based on an international literature review of PACS evaluation studies[1-14]. The objectives of the Assessment Study were (i) to identify positive and negative aspects of the PACS implementation, (ii) short and long term impacts on radiological services delivery and (iii) the overall impact on clinical service delivery.

2.1 Radiology department workloads

The operation of the RIS/PACS/CR was well received by the PAH radiologists. The time to report examinations has been reduced and this result has been achieved in a environment where the radiology workload is increasing in both volume and complexity.

The overall assessment found that the operation of the CR/RIS/PACS in the new PAH hospital has enabled the Radiology Department to improve the level of service to referring clinicians at a time of increasing workloads. In the PAH Radiology Department, there are eight radiologists, five Visiting Medical Officers, and up to 12 Registrars and a Radiology Fellow. As well as managing a workload of over 100,000 examinations a year (2002/20001 - 102,756 examinations on 85,346 patients) there is a substantial teaching component, as well as research activities.

Prior to the introduction of RIS/PACS in 1999, approximately 8000 radiology examinations a month were performed in the general areas shown in Table 1.

Modality	Number of examinations per month
CT	900
MRI	400
Ultrasound	500
Nuclear Medicine	250
Angiography	150
General X rays	2000
Emergency	2000
Orthopaedics	600
Venography	100
Mammography	50
Minor Procedures	250
Miscellaneous	50
Mobiles	900

Table 1 PAH Radiology Department - 1999 Monthly Workload

There was a high proportion of in-patients (approximately 45%) accounting for some 50% of examinations. Some 20% of examinations related to Casualty and the remaining 30% were Outpatients. It should be noted that this work load is typical of a public teaching hospital and is not therefore comparable in radiologist productivity terms with the workload of a private radiology practice.

Over the period of the RIS/PACS implementation (1999/2001), the nature of the radiology workload at PAH changed with a significant increase of 40 per cent in cross-sectional imaging. CT studies have increased from 900 to 1300 a month and MRI studies from 425 to 600 a month. This pattern of activity, involving increasing complexity and volume, is consistent with the experience of other PACS based hospitals.

©CARS/Springer. All rights reserved.

The introduction of the seven CR units producing digital images rather than film has been accepted, particularly in ED and ICU. A sample survey of the ED CR showed that the Reject Rate had been reduced to 4 per cent. Previously, the overall Reject Rate at PAH was 10 per cent. However, as noted by other RIS/PACS/CR assessments, the amount of radiographer time required to conduct examinations on patients using CR (linked to the HIS and RIS) is about the same as using conventional film/screen processing.

Following a Clinician Satisfaction Survey in August 2001, the immediate access storage (Web Cache) is to be upgraded to provide on demand sub-second retrieval to clinicians of six to twelve months of patients' images and reports. An interesting point is that some clinicians such as Urologists now refer their patients to the PAH Radiology Department for follow-up examinations, so that all the patient's images will be in digital form rather than on film and will be available for review on a Clinical Review Workstation.

One of the main findings of the RIS/PACS Assessment Study was the need for extensive training of both radiographers and radiologists in new systems and equipment. In conjunction with the suppliers Agfa/Cerner, the systems radiographers staff at PAH have taken on a training role that perhaps was not anticipated in the original discussions and planning.

3. Discussion

3.1 Workload

On balance, the findings of the introduction of RIS/PACS at PAH is that there has been an considerable workload in planning, system testing, training of staff and discussions with hospital administrators. A not unexpected finding from the Assessment Study conducted at PAH was that it is difficult to separate the effect of soft-copy reporting on radiologists' productivity from the effect of RIS and PACS on workflow in the Radiology Department and the effect of PACS on registrar teaching and research. The increase in radiology activity at PAH occurred during the introduction of RIS/PACS/CR and the relocation of the Radiology Department to a new hospital. As the number of Radiologists did nor increase, the view of Chairman of the PAH Radiology Department is that it would not have been possible for radiology services to be maintained to clinicians without the benefits of RIS/PACS facilitating reduced reporting times and improved turnaround of radiology reports.

On introducing PACS at Baltimore Veterans Administration Medical Center, Reiner et al [15] found that radiology staff did not increase at the same rate as the examination workload. Because of the nature of cross-sectional studies and the increase in the number of multiple images per study, Reiner estimated that a 40 percent increase in CT/MRI workload was equivalent to a 65 per cent increase in relative value workload units. The authors estimated that under PACS, BVAMC was 25 per cent more productive than national norms in 1995.

3.2 Radiologists' productivity

During the conduct of the PAH Assessment Study, it was obvious that there were a number of factors that impact directly on Radiologists' productivity. As these factors interact, a list of factors affecting Radiologists' productivity was prepared with assumptions as to the likely effect of RIS/PACS.

©CARS/Springer. All rights reserved.

1. **Request Form**
   (RIS/PACS will allow electronic order entry and follow up. May reduce interruptions to Radiologist.)
2. **Availability of historical information on patients**
   (RIS/PACS will pre-fetch relevant images prior to reporting. Potential to lengthen reporting process with more images for Radiologist to review.)
3. **Manual handling of films and reports**
   (RIS/PACS will eliminate this task.)
4. **Viewing of images on screen and making diagnosis**
   (RIS/PACS may lengthen this task, particularly for complex studies - window/level etc.)
5. **Dictation, review, sign and distribute report**
   (RIS/PACS may shorten this cycle, depending on ready access by Radiologists/Registrars to PC's.)
6. **Interruptions to reporting process**
   (Improved hospital procedures after RIS/PACS installation and move to new hospital may reduce interruptions and improve Radiologists' productivity.)
7. **Training of Registrars**
   (RIS/PACS and access to PC based Web Based Training has potential to reduce face to face training time and increase Radiologists' productivity)
8. **Effect of reporting environment**
   (Correct lighting required under RIS/PACS to minimise fatigue.)
9. **Ability to handle outside hospital films in PAH PACS environment**
   (Correct environment and procedures required - may lengthen reporting process, depending on number of cases.)

As it turned out, factors such as interruptions during the reporting process have a greater potential to effect Radiologists' productivity than any other event. The significance of interruptions in reducing the productivity of Radiologists has been noted in other assessment studies, particularly that of Bryan et al [16] on PACS at the Hammersmith Hospital, UK. The authors noted that radiology reporting time tended to be lengthened in addition to the time the Radiologist was actually involved in the interruption. It was assumed that the Radiologist required additional time to review the stage reached before interruption and then continue.

Such research findings would tend to reinforce the common sense suggestion that system designers should do everything possible to reduce interruptions to highly paid specialists performing a complex task. The use of receptionists for screening calls and the use of computer based radiology information systems in the wards would seem to be highly recommended. The operation of the RIS/PACS at the new PAH hospital, with changed workflow involving Radiologists' use the Cerner RadNet RIS to correct their own reports by typing corrections on computer screens after transcription, has led to a reduction in interruptions and an increase in Radiologists' productivity. This increase has been supported by the ability of the PACS to recall previous images and reports, so that the PAH Assessment Study has reinforced research findings on the importance of changed workflow and procedures to complement the introduction of new RIS/PACS systems [17].

An overview of the impact of RIS/PACS installed at Hammersmith Hospital in 1996 has been published by Bryan et al [18-19] indicating that PACS was almost universally preferred by users and brought many operational and clinical benefits. However, the authors noted that the older PACS came at a significant capital and net running cost. As well, there was a high non-capital implementation cost in terms of the time of hospital staff on PACS related business, often helping vendors to understand the hospital's requirements for PACS. Other hospitals planning similar activities would be advised to take these matters into account when planning a RIS/PACS/CR implementation.

©CARS/Springer. All rights reserved.

Further reports will address the aspects of costs and benefits of RIS/PACS/CR at PAH following the completion of the changeover period to filmless operation and the operation of a full year of filmless operation in 2002/2003 with a revised clerical and administrative structure.

Acknowledgement

The assistance of PAH personnel, including Dr K Siddle, Director of Diagnostic Imaging, Dr L Sim, PACS Project Director and Mr W Nuss, Director Radiography, in facilitating the conduct of the Assessment Study was greatly appreciated.

References

1. De Simone DN, Kundel HL, Arenson RL. Effect of a digital imaging network on physician behavior in an intensive care unit. Radiology.1988; 169: 41-44.
2. Straub W, Gur D. The hidden costs of delayed access to diagnostic imaging information; impact on PACS implementation. American Journal of Roentgenology. 1990; 155: 613-616.
3. Crowe B, Hailey D, Carter C. Assessment of costs and benefits in the introduction of digital radiology systems. International Journal of Biomedical Computing. 1992; 40: 369-373.
4. Horii S. Electronic imaging workstations: ergonomic issues and the user interface. Radiographics. 1992; 12: 773-787.
5. Breant CM, Taira R, Huang H. Interfacing aspects between the PACS, RIS and HIS. Journal of Digital Imaging. 1993; 6 (2): 88-94.
6. Bryan S, Weatherburn G, Keen J. Evaluation of PACS at Hammersmith Hospital: baseline assessment of costs and other resource-use parameters within the Radiology Department. Paper presented to CAR 93, Berlin, 1993.
7. Strickland NH. Cost-benefit considerations for PACS: a radiological perspective. British Journal of Radiology. 1996; 69: 1089-1098.
8. Bryan S, Keen J, Muris N. Issues in the evaluation of picture archiving and communications systems. Health Policy. 1995; 33: 31-42.
9. Keen J, Bryan S, Muris N. Evaluation of diffuse technologies: the case of digital imaging networks. Health Policy. 1995; 34: 153-166.
10. Bryan S, Weatherburn G, Watkins J, Buxton M. Explaining variations in radiologists' reporting times. British Journal of Radiology. 1995; 68: 854-861.
11. Kundel HL, Seshadri SB, Langlotz CP et al. Prospective study of a PACS: information flow and clinical action in a medical intensive care unit. Radiology. 1996; 199: 143-149.
12. Siegel E. Filmless radiology at the Baltimore VA. Diagnostic Imaging. 1997; 6: 54-66.
13. Flagel C. Economics of PACS: a cost benefit analysis. Jour. of Digital Imaging. 1998; 11 (3): Suppl 1, 237
14. Reiner B, Siegel E, Hooper F. Impact of filmless imaging on the frequency of the clinician review of radiology images. Journal of Digital Imaging. 1998; 11 (3): Suppl 1, 149-150.
15. Reiner B, Siegel E, Cox R. Changes in Radiology Department personnel requirements when transitioning from film-based to filmless imaging. Annual Meeting of the American Roentgen Ray Society. 100th Meeting, May 7-12 2000. 174(3): 20.
16. Bryan S, Weatherburn G, Watkins J et al. Radiology report times: impact of PACS. American Journal of Roentgenology. 1998; 170:1153-1159.
17. Wendler T and Loef C. Workflow management - integration technology for efficient radiology. Medica Mundi. 2001; 45(4): 41-48.
18. Bryan S,Weatherburn G, BuxtonM, Watkins J, Keen J, Muris N. Evaluation of a hospital picture archiving and communication system. Journ. of Health Services Res. and Policy. 1999; 4(4): 204-209.
19. Bryan S, Buxton M Brenna E. Estimating the impact of a diffuse technology on the running costs of a hospital. A case study of a PACS. Int. J. of Technology Assessment in Health Care. 2000;16(3);787-798.

CARS 2002 – H.U. Lemke, M.W. Vannier; K. Inamura, A.G. Farman, K. Doi & J.H.C. Reiber (Editors)
©CARS/Springer. All rights reserved.

Expressing DICOM SR constraints in XML

K. P. Lee[a]

[a]Philips Research, Briarcliff Manor New York 10501, USA, kp.lee@philips.com

Abstract

In using XML to encode DICOM Structured Reporting documents, it is desirable to mechanically enforce constraints expressed in natural language in the specification. XML Schema can be used to accomplish this partially but is not powerful enough to express all the constraints. We demonstrate how more complex constraints can be expressed in XML syntax using the Schematron language.

Keywords: Structured reporting, Schematron, electronic patient record

1. Introduction

The Digital Imaging and Communications in Medicine (DICOM) Structured Reporting (SR) standard [1], and the SR Documentation Model upon which it is based, improves the expressiveness, precision, and comparability of documentation about diagnostic images and waveforms. The DICOM SR Information Object Definition (IOD) supports the interchange of expressive compound reports in which the critical features shown by images and waveforms can be denoted unambiguously by the observer, indexed, and retrieved selectively by subsequent reviewers. Findings may be expressed by the observer as text, codes, and numeric measurements, or via location coordinates of specific regions of interest within images or waveforms, or references to comparison images, sound, waveforms, curves, and previous report information. The observational and historical findings recorded by the observer may include any evidence referenced as part of an interpretation procedure. Thus, DICOM SR supports not only the reporting of diagnostic observations, but can document fully the evidence that evoked the observations. This capability provides significant new opportunities for large-scale collection of structured data for clinical research, training, and outcomes assessment. This is a by-product of diagnostic image and waveform interpretation facilitating the pooling of structured data for multi-center clinical trials and evaluations. As is standard practice in DICOM, the SR specification is maintained in Microsoft Word format and published as a PDF file. This format is not amenable to machine processing and has the potential for misinterpretation, as is common in standards written in natural language.

Extensible Markup Language (XML) [2] is a set of technologies defined by the World Wide Web Consortium (W3C) [3] encompassing a universal data format for tree-based, hierarchical information. A number of new specifications extending its range and power, such as Extensible Stylesheet Language (XSL) [4], XML Schema [5], and XSL Transformations (XSLT) [4], have been developed. XML offers the advantages of platform independence and Web awareness, and many XML tools are open source and freely available. Thus XML technologies can provide a simple and low cost solution for enterprise-wide access to clinical information including medical reports. Having such reports in a formal notation allows them to be processed by machines more readily. There

©CARS/Springer. All rights reserved.

have been attempts [6] to produce an XML version of SR representing such reports as XML documents. Having such XML documents has the added advantage that they can be easily exported to non-DICOM environments such as Health Level 7 (HL7) [7]. Furthermore, as HL7 moves towards a specification of the Clinical Document Architecture (CDA) expressed in XML, it is important to have an XML version of SR to align these standards. How to produce an XML representation of DICOM SR is beyond the scope of this paper. Suffice it to say that it can be done in a fairly straightforward manner. Figure 1 shows an example SR document generated according to a schema we developed. The document is shown in the Enhanced Grid View of the XML Spy [8], a popular tool for developing XML, and shows the overall structure of the document. Note that the structure follows closely that of Section A.35 (Structured Report Document Information Object Definitions) in Part 3 of [1].

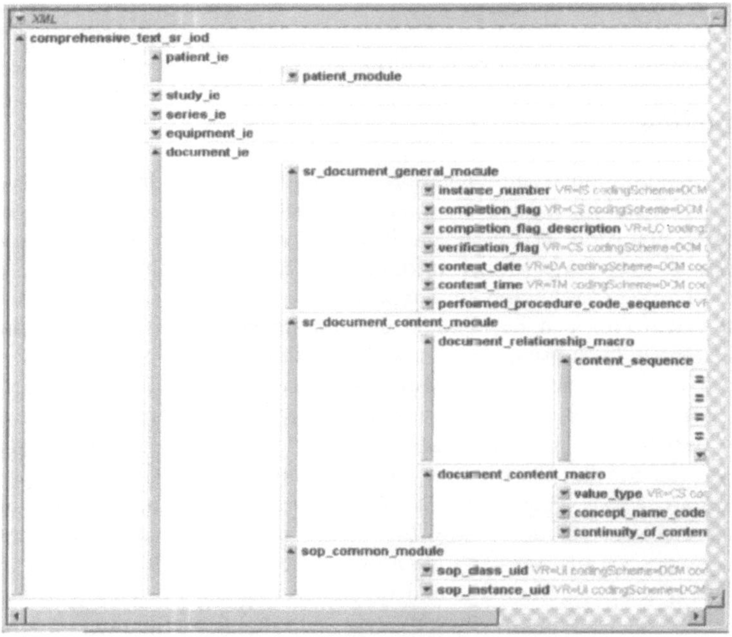

Figure 1. Partial view of a DICOM SR document

2. SR Constraints

An XML Schema can be produced to encode the syntactic structure of an XML SR document. However such a document must also satisfy a number of constraints expressed primarily in natural language in the standard. Some constraints are simple and others are more complex. Examples of simple constraints are that a numeric attribute must have a value between a given minimum and maximum, or that a string attribute cannot be more than 16 characters long. An example of a more complex constraint is that the Specimen Identification Module must be present if the subject is a specimen. Since these constraints are specified in natural language, they are subject to interpretation by the implementer and are hard to process by mechanical means. An important goal in expressing SR in XML is

©CARS/Springer. All rights reserved.

the expression of these constraints in XML syntax. Being able to express constraints systematically will ease the production of well-formed and valid DICOM SR documents.

2.1 Simple constraints

XML Schema provides mechanisms for constraining the structure and content of an XML SR document. It is relatively straightforward to express constraints involving a single attribute of a DICOM IOD using facilities of XML Schema. Such constraints are enforced when an XML SR document is processed with a validating XML parser. We give a number of simple examples (or simplicity, we ignore namespaces in this paper).

- The Patient ID (0010,0020) attribute must have a value which is a string of length no more than 64. This constraint is expressed in XML Schema by assigning a type deriving from the built-in type string using the maxLength facet:

```
<simpleType name="patient_id">
  <restriction base="string">
    <maxLength value="64"/>
  </restriction>
</simpleType>
```

- The Patient Age (0010,1010) attribute must have the form of three digits followed by one of the characters 'D' (day), 'W' (week), 'M' (month) and 'Y' (year). The type in this case is derived from string using the pattern facet:

```
<simpleType name="patient_age">
  <restriction base="string">
    <pattern value="[0-9]{3}[DWMY]"/>
  </restriction>
</simpleType>
```

- The Patient's Sex (0010,0040) attribute can only take on the values of 'M' (male), 'F' (female) or 'O' (other). This type is expressed using the enumeration facet:

```
<simpleType name="patients_sex">
  <restriction base="string">
    <enumeration value="M"/>
    <enumeration value="F"/>
    <enumeration value="O"/>
  </restriction>
</simpletype>
```

- Each DICOM attribute has a type. Type 1 attributes are required and must have a valid value. Type 2 attributes are required but may have zero length if the value is unknown. Type 3 attributes are optional. There are also Types 1C and 2C, which are the same as 1 and 2 respectively but only if certain stated conditions are met. An example of a Type 2 attribute is Patient ID (0010,0020). This is expressed by making the patient_id element nillable:

```
<element name="patient_id" type="patient_id" nillable="true"/>
```

In an instance document a missing Patient ID is expressed as:

```
<patient_id nil="true"/>
```

©CARS/Springer. All rights reserved.

- DICOM has sequence attributes which are ordered sets of repeating items. An example is the Admitting Diagnoses Code Sequence (0008,1084) in the Patient Study Module (Section C.7.2.2 of Part 3 of [1]). In the definition of such sequences there is always a condition stating how many items are allowed in the sequence. In our example the condition is that "one or more items may be included in this Sequence." This is expressed using the minOccurs and maxOccurs facets as follows:

```
<element name="admitting_diagnoses_code_sequence">
  <complexType>
    <sequence>
      <element name="admitting_diagnoses_code_sequence_item"
          type="admitting_diagnoses_code_sequence_item"
          minOccurs="1" maxOccurs="unbounded"/>
    </sequence>
  </complexType>
</element>
```

These examples show that XML Schema is powerful enough to express many of the DICOM constraints involving single attributes. Nevertheless, XML Schema is incapable of expressing certain common constraints in DICOM SR, in particular those involving multiple attributes such as a constraint that says the pregnancy status of a patient is irrelevant if the patient is male. Thus, there is a need for a way to express these complex constraints using the same XML syntax in a declarative manner.

2.2 Complex constraints

Schematron

We have selected a tool known as Schematron [9], which was designed to extend the expressive power of XML Schema in specifying constraints. Schematron is a declarative assertion language using XML syntax developed by Rick Jelliffe, a member of the W3C XML Schema Working Group, and consists of a set of rules using XPath [10] expressions, another W3C Recommendation, that specify relationships between different elements. While XML Schema is grammar-based, Schematron is rule-based. Thus Schematron has different strengths when compared to XML Schema and is complementary. The use of XPath means that in fact we can specify constraint relationships involving arbitrary elements in an XML SR document.

To use Schematron only a standard XSLT processor is needed. The two-step process is as follows: A set of Schematron rules is written to express complex constraints that cannot otherwise be specified with XML Schema. This set of rules is transformed automatically through a meta-stylesheet (a stylesheet that generates other stylesheets) to produce an XSLT stylesheet which can then be run in the second step against a given XML SR document to verify that the constraints expressed by these rules are satisfied. This is illustrated in figure 2.

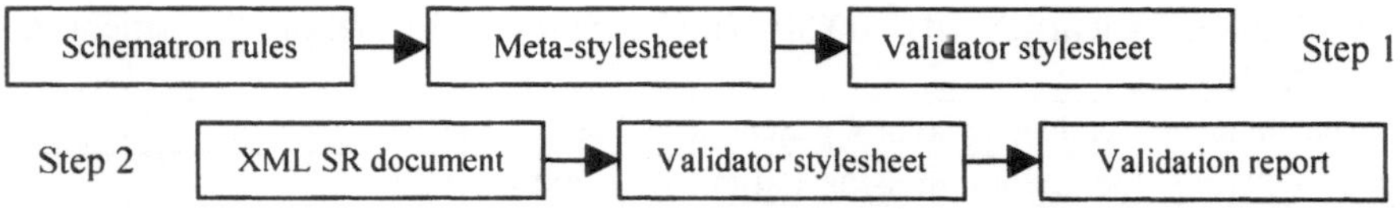

Figure 2. Using Schematron to validate an XML SR document

©CARS/Springer. All rights reserved.

Tools with graphical user interfaces are available, *e.g.*, Schematron Validator from Topologi [11], to combine the above into a one-step process. One only needs to supply the rules and an XML SR document and a report will be produced highlighting any detected violations. We will illustrate how complex constraints in SR can be specified using Schematron and show how such rules can be enforced.

Examples of complex constraints specified using Schematron

- If an SR document has been verified (i.e., the Verification Flag (0040,A493) attribute has the value 'VERIFIED'), then the Verifying Observer Sequence (0040,A073) must also be present. The following Schematron rule expresses this constraint:

```
    <rule context="sr_document_general_module">
       <report test="(verification_flag = 'VERIFIED') and (not
(verifying_observer_sequence))">
     Verifying Observer Sequence required if Verification Flag = VERIFIED</report>
    </rule>
```

This rule is applied in the context of the SR Document General Module (Section C.17.2 of Part 3 of [1]). The value of the test attribute in the report element is the condition to be checked and is specified using XPath. If the condition is not satisfied in an XML SR document, then a message stating the reason for violation is produced. Figure 3 shows the result of running the Topologi Schematron Validator using the above rule on an XML SR document where the Verification Flag has been set to VERIFIED but the Verifying Observer Sequence is absent. The upper window displays the message together with the XPath expression pointing to where the error occurs. The lower window shows a portion of the XML SR document.

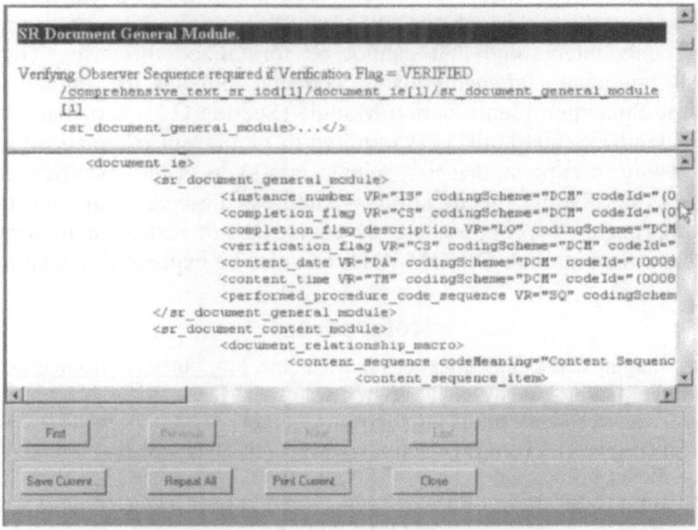

Figure 3. Error report for constraint violation in an XML SR document

- A second example is the constraint that the root item of the content item tree must have a type of CONTAINER (Section C.17.3 of Part 3 of [1]). Although this constraint involves only a single element, it applies only when that element is in a specific

©CARS/Springer. All rights reserved.

position in the document and is difficult to express in XML Schema. The following Schematron rule enforces the constraint:

```
<rule context="sr_document_content_module">
  <assert test="document_content_macro/value_type = 'CONTAINER'">
  Root Content Item must be of type CONTAINER</assert>
</rule>
```

- In an SR content item tree, relationships between a source content item and a target content item can be by-value or by-reference. In a by-reference relationship the target content item is denoted by the Referenced Content Item Identifier (0040,DB73). In such a case, the Document Relationship Macro and the Document Content Macro must not be present (Section C.17.3 of Part 3 of [1]). The following Schematron rule expresses this constraint:

```
<rule context="content_sequence_item/referenced_content_item_identifier">
  <report test="(../document_relationship_macro) or  (../document_content_macro) ">
    Document Relationship Macro and Document Content Macro shall not be present
    if the relationship is by-reference.</report>
</rule>
```

The above examples show how Schematron can address DICOM SR constraints that are beyond the capabilities of XML Schema.

3. Discussion

We have demonstrated that it is viable to use Schematron to express complex SR constraints in XML syntax. These can be enforced in XML SR documents using easily available tools. In working through the DICOM SR specification and trying to express constraints, we encounter some that cannot be formalized this way. These typically involve natural language statements using concepts outside the domain of SR. An example is in the Specimen Identification Module (Section C.7.1.2 of Part 3 of [1]). The attribute Slide Identifier (0040,06FA) is required to be present if the specimen is a slide. Yet there is no way to express that a specimen is a slide in the specification. We hope future updates of the SR IOD specification will address these cases in a more satisfactory manner. The approach we propose here of course is not restricted to formalizing SR constraints. Constraints in other DICOM IODs can also be expressed in a similar manner.

References

1. Digital Imaging and Communications in Medicine, http://medical.nema.org/.
2. Extensible Markup Language, http://www.w3.org/XML/.
3. World Wide Web Consortium, http://www.w3.org/.
4. Extensible Stylesheet Language, http://www.w3.org/Style/XSL/.
5. XML Schema, http://www.w3.org/XML/Schema/.
6. O. Baujard, J.C. Staub, D. Blot, D. Bandon, and Y. Ligier. *DICOM and XML: Union Makes Strength.* in Proceedings of *CARS 2001*. p. 773-776, 2001. Berlin: Elsevier.
7. Health Level Seven, http://www.hl7.org/.
8. XML Spy IDE, http://www.xmlspy.com/.
9. The Schematron Assertion Language 1.5, http://www.ascc.net/xml/resource/schematron/.
10. XML Path Language (XPath) Version 1.0, http://www.w3.org/TR/xpath/.
11. Topologi, http://www.topologi.com/.

CARS 2002 – H.U. Lemke, M.W. Vannier; K. Inamura, A.G. Farman, K. Doi & J.H.C. Reiber (Editors)
©CARS/Springer. All rights reserved.

A digital imaging network to facilitate a multi-center clinical trial for adrenoleukodystrophy

Mary Lou Ingeholm[a], Betty A. Levine[a], Ali Fatemi[b], Gerardo Jimenez-Sanchez[c], and Hugo W Moser[b]
[a]ISIS Center, Georgetown University, Washington DC
[b]Neurogenetics Research Center, The Kennedy Krieger Institute, Baltimore, MD
[c]Department of Pediatrics, Johns Hopkins University, Baltimore MD

Abstract

Finding a large enough patient population for performing clinical trials, especially for rare diseases, can be difficult. A multi-center clinical trial allows researchers to share information and interpretation of results from multiple institutions. Using a digital network and the Internet facilitates the sharing of acquired information between many locations and becomes key to establishing a successful multi-center clinical trial. A digital magnetic resonance imaging (MRI) network of clinical institutions to evaluate therapy outcomes in a multi-center clinical trial for adrenoleukodystrophy (ALD) has been created. The network uses the DICOM 3.0 standard to move MRI images securely over the Internet and Next Generation Internet (NGI) to a secure central clinical database. Virtual private network (VPN) technology is used to protect patient confidentiality and assure data integrity. 15 sites participate in the network; 160 ALD MRI studies have been stored in the clinical database and scored independently by two physicians.

Keywords: DICOM, digital imaging network, clinical trials

1. Introduction

X-linked adrenoleukodystrophy (ALD) is a rare neurological disorder, primarily affecting the nervous system white matter, adrenal cortex and testis. ALD has several phenotypes with the most severe phenotype affecting boys from ages 4 years to 10 years of age. In the childhood form of ALD, cerebral involvement occurs, resulting in the rapid decline of neurological functioning and death. Historically, the rarity of the disease in combination with its rapid progression has made it very difficult to efficiently evaluate promising potential therapies for childhood ALD. In the last few years however, researchers have found that cerebral abnormalities are present before the appearance of neurological dysfunction and that a brain magnetic resonance image (MRI) can best reveal these abnormalities. A brain MRI permits early detection of nervous system damage, and serves as a sensitive indicator of disease progression in individual patients [1,2]. For these reasons, it has become an indispensable tool for widening the window of opportunity for treatment and for evaluating the effectiveness of a particular therapy.

Nonetheless, finding a large enough patient population for performing clinical trials, especially for a rare disease like ALD, remains difficult. No one institution has enough

©CARS/Springer. All rights reserved.

patients to enroll in a clinical trial; thus, completion of the trial in a timely manner becomes an issue. Similarly, finding physicians trained to diagnose and treat rare diseases is often difficult, especially outside of large urban areas and away from large academic medical centers. A multi-center clinical trial eliminates both of these issues. Consolidating the data produces a sufficient patient pool for clinical trials while also enabling researchers to share information and interpretation of results from multiple institutions. Using a digital network and the Internet facilitates the sharing of acquired information between many locations and becomes key to establishing a successful multi-center clinical trial. We have established the infrastructure for a digital ALD MRI network. The network allows multiple institutions to send their ALD MRI cases via the Internet to a centralized clinical database. ALD-experienced physicians can independently summon up the ALD MRI cases remotely on softcopy display stations, review the study, and provide the therapy assessment.

Transferring MRI images to a central location using the Internet is significantly more efficient than any solution proposed in a film environment; however, with access to the Internet continuing to grow, the traffic and congestion on the Internet impacts the efficiency of the ALD MRI network. In order to optimize the capacity to transfer the MRI studies, the Kennedy Krieger Institute (KKI) has been given access to the Abilene network. Abilene is a very high-performance backbone network that is used by the Next Generation Internet (NGI) and Internet2 communities. Access to the Abilene network allows the KKI to communicate at high speed with other NGI participants. Most of the ALD MRI network sites are limited to standard Internet access; thus, their image transmissions occur over the standard Internet. For those sites that are NGI or Internet2 participants, image transmission is over a high-performance network to and from the KKI.

2. Methodology

The central ALD MRI database resides at the KKI. All images are sent to the KKI database for storage and retrieved from the database for evaluation. Implementation of the ALD MRI network takes into consideration the standard Internet and NGI environments, image transfer protocols that enable the images to be transferred to and from the KKI, and information assurance methods to protect patient confidentiality and data integrity. The implementation details are presented below with a network diagram shown in Figure 1. The mechanism for clinically evaluating and scoring the MRI studies is also discussed.

2.1 The network environment

The KKI has standard Internet connectivity; it also has access to the high-performance Abilene backbone network through the Mid-Atlantic Crossroads (MAX) network; MAX is a regional high-performance network that peers to Abilene. Any institution that has connectivity to one of the high-performance backbone networks such as Abilene or the very high-speed Backbone Network Service (vBNS) will communicate with the KKI using a high-performance network route. Institutions without connectivity to the NGI will use the standard Internet to send images.

©CARS/Springer. All rights reserved.

2.2 Image transmission

The Digital Imaging and COmmunications in Medicine (DICOM) version 3.0 standard [3] allows for the interchange of medical imaging data between vendors and modalities. The American College of Radiology (ACR) and National Electrical Manufacturers Association (NEMA) developed this standard jointly to facilitate digital medical image exchange. The ALD MRI network uses the DICOM 3.0 standard to move MRI images between the participating sites, central clinical database, and reviewing physicians' workstations. DICOM 3.0 provides standard connectivity and the best integration between the multiple devices. The use of the DICOM 3.0 standard, provides an increased capacity to seamlessly integrate each MRI scanner with the central clinical database.

A DICOM 3.0 server is installed at the Kennedy Krieger Institute (KKI) in Baltimore, Maryland. This server is a storage service class provider (SCP), query/retrieve SCP, and central database. Contributing sites use a DICOM storage service class user (SCU) to send their ALD-related MRI cases to the DICOM server at KKI while ALD trained physicians can remotely request the studies for review using a DICOM query/retrieve SCU. A variety of commercial DICOM SCUs are being successfully used over this network. Although the DICOM 3.0 messaging protocol is the image transmission method of choice, there are some instances where contributing sites cannot use a DICOM SCU for transmitting their images due to security concerns. To accommodate these concerns, an FTP server has been configured at the KKI to allow these sites to transmit the DICOM files via FTP. The files are then easily imported to the DICOM

2.3 Information assurance

To secure the data used in clinical trials, it is crucial to protect the privacy and confidentiality of the patient information and to ensure the integrity of the data. The ALD MRI network meets these criteria during storage of data in the central clinical database and transmission of data over the Internet. Firewall implementation protects the DICOM servers, providing protection for the clinical database. In addition, the specifications of the DICOM standard requires that the IP address, Application Entity Title (AET), and port number on which the device is listening be entered into the configuration database of both the sending and receiving DICOM devices. These features provide substantial control over who has permission to connect to the DICOM Server.

Many of the ALD studies arrive with the patient information intact. To preserve patient confidentiality, the patient-identifying information is stripped from the DICOM header and replaced with a unique identifying number generated by the software application MaskID. This masking technique protects the patient's confidentiality as well as blinding the ALD reviewing physician from the patient information. ALD-experienced physicians can only access the masked MRI studies.

To safeguard the privacy and confidentiality of patient information and to ensure the integrity of the data as it moves over the Internet or NGI, virtual private network (VPN) technology is used. A VPN uses encryption and message authentication to provide a secure channel through which data can be transferred. A VPN server has been installed at the KKI firewall and a VPN client is installed on the machine that will be communicating with the DICOM server at the KKI. Client encryption is used so that the data is encrypted

©CARS/Springer. All rights reserved.

before it leaves the remote machine, offering a secure solution for remote connections. The KKI VPN uses the Internet Protocol Security (IPSec) standard in conjunction with Internet Key Exchange (IKE) to provide IPSec-enabled devices a secure means to exchange the security parameters. IPSec provides two main functions; authentication to ensure that sending and receiving machines really are what they claim to be, and encryption to scramble data in flight so it won't be of any use if it is intercepted [4]. The Triple Data Encryption Standard (3DES) is the algorithm used to encrypt the data. A data integrity check is performed using the Security Hashing Algorithm 1 (SHA1). By applying the SHA1 hashing function to the data before and after it is sent, the hash results can be compared for any change in the data. The VPN also provides an access control mechanism by requiring user authentication with an eight-character user id/password mechanism.

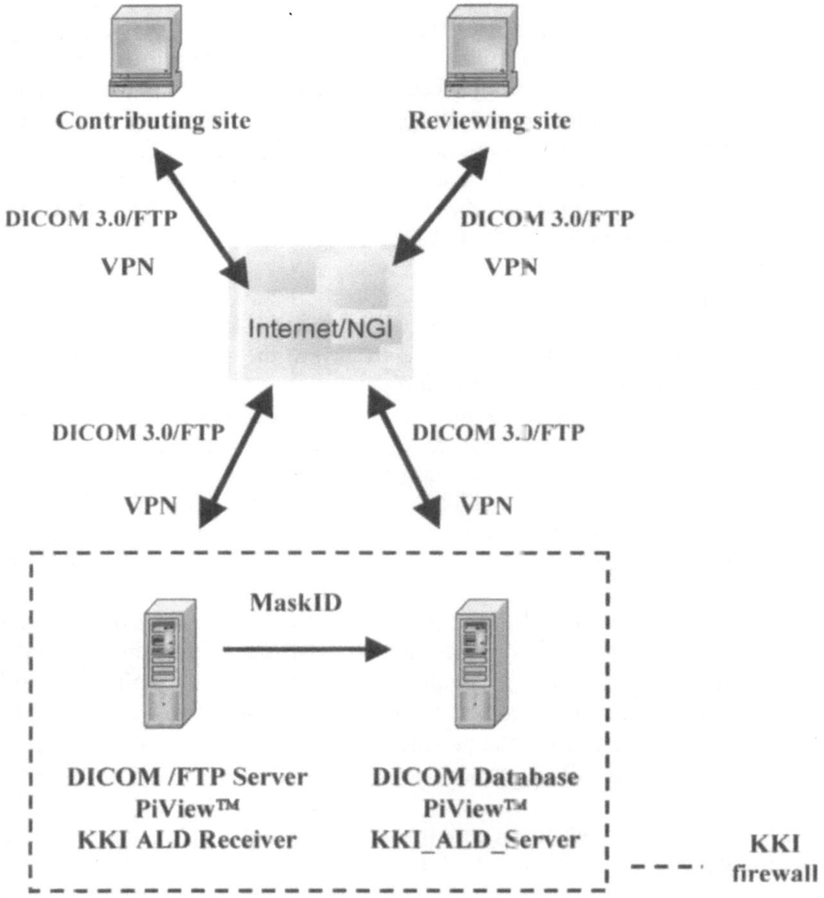

Figure 1. Digital ALD MRI Network

©CARS/Springer. All rights reserved.

2.4 MRI scoring mechanism

The Loes score sheet, a 34-point scoring system designed by Loes, et al [5] is an objective scoring mechanism of brain MRI abnormalities. ALD trained physicians use this tool to evaluate or score each MRI study submitted to the ALD database. The Loes score provides crucial information for tracking disease progression as well as predicting possible phenotype expression. A secure Web site has been developed allowing each physician to document the Loes score for a given patient. The resultant Loes scores are stored in a secure database. To enhance the validity of the interpretation, the MRI studies are independently read and scored by two ALD-trained physicians. The digital ALD MRI network in conjunction with the Web-based Loes score sheet allows physicians to review cases quickly and provide baseline and follow-up Loes scores to patients, parents, and their physicians.

3. Data

There are currently fifteen participating sites in the ALD MRI network. Twelve of the sites contribute images to the database sites; that is, they send their cases to KKI to be evaluated. Two sites both contribute studies to the database and request studies for review, and one site is only a review site. Nine different states in the U.S. and 5 different countries currently participate in the multi-center digital network. Of all the sites connected to the network, four out of the fifteen send or request studies using FTP, while the others use DICOM. Five of the fifteen sites access one of the high-performance computing networks like Abilene; the remaining sites connect using the standard Internet.

To date, 81 ALD patients with 160 MRI studies are stored in the KKI centralized database. At least two independent physicians have scored each of these exams using the Loes score sheet mechanism described above. Each physician reviews the studies independently and uses an on-line score sheet to record the results. We have seen a 98% correlation between the two scoring physicians and the Loes scores they have assigned to the different cases.

4. Results

For the participating sites, the ALD MRI network has proved to be invaluable. One of the reviewing physicians who previously made several trips a year to the KKI to score MRI studies of ALD patients now makes those assessments from home within a day of the MRI scan. The capacity to perform an immediate assessment has opened the window of opportunity for such therapies as bone marrow transplants. In a disease where the phenotypic expression is unpredictable, it is also of great social benefit to the patients and their families to receive the results of the MRI study in a timely manner.

We have found that those sites with high-performance network connectivity experience better integration of the ALD MRI network into the clinical environment. In addition, the capacity to transfer images at high speed consistently allows physicians to discuss the images, correlate them with other disease findings, measure disease severity, and request

©CARS/Springer. All rights reserved.

additional MRI studies in real-time permitting a more efficient clinical evaluation strategy.

From an implementation perspective, current technologies support the physical network infrastructure and its use, but we have found that while DICOM has become the standard for transferring digital imaging studies across a network, security concerns and the impending Health Insurance Portability and Accountability Act (HIPAA) regulations make the implementation of a large-scale DICOM network across the Internet more complex. Configuring DICOM clients and servers is straightforward; however, integrating DICOM with the security and confidentiality needs of the institution for transferring data over the Internet can be problematic.

5. Conclusion

Rare diseases such as adrenoleukodystrophy require a collaborative effort to identify and integrate pockets of disease and share clinical protocols. A multi-center digital MRI network provides the basis for exchanging and comparing the acquired digital images necessary for carrying out large-scale multi-center clinical trials. We have shown that such a network is technically feasible and enables accurate comparison on the reading of MRIs by physicians experienced in this particular disease. The use of standard transfer protocols like DICOM and FTP, wide area networks like the standard Internet and NGI networks, and security technologies like VPN and firewalls, have allowed for the creation of a secure digital network to facilitate multi-center clinical trials.

References

1. Moser, HW, "Adrenoleukodystrophy: phenotype, genetics, pathogenesis and therapy", Brain, 120:1485-1508, 1997.
2. Pouwels, PJW, Kruse B, Korenke GC, Mau X, Frahm J, "Quantitative proton magnetic resonance spectroscopy of childhood adrenoleukodystrophy", Neuropediatrics, 29:254-264, 1998.
3. American College of Radiology, National Electrical Manufacturers Association, Digital Imaging and Communications in Medicine (DICOM): Version 3.0 Standard. ACR-NEMA Committee, Working Group VI, Washington, DC, 1993.
4. Loes DJ, Hite S, Moser HW, Stillman AE, Shapiro E, Lockman L, Latchaw RE, Krivit W, "Adrenoleukodystrophy: A scoring method for brain MR observation", Am J Neuroradiology, 15:1761-6, 1994.
5. Newman D, Olewnick D, "IPSec VPNs: How Safe? How Speedy?", CommWeb.com., http://www.commweb.com/article/COM20000912S0009, 2000.

CARS 2002 – H.U. Lemke, M.W. Vannier; K. Inamura A.G. Farman, K. Doi & J.H.C. Reiber (Editors)
©CARS/Springer. All rights reserved.

ACRIN digital mammographic imaging screening trial informatics infrastructure

C.R. Welsh[1], B. Young[1], V. Gopalakrishnan[1], I Mahon[1], S. Sabina[1], C. Gatsonis[2], E. Pisano[3], M. Yaffe[4]

[1]American College of Radiology, Philadelphia, PA
[2]Brown University, Providence, RI
[3]University of North Carolina, Chapel Hill, NC
[4]University of Toronto, Canada

Abstract

The American College of Radiology Imaging Network (ACRIN) Digital Mammographic Imaging Screening Trial (DMIST) will enroll 49,500 women under a protocol that requires both digital and conventional film-screen examinations at 20 participating centers in North America during 18 months. A new clinical trials imaging infrastructure was developed to consolidate all of the digital mammographic images in a central archive at ACRIN headquarters in Philadelphia, PA. Each examination includes at least 4 views (2 of each breast) at 2K x 2.5K x 12 bit or higher resolution resulting in 10-64 Mbytes/image. Lossless compression resulted in 10:1 to 2:1 dataset reduction. Web-based forms are generated to acquire clinical information and the results of observations.

The central repository for this clinical trial includes a 1.5T byte RAID archive with DVD backup operating under Windows NT Server on a dual 1.3GHz Pentium IV host with 1 Gbyte RAM and 1 GHz Ethernet linked to a DS3 (15 Mbit/sec) dedicated line. Each remote site has a dedicated PC interfaced to one digital mammographic unit (Fuji, Lorad, GE and Fischer) that accumulates approximately 8 patient studies per day and transmits these overnight using the standard Ethernet to ACRIN HQ. In each case, special arrangements were made with each hospital or clinic's information technology departments to permit ftp transfer over existing network infrastructure. Data transmission speeds of 15-20 seconds/image were observed, with the performance goal of less than 2 minutes per image while receiving 200-300 images/night at peak utilization. In one instance, a DICOM wrapper was added to each digital mammographic image prior to transmission (since the imaging system was not DICOM compatible and no support was available from the manufacturer).

This clinical trial image archive system will ultimately manage an estimated 200,000 digital mammographic images that require 4-5 Tbytes of storage. All of these images will be independently interpreted by expert observers in a secondary analysis after the data acquisition phase of the trial has closed. As the images arrive, they are inspected for quality and comparison is made with the corresponding film images to assure that the patient identification is correct.

Importantly, this project was implemented on widely available and well supported "standard" platforms with generic database and operating system software, common

©CARS/Springer. All rights reserved.

networking components and inexpensive storage devices. Major savings were realized in comparison with more complex technologies, including commercially available PACS, storage area network (SAN) or network attached storage (NAS). No sacrifice in performance was made for this system, tailored to the specific needs of a large multicenter clinical trial.

This web-based system for clinical data acquisition and digital image archiving is unique in its size and complexity. Implementation was planned and completed in 6 months, with integration of 20 sites, training and testing before the end of the first year and initiation of the protocol. This system has accumulated 700 cases in the first month of operation with no downtime. Web-based data entry is time consuming for busy research coordinators and site research assistants, but allows quality and consistency checking of data and should ultimately reduce the number of errors in the final data set. The expected missing and erroneous data in the DMIST clinical trial is significantly less than 1%, justifying the additional time and effort needed for on-line entry procedures.

A new multicenter clinical trials imaging and information infrastructure was designed and implemented for the DMIST trial to handle unprecedented numbers of images (200,000+), sites (20), and overall size (4-5 Tbytes). This system sets a new standard for large scale clinical imaging trials and demonstrates that low cost, widely available technology and the public internet can suffice for most current and anticipated needs in these investigations.

Keywords: Digital mammography, clinical trial, observer studies

1. Introduction

The American College of Radiology has been actively conducting clinical research in the field of radiation therapy for over 25 years. This research has been conducted primarily from the ACR office in Philadelphia through the Radiation Therapy Oncology Group (RTOG). More recently, the ACR has become the recipient of a grant from the National Cancer Institute which has funded the establishment of the American College of Radiology Imaging Network (ACRIN), a new cooperative group formed for purposes of conducting clinical trials in diagnostic imaging related to cancer research. To date, ACRIN has X open and accruing trials and X in development, one example of which is a recently concluded trial focused on the evaluation of three dimensional colonography as a means of early detection of colon cancer. This involved the accumulation of approximately 80 cases, each of which were viewed and evaluated across three separate 3D diagnostic workstations by multiple reviewers in order to determine the efficacy of the 3D process. A more recent example and the focus of this presentation is a large clinical trial designed to compare more recent digital mammographic modalities with traditional screen film for purposes of breast cancer screening. ACRIN has over 100 institutions pre-qualified to enter patients on trial and has aggressive plans to expand the number of trials and participating institutions substantially over the coming years.

©CARS/Springer. All rights reserved.

2. Digital mammographic imaging screening trial overview

The Digital Mammographic Imaging Screening Trial (DMIST) is a large screening trial being conducted to evaluate digital mammography as compared to the traditional screen film technique for purposes of screening women for breast cancer. The trial has been designed to include 49,500 patients to be accrued over an 18 month period. There are 20 sites participating across 19 institutions which include large teaching hospitals as well as small hospitals and one free standing diagnostic imaging center, each responsible for recruitment of approximately 8 patients per day. The modalities included represent the 4 major manufacturers of digital mammography equipment, GE Medical Systems, Fuji, Fischer Imaging and Lorad. Each has provided 5 machines for purposes of the trial. During the period of the trial each patient will receive both a digital as well as screen film examination. The digital imaging along with the associated clinical information is being collected electronically at the sites and transmitted to ACRIN headquarters in Philadelphia on a daily basis. Screen films are being collected and sent by courier for storage and further use in the follow-up reader studies. The challenge with such a large trial was to develop an informatics infrastructure that could accommodate this volume of patients along with the associated data. It was anticipated that we would need to collect an average of 4 views both digital and film for each patient. Image file sizes for the digital exams range in size from 10 Mbytes to 65 Mbytes for each view. While digital image compression is being utilized, file reductions of only about 2 to 1 can be realized when using the required perfect, lossless technique. Equally important was to implement a reliable quality assurance and backup program that could insure data completeness and quality. This along with the need to collect and QA a significant amount of patient demographic and clinical information added to the complexity of the environment

2.1 Informatics infrastructure

It was determined during the design phase of the trial that timely collection of both imaging and clinical data would be critical to the success of the trial. It was then decided that extensive use of the Internet would be a key element in the design of the informatics system and a crucial goal for the informatics design team. Based upon previous experiences with other smaller trials, the ACR undertook an aggressive development effort designed to achieve this goal. The resulting system provides for the qualification, registration and randomization of patients as well as remote collection and transmission of images to headquarters in Philadelphia via the Web. Equally as important, the system needed to be developed using off-the-shelf hardware and software wherever possible in order to maintain economy and speed of deployment. As the result, the system was designed, developed and deployed in less than 6 months from date of inception of the project.

3. Network hardware and software

The DMIST informatics infrastructure consists of a local area computer network with high speed telecommunications links to remote sites where the mammographic images are acquired.

©CARS/Springer. All rights reserved.

3.1 Central server systems – hardware and software architecture
The central server systems include several Windows 2000 multi-processor servers organized to manage the Web based image and clinical data collection system, the main clinical database and the image repository. The current Microsoft BackOffice architecture utilized includes Microsoft SQL Serve 2000 used for both clinical data and image management databases. A Cisco Secure PIX Firewall has been implemented for the highest-performance as an enterprise-class firewall product in the Network. The integrated hardware/software within the Firewall delivers high security without impacting network performance, scaling to meet the entire range of ACRIN's project requirements.

The Firewall is a key element in the overall end-to-end security solution set for Image and Clinical data collection over the Web. The Web interface utilizes Silver Stream Version 3.7.5 which manages the browser based interactive forms for patient registration and clinical data entry along with specialized FTP server software for receipt of image files. The current storage architecture for the clinical database includes a 180 Gigabyte clustered RAID system. For the FTP site, a 1.5 Terabyte RAID has been implemented in conjunction with a 2.5 Terabyte RAID for the semi-permanent repository. As images mature they are indexed and moved to DVD off-line storage for future retrieval. Web access is accomplished through a DS3 (15 Mbit/sec) dedicated line. The central server systems are linked by a 1Gigabit Ethernet fiber network. This network also serves to connect to multiple display and film scanning workstations used for purposes of image review and quality assurance.

3.2 Central server systems – functions
The central clinical data storage is implemented by Microsoft SQL Server 2000 that acts as a complete database and query processor offering rapid delivery and scalable e-commerce and enterprise solutions. It has dramatically reduced the time required to open the ACRIN trials, while offering the scalability needed for the most demanding environments. The SQL Server stores the business logic and stored procedures that handle the web based registration and data collection operation. It constantly processes incoming data via the SilverStream Web and Application Server and dynamically generates web pages for various study forms. Upon an successful registration the database generates a patient calendar for the duration of the trial. SQL Server 2000 offers flexibility to take maximum advantage of our existing hardware investment and the agility to quickly adapt to our ever-changing business environment.

The diagnostic image collection and management system includes an FTP server, image database server and RAID repository, operating in conjunction with several imaging workstations providing various image management functions. Images are received into the FTP server from the remote client workstations. The FTP site is organized by study and institution. Images received are monitored by host management software which imports them into the permanent database by moving them through the firewall, de-encrypting and decompressing them into active RAID storage on the image database server. Separate management software runs on a scheduled basis to post received dates to the clinical database and perform first tier quality assurance by reading the DICOM header and comparing date of birth with the date entered into the clinical database when the patient was registered on study. DVD backup disks produced by the client systems at

©CARS/Springer. All rights reserved.

each site provide the second tier of quality assurance when received. The central image management software provides for checking each individual image file received on DVD with those received via FTP to insure completeness of data and image integrity.

3.3 Remote client systems – architecture and functions

The Online Patient Registration and data collection system allows the Research Associates (RA) on the field to download and enter new cases onto protocol 6652 (DMIST) using a standard browser such as Microsoft Internet Explorer or Netscape Navigator. Additionally the capability to accrue patients on this trial was extend to off-line registration in order to increase the usability, mobility and accrual of patients critical to the success of this trial. As a part of the initial study setup ACRIN provides the institutions with a block of 12 case numbers and hidden treatment option in advance. Additional case numbers are provided in blocks of 6 to a site when each previously assigned number has been used and patient data has been successfully submitted to the ACRIN website. Once a patient has consented, the RAs register them by logging onto the ACRIN website and selecting the link for Data Entry/Registration. The SilverStream Web Server then triggers an email with an attachment of Registration/Eligibility (A0) Data Entry form for these cases. These A0 forms can be utilized for randomising patients online or can be downloaded and saved onto a Notebook Computer for off-line registration. These Notebook computer are configured with MS Windows 2000 Professional and are equipped with a Java Application Server for processing registration information and converting the data format to XML. This XML file is utilized to upload the patient information to the ACRIN Website. For Online registration, the Java Classes in the SilverStream Server allows the RAs to complete the A0 form and reveals the Treatment Option to the RA after successful completion of the Form.

The Servlets running on the SilverStream Web Server checks every 2 minutes to monitor any uploaded patient data. Upon receiving the data the application server calls the SilverStream invoked Business Object to process the html or XML data and store it in the temporary table. Later the SQL database stored procedure generates a Patient Calendar and Migrates the A0 Form Data to the production environment. Ultimately the system sends an Email Confirmation to the RA with the Patient Calendar and A0 Form in a HTML format.

Each institution participating in the trial has been provided with a PC. These PC's are configured with MS Windows 2000 Professional on a hardware platform consisting of a 1.3 Ghz processor, 1 Gbytes memory, 63 Gbyte hard disk and 9.4 Gbyte DVD RAM drive. The PC is installed in the institution with access to the DICOM network as well as the internet gateway. The remote client software supports two functions. The first consists of DICOM server software running as an NT service client. This software provides for the remote DICOM C-Store functions. The PC is set up and identified on the digital mammography machine as a specific node on the DICOM network. When patients are imaged, images are "pushed" to the PC and is received by the DICOM server software and placed in a folder on the hard disk. The second function supported by the client software provides functionality for review of the images and transmission to ACRIN headquarters in Philadelphia. This is accomplished by the operator selecting a range of patients from a menu for transmission whereupon the software prompts for identification

©CARS/Springer. All rights reserved.

information in the form of ACRIN case, institution and study number. Once this information has been provided, the software automatically scrubs the patient identifying information from the DICOM header and replaces the corresponding tags with case, institution and study number. The image files are then encrypted and compressed in a perfectly lossless format. Temporary files are then prepared which will in turn be written to the DVD disk and subsequently transmitted to Philadelphia. In addition to the clinical images, phantom and physics QC images are collected and transmitted in the same manner.

4. Summary

As defined by the goals set forth previously, this system provides for an effective means of reliable and timely means of registering patients as well as acquiring and contributing clinical data and diagnostic images for the ACRIN Dmist trial. It also provides a reliable and reproducible model for submission of images for future clinical multi-center clinical trials.

Acknowledgements

Technical advice and encouragement of Michael Vannier, MD in reporting on this facility is gratefully appreciated. ACRIN is sponsored by a cooperative agreement with the Biomedical Imaging Program, National Cancer Institute at the National Institutes of Health, Bethesda, MD.

References

1. http://www.dmist.org/ - The DMIST website
2. http://www.acrin.org/ - The ACRIN website

CARS 2002 – H.U. Lemke, M.W. Vannier; K. Inamura, A.G. Farman, K. Doi & J.H.C. Reiber (Editors)
©CARS/Springer. All rights reserved.

Multicenter clinical trials of imaging workstations and methods

C.R. Welsh[1], V. Gopalakrishnan[1], J. Flaim-Spetsas[1], A. Toledano[2], C.D. Johnson[3]
[1]American College of Radiology, Philadelphia, PA
[2]Brown University, Providence, RI
[3]Mayo Clinic, Rochester, MN

Abstract

Infrastructure to support multicenter clinical trials of imaging workstations and methods in oncologic applications has been developed by the American College of Radiology Imaging Network (ACRIN). This infrastructure was assembled and tested in a retrospective trial of virtual colonography where 117 examinations from 8 centers were evaluated on 3 workstations (GE, Mayo, Vital Images) by 18 observers. The infrastructure consists of specialized applications to homogenize DICOM images from multiple manufacturers using an ACR-specific manufacturer code, data conditioning and archiving, observer-based rated response evaluation, and biostatistical analysis of results.

A group of networked (Fibre Channel) servers with Microsoft 2000 Server OS and Microsoft SQL Server software collectively acquire, manage, and process images and related clinical research data, including observations. A server is dedicated to document image management for paper forms and ancillary information (e.g., pathology reports) received from various sites, keyed to anonymized case records. In general, patient identifiers are removed and individual identities cannot be associated with specific data sets at ACRIN Headquarters. In some cases, site principal investigators may have the key lists that would permit this identification, but the information is not shared with ACRIN.

Keywords: Workstation, clinical trial, observer studies

1. Introduction

Multicenter clinical trials are essential to gather evidence used in medical decision making on specific instruments and methods. Imaging systems and their applications are studied in multicenter trials to determine their role in clinical practice. To satisfy the stringent requirements of evidence-based medicine, the design and quality of data in multicenter trials are of paramount importance. Few published trials of imaging methods and techniques meet these demanding requirements, however.

Clinical trials may be prospective or retrospective. Reported clinical trials of workstations have been predominantly retrospective, utilizing databases of previously acquired images presented to observers under controlled conditions. The design of trials to test for differences in diagnostic performance and operational parameters (such as the amount of time per case).

©CARS/Springer. All rights reserved.

The American College of Radiology (ACR) is a private, non-profit scientific and educational organization with headquarters in Reston, VA that represents diagnostic radiologists in North America. Since 1972, the ACR has operated a satellite office in Philadelphia, PA which manages clinical trials for the Radiation Therapy Oncology Group (RTOG) and ACR Imaging Network (ACRIN). The RTOG and ACRIN are cooperative groups which support hundreds of institutions that perform cancer clinical trials.

Recently, ACRIN has undertaken trials which test image post-processing (for virtual colonoscopy) on interactive workstations. These studies are important since ACRIN is a "neutral" organization (unaligned with any manufacturer), applies rigorous statistical experimental design methodology and conducts the trials under controlled conditions with a relatively large number of expert observers.

Specialized workstations are configured, as needed, for specific applications such as high resolution display, image segmentation and measurement, and interactive visualization. These workstations are connected to the local area network at speeds of up to 1GHz using fibre channel high speed Ethernet links. Images are maintained in standard DICOM format on a Microsoft SQL server and archive for future retrieval and review for ancillary research. In the case of the Virtual Colonography trial, archived CT image data sets (contiguous slices) were collected from 8 sites after IRB approval of the protocol and informed consent was obtained. Three workstations (one per manufacturer) were installed at ACRIN Headquarters and loaded with test data sets as needed. Each observer visited Philadelphia for a 3-day reading session where they were presented with 60 cases at 2 of the interactive workstations. All 18 observers completed the assigned 60 cases within a 2 month period. The observations were recorded on paper forms that were digitized and coded using the ACR document imaging system. The data sets were available for statistical analysis one month after the observations were complete.

2. Workstation evaluation

Post-processing of diagnostic images for screening (disease detection and characterization), staging, treatment selection and follow-up is increasingly common. The manipulation of images for visualization, computer aided diagnosis and measurement is done on workstations using specialized software. Several investigators have evaluated the application of workstations to diagnostic imaging tasks in multicenter, multireader clinical trials. The difficulty in testing post-processing methods and workstations motivated the creation of a technical infrastructure to perform these studies at ACRIN Headquarters.

3. Colonography trial

The purpose of the virtual colonography trial was to evaluate the accuracy of CT colonography (CTC) for the detection of colorectal polyps greater or equal to 1 cm using colonoscopy and pathology as gold standards, and to examine interpretation times for multiple readers using three different reader software platforms. In this protocol the accuracy of computerized tomographics colonography (CTC) as a potential new screening tool for colon cancer was evaluated retrospectively. CTC uses virtual reality technology to produce two- and three-dimensional images of the entire colorectal structure. This

©CARS/Springer. All rights reserved.

procedure is minimally invasive, yet permits a thorough evaluation of the entire colon. For these reasons, CTC may provide a safer, more cost-effective method of colon-cancer screening with a higher level of patient acceptance than colonoscopy. The accuracy of CTC across three different viewing platforms was evaluated using colonoscopy as a reference standard. This study used existing data, including CTC images and colonoscopy results, contributed by participating institutions from throughout the United States.

3.1 Motivation

Development of image display tools for interpretation of the CTC examination has focused on two types of display options: (2D) with supplementary 3D images for problem solving and 3D with supplementary 2D images for problem solving. Most experts in the field recognize that 2D and 3D images are complementary. Determination of optimal image display methods will be helpful in determining the image display features needed for a larger prospective study. In this study three image display systems were evaluated. All of these systems provide access to 2D and 3D images, but the manner in which these images are accessed and displayed differs substantially between them. Radiologists differ in their approach as to which type of image is reviewed first, and their need and use of multiplanar reformatted views, axial images, and 3D endoluminal views. This study assessed radiologist preferences for various types of image displays and the interpretation time differences across software platforms.

3.2 Retrospective colonography trial

One hundred and seventeen (117) colonoscopically-proven CTC examinations were collected from eight (8) institutions. Each case was assessed for quality with respect to CT technical specifications <=5 mm slice thickness, <=3 mm reconstruction intervals, <=2 pitch, entire colorectum coverage, prone and supine data sets) and patient preparation <=2 segments suboptimally distended or fluid filled, lack of large amounts of stool and/or respiratory artifacts). After these assessments, 94 cases (80.3%) remained for review. Case mix was constructed with 50% prevalence for colorectal neoplasms <=1 cm. Eighteen (18) radiologists with varying levels of experience interpreting CTC examinations were divided into three groups of six. Each group interpreted approximately 60 of the 94 cases using two of three software platforms in a counterbalanced design. Readings were conducted independently and blinded to the colonoscopy results. Interpretation time was recorded for each case.

3.3 Colonography trial results

The results of this trial showed that the diagnostic accuracy for the detection of polyps <=1 cm, as measured by the average area under the ROC curve, was 0.89 (range 0.78 – 0.94, 95% lower confidence bound > 0.80). Image interpretation times were similar across platforms. Average interpretation time was 15.9 min (range = 4 to 50 min, SD = 7.5 min, median = 14 min), with 78% of interpretations performed in <=20 minutes.

This multicenter, multireader evaluation of CTC (in a sample with 50% prevalence) demonstrates high accuracy for the detection of polyps <=1 cm. Most interpretations can be completed within 20 minutes.

©CARS/Springer. All rights reserved.

4. Future applications

The principal applications served by this infrastructure include post-processing image analysis for computer aided diagnosis, perfusion imaging, subtraction angiography (CTA or MRA), visualization, and virtual endoscopy.

A flexible and efficient infrastructure to support multireader multicenter clinical oncologic imaging trials has been developed. This was applied to the comparative evaluation in a retrospective investigation of observer performance in the screening of colon cancer. This infrastures may be adapted to investigate similar applications with virtually any modality, type of medical image, or oncologic application.

Acknowledgements

Technical advice and encouragement of Michael Vannier, MD in reporting on this facility is gratefully appreciated. ACRIN is sponsored by a cooperative agreement with the Biomedical Imaging Program, National Cancer Institute at the National Institutes of Health, Bethesda, MD.

References

1. CD Johnson, A. Toledano, B. Herman, A Dachman, E McFarland, D Lu, et al. CT Colonography: Performance Evaluation in a Multicenter Setting (American College of Radiology Imaging Network Study 6656), RSNA 2001 Annual Meeting.
2. CTC Protocol on ACRIN website, http://www.acrin.org/protocols/6656
3. multireader, multimodality studies
4. RL Arenson, DP Chakraborty, SB Seshadri and HL Kundel. The digital imaging workstation. Radiology, Vol 176, 303-315, 1990.
5. Wu C, van Kuijk C, Li J, Jiang Y, Chan M, Courtryman P, Genant HK.Comparison of digitized images with original radiography for semiquantitative assessment of osteoporotic fractures. Osteoporosis Intl 2000;11(1):25-30.
6. Redfern RO, Kundel HL, Polansky M, Langlotz CP, Horii SC, Lanken PN. A picture archival and communication system shortens delays in obtaining radiographic information in a medical intensive care unit. Crit Care Med 2000 Apr; 28(4):1006-13.

CARS 2002 – H.U. Lemke, M.W. Vannier; K. Inamura, A.G. Farman, K. Doi & J.H.C. Reiber (Editors)
©CARS/Springer. All rights reserved.

Detailed image classification code for image retrieval of medical images (IRMA)

Berthold B. Wein[a], Thomas Lehmann[b], Daniel Keysers[c], Henning Schubert[a], Michael Kohnen[a]
[a] Department of Diagnostic Radiology, Medical Faculty
[b] Institute of Medical Informatics, Medical Faculty
[c] Computer Science VI, Computer Science Department
Aachen University of Technology (RWTH), Aachen, Germany

Abstract

To support the automated classification of medical images an easy to use, tree-based, detailed examination code was developed. It consists of three parts: 1. technical code, 2. anatomical code, and 3. orientational code. The code was applied to about 6000 radiological images from daily routine, creating a well indexed database for testing of classifications. The code has been shown to be sufficient for the description of the images concerning image content.

Keywords: Image retrieval, medical images, detailed classification code.

1. Introduction

For real life medical use of Image Retrieval in Medical Applications (IRMA) different actions have to be undertaken in order to receive medical meaningful computer assisted analysis of images. The first of them are the classification of the image, the analysis of image patterns, the reasoning of deviations of the isolated patterns from normal, all under taking into account the location of the body region and the imaging technique. The last item will be the basis for the comparison of different feature vectors, resulting from the image recognition procedures, returning the most likely reference images. In daily routine this has to be done by an image analyzing program. The process of automated classification of medical images, which will result in the computerized extraction of the necessary information out of the image, should return a description code readable by man. This description code has to be as complete as possible and should be easy to use. To reach this goal, the reverse approach has to be performed, where the code is assigned to images by human readers and is used for assessment and improvement of the analyzing computer programs.

2. Methods

The methods describe the principals of the codification scheme and the rough layout of the supporting software-tool to manually enter the code data.

©CARS/Springer. All rights reserved.

2.1 The classification code

Starting with a systematical analysis of medical imaging procedures the technical code (part one of the classification code) was developed. It was specifically refined for radiological images. The description of this first part consists of a hierarchical code with a depth of 5 steps, naming the imaging system, modality, technique, subtechnique, and a modulator item. All of those technical items have an impact on image analysis or image interpretation. Every item of the code is represented by one digit or character.

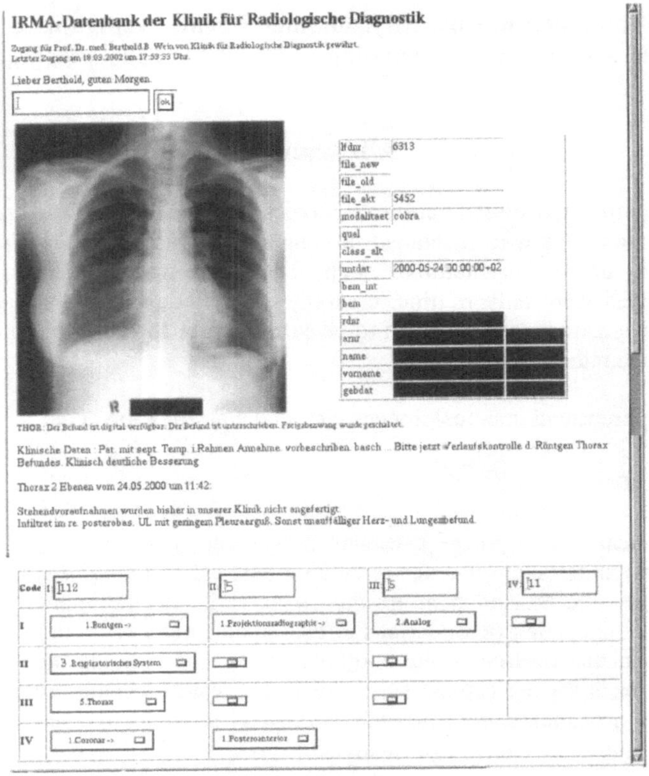

Fig. 1: A webbased system for assigning the classification code to the images in the cases database. For easy choise the pop-up menues are installed helping to compose the appropriate code. The radiological report is also available to judge for specific comments.

The next part of the code shows the anatomical codification. These codes have to consider that both an antomical region and a functional anatomical structure have to be identified for the examination. The region is derived from subsegmentation of the human body, the functional code shows hierarchical ordering of the organic systems of the body. Both techniques together allow systematic and complete description of the point of interest for the imaging procedure.

©CARS/Springer. All rights reserved.

The third part of the code consists of orientation, functional add-ons and external markers. This code was created in view of the existing DICOM orientations, but also of the variety of radiological examinations. This code is mainly used for the radiological examinations. Other medical disciplines have to create their own settings. This part of code allows to estimate deviations of the normal projections and may also explain the problems of the automated image classification.

2.2 The webbased system

Secondarily digitized images were converted to readable icons of about 200*200 pixels size and were labeled with the appropriate code by two professional readers, i.e. board certified radiologists. This was necessary for the assessment of the quality of computerized image categorisation and also to create a gold standard. The labelling tool was based on an SQL-database (postgres), an interface to a webserver (apache with built-in php-interpreter) and on client-site on an internet browser. All images were listed by their numbers, showing up one by one. The appropriate code was entered and remarks of the readers were collected (see Fig.1). The code could be entered directly into the appropriate field, if known by heart, or could be composed – making extensive use of javascripting in the HTML-file to enable modifying pop-up-menues according to the decision made at higher level (on lefthand side). This resulted in a stepwise refinement of the code.

The appropriateness and feasibility of the classification code was estimated on the base of the listed remarks.

3. Results

In the following examples for the code representations are given. The complete code will be available by the author.

The technical part of the five steps classification code has now 8 representations on the first level: 1. X-Rays, 2. Ultrasound, 3. Magnetic Resonance, 4. Nuclear Medicine, 5. Optical Techniques, 6. Biophysical Techniques, 7. Varia, 8. Secondary Captured Images. The first step is subdivided into 6 further entities, which distinguish different X-ray-modalities: 1. projection radiography, 2. fluoroscopy, 3. angiography, 4. computed tomography, 5. quantitative dual energy absorption measurement, 6. megavolt images (radiation therapy). The projection radiography is subdivided in the next step into digital and analog projection radiographs, X-ray stereometry and –graphy, and tomosynthesis. The digital projection radiography shows the following subdivisions: 1. tomography, 2. high-kV-beam, 3. low-kV-beam, 4. high-distance-imaging, 5. original size, 6. dual energy imaging. As modifier only small focus is available. Defined as such, the complete technical code consists of maximum 5 digits. At any position ‘0’, i.e. ‘not further specified’, can be used or omitted.

The organ system is also hierarchically organized: starting with the main topological order 1. total body, 2. head, 3. spine, 4. upper extremity, 5. chest, 6. breast, 7. abdomen, 8. pelvis, and 9. lower extremity further refinement is given in nearly every topic. Chest is subdivided into 1. bone, 2. lung, 3. hilum, 4. mediastinum, 5. heart, and 6. diaphragm.

©CARS/Springer. All rights reserved.

Bone is further subsegmented into 1. clavicula, 2. sternoclavicular joint, 3. sternum, 4. upper ribs, 5. lower ribs. This three-step approach guarantees a sufficient resolution of the anatomical code to be fine enough for the definition of imaging needs. Similarily the hierarchical order is organized for the functional structures. Starting on top with the division of the body into the main organisational components: 1. cerebrospinal system, 2. cardiovascular system, 3. respiration system, 4. gastrointestinal system, 5. uropoetic system, 6. reproductive system, 7. musculosceletal system, 8. endocrinal system, 9. immuncellular system, and 10. dermal system. Subdivision will be shown at the example of the gastrointestinal system, presenting 1. oropharynx, 2. oesophagus, 3. stomach, 4. small bowel, 5. large bowel, 6. appendix, 7. rectum/anus, 8. liver, 9. gallsystem, a. salivary gland. As third hierarchic step the small bowel is subdivided into duodenum, jejunum, ileum, and terminal ileum. All of those have their impact concerning diseases or radiological specificities. This hierarchical code could easily be extended towards substructures and subfunctionalities to even fulfil higher requirements concerning functional resolution or anatomical details.

The third code section describes the orientation, functional technique, and external markers. The orientation code has to be given in two signs, the first will be 1. coronal, 2. sagittal, 3. transversal, 4. oblique, and 5. RSA, the second will be a more detailed description of the first one. For example: sagittal orientation will be divided into the suborientations 1. "lateral, left first", 2. "lateral, right first", 3. "mediolateral", 4. "lateromedial". If no further specification is used, the number '0' has to be taken to fill up the two places completely.

The orientation will be accompanied by functional descriptors, which will describe the position of the patient regarding the examination technique and the action taken by the patient or the examinator. This position is an open list with 18 instances at the moment, where are 1. inspiration, 2. exspiration, 3. valsalva manoever, 4. Hitzenberg's sniffing, and 8. supine position, 9. prone position, a. lateral decubitus, and more. External markers will explain use of external forces like 1. external stress – subdivided to manual and mechanical stress – 2. drug application for heart frequency increase, 3. contrast administration.

Reviewing the complete code, it consists of four parts, combining digits or characters in each section and separation the sections by '-'. The example (Fig. 1) is represented by the following complete code: "1122 – 3 – 500 – 1110" meaning "high-kV conventional plain radiograph, depicting the respiratory system at the location chest, with posterior-anterior coronal view in inspiration without additional external markers", describing a normal pa-view of the chest.

The coding support was easy to use in so far on about 6000 single images, the loading time for the small images (max 200 pixels either direction) was short, the support of the javascripts in case of not known combinations of the codification scheme was helpful.

It turned out that rarely (less than 0,1%) the regional code is too limited to describe the body parts depicted on a radiograph. This is especially true for long extremity overviews.

©CARS/Springer. All rights reserved.

The extremity codes gives only the chance to make a very general or a highly specific localisation of a combination of two nearby regions.

4. Conclusion

Up to 6000 images have been classified so far with the complete detailed image classification code and are used to test classification programs for correctness of the prediction of the examination parameters. It could be shown that the code is sufficient to describe more than 99% of the X-ray images completely. Due to the tree structure of the code extensions are manageable, if a new method shows up, resulting in new parametric images. The code was an excellent help in assessment of the classification methods developed and used in the IRMA-Project.

Acknowledgements

This paper was granted by the Start-project / Aachen and the Deutsche Forschungsgemeinschaft / Bonn.

References

For references see the URL of the IRMA-project:
http://www.klinikum.rwth-aachen.de/webpages/MIB/mbv/projects/irma/irma.html

Computer Assisted Radiation Therapy

CARS 2002 – H.U. Lemke, M.W. Vannier; K. Inamura, A.G. Farman, K. Doi & J.H.C. Reiber (Editors)
©CARS/Springer. All rights reserved.

Dynamic reconstruction for radiotherapy planning

Anne Koenig [a], Pierre Grangeat [a], Stéphane Bonnet [a], Patrick Hugonnard [a]
[a] LETI/DSIS/SSBS, Commissariat à l'Energie Atomique (CEA-Grenoble),
17, rue des martyrs, 38054 Grenoble cedex 9, France

Abstract

Dynamic cone-beam reconstruction algorithms are required to reconstruct 3D image sequences on dynamic 3D CT combining multi-row 2D detectors and sub-second scanners. In order to compensate for time evolution and motion artefacts, we propose to use a dynamic particle model to describe the object evolution. One main interest is to process data acquisition on several half-turns in order to reduce the dose delivered per rotation with the same signal to noise ratio. In this article, we first briefly explain the principle of the proposed dynamic cone-beam reconstruction algorithm. Then we present results obtained on both simulated and clinical data for radiotherapy planning demonstrating that motion compensation and temporal filtering allow to reduce radiation dose and is robust against appearance and transition within the region of interest.

Keywords: Dynamic Computed Tomography (CT), radiotherapy planning, particle model

1. Introduction

The purpose of dynamic Computed Tomography (CT) is to reconstruct tomographic image sequences of dynamic organs in order to take into account the dynamic nature of a living human body. This dynamic nature includes both time evolution and motion. In this paper, we mainly focus on dynamic 2D CT and radiotherapy planning application. Traditionally, radiotherapists count with static images acquired during a patient breath hold. But motion is a key issue during dose delivery. That is why they need to "guess" from their experience the margins induced by physiological motion. The use of active breathing control to reduce margin for breathing motion is described in [1]. A method is proposed to analyze the reliability of tumors position during radiotherapy treatment in [2].

We propose here to reconstruct off-line a 2D image sequence covering a full breathing cycle. The aim of the reconstruction is to estimate the envelop of moving targets or vital organs. Knowing this envelop, the radiotherapist can plan his intervention targeting the tumors and avoiding the healthy organs. He can also choose precisely the control position within the breathing cycle without asking the patient to hold his breath. The main issue is to avoid blurring linked to breathing motion during the reconstruction process.

LETI is involved in the European project DynCT (IST-1999-10515) dedicated to both real time and off-line motion compensated reconstruction and visualization for dynamic CT. The main issue to go from static to dynamic CT is the radiation dose. LETI has proposed a new framework for a dynamic cone-beam algorithm based on a dynamic particle model. In this new framework a spatio-temporal averaging along the particle trajectories on partial back-projected images allows to smooth the noise and thus to reduce the dose up to a factor 4. We present here only the 2D off line case according to the theoretical

©CARS/Springer. All rights reserved.

framework described in [3] and [4].

2. Methodology

In radiotherapy, the user needs to know the envelop of moving targets and vital tissues during a physiological motion. To get this information (a common case is breathing motion), the most straightforward idea is to sample the motion period to be analyzed and to take an image of moving organs at each time sample. The processing principle is then to extract the outlines of target and vital organs on each frame, and to compute the envelop of each of these outlines over all the frames. Here, the acquisition is done continuously over the whole breathing cycle for each axial position. In order to cover the whole region of interest, we proceed sequentially, slice by slice. We now consider the new method we designed to reconstruct each image sequence.

2.1 The sliding window principle

The proposed reconstruction algorithm is based on block image reconstruction with both motion and temporal compensation. The scanner rotation angle β is split into several angular regions, equal to the full fan angle $2\gamma_m = \pi/3$. That means that $\Delta\beta=\pi/3$ is the angular step of the gantry between two reconstructed frames. Furthermore, as we work off line, these frames are reconstructed at a time t_i corresponding to the middle of the angular range. The sliding window principle is that a new frame is computed for each new t_i value. corresponding to a shift of the β sliding window from $\Delta\beta=\pi/3$. The reconstructed images are updated each 0.12 s for a typical scanner rotation of 0.7s.

2.2 The fan-beam to parallel-beam rebinning and block reconstruction

In order to reconstruct with the same modules acquisitions done on different angular ranges, we have chosen to rebine the fan-beam acquisition (β, γ) into parallel beam geometry (φ, p) and to perform the filtered backprojection (FBP) in this new geometry. This allows to avoid applying weighting coefficients (varying both with β and γ angles) on the projections, and to compute the backprojection of each projection direction only once.

We neglect the intra block motion, and achieve standard FBP reconstruction within each block. Inter-frame motion is estimated over images separated from π, on a first list of low resolution images reconstructed over a half turn range. To get each final image, we need to average the images associated with each block over the period chosen for compensation, which represents 1, 2, 3 or 4 half turns. Motion compensation is carried out during this averaging process, in order to avoid blurring.

We represent by $f(M,t) = f(x,y,z,t)$ the function f value we consider (X-ray linear attenuation coefficient), at the point M of coordinate (x,y,z), at the time instant t. We define the trajectory $\Gamma(M,t)$ associated with the point M. We denote $BHDYf(\Gamma(M,t),t,\varphi_i)$ the partial block backprojection over the projection angular range $[\varphi_i, \varphi_i+\Delta\varphi]$:

$$BHDYf(\Gamma(M,t),t,\varphi_i) = \int_{\varphi=\varphi_i}^{\varphi_i+\Delta\varphi} HDYf\left(\varphi, A\left[\Gamma(M,t)\right], t\right) d\varphi \qquad (1)$$

We assume we want to reconstruct the function at the instant $t = t_0$. Since $\Delta\varphi=\pi/3$, we decompose this continuous integral into 3 terms associated with 3 partial block backprojections sectors, $[0, \pi/3]$, $[\pi/3, 2\pi/3]$, $[2\pi/3, \pi]$:

©CARS/Springer. All rights reserved.

$$f(M,t_0) = \sum_{i=0}^{2} BHDYf(M,t_0,\varphi_i) \qquad (2)$$

2.3 Dynamic evolution compensation

We introduce here the cartoon like step-by-step motion law assuming no dynamic evolution takes place during the time period associated with each block. So, the prediction principle described here-after can be applied on each partial block backprojection with a $\Gamma(M,t)$ trajectory piecewise constant : $\Gamma(M,t) = \Gamma(M,t_i)$ for $t_i \leq t < t_{i+1}$.

For each angular sector i, let us take a set of N_b block projection intervals $[\varphi_{ij}, \varphi_{ij}+\Delta\varphi]$, included in the angular sliding window $[\varphi_d, \varphi_f]$, associated with φ_0 and t_0 :

$$\varphi_{ij} \equiv \varphi_i \quad (\text{modulo}\,\pi) \qquad j \in \{0,\ldots,\text{Nb}-1\} \quad i \in \{0,1,2\} \qquad (3)$$

We get for each M point a set of values along the $\Gamma(M,t)$ trajectory, for each associated block instant : $BHDYf(\Gamma(M,t_{ij}),t_{ij}\ \varphi_{ij})$, where t_{ij} is the time associated with φ_{ij}.

For dynamic compensation, we introduce a first order prediction model to describe the time evolution along the particle trajectory. Under the piecewise constant motion hypothesis, as no motion occurs during the block angular range, the same model holds for the partial backprojection :

$$BHDYf(\Gamma(M,t_{ij}),t_{ij},\varphi_{ij}) \approx BHDYf(M,t_0,\varphi_i) + a(M,\varphi_i)\cdot(t_{ij}-t_0) \qquad (4)$$

Thus, the terms $BHDYf(M,t_0,\varphi_{i0})$ and $a(M,\varphi_{i0})$ can be computed by linear regression on the discrete sample set: $\{BHDYf(\Gamma(M,t_{ij}),t_{ij},\varphi_{ij})\}\ j \in \{0,\ldots,\text{Nb}-1\}$. The dynamic evolution compensation takes place in the prediction of each partial block backprojection at the instant $t=t_0$. The final image is computed by the accumulation of the three predicted partial block backprojection $BHDYf(M,t_0,\varphi_i)$ as described in the formula (2).

2.4 Motion estimation

In the previous sections, we have assumed that we knew the particle trajectory $\Gamma(M,t)$. However, such motion field is a priori unknown and motion estimation techniques are therefore needed. The computation of motion could be obtained using several types of information : projection dataset, sequence of partial block images, sensors… We adopt a more general framework with the introduction of an additional dataflow : a sequence of reconstructed images obtained in a fast mode with the minimum latency and the minimum acceptable spatial resolution.

Because of its simplicity and regularity, we use a block matching algorithm (BMA) for the estimation of particle trajectories. This algorithm is massively used in all video compression standards (MPEG, H.261…) and has proven to be useful to remove temporal data redundancy in video compression. Motion vector fields obtained using plain BMA may differ largely from the true displacement field and may lead to wrong results in homogeneous areas. To achieve higher reliability and insure vector smoothness, we post-process the vector field obtained by BMA, using a temporal and spatial regularization [5].

One other important issue is the ability to detect motion when the particle trajectory goes outside the region of interest or when a particle appears in the scene. To manage this issue, we introduce, for each motion vector, a confidence coefficient, associated with the estimation criterion [6]. This coefficient is taken into account within the estimation of the prediction rule coefficients given by the equation (4).

©CARS/Springer. All rights reserved.

3. Data

We present in the following section several results obtained on both simulated data generated with the LETI Sindbad software [7] and clinical data.

Three different motions are simulated. In the first "appearance" case, the phantom appears instantaneously in the image. In the 2nd "X-motion" case, the phantom is instantaneously moved along x axis from one position to another. These two motions are used to validate extreme use conditions of the software. The normal use is validated by the third "periodic motion" case where the phantom is animated with a periodic motion along the x axis with an amplitude of 40mm, a period of approximately 3.5s that is 5 times the scanner period.

4. Results

We show on Figure 1 the reconstruction of the phantom animated with a periodic motion without motion compensation with the three temporal prediction possible modes : π, 2 π, 4 π modes. It outlines the blurring effect on the spheres, increased in mode 2 π and 4 π were the spheres are doubled or quadrupled. This effect is suppressed when motion compensation is used, as shown on images of the right.

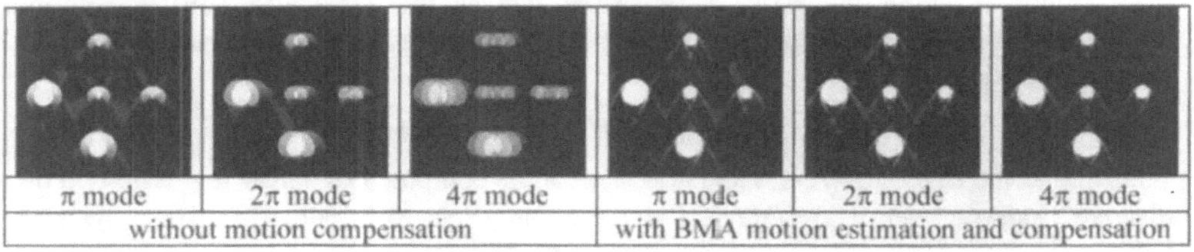

Figure 1 : Comparison of prediction modes for motion compensation.

Quantitative results : center of mass value of the central sphere for the Appearance case is plotted on Figure 2, central sphere x-position for X-motion case is plotted on Fig. 3.

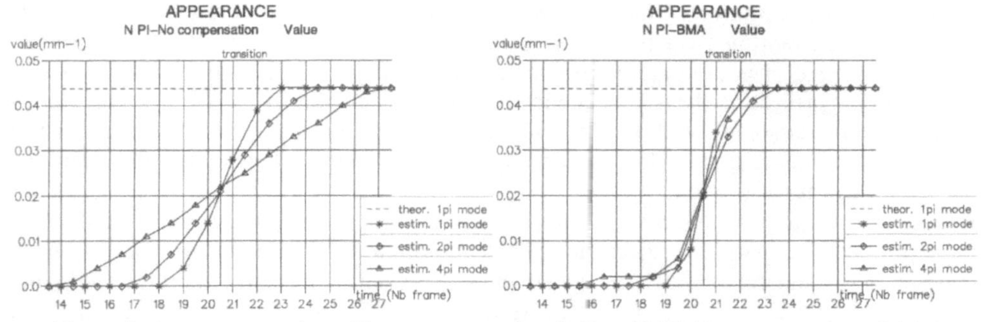

Figure 2: Appearance, value without compensation (left), with BMA compensation (right).

We can compare the temporal resolution of the three temporal prediction modes : π, 2 π, 4 π modes as explained in [8]. On Figure 2 left, without motion compensation this temporal resolution is increased in 4 π mode up to 13 frames. It is reduced to 3 frames on right with BMA motion estimation. On Fig. 3 (left), without motion compensation the error on position is about 15% whereas with motion compensation (right), this error is suppressed.

©CARS/Springer. All rights reserved.

These two tests clearly state that the appearance and transition temporal range in 2 π and 4 π mode with compensation is nearly the same as the one in π mode. This temporal range is doubled in the 2 π mode and quadrupled in 4 π mode when no compensation is applied.

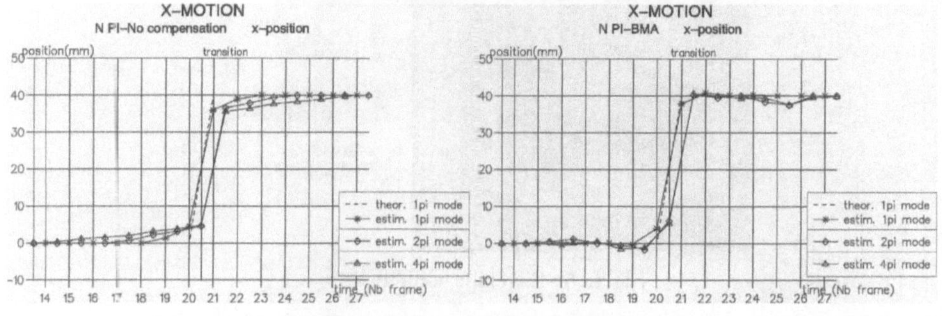

Fig. 3 : X-motion, x-position without compensation (left), with BMA motion compensation (right).

The following test on the dose verifies that the 4 π mode with a dose reduced by a factor 4 gives the same results in terms of signal to noise ratio as a full dose in the π mode. The dose reduction is performed by the temporal compensation on a longer period.

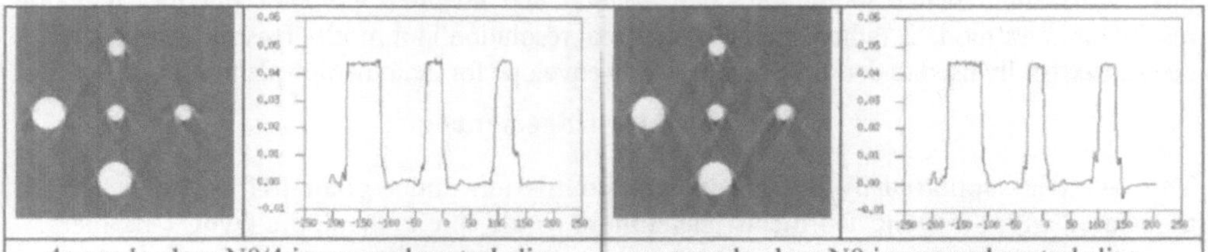

4π mode, dose N0/4 image and central slice	π mode, dose N0 image and central slice

Figure 4 : Dose comparison.

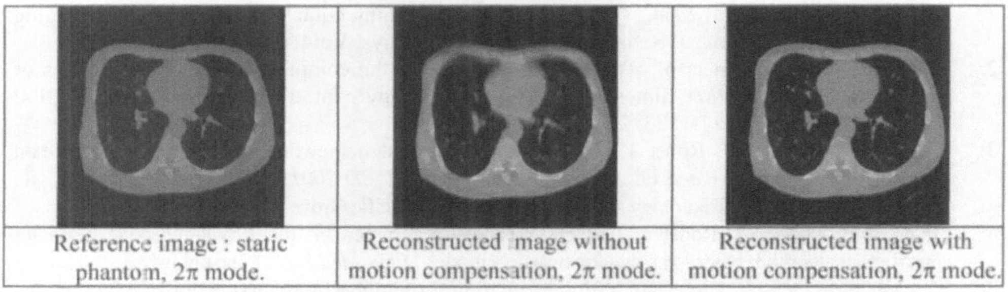

Reference image : static phantom, 2π mode.	Reconstructed image without motion compensation, 2π mode.	Reconstructed image with motion compensation, 2π mode.

Figure 5 : Reconstruction of animated phantom with or without motion compensation.

Last results concern a human thorax (see Figure 5). Left image presents the reconstruction of the static phantom as a reference. Using Free Form Deformation (FFD) [9], we animate the phantom in order to simulate breath and re-project it using the Sindbad software[7]. We see the reconstruction of this animated phantom without motion compensation in the middle image. We can see the blurring effect, particularly visible in the plexus zone. And finally, we compare it to the reconstruction using motion compensation (right). There is much less blurring and the image can be easily compared to the reference one. We show on Figure 6 the envelope of motion calculated on this image sequence, using motion

©CARS/Springer. All rights reserved.

vectors estimated by the algorithm. The envelope of the right lung is represented using a software developed by Schlumberger–Sema (Spain) and UPCT (Spain).

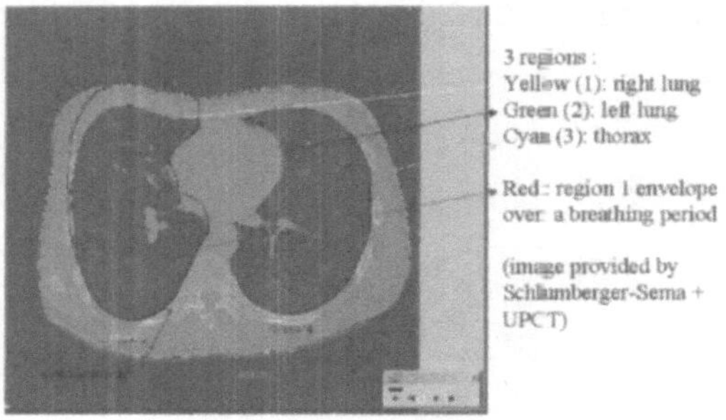

Figure 6 : Envelope computation

5. Conclusion

In conclusion, we can say that the algorithm used in 4π mode can work with a dose reduced by a factor 4 in comparison to the dose used in the π mode. Motion compensation and temporal compensation are then necessary in order to reduce the artefacts in the images. We then verify that, thanks to motion compensation and adaptive temporal filtering, temporal resolution in 4π mode is rather similar to temporal resolution in π mode. This reconstruction has been successfully used to compute organ motion envelope for radiotherapy planning.

Acknowledgements

This work is supported by the European Commission under grant IST - 1999 - 10515, associated with the DynCT project. The authors would like to thank the DynCT partners.

References

1. Wong J.W., Sharpe M.B & al., "The use of active breathing control (ABC) to reduce marging for breathing motion", Int. J. Radiation Oncology Biol. Phys, Vol44,N°4,pp.911-919, 1999.
2. Shimizu S, & al., "Impact of respiratory movement on the computed tpmographic images of small lung tumors in three-dimensional (3D) radiotherapy", Int. J. Radiation Oncology Biol. Phys, Vol46,N°5,pp.1127-1133, 2000.
3. Grangeat P., Koenig A., Rodet T., Bonnet S., "Theoretical framework for a dynamic cone-beam reconstruction algorithm based on a dynamic particle model",*3D 2001*, 6th Int. Meeting on fully 3D Image Reconstruction in Radiology and Nuclear Medicine, Pacific Grove, USA, 30/10-2/11 2001.
4. Grangeat P, Koenig A, Rodet T, Bonnet S,"Theoretical framework for a dynamic cone beam reconstruction algorithm based on a dynamic particle model", *Phys.Med.Biol.*, to be published, 2002.
5. T. Aach and D.Kunz, "Bayesian motion estimation for temporally recursive noise reduction in X-ray fluoroscopy", *Philips Journal of Research*, 51(2):231-251, 1998.
6. M.K. Ozkan, I. Sezan and A.M. Tekalp, "Adaptive motion-compensated filtering of noisy image sequences", *IEEE Trans. On Circuits and Systems for Video Technology*, 3(4):277-290, Aug 1993.
7. A.Glière, "Sindbad: From CAD Model to Synthetic Radiographs." *Review of Progress in QNDE*, ed. By D.O.Thompson and D.E.Chimenti, Vol. 17, pp 387-394, 1998.
8. Hsieh Jiang., "Analysis of the temporal response of computed tomography fluoroscopy", *Medical physics*, Vol 24, N°5, May 1997, Pp. 665-675.
9. Clarysse P. & al, "Un modèle de thorax respirant pour l'évaluation d'algorithmes de reconstruc-tion d'organes en mouvement par tomographie virtuelle", GRETSI'01, 10-13 Sep 2001, Toulouse.

CARS 2002 – H.U. Lemke, M.W. Vannier; K. Inamura A.G. Farman, K. Doi & J.H.C. Reiber (Editors)
©CARS/Springer. All rights reserved.

Registration of 3D U/S and CT images of the prostate

Evelyn A. Firle[a], Wei Chen[a], Stefan Wesarg[a]
[a] Fraunhofer Institute for Computer Graphics, Darmstadt, Germany
email: {Evelyn.Firle, Wei.Chen, Stefan.Wesarg}@igd.fhg.de

Abstract

Radiotherapy is a rapidly growing cancer treatment technique. In brachytherapy – one radiotherapy treatment technique – pre- and post-planning is usually carried out using CT imaging. As CT scanners cannot easily be moved from one operation room to an other and as CT does not have real-time imaging capability, alternative imaging modalities are needed to realize the vision of image guided surgery. Ultrasound (U/S) is such an alternative imaging modality. For the comparison of U/S and CT image fusion is very useful. After volume segmentation (see ref. 1) the volumes have to be registered, and afterwards the fused volume can be displayed. In this paper we investigate the registration part. We present two different approaches for the 3D registration of CT and U/S volumes. They are compared regarding accuracy and speed of calculation. The resulting fused volumes are visualized using the "InViVo" software where the registration routines have been integrated into.

Keywords: Registration, 3D ultrasound, brachytherapy

1. Introduction

Cancer is a growing concern all over the world. One out of five men is expected to develop prostate cancer sometime in his life.
The traditional treatment for cancer is surgery. A modern and very rapidly growing alternative is radiation treatment. Brachytherapy radiation procedures are divided into LDR (Low Dose Rate), where a number of weak radioactive seeds are permanently implanted around the tumor, and HDR (High Dose Rate), where hollow needles (catheters) are temporarily placed in the tumor and very intense radioactive sources are driven through them. Since in both variants imaging is critically important to the safe delivery of the therapy, modern CT and MRI scanners allow minimally invasive procedures to be performed under direct imaging guidance. However, conventional CT does not have real-time imaging capability, and both CT and MRI are expensive technologies requiring a special facility. Ultrasound (U/S) is a much cheaper and more flexible imaging modality. Unlike CT or MRI, who are often located in dedicated suites, U/S machines can be moved to the application room as needed. Moreover, with U/S, the physician sees in real-time what is happening as it occurs.

In several cases where a CT device is available a combination of the information provided by CT and 3D U/S images offers advantages in recognizing the borders of the lesion and delineating the region of treatment. For these applications the CT and U/S scans have to be registered and fused in a multi-modal data set. Furthermore a comparison of CT and

©CARS/Springer. All rights reserved.

U/S - by registering the modalities – can show the equivalence of using only U/S in Brachytherapy for the prostate instead of CT.
Purpose of the present development is to register and fuse available CT volumes with 3D U/S images of the same anatomical region, i.e. the prostate. Firstly we developed these algorithms using an U/S Phantom of the prostate, i.e. CT and 3D U/S data sets acquired with this phantom.

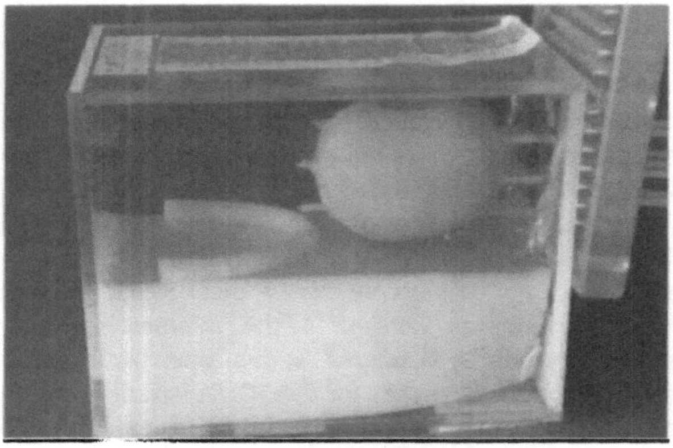

Fig. 1: The prostate phantom with inserted catheters.

The working steps of the whole procedure are:

- Acquisition of the CT and 3D US data: A CT and US data set of the prostate of the patient is acquired for the treatment planning.
- Volume delineation: The Region of interest (i.e. the prostate) and critical organs (e.g. the urethra) are manually contoured or automatically detected in both data sets [1].
- Registration: Calculation of the registration matrix between the two modalities.
- Visualization: The fused data sets are visualized and can be used for the treatment planning respective to validate the equivalence of using CT and US.

In the following we will first describe the overall system, the contouring and registration methods and the visualization. Here our main focus lies in the registration methods. In the 3rd section we will then summarize the results and give a short outlook about the future work.

2. Materials and Methods

Objective of the developed system is a registration of CT images and 3D U/S. The combination of these two imaging modalities interlinks the advantages of the high cost CT imaging and low cost U/S imaging and offers a multi-modality imaging environment for further target and anatomy delineation.
The visualization software is based on the "InViVo" system that has been developed over several years in Fraunhofer IGD in Darmstadt (s. [7],[8],[9]). It is mainly used for visualization of medical volume data, such as CT, MRI or 3D ultrasound data and has been extended for this development. The CT data available in DICOM format can be read

©CARS/Springer. All rights reserved.

directly and can be displayed as 2D CT slices and 3D reconstruction. The 3D U/S images can either be acquired using the system or already available scans can also be read. These can then be displayed parallel to the CT data as 2D slices and 3D reconstruction.
The process of image registration can be formulated as a problem of minimizing a cost function that quantifies the match between the images of the two modalities. In order to find this function different common features of these images can be used such as: points visible in both (fiducial markers or landmarks), outer contours of different structures (e.g. organ or outer body contour) or the voxel intensity.

2.1 Contouring

In our situation the registration algorithms are based on the geometry of the urethra. So our first step after loading both images is to segment the anatomy of the urethra in both modalities. This segmentation step can be performed semi-automatically using an active contouring model (s. [1]) or manually using the contouring tools available in the system (s. [2],[3]). These algorithms are also used for acquiring the prostate boundary semi-automatically.

2.2 Registration

Using the resulting two sets of points for the urethra (one for each modality) we calculate a transformation matrix that reflects the correlation between the two modalities. Here we used and compared two different approaches. The first one was based in the Iterative Closest Point (ICP) principle and the second one is using the distance maps calculated from the contoured volumes in both modalities.

Iterative Closest Point

The first one is an iterative process using the point sets of the contour from each modality:

a. For each contour point of modality A we search for the closest point on the contour of modality B using the starting transformation.
b. From this correlation we calculate then a new transformation matrix using the least square fitting.
c. With that transformation we receive a new set of points which is the used during the next iteration (i.e. repeat a-c).

In each step we calculate the mean distance between all points and repeat the whole procedure until the difference of two successive distances under-runs a user defined tolerance. This procedure converges to a minimum distance.

Distance Map

The second method uses the distance map to calculate the transformation matrix. I.e. given the 3D distance map DM_{ijk} with respect to the contoured volume of modality A, we consider the Similarity Measure Value defined by

$$SMV = \frac{1}{N}\sum_{n=1}^{N} DM_{i'j'k'},$$

where N is the amount of points belonging to the contoured volume of the modality B and (i',j',k') correspond to (i,j,k) using the transformation matrix. Employing the optimization method Simulated Annealing (SA) we minimize that function to calculate the best transformation matrix between the two modalities.

©CARS/Springer. All rights reserved.

2.3 Visualization

The last step in our registration pipeline is the visualization of the transformed and fused images. Here we treat one of the volumes as reference modality and the other one is fused into that reference image. The choice of the reference modality can be changed interactively and a weighting factor of the display (defining the mixture of the two modalities) can be determined by the user. We realized a 2D Image fusion of corresponding 2D cutting images (s. fig. 2) as well as a 3D fusion (s. fig. 3) of the volumes. For the 2D Fusion, for each slice through the reference volume, the oblique cut through the registered modality is calculated and displayed in real time. Thereby the user is given the possibility to delineate regions of interest within one volume and is immediately given the right position of that region in the other modality.

3. Results and Discussion

We evaluated the registration methods specified in section 2 for 3 different datasets (each acquired with CT and U/S). The results with respect to final distance and time required for the calculation are listed in Table 1.

In Fig. 1 you can see the results of the registration for one dataset using the Distance Map calculated for the urethra and as Optimization method the Simulated Annealing. It shows furthermore exemplarily the user interface of the software.

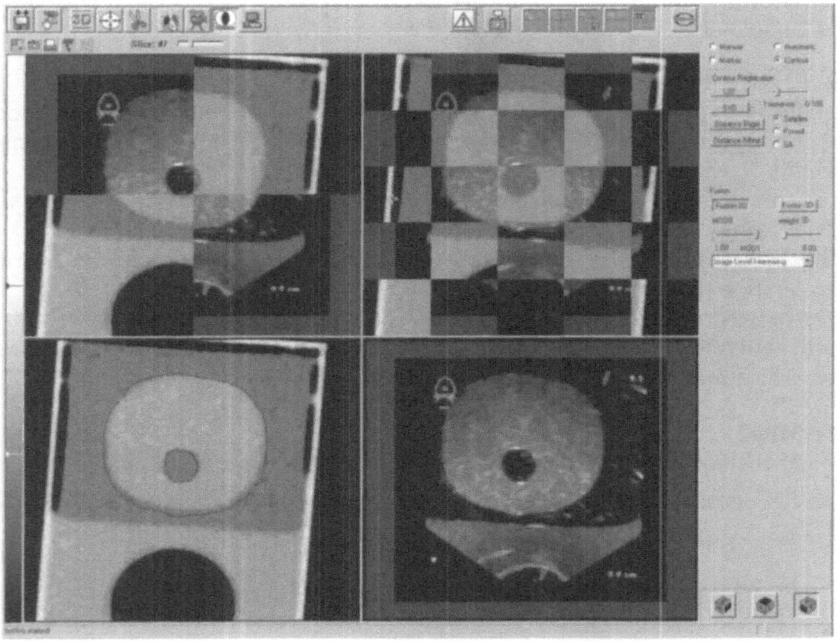

Fig. 2: Registration Results of a cut through the fused volumes in axial direction (lower right: US slice, lower left: corresponding oblique cut through the CT volume with respect to the final transformation.

©CARS/Springer. All rights reserved.

The next figure depicts the 3D fusion of the two volumes.

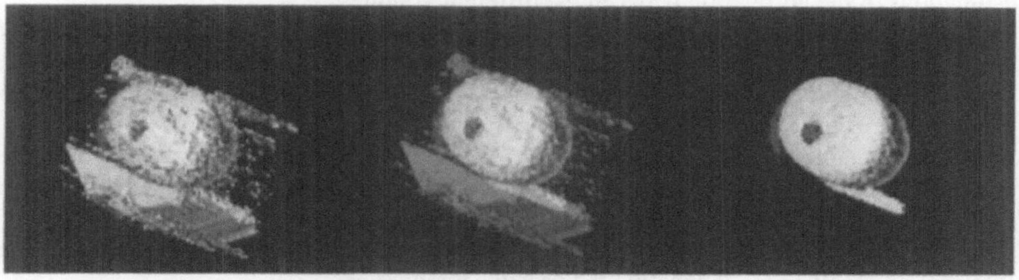

Fig. 3: 3D Fusion of a CT and US data set (left: US volume, right: CT volume, middle: mixture of both volumes).

In figure number 4 you can see the contoured objects, i.e. the urethra (left image) and the prostate (right image) of both volumes after registration.

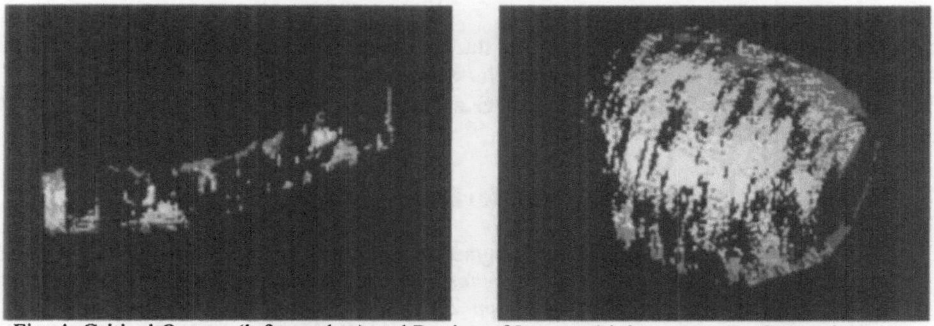

Fig. 4: Critical Organs (left: urethra) and Region of Interest (right: prostate) after registration.

Comparing the results of the two approaches we can conclude that, as expected, the second method works more accurate than the first method but is also more time consuming.

Volumes	Registration Method	Time (sec)	final Distance (mm)
1	ICP	2.7603	0.91812
1	SA	24.8900	0.69063
2	ICP	1.1560	1.66551
2	SA	23.6870	0.83005
3	ICP	2.0904	0.95692
3	SA	23.3750	0.55267

Table 1. Comparison ICP and Distance Map using SA.

The introduced system offers a fast methods for segmenting and registering CT volumes with 3D U/S images of the prostate using the geometry of the urethra visible in both modalities. The segmentation is realized semi-automatically using an active contouring

©CARS/Springer. All rights reserved.

model and the registration algorithms based on the chosen geometry provide two different estimations of the correlation between the different volumes.
Finally we developed a fusion software for a quick display of fused images from any modality. Apart from the semi-automatically segmentation of the urethra in ultrasound, our current method is absolutely independent of the chosen imaging source. We also tested the procedure using MR and CT patient data [6].
The developments were at first carried out using an U/S phantom. In a next step the system will be evaluated using real patient data. Here the urethra will be made visible in the 3D ultrasound volumes using a catheter during acquisition.
The future developments will include methods for validating the results using also the information received by delineating the prostate boundaries.
In addition we are working on registration algorithms for CT and U/S based on the pure voxel information. These advancements will also include region based elastic registration methods.

Acknowledgements

Evaluating the system using real patient data will be done in cooperation with the clinical partners at the Clinical Complex Offenbach / Strahlenklinik.
This work is partially funded by MITTUG a project of the European Commission. The project number is IST-1999-10618.

References

1. E. A. Firle, "Semi-automatische Segmentierung der Prostata mit Hilfe von 3D Ultraschallaufnahmen", *Proc. Bildverarbeitung für die Medizin 2001*, Handels, H., Horsch, Alexander, Lehmann, T., Meinzer, H.-P., pp. 262-266, Springer, Heidelberg, Germany, 2001
2. G. Karangelis, S. Zimeras, E. A. Firle, et al.: "Volume Definition Tools for Medical Applications". *Proc. Medical Image Computing and Computer-Assisted Intervention - MICCAI 2001*, Wiro J. Niessen and Max A. Viergever, Vol. 2208, pp. 1295-1297, Springer, Utrecht, The Netherlands, 2001.
3. S. Zimeras, G. Karangelis, E. A. Firle. "Object Segmentation and shape reconstruction using computer-assisted segmentation tools". To appear in: *SPIE International Symposium on Medical Imaging*, Seong K. Mun, Vol. 4681, 2002
4. Großkopf S, Park SY, and Kim MH: "Segmentation of Ultrasonic Images by Application of Active Contour Models", *Proc. CAR 98 – Computer Assisted Radiology and Surgery*, Lemke, Heinz U. u. a., p. 871, Elsevier, Amsterdam, Lausanne, The Netherlands, 1998.
5. P. Besl, N. McKay, "A method for Registration of 3-D Shapes", *IEEE Trans. Patt. Anal. And Mach. Intell.*, Vol. 14. No. 2, pp. 239-255, Feb. 1992.
6. Firle, Evelyn; Chen, Wei, "Semi-Automatic Registration for MR and CT Datasets", *Proc. Third Caesarium on Computer Aided Medicine*, International Workshop on Deformable Modelling and Soft Tissue Simulation, Bonn, 2001.
7. G. Sakas, S.Walter, "Extracting Surfaces from Fuzzy 3D Ultrasonic Data", *ACM Computer Graphics*, SIGGRAPH '95, Los Angeles, USA, pp. 6-11, 1995.
8. G. Sakas, L.A.Schreyer, M.Grimm, "Case Study: Visualization of 3D Ultrasonic Data", *IEEE Visualization '94*, Washington D.C., USA, pp. 369-373 1994.
9. G. Sakas, S. Walter, W. Hiltmann, A.Wischnik, "Foetal Visualization Using 3D Ultrasonic Data", *Proc. CAR 95 – Computer Assisted Radiology and Surgery*, Lemke, Heinz U. u. a., p. 241-247, Springer, Berlin; Heidelberg, 1995

CARS 2002 – H.U. Lemke, M.W. Vannier; K. Inamura, A.G. Farman, K. Doi & J.H.C. Reiber (Editors)
©CARS/Springer. All rights reserved.

Interferometric measurement of patient surface topology changes during therapy irradiation

Moore Christopher[a], Woods Katherine[b], Sharrock Philip[a]
Lilley Francis[c], Lalor Michael[c] and Burton David[c].
[a] N W Medical Physics, Christie Hospital, Withington, Manchester, UK
[b] Department of Radiotherapy, Christie Hospital, Withington, Manchester, UK
[c] CEORG, Liverpool John Moores University, Byrom Street, Liverpool, UK

Abstract

Hampered by the lack of technology, detailed patient surface topology changes during radiotherapy have not been determined. This paper describes a structured light solution to dynamic surface measurement with an interferometer producing a fringe pattern across a treatment couch. Body surface topology alters the relative spatial phase content in the pattern, which can be used to generate relative surface heights. Triangulation of one surface point allows conversion to an absolute scale with half-millimetre resolution. By capturing fringe images at 25Hz, dynamic sequences of 898, 440x440 point height maps have been computed. For an example patient being treated for rectal carcinoma, standard deviations of surface heights are predominantly below 1mm, with 1% up to 2mm and occasional points as high as 6mm. Statistical summaries show movement concentrated along the arch of the back and within 3mm of the mean surface. Despite the prone position of the patient, the distance of the treatment site from the diaphragm and the small scale of motion , periodic breathing is clearly revealed.

Keywords: Radiotherapy, topology, measurement

1. Introduction

Radiotherapy dose computation is predicated on unchanging body surface topology and patients are positioned using skin markers complemented by radiography of rigid bony anatomy. Hitherto it has not been possible to measure surface topology changes during treatment, and so the magnitude of any topological problem could not be assessed. In the mid-1990s ICRU-50 guidance [1] implicitly acknowledged this deficiency by statistically subsuming complex body surface variations into margins that relate the planning target volume, PTV, to the gross tumour volume, GTV. In this approach the PTV lies within an unchanging CT body surface. At treatment time the body surface topology is replaced by a handful of manually defined skin marks, which guide repeated patient positioning and radiation beam aiming over many weeks of treatment. Both intra-fraction and inter-fraction it is not known if this approach reliably reproduces the same planning surface topology, or if invariant statistical estimates of motion are appropriate for individuals. Until now these questions could not be answered.

©CARS/Springer. All rights reserved.

Stereophotogrammetry exploits feature correspondence in separate views of an object to determine the spatial position of points across a surface. The technique can work well where there are strong, detailed features on the surface being examined. For radiotherapy the surface in question is the body. Apart from the head, there are few grey-level or topologically rich surfaces. Consequently the stereophotogrammetric literature has focussed on head and neck imaging with at least one radiotherapy application targeted at face mask investigations [2]. Since stereophotogrammetric techniques rely on the presence of natural markers, which suggests that artificially creating correspondence will facilitate the measurement of smooth surfaces.

Attaching artificial markers to a surface has spawned the field of marker tracking. Here 'passive' and 'active' markers either reflect or emit light respectively. Because the markers are few in number and have pre-designed properties, establishing correspondence between two views is mathematically if not technically trivial. Effective markers have large physical profiles, introducing a displacement from the underlying surface point. Nevertheless, Gerig et al [3] reported patient set-up verification for broad beam radiotherapy using a small number of markers. This study, ad many others, are machine assisted adaptations of set-up by conventional body tattoo points. Baroni et al [4] have reported the use of ten, half-centimetre passive infra-red markers attached to the torso. If the limits to packing density and integrity of attachment could be overcome a crude estimate of body surface topology could be obtained in less than a second by using several thousand body markers. In a recent paper Baroni et al [5] have explored a potential solution by supplementing two physical markers with a 3x3 array of infra-red laser spots, and testing the approach on the breast of a volunteer.

Instead of adding physical markers to provide detail a light pattern can be projected onto a surface and structure determined from changes to the pattern. Early radiotherapy applications had limited goals, namely automating routine body contour generation. Berry and Aldrich [6] demonstrated that multi-slit line projection could be used to compare structures. Wilks [7] tiled measured contours to generate an approximation to the underlying body surface. Modern methods now include laser stripe triangulation [8]. However, motion and deformation of surface topology are obstacles to the use of these techniques. Recently, Moore et al [9] and MacKay et al [10] reported the use of complex structured light projection in which true surface topology, consisting of $2x10^5$ body surface points, can be measured from a single sub-second video frame.

This paper describes and analyses dynamic measurement of 3D-surface topology at sub-millimete resolution, with a specific example of small scale periodic motion detected in a patient being treated for carcinoma of the rectum.

2. Theory

Interference fringes are produced when coherent light from a laser beam is split and fed into twin optical fibres and then recombined at projection with fractional wavelength optical path difference. The fringes have sinusoidal intensity profile, period T_i, when projected onto the plane of a treatment couch with angle of incidence θ_i . They appear to

©CARS/Springer. All rights reserved.

have spacing T_r when observed at angle $(\theta_r + \theta_i)$ to the line of projection. A surface some vertical height Z above the couch will intercept the projected fringes and shift them by distance d from their originally observed position, corresponding to a spatial phase change $d\phi=2\pi.d/T_r$. Using simple geometry the relationship between the vertical height and spatial phase of a point can be shown to be $Z=T_i.d\phi / [2\pi(\tan\theta_i+\tan\theta_r)\cos\theta_i]$.

Takeda [11] described the extraction of spatial phase information from the Fourier transform of a modulated fringe image. The transform is band-pass filtered to isolate the fringe spectral maxima, reduce harmonics, noise and grey-level background detail. The inverse Fourier transform then produces a new image that is mathematically complex. The spatial phase ϕ at each point on the original surface image is then given by the arctangent of the ratio of the imaginary and real components of each new pixel value. It is then possible to determine the relative heights of all points across the surface of interest using the equation relating Z to ϕ. The conversion of this height map to absolute heights only requires that a single point on the surface be determined by some other method. In this study a single laser spot aimed at the surface provides the required height by triangulation.

3. Methods

A He-Ne laser interferometer is mounted at one end of a rigid section of tubing held securely just below ceiling level in a treatment room. This provides a divergent fringe beam with a path length to isocentre of over 3 metres. A laser diode spot source is mounted adjacent to the interferometer for triangulation purposes. A Pulnix TM-6CN CCD observation camera, with zoom lens and filter, is mounted at the opposite end of the tube. A volume of 40x40x40cm about the isocentre is calibrated for surface sensing using the techniques described by Lilley et al [12]. This volume matches the maximum irradiation field size of the treatment machine and takes into account the positioning of a large patient. Fringe projection, triangulation spot computational and phase-to-height processing are performed on a dual Pentium-III PC equipped with Matrox Meteor_II framegrabber, 1Gbyte of main memory, 92Gbyte RAID array and separate system disk. Software is written in C and IDL v5.4. This clinical system is a robust copy of a faster laboratory system, and can processes fringe data at an average rate of 61,000 points/second. For this study 440x440 pixel fringe images are captured at 25Hz for 36 seconds and pipelined into an 'avi' file for off-line processing. The observation time is matched to the clinical irradiation time for a single beam and the need to limit data volumes for archive data to a single CD-ROM.

Resolution and reproducibility of the sensor was checked using a RANDO anthropomorphic phantom before subsequent, weekly use to follow dynamic changes in the surface topology of a patient with rectal carcinoma and receiving treatment by chemotherapy and 5000 cGy of X-ray therapy at 6MV delivered in 25 fractions. The patient was positioned prone during the delivery of four fields from the anterior, posterior, left and right lateral directions at each fraction. Before and after irradiation the optical sensor was used to capture single fringe frames as a check on system integrity. During treatment 36 seconds of surface data were collected in a 389 Mbyte avi file. The avi file was then stripped and processed off-line to produced 898 consecutive 3D surface height

©CARS/Springer. All rights reserved.

maps, each of size 387kBytes. The height maps were then analysed and combined into a 4.3MByte 'mpeg' rendered-surface animation.
The 898, 440x440 point surface height files were used to compute a mean body surface with associated statistics. Each height map was then subtracted from the mean surface to produce a surface deviation image. Since underlying, small scale systematic surface motion is of particular interest, both in terms of proving the technology and determining the limits to clinical application, it is necessary to ameliorate resolution effects in the any dynamic visualisation. Hence, surface data were reduced by local averaging to produce dynamic 44x44 point, deviation-surface animations, again stored as small mpeg files.

4. Results

Laser triangulation, which determines the conversion to absolute height, is also the limiting technology in the optical surface sensing system. Using a Pulnix TN-6CN the limit to absolute height resolution by triangulation is 0.55mm, which has been confirmed in previous experiments using repeated static imaging [12]. Dynamic RANDO phantom imaging using avi-file imaging in the clinic confirm this resolution and establish the reproducibility of point measurement, via point-height standard deviations, at 0.05-0.25mm. The spacing between the 440x440 measurement points depends on the CCD array and the field of view set using the camera lens. In this study it is 0.5mm.

Static, intra-fraction height maps used for set-up verification show that 62% of points across the monitored patient surface exhibit *absolute* changes that are less than 1mm, with 28% between 1-2mm and 10% between 2-5mm. Notable deviations from these averages were observed during the first weekly imaging session where 1% of surface points lay between 5-10mm, 35% changed height by 2-5mm, 30% lay in band 1-2mm and 33% less than 1mm. In week four there were no points showing changes greater than 5mm, but 18% lay in the 2-5mm band. The set-up height maps appear to be random samples of the wider ranging and varied motion observed by dynamic optical sensing during radiation delivery. Statistical summaries computed using the entire 898 consecutive, 40msec, 3D height maps in show that the parent standard deviations of 99% of the 193,600 measured surface points are less than or equal to 1mm. Most of the remaining 1% of points have standard deviations less than 2mm with a few extending up to 6mm. Figure-1 shows the mean surface computed from a dynamic sensing sequence of fringe frames. Figure-2 shows the corresponding standard deviations. From this it is quite clear that the larger changes are concentrated along the small of the patient's back with some between the buttocks.

Observation of the mpeg animations of the patient surface invite a search for evidence of small scale periodic motion. After processing the data to ameliorate the effects of the 0.5mm resolution limit (see Methods) and subtracting the instantaneously measured patient surface from the mean surface, clear periodic breathing is revealed. This is despite the prone position of the patient and the distance of the treatment site from the diaphragm. The image sequence in Figure-3 shows side elevations of the deviation-surface for frames 11, 31, 43 and 57. The motion visible in these images has an approximate period of 2.5 seconds and is consistently reflected in the entire fringe frame sequence.

©CARS/Springer. All rights reserved.

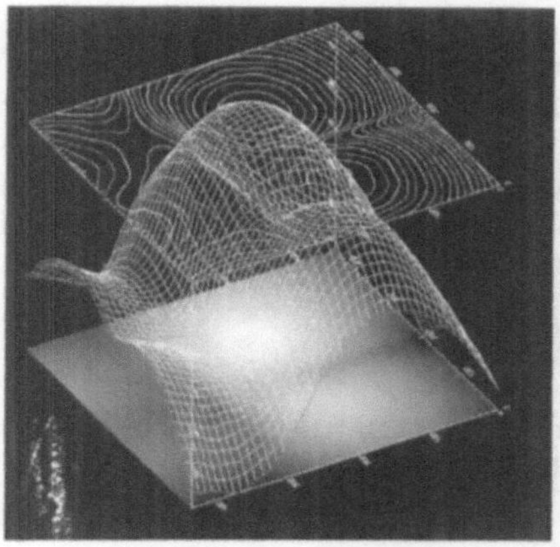

Figure-1. Mean surface height map in grey level, mesh and contour representations.

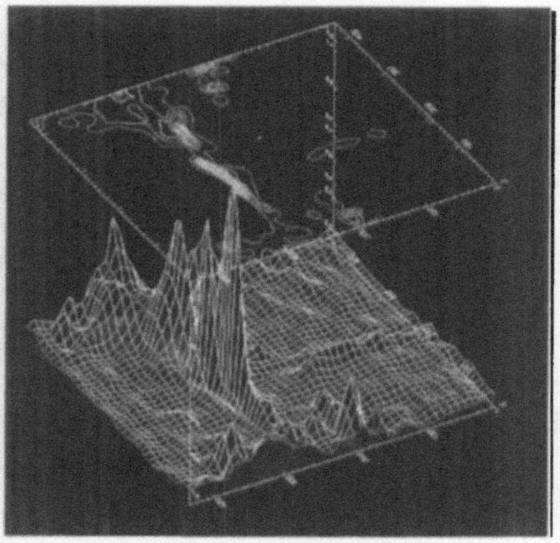

Figure-2. Mean surface height standard deviations on a vertical scale 0.2-1.6 mm.

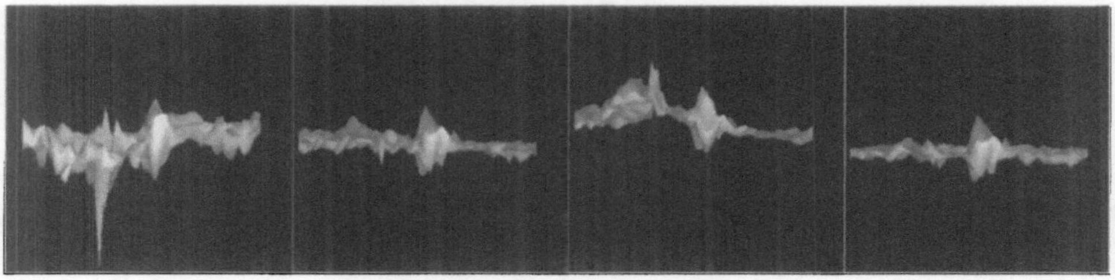

Figure-3. Height deviations from mean surface (Figure-1), seen in side elevation, for frames 11, 31, 43 and 57 of the 898 frame, 35 second sequence. The vertical scale is 6mm, the horizontal scale 22cms.

5. Discussion and conclusions

Patient surface motion sensing using phase extracted from interferometer fringe projection has been shown to be practical for assessing the stability of patient set-up and in-treatment monitoring in a radiation environment. In the treatment room it is necessary to ensure that clothing and bedding are outside the field of view of the CCD camera. Both the camera and fringe projection interferometer are susceptible to shadows cast by these objects. It is particularly important to mask any highly reflective metallic objects, such as the treatment couch side rails, and stow away the ceiling mounted treatment machine control-pods used by radiographic staff during patient set-up. Body surface monitoring prior to irradiation adds a minute or two to treatment time, whereas surface sensing during irradiation incurs no time penalty. Fringe images captured during irradiation are only minimally contaminated by electromagnetic speckle interference from the treatment machine during irradiation. Speckle contamination is highly characteristic and so can be filtered out prior to phase extraction. The use of shielded cabling would entirely eliminate the speckle at source. Surface changes measured for a patient undergoing treatment for rectal carcinoma are most likely to be within 3mm during irradiation. Periodic motion in the surface, even

©CARS/Springer. All rights reserved.

though small scale, is clearly and consistently visible. From a clinical viewpoint, given the presence of re-entrant surface sections that have large gradients, it is gratifying that the effects of breathing and the discomfort of lying prone are not evidenced as much larger changes. In 36 seconds the raw fringe data that is created requires just under 350 Mbytes of storage. After processing into 3D height maps this figure is more than doubled, taking it beyond the capacity of a CD archive disc. This highlights the need for high bandwidth networking infrastructure in the clinic to support dynamic measurement.

Acknowledgements

This work was supported in part by EC Biomed-II contract BMH4-98-3660 project name ARROW (Animated Real-time Radiation Oncology Worktools).

References

1. ICRU, Report 50, Prescribing, Recording and Reporting Photon Beam Therapy, *Intl Com on Radiation Units and Measurements*, Washington DC, USA, 1996.
2. 3dMD Company Internet Site January 2002: http://www.3dmd.com/rd.htm
3. Gerig l H, El-Hakim S F, Szanto J, Salhani D and Girard A, "The development and clinical application of a patient position monitoring system", *Procs SPIE Videometrics III*, 2350, 59-75, 1994
4. Baroni G, Ferrigno G, Orecchia R and Pedotti A, "Real-time three dimensional motion analysis for patient positioning verification" , *Radiation Oncology*, 54, 21-27, 2000.
5. Baroni G, Troia A, Orecchia R and Pedotti A, "Opto-electronic techniques and 3D surface reconstruction for the control of patient positioning in the radiotherapy of breast cancer" , *La Radiolgia Medica*, 102, 168-177, 2001
6. Berry J A and Aldrich J E, "Surface topography for patient repositioning" , *Medical Dosimetry,* 16, 71-77, 1991.
7. Wilks R J, "An optical system for measuring surface stripes for radiotherapy planning" , *British Jnl Radiology*, 66, 351-359, 1993.
8. PROFA, Duncan Hynd Associates Ltd, UK, http://www.dha.co.uk/
9. Moore C J and Graham P A, '3D Dynamic Body Surface Sensing & CT-Body Matching A Tool for Patient Set-up & Monitoring in Radiotherapy", *Jnl Computer Aided Surgery*, 5(Number 4), 234-245, 2000.
10. MacKay R I, Graham P A, Logue J P and Moore C J, "Patient Positioning using detailed 3D Surface Data for patients undergoing Conformal Therapy of the Prostate: A feasibility Study" , *Intl Jnl Radn Onc Biol Phys*, 49(1), 225-230, 2001.
11. Takeda M, Ina H and Seji K, "Fourier Transform method of Fringe Pattern Analysis for Computer Based Topography and Interferometry", *Jnl Optical Soc America,* 72(1), 156-160, 1982.
12. Lilley F, Lalor M J and Burton D R, " A Robust Fringe Analysis System for Body Shape Measurement", *Optical Eng*, 39(Number 1), 187-195, 2000.

©CARS/Springer. All rights reserved.

Adaptive filtering to predict lung tumor motion during free breathing

Martin J. Murphy[a], Marcus Isaakson[b], Joakim Jalden[b]
[a]Department of Radiation Oncology , Stanford University
[b]Department of Electrical Engineering, Stanford University

Abstract

Breathing-induced tumor motion during radiation therapy can be compensated either by gating or correcting the pointing of the radiation beam, but these techniques involve time delays in the corrective response. We have analyzed the accuracy of adaptive filter algorithms in predicting tumor positions with sufficient lead time to compensate for these systematic delays. Tumor and chest motion during respiration has been recorded fluoroscopically for lung cancer patients, using gold fiducials implanted in the tumors to enhance visibility. The motions been analyzed for predictability up to 1.0 second in advance using tapped delay line, Kalman filter, and neural network filter algorithms. Breathing patterns are not stationary in time. Both internal tumor and external chest movement can show amplitude and period modulations during a 30 second interval. Tapped delay line and other stationary filters cannot compensate for the changes and consequently have poor predictability. The predictive accuracy of adaptive filters has little dependence on the type of algorithm, but depends mainly on the frequency of updating and deteriorates rapidly when predicting more than 0.2 seconds in advance of the breathing signal. Longer-period (e.g., 30 seconds) variability in breathing requires frequent adaptation of the filter parameters.

Keywords: Breathing motion, breathing compensation

1. Introduction

Many internal tumor sites move with breathing. Lung tumors have been observed to move by 5 mm to 25 mm during regular breathing; the pancreas is known to move by up to 35 mm. If breathing motion is not restricted or compensated, dose margins must be enlarged to ensure complete irradiation of the target volume. This increases the exposure of healthy tissue and limits the total dose to the tumor.

The approximately regular pattern of normal breathing suggests it may be possible to devise tracking schemes to monitor the tumor position during free breathing and make continuous adjustments in the alignment of the radiation beam. This could be done by shifting the aperture of a multileaf collimator or moving a robotically mounted linear accelerator in synchrony with the breathing cycle. However, any adaptive response in beam delivery will be delayed with respect to the signal of the tumor's position. The delay can range from 50 ms for a signal to interrupt the beam cycle [1] to as much as 0.8

©CARS/Springer. All rights reserved.

seconds to mechanically reposition a linear accelerator. [2] This represents a familiar problem in adaptive signal processing for closed-loop control systems.

If a tumor's breathing-induced cycle of movement were perfectly uniform and regular, so that its time average over any interval was independent of the averaging interval (i.e., the time series was stationary) then simple fixed delay-line filters would be able to predict the motion arbitrarily far into the future after sampling a short interval. Unfortunately, decades of research into breathing behavior show that breathing is not stationary. [3] One consequence of this is that the simultaneous movement of different anatomical structures does not settle into an equilibrated state of coupled simple harmonic motion, but instead shows a sometimes complex pattern of phase differences and time-changing temporo-spatial correlations. Conversely, the presence of phase differences and complex correlations is a signal of instability in the breathing cycle.

We have begun a study of this problem by addressing three questions -

(1) what is the motion pattern of the tumor like during free breathing, and how does it relate to the motion of other anatomical structures?
(2) what signal processing concepts can be used to predict breathing motion with enough lead time to accomodate typical delays in adaptive response?
(3) how accurately can one predict the internal tumor position, as a function of lead time?

These questions impact all strategies for detecting and adaptively compensating breathing motion, including continuous monitoring of the tumor via fluoroscopy [4], monitoring via external breathing signals [5], or some combination of the two [2].

2. Method and materials

2.1 Clinical breathing data

Four radiosurgery patients were imaged fluoroscopically during free breathing to record the respiratory motion of the treatment target. Three of the patients had lung tumors and one patient had pancreatic cancer. All four treatment sites were marked by small gold fiducials implanted in the tumor, making the tumor motion easily visible under fluoroscopy. Each patient also had external radio-opaque markers attached to the chest to record external breathing motion synchronously with the tumor. The pancreatic cancer patient and one lung patient were imaged continuously for 60 seconds. The other two lung patients were each imaged continuously for three consecutive 60 second periods separated by three-minute intervals, to sample breathing motion over a time span of nine minutes. The fluoroscopic sessions were recorded on videotape for later analysis.

Each fluoroscopic study was analyzed frame-by-frame to extract the *(x,y)* coordinates of each internal fiducial and each external chest marker. The resulting data for each patient comprised simultaneous time series for the motion of the internal and external markers. This provided data to document the internal motion pattern of the tumor, the temporal and spatial relationships between the tumor's motion and other breathing indicators, and the temporal characteristics of the respiratory cycle.

©CARS/Springer. All rights reserved.

For each patient the temporal relationship between the tumor and external marker motion was graphed to display the phase difference between the two moving sites. The data for the two longest fluoroscopic studies were analyzed further to detect long-period changes in the breathing pattern and to test the predictability of the motion patterns.

2.2 Motion prediction and correlation filters

The conventional tool for predicting a signal based on its past behavior, or based on another correlated signal, is the adaptive filter. A linear stationary filter models the output signal as a linear combination of samples of the input signal, using a fixed set of coefficients to weight the input samples. A linear adaptive filter models the output signal as a linear combination of input signal samples using an updating algorithm to continuously adjust the weighting coefficients to adapt to changes in the input signal pattern. A nonlinear neural network filter models the input/output transfer function as a network of adaptable neurons that are trained from past input/output data to predict future or correlated signal behavior.

Using data from the fluoroscopic studies, the internal tumor motion was analyzed for temporal predictability using two methods: (1) a linear adaptive filter updated by the Least Mean Squares (LMS) method and a neural network adaptive filter. Then the correlation between external and internal motion was analyzed for predictability using a stationary linear filter, a linear adaptive filter updated by the LMS method, a linear adaptive filter updated by the Sequential Regression (SER) algorithm, and a neural network filter. Finally, the combined problem of predicting the respiratory motion of the external marker ahead in time and then using that result to predict the internal target position (also advanced in time) was analyzed, again using linear LMS and neural network filter algorithms.

The accuracy of the prediction and correlation filters was quantified by the normalized Root Mean Square Error (nRMSE). If x_i is the signal sample we wish to estimate, and x_i' is the filter's estimate of the signal sample, then *nRMSE* is defined as

$$nRMSE = \frac{\sum(x_i - x_i')^2}{\sum(x_i - \mu_i)^2}$$

©CARS/Springer. All rights reserved.

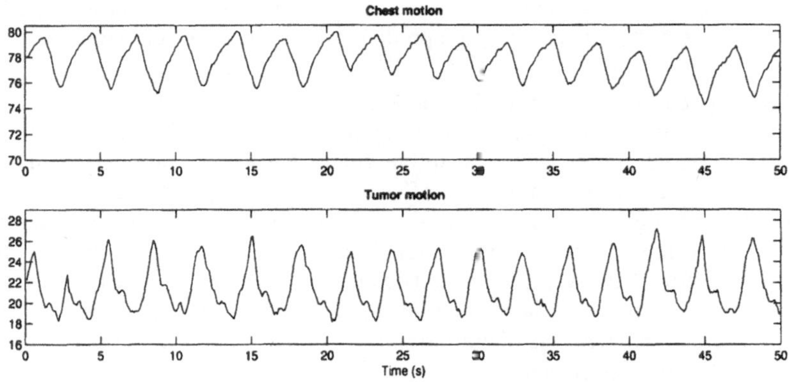

Figure 1 - The time series for the motion of a lung tumor in the inferior/superior direction (top plot) and the motion of the external chest surface in the anterior/posterior direction during a 50 second fluoroscopic imaging study.

where $\mu_i = (1/N) \sum x_i$

Thus *nRMSE* = *100%* corresponds to a fixed prediction at the mean of the signal - i.e., a prediction that aims at the average position of the moving target. If the predictor is tracking the tumor to within 10% of the maximum displacement during free breathing, then *nRMSE* = *28%*.

3. Results

We will present here the observations for one lung cancer patient. Figure 1 shows the recorded position of the external chest surface (top trace) and the lung tumor (bottom trace) for a period of 50 seconds of free breathing. There is 20% variability in the period and up to 60% variability in the amplitude of the chest and tumor motion. The relative phase of the two motions fluctuates systematically in time with approximately a 30 second cycle. This indicates that the breathing cycle is not in simple harmonic equilibrium and is not stationary. Therefore tracking it will require a filter that can continuously adapt to the changing temporal relationship.

We have analyzed the predictability of the chest motion up to 0.8 seconds in advance using various adaptive filters as signal predictors. We have analyzed the predictability of the tumor position given the chest surface position using adaptive filters as correlators of the two signals. Finally, we have analyzed the combined process of predicting the external chest motion and then correlating it with the internal tumor position. The results of these tests are presented in Table I. For comparison, we note that if one uses a pure sinusoidal breathing pattern, the error *nRMSE* is zero for the sampling frequency and observation period used in these measurements.

©CARS/Springer. All rights reserved.

Figure 2 illustrates the combined prediction and correlation result by showing the predicted tumor position in parallel with the known tumor position, with the error in the predicted position indicated by the shaded region between the two curves.

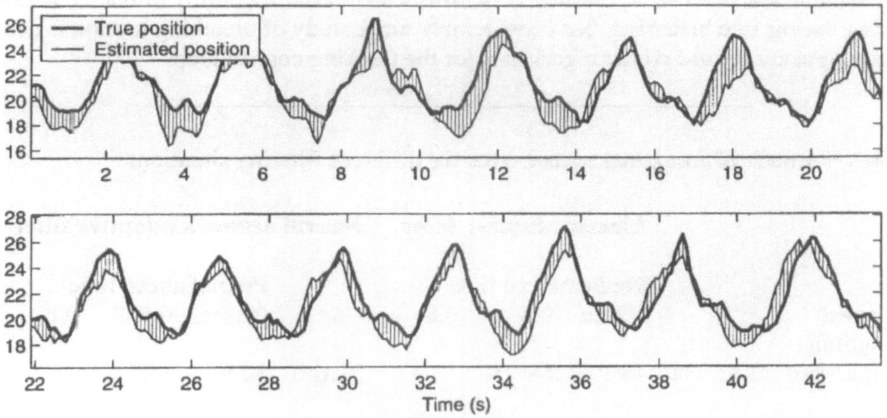

Figure 2 - The predicted (thin line) and actual (thick line) positions of a lung tumor for a 32 second period, using the LMS linear adaptive filter algorithm to predict the external marker position ahead by 0.8 seconds and then to predict the tumor position from the anticipated external marker position. The error in the prediction is highlighted by the shaded area between the two time series and corresponds to *nRMSE* = 39.6%.

4. Discussion and conclusions

This study has documented the potential variety and complexity of tumor motion during free breathing, paying attention to three fundamental characteristics - (1) the temporal pattern of the breathing cycle over time periods relevant to conventional and hypo-fractionated radiotherapy; (2) the spatial relationship between the tumor position and external signals of breathing that might be used as surrogates to predict the tumor position; and (3) the timing relationship between external breathing indicators and the internal tumor's motion. Secondly, it has tested prospective schemes to predict tumor motion while accomodating the inevitable delay between detecting and responding to a change in tumor position. From the early data we observe that:

(1) During free breathing, different parts of the anatomy can move with different temporal and spatial relationships. These relationships can change with time. Thus tumor motion cannot be expected to have a linear and stationary relationship with external breathing indicators. A stationary linear filter predicting ahead in time or correlating tumor with chest wall motion gives a poor result because it is unable to adapt to the changing patterns of breathing.

(2) Breathing is not strictly periodic. Therefore (in contrast to a true periodic motion) it cannot be predicted exactly even when using adaptive filters.

(3) When adaptive filters are used to predict breathing, the performance deteriorates sharply beyond about 0.2 seconds.

©CARS/Springer. All rights reserved.

(4) When adaptive filters are used to correlate tumor with chest wall motion, the accuracy depends less on the type of filter than on the frequency of updating the filter parameters.

We conclude that one can be cautiously optimistic about the feasibility of real-time tumor tracking during free breathing, but considerably more study of breathing motion is needed to develop accurate and robust algorithms for the tracking control loop.

Table - Normalized root mean square error for different filtering situations

		Linear adaptive filter			**Neural network adaptive filter**			
		Predict ahead time				Predict ahead time		
Temporal Prediction		0.2sec	0.5	0.8		0.2sec	0.5	0.8
(using LMS)	23.1%	48.1%	68.7%		21.6	50.8	61.3	
		Time between updates				Time between updates		
		0.1s	1.0	5.0		0.1s	1.0	5.0
Spatial Correlation fixed		39.4%	39.4	39.4		--	38.1%	39.5
	LMS	25.2	33.1	35.6				
	SER	28.8	35.9	38.4				
		Predict ahead time				Predict ahead time		
		0.2s	0.5	0.8		0.2s	0.5	0.8
Prediction plus 0.1s	26.6%	37.3	39.6		--	--	--	
correlation 1.0	40.4	54.9	60.7		45.0%	47.4	64.9	
(using LMS) 5.0		41.1	55.2	71.1		47.4	50.3	64.4

References

1. Ohara K, Okumura T, Adisada M, *et al. Irradiation synchronized with respiration gate.* Int J Radiat Oncol Biol Phys 17: 853–857 1989).
2. Schweikard A, Glosser G, Bodduluri M, *et al. Robotic motion compensation for respiratory movement during radiosurgery.* Comput Aided Surg 5: 263-277 (2000).
3. Priban IP. *An analysis of some short-term patterns of breathing in man at rest.* J Physiol 166: 425-434 (1963).
4. Shirato H, Shimizu S, Kunieda T, *et al. Physical Aspects of a real-time tumor-tracking system for gated radiotherapy.* Int J Radiat Oncol Biol Phys 48 1187-1195 (2000).
5. Keall PJ, Kini VR, Vedam SS, *at al. Motion adaptive x-ray therapy: a feasibility study.* Phys Med Biol 46: 1-10 (2001).

CARS 2002 – H.U. Lemke, M.W. Vannier; K. Inamura A.G. Farman, K. Doi & J.H.C. Reiber (Editors)
©ARS/Springer. All rights reserved.

Protocol conversion by automatic pattern matching for the on-line linkage between multi-institutional radiation oncology databases

Kumazaki Yuu[a], Harauchi Hajime[b], Haneda Kiyohumi[c], Kou Hiroko[a], Kondou Takashi[a], Ishibashi Masatoshi[a], Numasaki Hodaka[a], Shimizu Keiji[a], Umeda Tokuo[d], Takemura Akihiro[e], Inamura Kiyonari [b]

[a] Graduate School of Medcine, Course of Health Sciences, Osaka University, Yamadaoka 1- 7, Suita- city, Osaka, 565- 0871, Japan,

[b] School of Allied Health Sciences, Osaka University

[c] Dept. of Radiological Sciences,Hiroshima Prefectural College of Health Science

[d] School of Allied Health Sciences, Kitasto University

[e] School of Allied Health Sciences, Kanazawa University

Abstract

We developed method of collecting clinical records of radiotherapy for ROGAD (Radiation Oncology Greater Area Database) which is a multi-institutional type database developed for the purpose of grasping the actual situation of the radiotherapy in Japan and aiming at improvement of results of radiotherapy. The method employs a data import system which convert automatically clinical records of different protocol to those of ROGAD protocol by using the Internet and by taking advantage of its higher interactivity. Also improvement in data link efficiency was aimed at. By comparing contents of registrated data in a facility with those of ROGAD and by recognizing pattern of the histogram of registrated data, we create a code conversion table automatically. In this way, we convert clinical records of protocol in existed database in a facility into data of ROGAD protocol by employing the conversion table. This system is expected to be a method for mutual on-line linkages between plural number of radiation oncology databases.

Keywords: Radiotherapy database, on-line linkage, protocol conversion

1. Introduction

We have three methods of collecting clinical history records of radiotherapy for ROGAD(Radiation Oncology Greater Area Database) of multi-institutional type for the purpose of grasping the actual situation of the radiotherapy in Japan and aiming at the improvement of results of radiotherapy. First collection method is by running data registration program. Second collection method is by hand-write filling of worksheet. Third collection method is by off-line linkage with an existed database in a facility. In case of the third method, it is difficult to collect clinical record by the off-line linkage with an existed database in a facility which has different data form from that of ROGAD. Therefore, it was necessary to convert data with protocol of an existed database in a

©CARS/Springer. All rights reserved.

facility into data with ROGAD protocol. The above-mentioned off-line conversion programs were developed and have been used in ROGAD office. In this off-line system, each facility firstly mails clinical records to ROGAD office by floppy disks. The mailed clinical records are converted to those of ROGAD form by using a conversion software on the basis of a conversion table which has been discussed and created by both facility side and ROGAD side beforehand. (fig.1) Then data are stored in ROGAD. The conversion table describes method of translation or correspondence between both forms in semantics as well as syntactics. However, each facility and the ROGAD office needed to minutely examine difference of both forms. Fig.1 shows an example of conversion table.

conversion table : テーブル

U_Treatment method	R_Treatment method	U_Treatment basis	R_Treatment basis	U_Irradiation policy	R_Irradiation policy
Treatment method	Treatment method	Treatment basis	Treatment basis	Irradiation policy	Irradiation policy
Operation	1	Outpatient	1	Symptomatic	1
Irradiation	2	Inpatient	2	Palliative	2
Operation+Irradiation	3	Others	8	Full dose, cure not intended	3
Chemotherapy	4	Unknown	9	Full dose, curative intent	4
Thermotherapy or BRM etc.	5			Pre-oparative	5
Chemotherapy+Irradiation	6			Post-oparative	6
Operation+Chemotherapy+Irradiation	7			intra-opetrative	0
Irradiation+Thermotherapy or BRM etc.	0			Preventive	7
Others	8			Others	8
Unknown	9			Unknown	9

Fig.1 Conversion table

In Fig.1, the column of the "U_Treatment method" is according to protocol of data element which corresponds to " Treatment method " on the side of each facility. The column of "R_ Treatment method " is according to protocol of item of " Treatment method " on the side of ROGAD. Both codes are 1 to 1 correspondence. That is, registration of "1" means the " Treatment method " of ROGAD corresponding to "Operation" .

2. Purpose

In order to save time and labor for linkage, a data import system which convert automatically clinical records of different protocol to those of ROGAD protocol was developed by using the Internet and by taking advantage of its higher interactivity. Also improvement in data link efficiency was aimed at. Also for the purpose of accuracy maintenance, an operator simply enter codes of an existed database in a facility and create a conversion table by automatic pattern recognition.

3. Materials

Ten years have passed since ROGAD firstly collected clinical data, and 325 facilities, and 13,448 effective cases have come to be registered to ROGAD. We sent questionnaire last year to all 723 radiotherapy facilities in Japan to get information on operation status of databases, and 125 facilities responded. Number of users who will apply our developed method by this study is estimated to be about 90. This number is 73% of 125 facilities which are operating their own database.

©CARS/Springer. All rights reserved.

4. Methods

We created a software equipped with the following functions. First function is to customize each protocol of a facility into ROGAD form. Second one is to make a histogram of frequency versus values of a data element of the existed database in a facility. Horizontal axis of the histogram is values of a code such as ICD-O code or topographical regions, and the vertical axis is frequency or number of clinical cases for each value. The histogram is made for each data element. The third is as follows. For the purpose of comparing contents of registrated data in the facility with those of ROGAD and by means of recognizing pattern of the histogram, we create a code conversion table automatically. For an example, the histogram of contents of registrated data of cases of breast in an existed database in a facility was first compared with those in ROGAD by using non-parametric test. By this method, the histogram was brought to be close to that of ROGAD by replacing value items on the horizontal axis so that P value became the maximum. By making those histograms close to each other, a table of the value items of the facility corresponding to the value items of ROGAD was displayed to a radiation oncologist. and the table was approved by him. Fourth function is to convert clinical records of the protocol in the existed database in the facility into data of ROGAD protocol by employing the conversion table. Fifth one is that an operator can check the converted contents after conversion. Sixth function is to append the contents of clinical records in the facility to an E-mail automatically, and to send the E-mail to ROGAD server by enciphering it specifically to the facility and by using SSL (Secure Sockets Layer). Seventh function is to perform collation of file structure and to carry out data import to ROGAD after mailing to ROGAD server. Fig.2 shows flow-chart in our on-line data import system.

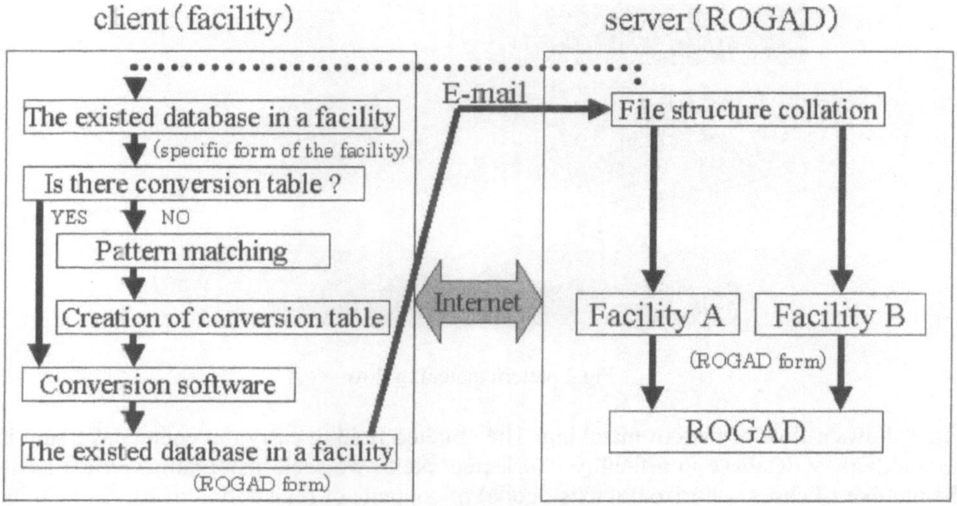

Fig.2 On-line data import system

©CARS/Springer. All rights reserved.

In Fig.2, a conversion table is first generated by this software. Before converting clinical data of a existed database in a facility into clinical data of ROGAD form, the software checks whether a conversion table exists. If a conversion table does not exist, a conversion table is generated on PC by a client side. Clinical data of the existed database in the facility is converted into clinical data of ROGAD form by using the conversion software of our make at the client side. They are sent to the ROGAD server using E-mail. The server checks file structure whether the sent file is damaged or not, and whether it is a designated file or not. When the file is damaged, or it is not a designated file, the information is reported to the facility. After the file collation is completed, the file was judged to be the right one for the facility, and the data are stored in ROGAD.

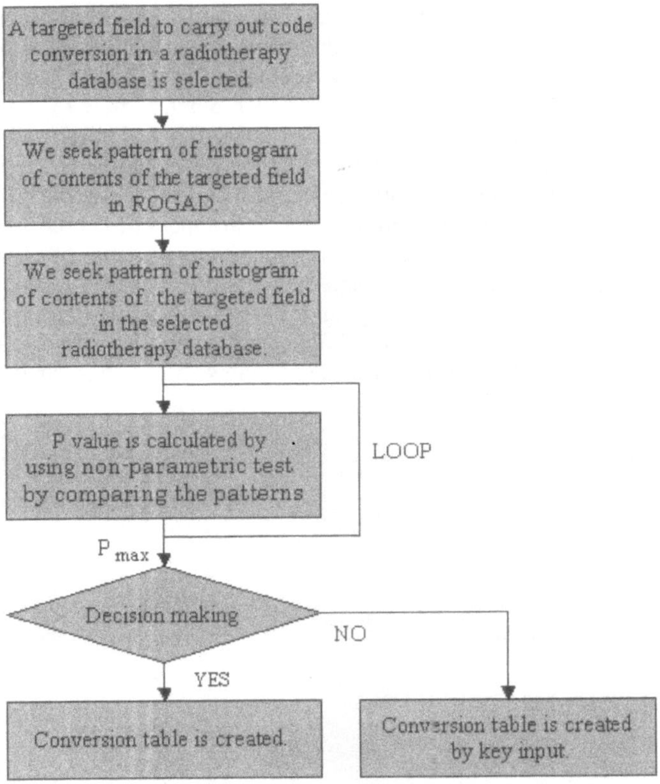

Fig.3 pattern matching flow

Fig.3 shows a flow of pattern matching. The targeted field to carry out code conversion in a radiotherapy database in a facility is selected. Next, we seek histogram (vertical axis : the number of cases, a horizontal axis : code) of contents of registration of ROGAD in the field. Next, we seek histogram of contents of registration of the facility. The order of code of histogram by the side of an institution is replaced and repeated. Comparison and non-parametric test is carried out with the pattern of ROGAD, and P value is calculated. A temporary input is tried in each code corresponding to the code of ROGAD with the

©ARS/Springer. All rights reserved.

pattern of the maximum in P value. Then, an operator checks a temporary input, corrects it, if required, a conversion table is created by key entry.

5. Results

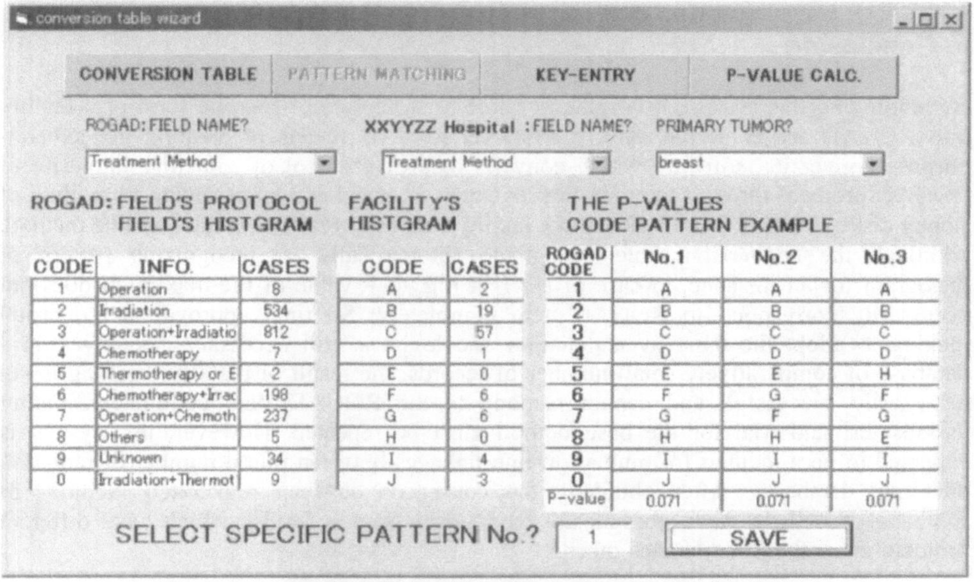

Fig.4 An example of wizard for generating conversion table

Fig.4 shows an example of wizard for generating a conversion table by using pattern matching. A field name in ROGAD, each institution and primary tumor are selected. P value is calculated by pushing the button "P-VALUE CALC.". Only No.1, No.2, and No.3 candidates are displayed in an order from the maximum of P value. An operator chooses a candidate in them and pushes the "SAVE" button. Then they are written in conversion table. If correction is required, he pushes the "KEY-INPUT" button and a conversion table are made by key entry.

An example of pattern matching is as follows. In case of a data element named “treatment method” in ROGAD protocol, we have 10 items of value (1:Operation, 2:Irradiation, 3:Operation+Irradiation, 4:Chemotherapy, 5:Thermotherapy or BRM etc., 6:Chemotherapy+Irradiation, 7:Operation +Chemotherapy +Irradiation, 0:Irradiation+Thermotherapy or BRM etc., 8:Others, 9:Unknown). We had 13,448 effective cases in ROGAD. There were 750 cases of breast in university hospitals in Japan. The order of number of cases of breast in ROGAD was, (3:Operation+Irradiation, 2:Irradiation, 7:Operation+Chemotherapy+Irradiation, 6:Chemotherapy+Irradiation, 9:Unknown, 0:Irradiation+Thermotherapy or BRM etc., 4:Chemotherapy, 1:Operation, 8:Others, 5:Thermotherapy or BRM etc.). While, There were 315 effective cases, and 98 cases of breast in one University Hospital. The order of number of cases of breast in that Hospital was, (C:Operation+Irradiation, B:Irradiation, F:Chemotherapy +Irradiation,

©CARS/Springer. All rights reserved.

G:Operation+Chemotherapy+Irradiation, I:Unknown, .:Irradiation +Thermotherapy or BRM etc., A:Operation, D:Chemotherapy, H:Others, E:Thermotherapy or BRM etc.).
The order matching, namely histogram matching was carried out. The conversion table was completed to convert data of "Treatment method" between the facility and ROGAD in cases of breast.

6. Conclusion

By employing this system, it became possible to store data of specific form of a facility into ROGAD server as the data of ROGAD form by means of creating the general-purpose conversion software which converts data of protocol of a facility into data of ROGAD protocol through Internet. Improvement in speed and labor saving in mailing of floppy disks at both ROGAD side and a facility side were realized by this on-line method. Although the conversion table was made automatically by recognizing pattern of histogram for an instance, in case of No.1 in Fig. 4, P value of the maximum does not necessarily correspond to ROGAD item completely. So final approval and decision making to adopt the table by a radiation oncologist is still necessary. Moreover, in a database of comparatively small number of records, the result of pattern matching is not necessarily successful, and cannot respond to the ROGAD item completely. Futher various test and trial for the best method must be repeated. However, this system is expected to be a method for mutual on-line linkages between plural number of radiation oncology databases. After obtaining the consensus between registrated facilities of ROGAD, it will be made possible to export data from a facility which have different protocol to another facility each other.

CARS 2002 – H.U. Lemke, M.W. Vannier; K. Inamura, A.G. Farman, K. Doi & J.H.C. Reiber (Editors)
©CARS/Springer. All rights reserved.

Photon radiosurgical system for treating brain tumors

Kintomo Takakura, Osami Kubo
Yoshihiro Muragaki, Hiroshi Iseki and Madoka Sugiura
Institute of Advanced Biomedical Engineering and Science and
Department of Neurosurgery, Tokyo Women's Medical University,
8-1 Kawada-cho, Shinjuku-ku, Tokyo 162-8666, Japan

Abstract

A small, handy portable X-ray generator, photon radiosurgical system (PRS) was evaluated its efficacy to treat malignant brain tumors. Most of the tumors were treated by intraoperative radiation with PRS to the residual tumors. Some tumors were treated by stereotactically applied PRS after the biopsy of the tumor without craniotomy. The accurate position of the tip of the PRS probe into the brain tumor was decided by using the operative navigator with an open MRI in the operating theater. Seventyeight cases of malignant brain tumors were treated from 1995 to 1999. All cases were completely followed up for more them 2 years after the treatment. The radiation by PRS decreased the size of the tumor very quickly. The post surgical 2 years survival rate of primary glioblastoma was 40 percent and it of anaplastic astrorytoma was 90 percent. The data were the best survival rates ever reported for those malignant gliomas. PRS can give locally focussed strong radiation effect with quite localized hyperthermia at the site of the tip of the PRS probe. PRS can be used safely without any serious complications and it is anticipated to be used also for treating various malignant tumors other them brain tumors.

Keywords: Radiotherapy, photon radiosurgery system (PRS), brain tumor

1. Introduction

The Photon Radiosurgery System (PRS) is a low voltage powered miniature X-ray generator for single fraction interstitial radiosurgery (1, 2). The X-ray dose administered by this unit falls off sharply with distance from the tip of the probe, making it possible to expose localized areas of a tumor to concentrated X-rays. Although the basic concept of treatment using the PRS is similar to that of brachytherapy, the PRS does not involve the use of radioactive isotopes. It can, therefore, be used easily and safely, with less of a burden on the patient and offers the advantages of an adjustable dose rate and a safer dose gradient minimizing the radiation dose to normal brain tissue outside the target volume.

Initial clinical experiences with the PRS treatment of brain tumors was reported by Yanch, Zervas, Hakim, Cosgrove et al (3-5). They treated 14 metastatic brain tumors. During a follow up period, 3 patients showed radiographic progression and only one patient showed symptomatic recurrence. No adverse effects were observed. We have treated 78 malignant brain tumors from June 1995 to September 1999, and followed up all cases for more than 2 years. The tumor suppressive effect was analyzed in this study and the

©CARS/Springer. All rights reserved.

mechanism responsible for the high level control effect and the clinical applications of PRS in future are discussed.

2. Materials and methods

PRS (Photoelectron Corp. Lexington MA), a portable small X-ray generator (Fig. 1) was used for intratumoral local irradiation. PRS consists of 3 parts: an X-ray generator with a needle-like probe (3 mm in diameter, 10 cm in length), an electrical power supply unit and a treatment control unit. The X-ray generator is about 1 9 kg of weight and works by 12

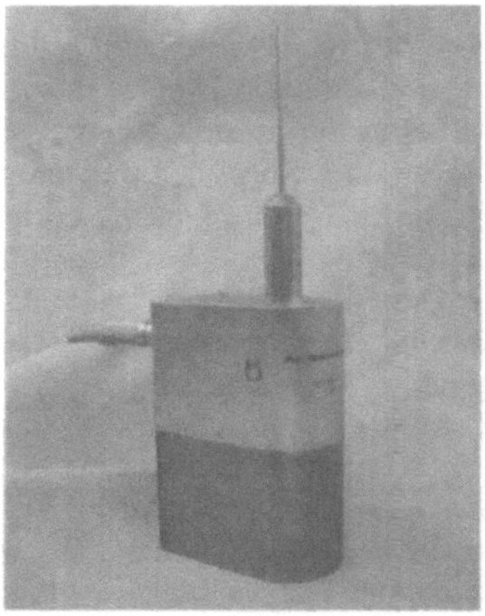

Fig.1: X-ray generator of Photon Radiosurgical System (PRS).

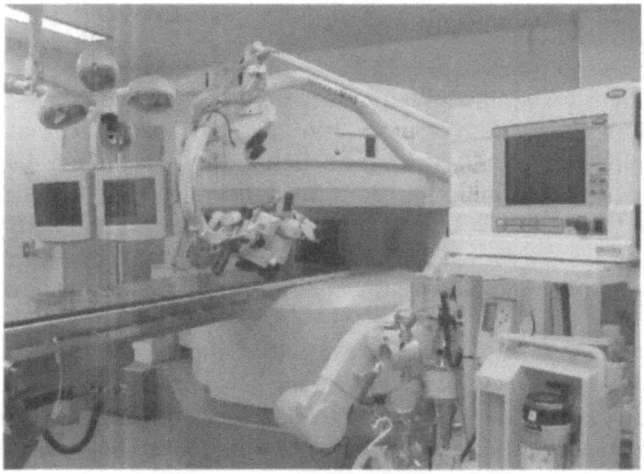

Fig.2 : Open MRI(AIRIS II, Hitachi) in the operating theater.

©CARS/Springer. All rights reserved.

Volts electrical current. Two therapeutic techniques are used for performing PRS treatment of brain tumors. In one technique, the tip of the probe is inserted stereotactically into the tumor tissue by using a CRW head frame (Radionics, Inc. Burlington, MA) and a PRS holder, after the stereotactic biopsy and histological confirmation of the malignant brain tumors. In the other technique, the tip of the probe is placed into the residual tumor tissue intraoperatively following the craniotomy and partial removal of the tumor. The morphological figure of the residual tumor is monitored by the open MRI (0.3 Tesla, Iris□, Hitachi) in the operating theater. The position of the tip of the PRS probe is guided to the most suitable place by the real time monitoring system with the open MRI (Fig.2). The radiation dose planning is made by a computer system in the operating theatre. The average marginal dose of X-ray was 15 Gy (8-18 Gy) and the average radius of irradiation was 13.6 mm. The irradiation time Gy (8-18 Gy) and the average radius of irradiation was 13.6 mm. The irradiation time ranged from 5 to 60 min.

2.1 Patients

Seventy-eight patients were treated by PRS. There were 56 gliomas, 11 metastatic brain tumors, 5 malignant lymphomas, and 6 other malignant brain tumors. All but 4 patients underwent PRS treatment in a single time. One glioblastoma patient underwent 5 successive PRS treatment and 3 patients underwent 2 PRS treatment each for the residual tumors. Eighty-one tumors were treated by using intraoperative technique and 4 tumors were treated by using stereotactic surgical technique. All 37 primary gliomas received post-surgical conventional radiotherapy (55gy) after PRS treatment with a linear accelerator for medico-ethical reason, because surgery plus post-surgical radiotherapy using linear accelerator is the only EBM based accepted therapeutic modality for malignant gliomas in Japan today. No specific tumor treatment were used in combination for the other 44 brain tumors including recurrent gliomas. This clinical study was approved by the review board of the Ethical Committee of our University. Written informed concent was obtainsed from the patient or the patients legal gurdian. The effectiveness of PRS treatment was evaluated by the actuarial survival rate of the patients. The survival rate were compared with the data accumulated by the Japan Brain Tumor Registry (6). Any adverse effects in terms of neurological signs and symptoms or changes in laboratory examinations as well as any evidence of brain edema, hemorrhage or other changes identified in CT or MRI after PRS treatment were recorded in order to evaluate the side effects of this treatment.

3. Results

The navigation system with the open MRI worked quite well and we could irradiate accurately to the residual brain tumors. The radiation by PRS decreased the size of the tumor very quickly and strongly. The example case of the shrinkage of the tumor by PRS treatment is shown in Fig. 3. The post surgical 2 year survival rate of primary glioblastoma (19 cases) was 40 percent, whereas the average survival rate reported by Japan Brain Tumor Registry (JBTR) was 19 percent. The 2 year survival rate of primary anaplastic astrorytoma (18 cases) was 90 persent, whereas it was 40 percent by JBTR. The data were the best survival rate ever reported for those malignant brain tumors (5 lung, 4 gastrointestinal and 2 other cancers) was 82 percent and the average post surgical

©CARS/Springer. All rights reserved.

survival time was more them 13 months. The local control of malignant lymphoma was 100 percent and the PRS treatment showed the excellent result.

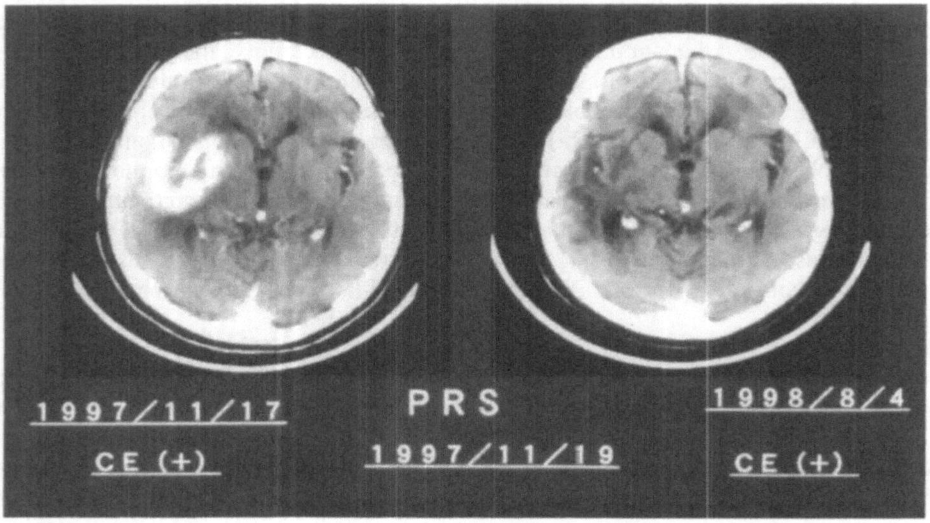

Fig.3: Effect of PRS on malignant lymphoma(52 years old, female). CT scan before and 9 months after PRS treatment.

4. Discussion

The PRS can deliver a strong single fraction of radiation to a strictly circumscribed area of the tumor, with minimal exposure to surrounding normal brain tissue. As the radiation dose at the tip of the PRS probe is very high, the local temperature of the tumor tissue rises substantially but the distribution of the increased temperature is quite localized and decreases sharply in distance from the tip of the probe. We have performed the animal experiment using pig brains to see the distribution of increased temperature and the result indicated that the tumor tissue was irradiated very strongly with hyperthermic state, but the brain tissue outside of the tumor was not irradiated significantly and maintained normal brain temperature. The very strong tumor suppressive effect of PRS is considered to be the synergistic effect of localized strong radiation energy with local hyperthermia which induce apoptosis of the tumor cells.

The basic concept of PRS treatment is similar to that of brachytherapy using radioactive isotopes. The effectiveness of brachytherapy on malignant brain tumors has also been reported by several investigators. PRS does not, however, require any special facilities or management procedures to protect against the leakage of radiation outside the patient as in cases of brachytherapy using isotopes. PRS can be used safely for the patients and medical stuffs.

©CARS/Springer. All rights reserved.

Treatment with PRS for glioblastoma, anaplastic astrorytoma, metastatic brain tumors and other brain tumors was quite effective. The intraoperative radiotherapy by PRS for malignant brain tumors is thus recommended to improve the outcome. It is anticipated that PRS will be used safely and effectively for treating various cancers other than brain tumors in future.

Acknowledgements

We thank to Photoelectron Corp. and Toshiba Co. for providing the PRS devices.
This study was supported by the Research Grant for Cancer Research from the Sharyo Foundation Japan.

References

1. Dinsmore M, Yanch JC, Sliski AP, Harte KJ: New X-ray generator for interstitial radiotherapy. Transact. Amer. Nuclear Soc. 70: 24-25, 1994
2. Biggs DJ, Thompson ES: Radiation properties of a miniature X-ray device for radiosurgery. Brit. J. Rad. 69: 544-547, 1996
3. Yanch JC, Zervas NT: The photon radiosurgery system. Scientific Amer. Science and Med. 1: 38-47, 1995
4. Hakim R, Zervas NT, Hakim F, Butler WE, Beatty J, Yanch JC, Biggs PJ, Gall KP, Sliski AP: Initial characterization of the dosimetry of a device for administering interstitial stereotactic radiosurgery. Neurosugery 40: 510-517, 1997
5. Cosgrove GR, Hochberg FH, Zervas NT, Pardo FS, Valenzuela RF, Chapman P: Interstitial irradiation of brain tumors, using a miniature radiosurgery device: Initial experience. Neurosurgery 40: 518-525, 1997
6. Committee of Brain Tumor Registry of Japan: Special Report of Brain Tumor Registry of Japan, Neurol. med. Chirurgica 39: 59-107,1999.

Towards a World Engineering Anthropometry Resource

CARS 2002 – H.U. Lemke, M.W. Vannier; K. Inamura, A.G. Farman, K. Doi & J.H.C. Reiber (Editors)
©CARS/Springer. All rights reserved.

Shape modeling driven by the product design

R. Mollard
Laboratoire d'Anthropologie Appliquée
45 rue des Saints-Pères
75270 Paris Cedex 06 - France

Abstract

After a review of the main characteristics of databases in anthropometry and ergonomics, and a short overview of the WEAR project, different approaches are presented to provide well-adapted information on human shape variability for the design of industrial products.

Keywords : Biostereometrics, database, ergodata.

1. Introduction

With the development of extensive networks like INTERNET, large databases have been developed in the different fields of technical and scientific information. Concerning ergonomics, the first steps concerned bibliographical databases gathering large amount of references. Simultaneously the development of more specific databases related to anthropometry and biomechanics was achieved. The purpose of these data systems was to create a tool for extracting main anthropometric data in a variety of useful forms and customizing the information to many different user needs. Pioneer works in the seventies were mainly the fact of the Human Engineering Laboratory from US-AMRL, USA [1] and the Laboratoire d'Anthropologie Appliquée from Université Paris V in EUROPE [2]. Based on a mutual exchange of surveys in anthropometry, these two teams created two international databases related to analysis of human morphology. Next steps for both parties and now for the World Engineering Anthropometry Resource (WEAR) Group are the data processing of 3-D anthropometry and biomechanics, and the development of more specific tools connected with Computer Aided Design softwares to provide well-adapted information for the design of industrial products.

This paper reviews general concepts for population databases in Ergonomics, with the example of ERGODATA, and some principles for the modeling of human shapes to include in a database system as proposed in the WEAR project.

©CARS/Springer. All rights reserved.

2. Population databases in ergonomics

2.1 Principles for databases in anthropometry and ergonomics

A review of the needs in this field leads to an organization of the databases in nine main sections as shown in figure 1. Basically, traditional 1-D anthropometry is the most documented, thanks to the large amount of surveys available all around the world. Nowadays the other sections concern more limited samples, due to the difficulty of collecting experimental data, or to the lack of standardization in the methods for measurement or for data processing. Further to this classification, two kinds of databases can be applied to section 1 up to section 8 which are concerned with numerical data; section 9 being more related to bibliographical references. Those two kinds of databases are described in their principles in figure 2. The main differences originate in the types of input data:

- Individual Data (ID) using raw measurements on individual subjects from small or large surveys,
- Aggregate Data (AD) coming from results taken from articles, reports...

Both ID and AD databases are able to use a common dictionary for the definitions of measurements and are able to lead to the same results: statistical models of population. However one important point has to be mentioned concerning ID and AD databases:

- AD can easily be obtained from articles, proceedings, technical reports in the field of ergonomics. The results, then, only concern statistics, and post data processing is still limited.
- ID are more difficult to collect, but more powerful due to the possibilities to create new samples, using different criteria for sorting of data: age, sex, origin,... and to apply new processing adapted to a specific question. For example, sizing systems can be derived with quite a good accuracy from such data processing on ID, which is not possible with AD. Moreover, estimate of missing measurements can be obtained by using correlation matrix computed on ID. New measurements and indexes can also be calculated from ID.

ERGODATA was developed using this structure to provide basic data in the fields of anthropometry, biomechanics, and more generally ergonomics as well as statistical models of populations, with for instance a prediction of change in morphologies in the next 10-20 years [3],[4]. Individual Database (ID) and Aggregate Database (AD) in anthropometry contain worldwide surveys on various samples of subjects: males and females, civilians and military,... Specific databases were linked with ID and AD to collect and process experimental results on inertial properties, human strengths, as well as upper limb reach capabilities and movements for seated operators. Bibliographic data and documentary sheets on norms and recommendations in ergonomics are also available. A new database focused on 3-D surface anthropometry is now available. All this information may be used to create and animate digital human models. ERGOMAN was developed for this purpose. This digital man-model is dedicated to ergonomic analysis in a workplace design process: postural assessment, visual field, reach area capabilities. Shape modeling is also possible using dedicated softwares [5].

©CARS/Springer. All rights reserved.

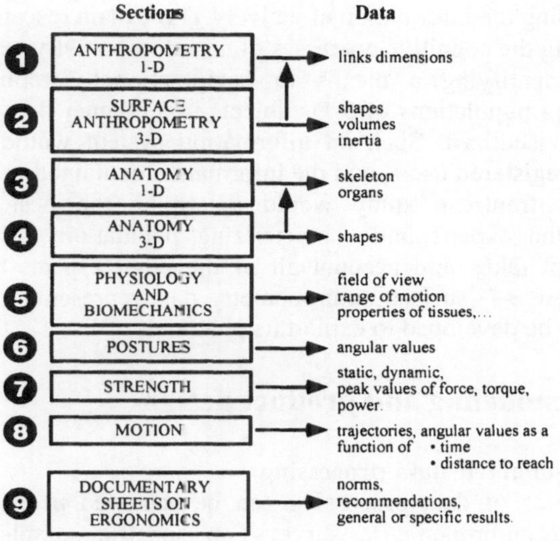

Figure 1. Main sections for population databases in ergonomics.

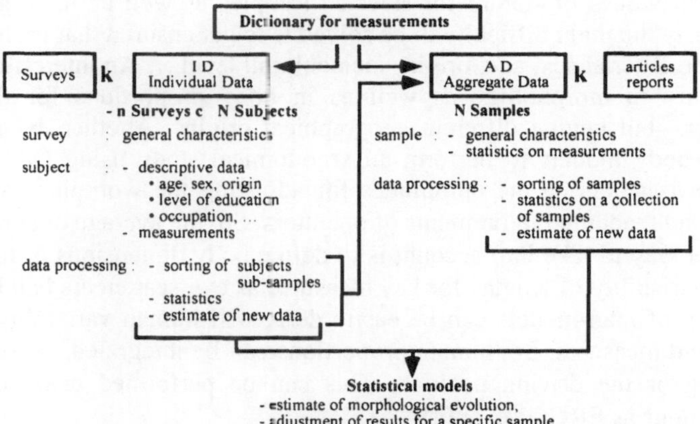

Figure 2. Principles used for Individual and Aggregate Databases.

©CARS/Springer. All rights reserved.

2.2 WEAR project

The objective of the WEAR project is to identify and develop data models and software tools that support the development of an on-line world-wide information system for utilizing the latest anthropometry databases in engineering environments. This system would include not only the latest 3D surface anthropometric data from all over the world, but also traditional anthropometric data contained in existing databases, fit and accommodation information, analytic and software tools, and guidance or intelligent agents for using the information effectively.Three main research issues must be addressed: understanding the cognitive processes of an anthropometry expert when dealing with such databases, identifying a means to computationally replicate these processes, and characterizing populations of 3-D subjects in a manner that can be effectively searched, mined and visualized. Such an information system would be able to be continually updated by registered users, and the information contained in it distributed throughout the world. This front-end study would determine the best potential technologies for replicating the experts and characterizing populations of 3-D objects in a systems approach that takes into account all of the other aspects and requirements of such a resource. New 3-D surface anthropometry data represents a valuable global resource if methods can be developed to exploit its potential.

3. Shape modeling and product design

3.1 Anthropometric data processing

Different kinds of data processing can be achieved using, for instance, retrospective results from anthropometric surveys on specific samples or populations. A well documented example concerns the increase of the stature since the last 40-50 years. Based on the results taken from ID and AD databases, it is possible to determine the evolution of the mean values of stature for selected samples as well as for a global population [6]. Obviously the main difficulty to be solved is to get ensured that each sample is defined by the same criteria: sex, age, origin, sociocultural level,... An interesting result concerns the variability in morphology as well as in body proportions for the same samples of operators, but having different geographical origins. Another example is the choice of human body models to perform an ergonomical study using CAD technics. The main purpose is to define the amplitudes for adjusting the workplace according to postural, visual and reaching requirements of operators. So, the average operator is without interest. A better way to take into account is to define body dimensions of man-models according to the variability of lengths for key measures as eye-seat erected and buttock-knee length. A group of man-models can be easily derived if human variability can be modeled for these two measures. So, human proportions can be integrated as a criterion to define the working or the driving position. This can be performed using different man-models applications as ERGOMAN [4].

©CARS/Springer. All rights reserved.

3.2 Biostereometric (3-D) data processing

With the availability of 3-D automatized measurement systems, new kinds of large surveys are now achieved by different teams all around the world. So, using 3-D data shape analysis is theoritically available. But in a practical manner, summarizing shape, for example for sizing, still remains a challenge [7, 8]. Other difficulties to be solved concern the relations with classical 1-D anthropometric data and the definition of reference postures and landmarks for 3-D data capture. In fact, we first have to face a standardization problem with 3-D measurements. Then, it is necessary to define a common manner to store these data and how to process them. This goal needs to be attained very rapidly in order to preserve some opportunities to compare results from surveys based on 3-D capture as CAESAR [9]. A proposal for standardization of procedure for databases on this specific topic have been pointed out during the workshop held in Paris last June (1998) (Workshop on 3-D Anthropometry and Industrial Products Design) but more work needs to be completed on this topic.

4. Shape modeling driven by the product

Modern rapid prototyping is marked by a large amount of creating procedures which can be done computer aided. However, to create a new product or to define a new workplace when man-machine-interface is a key issue, we need to describe human shapes related to the interface. Based on 3-D as well as 1-D anthropometric data, digital models can be derived. The main difficulties are to summarize human shapes in terms of variability. Sizing determination is necessary with generally "small", "medium" and "large" models. The main question is to select the criteria that characterize the small, medium or large models. For example, the design of an oxygen mask or a fore-face requires the determination of digital models of face and heads. As dimensions describing height, width and depth of the head are not related together (r less than .4), it is not possible to define a global model including, for instance, the 5th percentile values for all measures.

One of the way to solve the problem is to identify the key dimensions related to the product. This is the real first step for an ergonomical study. These key dimensions are retained as constraints and provide the range of variation for the anatomical area concerned by the interface with the product. Then the other criteria can be defined as a function of the fixed constraints. For example, in the design of a fore-face, the shape modeling will not necessarily concerns all the face. The frontal and lateral areas are more critical than the central area (eye, nose, month) and the digital model can be reduced (and simplified) to the anatomical areas related to the interface with the profile of the fore-face. Due to the constraints of stability and of protection, the frontal width and the curvature of the associated frontal anatomical area are the key dimensions, and the range of variations are provided by the deformability of the material retained by the designer to elaborate the product.

To summarize this approach, the main issue is to identify the geometrical zones of the product that will create the constraints. The digital model will necessary fit these constraints. The other areas are less critical. However the same approach needs to be replicate for these areas to identify the amplitude of variation which can be compensated

©CARS/Springer. All rights reserved.

or not by the profile. So, the number of sizes to fit the variability of the population will depend of these constraints.

The result of this methodology is the determination of simplified, but well-adapted, digital models of human shape, according to the identified needs of the users and the technical constraints of the designers.

References

1. Churchill, E, Churchill, T, Kikta, P.- AMRL Anthropometric Data Bank Library : Volumes I-V (AMRL-TR-77-I, AD A047 314) 1977.
2. Coblentz, A.- Une Banque de Données de Biométrie Humaine.- Conférence "On Advancements in Retrieval Technology as related to information systems". Arlington. 20-21 Octobre 1973.- Neuilly-Sur-Seine : AGARD.- pp. 8.8-8.14.- (AGARD C.P.P. 207).
3. Coblentz, A., Mollard, R., Hennion, P.Y., Vernay, J.- Ergodata: databases in anthropometry and ergonomics.- In: Proceedings of the International Conference on Occupational Safety Health Ergonomics & Environment, Wuhan (China) , September 9-15, 1997, pp. B47-B53.
4. Mollard, R., Hennion, P.Y., Vernay, J., Coblentz, A.- ERGODATA: a dedicated database system for digital human modeling and ergonomics studies.- SAE International "Digital human modeling for design and engineering. The Hague (Netherlands) 18-20 May, 2000, 8 p. (CD-ROM).
5. Coblentz, A., Mollard, R., Renaud, C.- ERGOMAN : 3-D representation of human operator and man-machine systems.- International Journal of Human Factors in Manufacturing, 1991, pp. 168-178.
6. Mollard, R, Hennion, P.Y., Coblentz, A.- Morphological evolution of French military personnels.- In: 44th Annual Meeting of the Human Factors Society, San Diego, July 30-August 4, 2000, pp. 6.774-6.747.
7. Coblentz, A., Mollard, R., Ignazi, G.- Three dimensional face shape analysis of french adults. Application for the conception of protective equipment.- Ergonomics, 34, 4, 1991, pp. 497-517.
8. Mollard, R.- Analyse des formes de la face à l'aide de mesures 1-D et 3-D.- In : Journées d'études Anthropométrie 3-D et Conception de produits industriels, Paris, 25-26 Juin 1998, pp. 16-1/16-8.
9. Robinette, K.M.- CAESAR 3-D Anthropometric Database. The Civilian American and European Surface Anthropometry (CAESAR) project.- In : Proceedings of Workshop on 3D anthropometry and Industrial Products Design, Paris (France), June 25-26. 1998, pp. 18-1/18-3.

CARS 2002 – H.U. Lemke, M.W. Vannier; K. Inamura, A.G. Farman, K. Doi & J.H.C. Reiber (Editors)
©CARS/Springer. All rights reserved.

Medical image archives – present and future

Michael W. Vannier[1,2], Edward V. Staab[2], Laurence C. Clarke[2]
[1]University of Iowa, Iowa City, IA
[2]Biomedical Imaging Program, National Cancer Institute, Bethesda, MD

Abstract

Repositories, data warehouses, public archives, and multimedia databases, especially those containing images, are important for clinical practice, education, and research in medicine. Imaging modalities, such as digital radiography, computed tomography, ultrasonography, nuclear medicine, digital angiography and magnetic resonance imaging produce large amounts of data that are managed, archived, and reported using picture archiving and communications systems (PACS) in an integrated healthcare enterprise (IHE) infrastructure. The technology and applications of PACS and IHE are well understood and widely available worldwide.

However, typical PACS and IHE systems are closed to ensure privacy, security and confidentiality. Sharing of medical image databases is relatively new, despite the widespread prevalence of open public archives for other types of biological data, especially in genomics and proteomics. Bioinformatics often implies that sequence and not image information is the focus of interest. Medical image visualization, analysis and measurement are widely used, and should continue to grow in importance as computer and display technology continues to evolve.

The principles of medical image archives, repositories, data warehouses, and multimedia databases will be reviewed. The applications of publicly available data sets include research, both basic and clinically applied, on the development, testing and standardization of algorithms and heuristics for computer assisted diagnosis, for example. Data mining of clinical databases, especially those richly invested with images, may be beneficial in producing quantitative image-based metrics and biomarkers for disease presence, staging, treatment selection and planning, prognosis, and monitoring. The technical requirements for construction of publicly accessible medical image archives that are well suited to exploratory data analysis, synthesis and testing of diagnostic and prognostic quantitative image analysis methods, biomarker and surrogate endpoint testing, and computer aided diagnosis will be outlined.

Regulatory requirements for testing of quantitative medical image-based analysis methods are in development. The FDA requirements for electronic submission and review of medical image analysis devices will be described, and their impact on the technical requirements for publicly accessible medical image archives will be delineated.

Keywords: Archive, image database, research resource

©CARS/Springer. All rights reserved.

1. Introduction

Public libraries of printed works have evolved into open access repositories of documents, images, and media, sometimes known as digital libraries. [1] Molecular biologists share genome and related data in digital form on open access servers with portable open source software tools. [2] Biomedical signal databases have been constructed for open access to the academic community. [3] Recently, the concept of shared results from medical research has expanded beyond sequence information to include all forms of data that may be reused by other investigators. The successes of the molecular biology infrastructure are well known. It has provided the means for experts in computer science, mathematics and statistics to make significant contributions to this field from which, without the infrastructure, most of them would have been excluded. These successes are not necessarily unique to molecular biology, and the Biomedical Informatics Research Network (BIRN) initiative is aimed at building upon them and extending them to a wider set of biomedical research arenas. [4] In March 2002, the National Institutes of Health announced its data sharing policy, scheduled for implementation in 2003. [5] There are numerous shared medical image archive projects underway, notably the National Cancer Institute's Lung Image Database Consortium (LIDC) [6], RSNA Medical Imaging Resource Center (MIRC) [7], and other image repositories that will be introduced in this paper.

2. Medical image access policy

Access to medical images stored in repositories is essential for investigators who do not possess the resources to collect data of their own, for standardized comparisons of image analysis methods tested with the same input data, for regulatory approval of new medical devices, to develop new methods, and potentially for use in clinical decision support. Recently, new data sharing policies have been developed that govern access to medical data, including images.

2.1 NIH data sharing policy

Data sharing promotes many goals of the National Institutes of Health's (NIH) research endeavor. It is particularly important for unique data that cannot be readily replicated. Data sharing allows scientists to expedite the translation of research results into knowledge, products, and procedures to improve human health. The NIH is developing a statement on data sharing that expects and supports the timely release and sharing of final research data from NIH-supported studies for use by other researchers. Investigators submitting an NIH application will be required to include a plan for data sharing or explain why data sharing is not possible. This statement will apply to extramural scientists seeking grants, cooperative agreements, and contracts as well as intramural investigators. [5]

2.2 Background

There are many reasons to share data from NIH-supported studies. Sharing data reinforces open scientific inquiry, encourages diversity of analysis and opinion, promotes new research, makes possible the testing of new or alternative hypotheses and methods of

©CARS/Springer. All rights reserved.

analysis, supports studies on data collection methods and measurement, facilitates the education of new researchers, enables the exploration of topics not envisioned by the initial investigators, and permits the creation of new data sets when data from multiple sources are combined. By avoiding the duplication of expensive data collection activities, the NIH is able to support more investigators than it could if similar data had to be collected de novo by each applicant.

NIH-supported basic research, clinical studies, surveys, and other types of research produce data that may be shared. However, NIH recognizes that sharing data about human research subjects presents special challenges. The rights and privacy of people who participate in NIH-sponsored research must be protected at all times. Thus, data intended for broader use should be free of identifiers that would permit linkages to individual research participants and variables that could lead to deductive disclosure of individual subjects. Similarly, NIH recognizes the need to protect patentable and other proprietary data and the restriction on data sharing that may be imposed by agreements with third parties. It is not the intent of this statement to discourage, impede, or prohibit the development of commercial products from federally funded research.

There are many ways to share data. Sometimes data are included in publications. Investigators may distribute data under their own auspices. Some investigators have placed data sets in public archives while others have put data on a web site, building in protections for privacy through the software while allowing analysis of the data. Restricted access data centers or data enclaves facilitate analyses of data too sensitive to share through other means. All of these options achieve the goals of data sharing. A web-based image archive was developed at the NIH Center for Information Technology to support data sharing. [8] However, the NIH also recognizes that in some particular instances sharing data may not be feasible. For example, studies with very small samples or those collecting particularly sensitive data should be shared only if stringent safeguards exist to ensure confidentiality and protect the identity of subjects while recognizing the contribution of the investigators who designed the protocol and collected the data.

2.3 National Cancer Institute - Biomedical Imaging Program (BIP)

The National Cancer Institute (NCI) is the component of the NIH that investigates, develops and applies new methods for patients with cancer. The Biomedical Imaging Program (BIP) in the Division of Cancer Treatment and Diagnosis at NCI is the principal resource for oncologic imaging for the full range of applications from the molecular level to intact patient. The NCI BIP funds the American College of Radiology Imaging Network (ACRIN) to conduct multicenter trials of cancer imaging.

2.3.1 ACRIN image access policy

ACRIN archives the images collected in cancer clinical imaging trials under its protocols. For example, the Diagnostic Mammographic Imaging Screening Trial (DMIST, http://www.dmist.org) will collect digital mammograms from almost 50,000 patients and place all of the data in an electronic archive. ACRIN has developed a policy under NCI guidance for sharing data after completion of its clinical trials, by allowing access to qualified investigators who were not involved in recruiting subjects or performing examinations. [9]

©CARS/Springer. All rights reserved.

2.3.2 Lung Imaging Database Consortium (LIDC)

Preliminary clinical studies show that spiral CT scanning of the lungs can improve early detection of lung cancer in high-risk individuals. However, more clinical data are needed before public health recommendations can be made for population-based screening. Image processing algorithms have the potential to assist in lesion detection and characterization on spiral CT studies, and to assess the stability or change in lesion size on serial CT studies. The use of such computer-assisted algorithms could significantly enhance the sensitivity and specificity of spiral CT lung screening, as well as lower costs by reducing physician time needed for interpretation. The LIDC initiative [6] receives BIP support for a consortium of five institutions to develop consensus guidelines for a spiral CT lung image resource and to construct a database of spiral CT lung images. The investigators funded under this initiative will create a set of guidelines and metrics for database use and develop a database as a test-bed and showcase for those methods. The database will be available to researchers and users through the Internet and will have wide utility as a research resource.

2.3.3 BIP image archive advisory committee and workshops

An advisory committee met for workshops in 2000 and 2001 [9,10] to advise the BIP on the need, feasibility and approach to a common archival system for storing and accessing imaging databases by the broad scientific community. This work continues with open communications to all interested parties through a public moderated listserver, archive-comm-l at http://list.nih.gov. Comments on this paper and related matters are encouraged and may be entered in the listserver by sending e-mail to archive-comm-l@list.nih.gov

3.0 Medical image archives

Several important initiatives are underway to assemble and distribute medical image data to investigators to develop and test new post-processing and visualization methods. A searchable list of websites for archives is available through the University of California at San Diego at http://odwin.ucsd.edu/idata/

3.1 BIRN – Biomedical Imaging Research Network

The BIRN is an NIH National Center for Research Resources (NCRR) initiative aimed at creating a testbed to address biomedical researchers' need to access and analyze data at a variety of levels of aggregation located at diverse sites throughout the USA. [4] The BIRN testbed will bring together hardware and develop software necessary for a scalable network of databases and computational resources. Issues of user authentication, data integrity, security, and data ownership will also be addressed.

The plan for the testbed is to focus on research involving neuroimaging to take advantage of the relatively advanced level of sophistication of this community in the use of information technology. An essential feature of the testbed will be creation of infrastructure that can be deployed rapidly at other research centers throughout the country, that may have research emphases outside of neuroimaging. This means that in addition to scalability, the software/hardware must be reusable and extensible.

The BIRN testbed will draw heavily on resources of the next generation internet that is funded by the National Science Foundation for both design and implementation. The

©CARS/Springer. All rights reserved.

initial awards join General Clinical Research Centers and co-located Biomedical Technology Research Resources to establish the necessary infrastructure in the context of ongoing neuroimaging research projects. Support for "system integrators" that coordinate network, grid, and data mining software development as well as hardware configurations will be awarded to a recognized leader in such technical development and service efforts.

To contain the scope of the testbed, the BIRN initiative is initially focused on neuroimaging and is supporting several virtual neuroimaging research centers, each of which spans multiple leading academic and clinical institutions.

3.2 Craniofacial image archive

The Craniofacial Imaging Laboratory at the Cleft Palate and Craniofacial Deformities Institute, St. Louis Children's Hospital, Washington University Medical Center, has developed an electronic archive for the storage of computed tomography image digital data that is independent of scanner hardware and independent of units of storage media (i.e., floppy disks and optical disks). [12] The archive represents one of the largest repositories of high-quality computed tomography data of children with craniofacial deformities in the world. Archiving reconstructed image data is essential for comparative imaging, surgical simulation, quantitative analysis, and use with solid model fabrication (e.g., stereolithography). One tertiary craniofacial center's experience in the establishment and maintenance of such an archive through three generations of storage technology is reported. The current archive is housed on an external 35-GB hard drive attached to a Windows-based desktop server. Data in the archive were categorized by specific demographics into groups of patients, number of scans, and diagnoses.

The Craniofacial Imaging Laboratory archive currently contains computed tomography image digital data for 1827 individual scans. Storage of CT image data in a digital archive allows for continuous upgrading of image display and analysis software and facilitates longitudinal and cross-sectional studies. Internet access for clinical and research purposes is feasible, contingent on protection of patient confidentiality and investigator's rights or recognition.

3.3 Radiology teaching files and RSNA's MIRC

The importance of electronic images for teaching medicine and especially radiology has been enhanced by linkage to PACS [13] and the AFIP collection. [14] The Radiological Society of North America (RSNA) is developing a Medical Imaging Resource Center (MIRC). The goal is to develop a central repository for medical images, as well as related text, in support of projects related to research, education, and clinical care. PACS vendors should provide much more sophisticated tools to create and annotate teaching file images in an easy to use but standard format (possibly RSNA's MIRC format) that could be exchanged with other sites and other vendors' PAC systems. The privilege to create teaching or conference files should be given to the individual radiologists, technologists, and other users, and an audit should be kept of who has created these files, as well as keep track of who has accessed the files. Vendors should maintain a local PACS library of image quality phantoms, normal variants, and interesting cases and should have the capability of accessing central image repositories such as the RSNA's MIRC images.

©CARS/Springer. All rights reserved.

4. Conclusion

Sharing medical image data on public repositories is expected to facilitate the development of image analysis tools and results. Several examples of new policy guidelines for electronic access to images from repositories were given to illustrate how these archives are organized and operated. Many more examples exist, and new medical image archive initiatives are announced each year. In time, we can measure the impact of this fundamental change in the culture of medical imaging research. Importantly, the current format standard for this data is DICOM [15], and electronic images may be useful for regulatory purposes in FDA review of new drugs and devices. [16]

References

1. Nadkarni PM. Information retrieval in medicine: overview and applications. J Postgrad Med 2000 Apr-Jun;46(2):116-22.
2. Entrez at http://www.ncbi.nlm.nih.gov/Database/
3. A. Cohen and I. Korhonen, eds. Biomedical Signal Databases, special issue of IEEE Engineering in Medicine and Biology Magazine (20) 3: 2-85, 2001.
4. http://birn.ncrr.nih.gov/
5. NIH data sharing policy at http://grants.nih.gov/grants/policy/data_sharing/
6. Clarke LP, Croft BY, Staab E, et al. National Cancer Institute initiative: Lung image database resource for imaging research. Acad Radiol 2001 May;8(5):447-50
7. http://mirc.rsna.org/ and http://rsna.org/mirc/
8. E B. Suh, S Warach, H Cheung, et al.. A Web-Based Medical Image Archive System. SPIE Medical Imaging Conference, San Diego, CA. 2001.
9. ACRIN archived images access policy, http://www.acrin.org/archivepolicy.html
10. National Cancer Institute, Biomedical Imaging Program. Image archive workshop report (2000) at http://cancer.gov/bip
11. Staab E, Clarke LP, Baker H, Sullivan D. NCI image archive management workshop: a preliminary report. Acad Radiol 2001 Jul;8(7):690-1.
12. Perlyn CA, Marsh JL, Vannier MW, et al. The craniofacial anomalies archive at St. Louis Children's Hospital: 20 years of craniofacial imaging experience. Plast Reconstr Surg. 2001 Dec;108(7):1862-70.
13. Siegel E, Reiner B. Electronic teaching files: Seven-year experience using a commercial picture archiving and communication system. J Digit Imaging 2001 Jun;14(2 Suppl 1):125-7.
14. Williams BH, Mullick FG, Becker RL, Kyte RT, Noe A. A national treasure goes online: The Armed Forces Institute of Pathology. MD Comput 1998 Jul-Aug; 15(4):260-5.
15. DICOM website at http://medical.nema.org/
16. FDA Center for Drug Evaluation and Research's Electronic Regulatory Submissions and Review (ERSR) web page at http://www.fda.gov/cder/regulatory/ersr/

CARS 2002 – H.U. Lemke, M.W. Vannier; K. Inamura, A.G. Farman, K. Doi & J.H.C. Reiber (Editors)
©CARS/Springer. All rights reserved.

3D description of the human body shape: application of Karhunen-Loève expansion to the CAESAR database

Zouhour Ben Azouz [a, b], Marc Rioux [a], Richard Lepage [b]
[a] Visual Information Technology Group
Institute for Information Technology, National Research Council
[b] Laboratoire d'imagerie de vision et d'intelligence artificille
École de Technologie supérieure de Montréal

Abstract

In this Paper, the Kurhunen-loève expansion is used for a compact 3D description of the human body shape. A set of eigenvectors is extracted from the CAESAR (Civilian American and European Surface Anthropometry Resource) database to define a basis for the human body shape space. Experimental results including the variation of the eigenvectors number with the size of the training set are presented.

Keywords: 3D Anthropometry, Karhunen-loève expansion

1. Introduction

The measurement of the human body (Anthropometry) is an essential part of the engineering design of cars, aircraft, workspaces, and clothing, to name a few. Traditionally such measurements involve the linear distances between anatomic landmarks and the circumference values at predefined locations. Practically, such measurements are limited to a set of about 100 values.

The main limitations of the traditional approach are the following:
- The set of values collected is so small that the only valid attempt to reconstruct the original shape is limited to very simple geometries.
- In most cases the set of unconnected (unregistered) values does not provide an accurate reconstruction of the original subject. Reconstruction ambiguities are due to the lack of a coordinate reference system.
- Surface shape is lost, and all attempts to reconstruct it from model-based approaches have yet to be validated.

A recently developed technology (Full body 3D digitizing [1]) allows increasing the number of measurements from a hundred to a million, and, in a small fraction of the time required by traditional measurement method. Furthermore each value in the data set is related to a common coordinate system, allowing an accurate and detailed 3D reconstruction.

The challenge now is to analyze the human body shape variability using statistical methods applied to a very large data set. This paper is proposing a method to achieve this goal. A number of methods have been proposed in the literature to represent 3D shapes. As an example, the wavelet transform allows multi-resolution description of 3D shapes [2]. However, the huge number of generated coefficients makes this tool far from

©CARS/Springer. All rights reserved.

providing a compact description. Superquadrics and hyperquadrics [3] have also been used for very compact description of 3D shapes but the complexity of the human body topology is too high for such a representation.

In the approach presented in this paper we consider the fact that the analysed 3D objects belongs to the same family. Intuitively we can think that the family is low dimensional. It follows that any member might be represented by a small number of parameters. The Karhunen-Loève expansion [4] is used to extract a small set of shapes, which allow the reconstruction of any of the shapes contained in the data set. The basic approach is similar to the one used in face recognition [5]. The data set here is three-dimensional data and the extracted shapes will be named "eigen-persons" equivalently to the "eigenfaces" obtained in face recognition experiments.

2.Method

2.1 CAESAR

The data used in this work has been collected within the CAESAR project (Civilian American and European Surface Anthropometry Resource) [6]. It is the first 3-D surface anthropometry survey performed in both U.S. and Europe. The CAESAR project is a collaborative effort with partners from several countries such as the Air Force Research Laboratory (AFRL) in Ohio, the Society of Automotive Engineers (SAE), the Netherlands Organization of the Applied Scientific Research (TNO) and the National Research Council of Canada (NRC).
During this project, body measurements have been taken for people between the ages of 18 and 65 in three countries: U.S, The Netherlands, and Italy, The most important data recorded are full body 3-D scans of people in three postures. Two scanners were employed, a Cyberware WB4 scanner in the United States and Italy, and a Vitronic scanner in The Netherlands.

2.2 Data pretreatment

For the purpose of this work we assume that the height of the human body is uncorrelated with its shape. In other words a short person and a tall person could have the same shape even though they don't have the same height.

Although within the traditional anthropometric studies, the human height is a measure that has been largely investigated, the description of the human shape is still a challenge. That is why in this work we eliminated the variability related to the height by normalizing the height of all the persons in the database.

Before the normalization though, it is important to align all the persons in order to have a common center of gravity. After alignment and normalization, the variability in the 3D data corresponds only to the variability of shape.

We adopted a voxel description of the 3D data. In this case a cube of 1m of dimensions has been sampled to n voxels, where $n = (200)^3$. A function describing the occupancy of those voxels is equal to one if the voxel contains at least one point, and zero otherwise.

©CARS/Springer. All rights reserved.

2.3. Karhunen-Loève expansion

We consider the use of the Karhunen-Loève expansion, also known as Principal Component Analysis (PCA) [7] on the 3D data. The main idea of the approach is to find vectors which best account for the distribution of the body shape within the entire shape space.

Each 3D person is converted into a vector form $\vec{\Psi}_i$ describing the occupancy of the n voxels. The mean person over a set of N persons is given by:

$$\overline{\Psi} = \frac{1}{N}\sum_{i=1}^{N}\vec{\Psi}_i \qquad (2.1)$$

Deviation vectors $\vec{\Phi}_i$ are generated (Equation 2.2) and arranged in a data set matrix A (Equation 2.3).

$$\vec{\Phi}_i = \vec{\Psi}_i - \overline{\Psi} \qquad (2.2)$$

$$A = \left[\vec{\Phi}_1\,\vec{\Phi}_2\,\ldots\ldots\ldots\vec{\Phi}_N\right] \qquad (2.3)$$

The eigenvectors of the covariance matrix C form the orthonormal basis that optimally spans the subspace of the human shape.

$$C = A^T A \qquad (2.4)$$

The eigenvectors, and their corresponding eigenvalues, of this n x n symmetric matrix C are ranked such that $(\lambda_i > \lambda_j)$ for $(i < j)$.

The magnitude of λ_j is equal to the variance in the data set spanned by its corresponding eigenvector $\vec{u}_j$ as shown in Equation 2.5.

$$\lambda_j = \sigma_j^2 = \frac{1}{N}\sum_{i=1}^{N}\vec{\Phi}_i . \vec{u}_j \qquad (2.5)$$

It then follows that any vector $\vec{\Phi}_i$ in the data set, A, can be optimally approximated as shown in Equation 2.6. Thus, the n-dimensional body shape deviation vector can be re-defined as a linear combination of eigenvectors determined by M coefficients denoted by c_{ij} (computed using Equation 2.7).

$$\vec{\Phi}_i \approx \sum_{j=1}^{M} c_{ij}\,\vec{u}_j \quad 0 \le M \le n \qquad (2.6)$$

$$c_{ij} = \vec{\Phi}_i . \vec{u}_j \qquad (2.7)$$

Computing the $(n = 200^3)$ eigenvectors and eigenvalues of C is however impractical. Determining the eigenvectors $\vec{u}_i'$ and eigenvalues λ_j' of the $N \times N$ matrix given by Equation 2.8 represents a computationally feasible alternative to resolve the problem.

$$C' = AA^T \qquad (2.8)$$

In fact, since the number of persons is less than the number of voxels $(N < n)$, there will be only N meaningful eigenvectors rather than n. Moreover, the first N eigenvalues and eigenvectors of C are directly computed as given by Equations 2.9 and 2.10.

©CARS/Springer. All rights reserved.

$$\lambda_i = \lambda_i^{'} \; \forall i \in [0, N-1] \qquad (2.9)$$

$$\vec{u}_i = \frac{1}{\sqrt{\lambda_i}} \vec{u}_i^{'} \; \forall i \in [0, N-1] \qquad (2.10)$$

The quality of the reconstruction is dependant on the fraction of the total variance contained in the M eigenvectors used in the reconstruction. This fraction is given by the equation 2.11

$$q_M = \sum_{i=1}^{M} \lambda_i \Big/ \sum_{i=1}^{N} \lambda_i \qquad (2.11)$$

Thus each 3-D body scan will be characterized by a set of M coefficients, which represent a compact and reliable description.

3. Results

3.1 Reconstruction of human body using a set of eigenpersons

We applied the above method on a subset of the CAESAR database. Three hundred scans of male subjects in the standing posture have been used to extract a set of eigenpersons. The experimental results show that 185 eigenpersons span a space representing 80% of the variability induced by the training set. The first 5 eigenpersons are shown in the figure1. Only voxels corresponding to positive values are visualized.

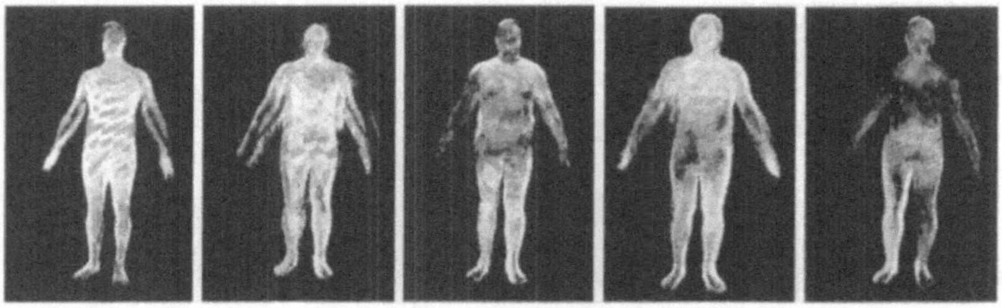

Figure 1. The first 5 eigenpersons. The visualized points correspond to voxels having positive values.

Figure 2 illustrates the original scans of two subjects included in the training set (2a and 2d), their corresponding sampled data (2b and 2e) and their reconstructed shapes (2c and 2f). Note the precise reconstruction of those two scans.

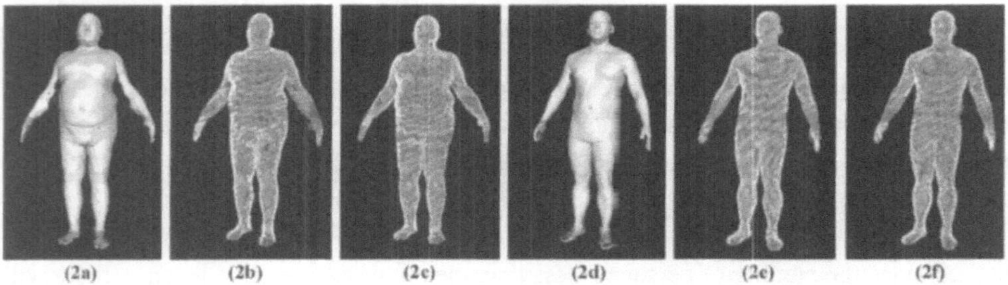

Figure 2. Original scans of subjects included in the training set (2a and 2d), corresponding sampled data (2b and 2e) and reconstructed shapes (2c and 2f).

©CARS/Springer. All rights reserved.

The reconstruction of the subject illustrated in figure 3a is less precise using only 185 eigenpersons. We notice though the improvement (figure 3.c) using 260 eigenpersons. The fraction of variability spanned by those eigenpersons is 95% of the total variability.

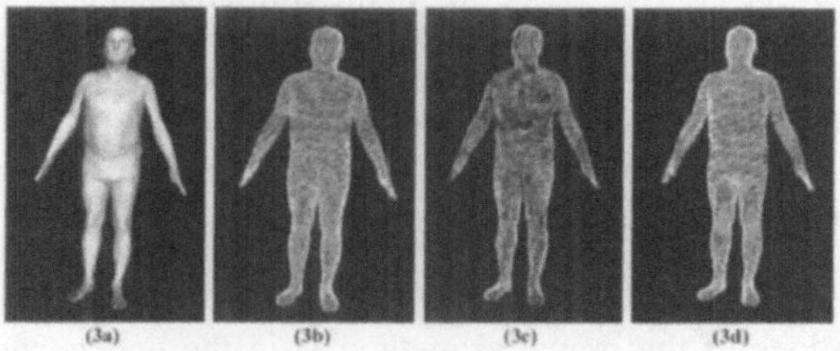

Figure 3. Reconstruction of a subject included in the training set using different numbers of eigenpersons. Original scan (3a), sampled data (3b), reconstruction with 185 eigenpersons (3c) and reconstruction with 260 eigenpersons (3d).

The reconstruction of the two persons non-included in the training set (figure 4c, 4f) is quite precise. The reconstruction could be improved with an appropriate choice of the training set.

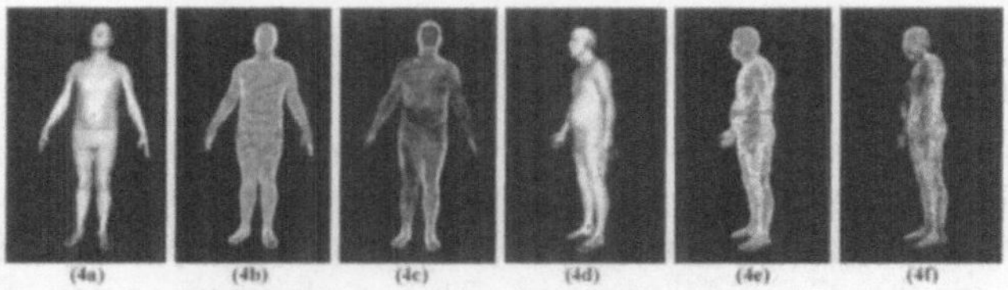

Figure 4. Original scans of 2 subjects non-included in the training set (4a and 4d), corresponding sampled data (4b and 4e) and reconstructed shapes (4c and 4f).

3.2 Variation of the eigenpersons number with the size of the training set

The proposed approach was applied to different embedded sets of human body scans in order to study the variation of the number of the eigenpersons required to span 80% of the variability induced by the training set.

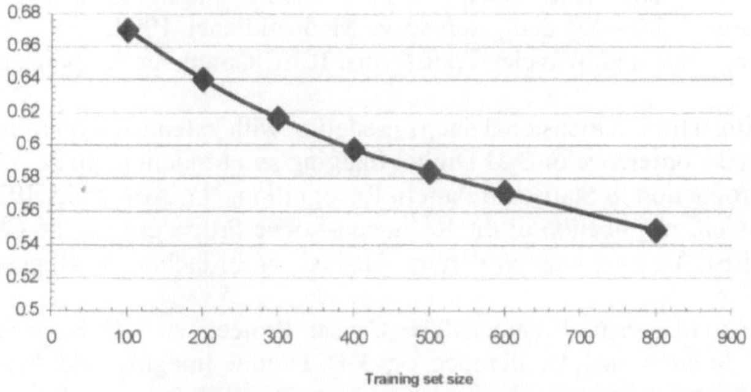

Figure 5 Variation of the ratio of the eigenpersons number needed to span 80% of the variability and the size of the training set

©CARS/Springer. All rights reserved.

The decrease of the ratio of the eigenpersons number and the size of the training set (figure 5) prove that the increase of the eigenpersons number will be insignificant from a certain training set size. Which mean that we can extract from this training set a group of eigenpersons that can span a wide variability in the entire human body shape space.

During this preliminary study, the 3-D scans used represent a reduced number of polygons(20000). We expect that using models of full resolution(300000 polygons) will reduce the number of the required eigenpersons and so enhance the compactness of the developed description of the human body.

4. Applications

One of the applications of the proposed method is in the understanding of the human shape variability and its distribution for a given population in the design of products such as seats, workstations and clothing. In clothing applications for example, a better understanding of the human shape variability should lead to an improved sizing strategy reducing inventory and unsold items. In computer simulation for the design of automobiles, the method should allow the validation of human models and help in the selection of cases representative of the target population to which such car models are designed.

5. Conclusion

This paper presented an approach to describe the human body shape which allows 3D reconstruction for visual evaluation of human models, either real or computer generated. It also gives a new tool for the statistical analysis of 3D anthropometric data such as the ones collected in the CAESAR project. This preliminary study shows that the representation is compact since a 3D model of human body containing thousands of polygons could be characterized by a few hundred coefficients.

References

1. K..M. Robinette, M.W. Vannier, M. Rioux, and P.R.M. Jones, 3-D Surface Anthropometry : Review of Technologies (L'Anthropométrie de surface en trois dimensions: examen des technologies). Neuilly-sur-Seine: North Atlantic Treaty Organization Advisory Group for Aerospace Research & Development, Aerospace Medical Panel, 1997.
2. S.Muraki. Volume Data and Wavelet Transforms. IEEE Computer Graphics and Applications, pp.50-56, 1993.
3. M.Ohuchi, T.Saito. Three-dimensional shape modeling with extended hyperquadrics.
4. Third International Conference on 3-D Digital Imaging and Modeling, pp 262-269, 2001.
5. K.Fukunaga, Introduction to Statistical Pattern Recognition. NY Academic, 1972.
6. M.Kirby, L.Sirovich. Application of the Karhunen-Loève Procedure for the Characterisation of Human Faces. IEEE Transactions on Pattern Analysis and Machine Intelligence, (1): 103-108, 1990.
7. K. M. Robinette, H.Daanen, E.Paquet The Caesar Project: A 3-D Surface Anthropometry Survey. Second International Conference on 3-D Digital Imaging and Modeling, pp. 380-386,1999.
8. L.Lebart, A. Morineau, M.Piron. Statistique exploratoire multidimensionnelle. Dunod 1995.

CARS 2002 – H.U. Lemke, M.W. Vannier; K. Inamura, A.G. Farman, K. Doi & J.H.C. Reiber (Editors)
©CARS/Springer. All rights reserved.

Recent advances in Korean anthropometry

Youngsuk LEE
Chonnam National University, Youngbongdong 300, Gwangju, Korea

Abstract

Anthropometry deals with the measurement of human body by 2D data and certain other physical characteristics of the human body by 3D data such as volumes, proportions, body contours and body silhouette. Here we would like to introduce part of what has been done in Korea, concerning anthropometric surveys and their applications to provide informations for products design.

Keywords: Anthropometry, products, design, body

1. Introduction

It has become generally recognized that both workplaces and products which are related to the human body, must be designed with reference to body measurements and the range of movement of the people concerned in mind. In the new trend of globalization, one may think that all humans may one day finally not be very different from each other, eating other country dishes, dressing more or less all in the same manner, behaving along a more unified way of thinking. This is already true to a certain extent, and the trend with several pauses and reactional short periods, will probably continue. But, interestingly one of the most important element of globalization (beside profit), the ever widespreading of information all over the world, seems to contain in itself the necessity of taking more and more in account the characteristic of individuals. Indeed, the technological information age means also that every producer and market researcher looks more and more towards any information he can get about his customers (behavior, society, cultural and physical features), to try to maximize his market. He may try to do without, but then may risk much, for others will probably not do so. Another aspect of the dissemination of information and knowledge is also that consumers all over the world become at the same time more educated and will no doubt be more and more choosy. The average individual will probably not be too dissatisfied to have more or less an average product, as long as it fits well its desire and also his physical features. In one word, products will have to suit much more individuals. In the field of clothing as in many others, advertisement will have to be paired increasingly with quality and suitably and rely somewhat less on consumer psychology. Individuals, even those who follow fashion trends, will give their preference to those producers who can produce garments which suit most their physical features. The importance of good physical statistics, by countries, ages, sexes and in multiracial societies, races or interracial types must be then emphasized. Indeed such statistics allow to define some virtual individual average shape for each classes, to recognize the growing importance of them and changes occuring with the passing of time. Here we would like to introduce part of what has done in Korea, concerning anthropometric surveys and anthropometric applications.

©CARS/Springer. All rights reserved.

2. Methods

2.1 Korean national survey

The first national anthropometry survey in Korea was conducted in 1979 by the Korean government division, the National Institute of Technology and Quality. It collected at the time, data concerning 17,000 samples residing in various parts of the country from the age of six to fifty. A number of 117 measurement dimensions were taken, using calipers and tape measure. Thanks to these data, the NITQ established 46 items defining Korean standards concerning clothes, furniture, desk and chairs. 41 of them (KS0035 to KS0096) concerned the size designations of men's wear, women's wear, brassieres and socks. After this survey, the Korean government presented a national anthropometric survey every 5 or 6 years. In 1997, the 4th rather large-scale anthropometric survey was carried out throughout the country and samples were selected more randomly to get better representative anthropometric data. Surveys showed how much Korean individual's physical features had changed during these last 10 years: with economic development and better health facilities, height, body proportion and even face shapes had evolved and were still changing. A new need for re-examination of some Korean standards was again acknowledged, specially those relating to body size: clothes, shoes, headgear and the like. Thus, 1998 has been thus the year of data analysis research conducted for the definition of a new body size classification updating the garment sizing system for Koreans, the year 1999 concerned with the standardization of shoe sizing system, and the year 2000 concerned with the headgear sizing and the table sizing . The 5th survey will be performed in 2003 using 2D and 3D method. The basic informations for the Korean national surveys are shown in Table 1.

	1st survey	2nd survey	3rd survey	4th survey	5th survey
Year	1979	1986	1992	1997	2003
Age	6-50yrs	6-50yrs	6-50yrs	1-70yrs	1-0yrs
Samples	17.000	21.650	8.800	13.000	20.000
Dimension	117	80	84	120	200
Method	2D	2D	2D	2D	2D+3D
Application	Establish 46 korean standard (KS K 0031 etc)	Updated 41 Korean standard (KS K 0034 etc)	Updated 44 Korean standard (KS G 2016 etc)	Updated Korean standard (KS K 0051, KS G 3405 etc)	

Table 1. Korean national surveys

CARS 2002 – H.U. Lemke, M.W. Vannier; K. Inamura, A.G. Farman, K. Doi & J.H.C. Reiber (Editors)
©CARS/Springer. All rights reserved.

2.2 Human modelling by age

With the data which were obtained from national survey, we compared the body shape by age. Figure 1 and 2 show the comparison of the body shape between different age groups. We found that there were few significant differences in body depth between young and middle age groups. All these differences need to be reflected to design products.

Human Modeling (Korean Man)

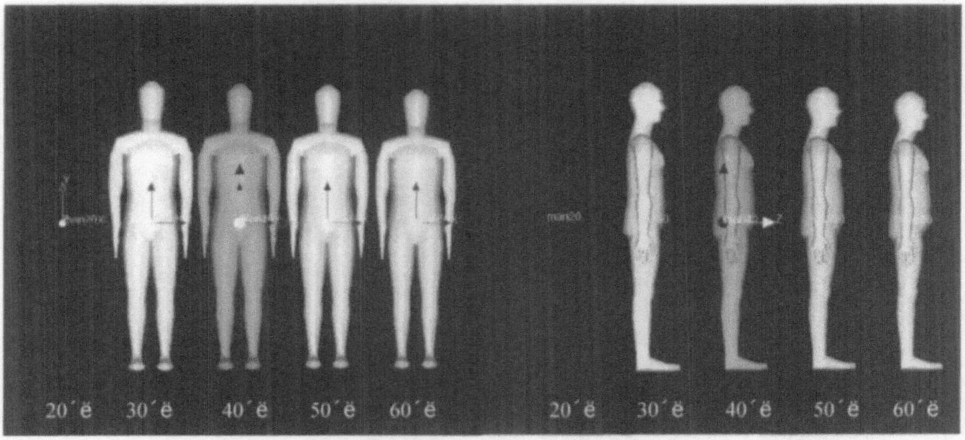

Chon-nam National Univ.Lee.Y.S

Human Modeling (Korean woman)

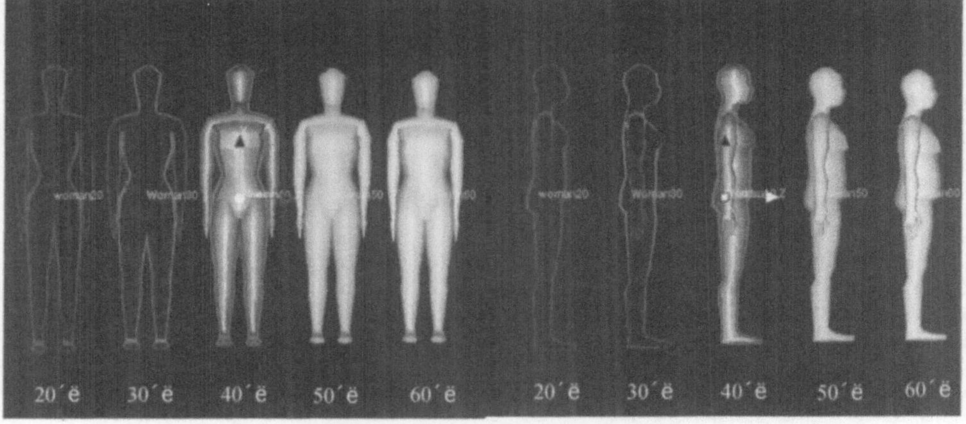

Chon-nam National Univ.Lee.Y.S

©CARS/Springer. All rights reserved.

2.3 Human sensibility ergonomics for products design

The human sensibility concept originated in Japan with professor Nagamachi, who measured a large range of human senses using the SD method, intending to take advantage of all the data he could get to help the industry, makes better products fitting the human individual and its never ending desire for comfort. In this study we also tried to analysis the breast shape to provide the wearing comfort when women wear innerwear. The breast shapes were measured by 2D and 3D method. Several breast shapes are shown in Figure 3. From these figures we can see the different breast lines and shapes. The elements of the shape should be considered for design concept.

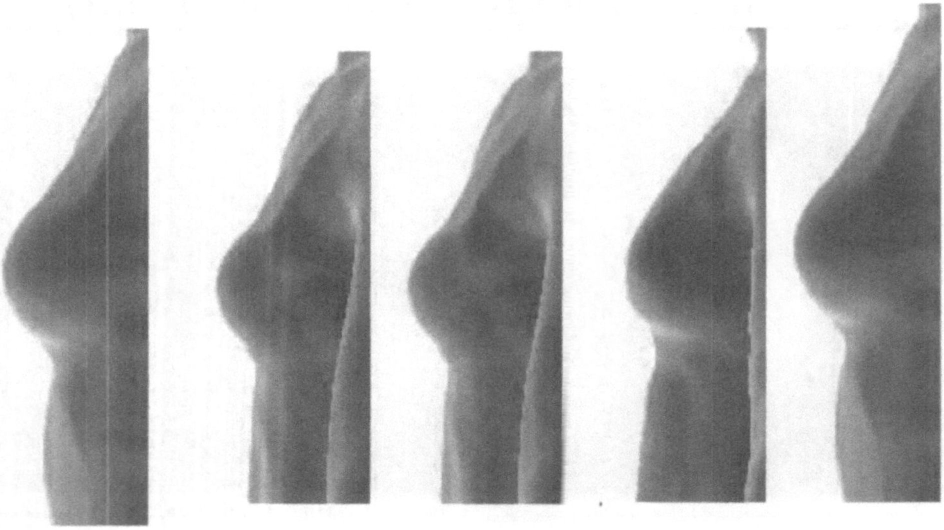

Figure 3 The comparison of different breast shapes

Figure 4 and 5 show the Korean women model in average size.

Acknowledgement

This research was supported in part by a grant-in-aid for G7 research project from the ministry of Korea science and. Engineering foundation.

References

1. Youngsuk LEE : Anthropometry I, The measure of man, korea, 1999..
2. Youngsuk LEE : Anthropometry II, The measure of woman, korea, 1999..
3. Youngsuk LEE : Anthropometry III, The measure of youth, korea, 1999..
4. Youngsuk LEE : Anthropometry IV, The measure of infant, korea, 1999..

CARS 2002 – H.U. Lemke, M.W. Vannier; K. Inamura, A.G. Farman, K. Doi & J.H.C. Reiber (Editors)
©CARS/Springer. All rights reserved.

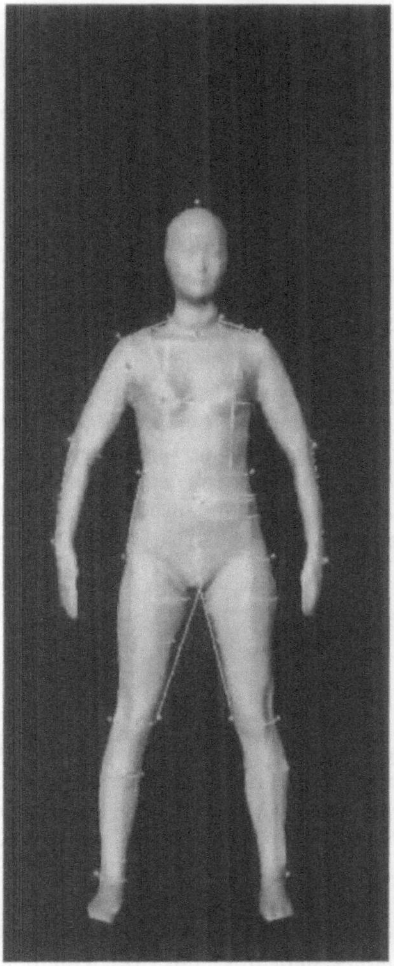

Figure 4 3D scan data

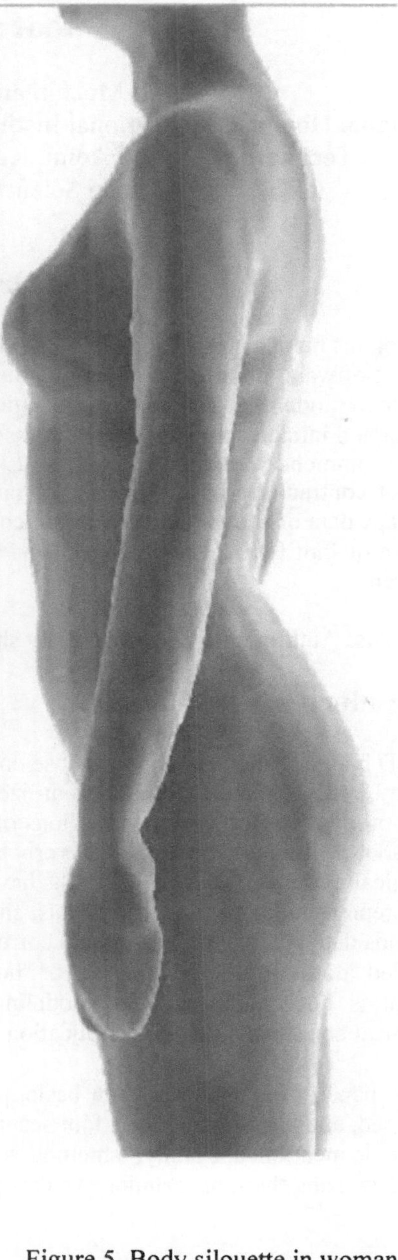

Figure 5 Body silouette in woman

©CARS/Springer. All rights reserved.

Automatic shape modeling of the foot: towards a database of foot shapes

Masaaki Mochimaru[a,b], Makiko Kouchi[a,b]
[a] Digital Human Lab., National Institute of Advanced Industrial Science and Technology, 2-41-6 Aomi, Koto-ku, Tokyo 135-0064 JAPAN
[b] CREST, JST (Japan Science and Technology Corporation)

Abstract

Homologous human shape modeling is critical to utilize 3D human body data for product design. Software libraries for homologous modeling were developed and application software to model the foot form was also developed using the libraries. This software was incorporated into a compact low-cost foot scanner. With the scanning system, retailers can select/recommend well-fitting shoes to customers. By storing a copy of scanned data that does not contradict with the privacy of customers, customers can enjoy browsing their foot shape data or shopping in electronic commerce. This system is useful to make a large database of foot forms. Possible problems in making a large database in this manner are discussed.

Keywords: Anthropometry, human body shape, foot

1. Introduction

With 3D body scanners, a large database on body dimensions and forms can be developed efficiently. It is difficult, however, to utilize the information on the 3D human body forms for the product design only with millions of surface data points and dozens of anatomical landmarks. Millions data points are verbose to describe a body form, and they have no anatomical correspondence. Landmarks have anatomical correspondence, but they are too few to represent the surface form. Thus, shape representation methods using hundreds to thousands data points with anatomical correspondence have been proposed. Such methods are called "normalized modeling" [1] or "homologous shape modeling" [2]. The modeling protocol is not unique, but the modeling guideline is defined reasonably based on anatomical correspondence and application purposes of the models.

In this paper, the common and basic protocols for the homologous modeling are mentioned, and development of a foot scanning system with an automatic shape modeling software is mentioned. Finally, a method is proposed for collecting a large amount of foot shape data using the foot scanning systems installed in shoe retailers.

CARS 2002 – H.U. Lemke, M.W. Vannier; K. Inamura, A.G. Farman, K. Doi & J.H.C. Reiber (Editors)
©CARS/Springer. All rights reserved.

2. Homologous shape modeling

2.1 Basic modules designed for homologous shape modeling

We have developed several homologous shape models for different body parts. Fig. 1(a) shows a torso model for developing a dressmaking dummy [3]. It consists of 547 data points (1039 polygons) defined based on 25 landmarks. Fig. 1(b) is a face model for designing a spectacle frame, which consists of 211 data points (366 polygons) based on 61 anatomical landmarks [4]. A foot model for shoe last design is shown in Fig. 1(c). This model has 295 data points (586 polygons) defined based on 9 landmarks [2]. Common and basic protocols for the geometrical processing to generate homologous models are as follows:

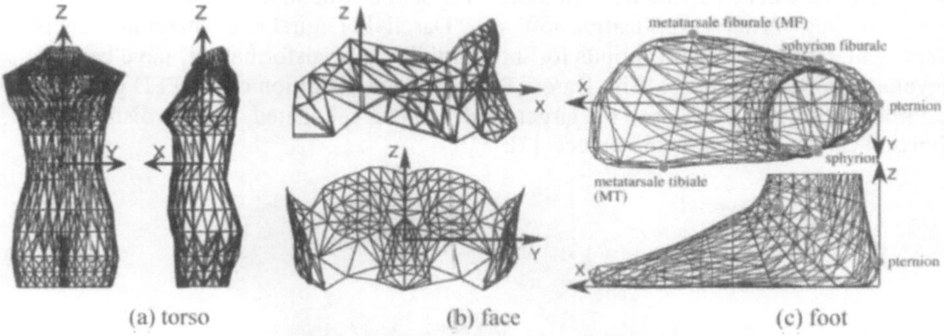

Fig. 1: Homologous shape modeling.

A. Generation of an interpolated point: calculate equidistant dividing points of a shortest surface distance between two landmarks.

B. Generation of a cross section

(b-1) The cross section is defined by three landmarks.

(b-2) The cross section is perpendicular to the coordinate plane and contains two landmarks.

(b-3) The cross section is parallel to the coordinate plane and contains one landmark.

C. Generation of dividing points on a cross section

(c-1) The center of the cross section is defined as the centroid or a uniquely defined point such as the midpoint of two landmarks. The contour of the cross section is divided into segments by the same angular interval. The starting point on the contour is defined by the axis of coordinates.

(c-2) The contour of the cross section is divided into segments by the same distance interval of contour line instead of the same angular interval.

(c-3) The whole contour of the cross section is divided into segments by the lines connecting the center of the cross section and landmarks projected on the plane. The center of the cross section is defined as stated in (c-1). Each segment contour is divided according to the process (c-1) or (c-2).

2.2 Foot shape modeling software "Di+"

Software libraries for generating interpolated points, cross sections and dividing points were developed to do the basic geometrical processing. Application software "Di+" to

©CARS/Springer. All rights reserved.

generate a homologous foot model was developed using the software libraries. The software was coded by I-Ware Laboratory Co, Ltd.

3. Application of homologous shape models

3.1 Representation of shape difference

When two body forms were represented by homologous shape models, the difference between two forms can be represented by the spatial distortion of the control lattice points (Fig. 2). This is the Free Form Deformation (FFD) technique [5]. With the original FFD technique, a 3D shape is deformed smoothly by moving the control lattice points. When two body forms were represented by homologous shape models, the optimal distortion of the FFD grids can be calculated to minimize the sum of Euclidian distances between corresponding vertices. Application software "Darcii-T: Digital and Anatomical shape Representation with Control-points for Inter Individual Transformation" have been developed for this purpose. With Darcii-T, the optimal distortion of the FFD grid to deform the original model into the target model can be calculated, and the distortion function can be applied to any objects [2].

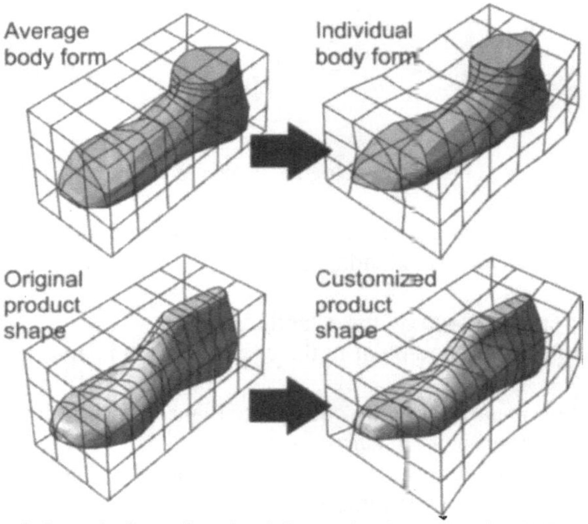

Fig. 2: Last design using the deformation based on the FFD grid.

3.2 Designing a well-fitting shoe last

The average form can be calculated easily for homologous models. An average foot form is calculated for the panels for whom the same existing shoe fits well. The average foot form and the last shape for the shoe is the master pair with good fitting comfort. The shoe does not always fit to a customer even if his/her foot length is the same with the panels because of the foot shape differences. Thus, the customer's foot is modelled by Di+ and the difference between the average foot form and the customer's foot form is represented as the FFD grid distortion by Darcii-T (Fig. 2, top). The distorted FFD grid has the information on the differences in the foot size and shape. Then the distorted FFD gird is applied to the last shape for the existing shoe, and a new last shape for the customer is

©CARS/Springer. All rights reserved.

calculated (Fig. 2, bottom). The digital last can be materialized by an NC lathe, and a shoe manufactured using the last.

4. Foot database by foot scanning systems in retail shops

4.1 Foot scanning system "INFOOT"

A foot scanning system "INFOOT" has been developed with I-Ware Laboratory Co. Ltd (Fig. 3(a)). This system consists of a compact and low-cost foot scanner, automatic foot modeling software (Di+), and FFD software (Darcii-T). Eight cameras and four laser line projectors were installed in the scanner. Using a glass plate for the standing plane, complete shape including the sole can be measured. The accuracy and the resolution of this scanner was 1.0 mm [6].

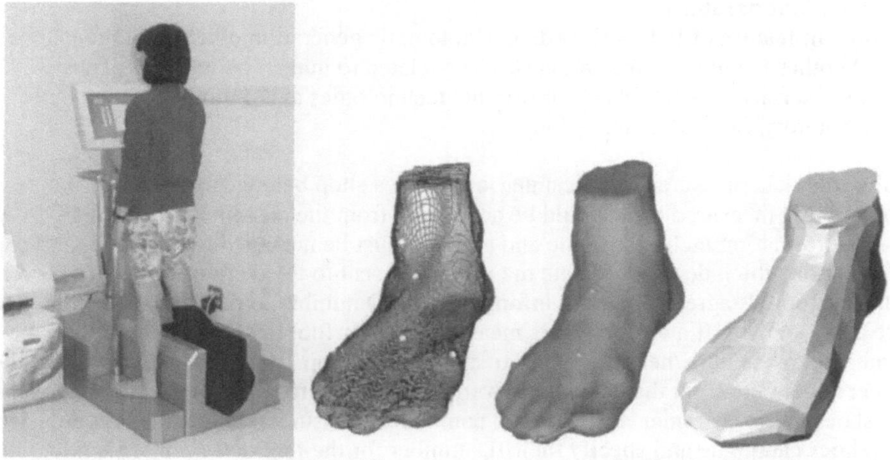

(a) foot scanner (b) millions data points and landmarks (c) homologous model

Fig. 3: Foot scanning system "INFOOT".

Special marker seals are pasted on the following 5 landmarks: (1) Metatarsale tibiale (MT), (2) Metatarsale fibulare (MF), (3) Sphyrion fibulare: the tip of the lateral malleolus, (4) Sphyrion; the tip of the medial malleolus, (5) the lateral junction point; a point at the junction between the leg and foot on the lateral aspect of the dorsum pedis. It is defined as the crossing point of the tendon of M. extensor digitorum longus leading to the 5th toe and the crease which appears when the subject flexes his/her knees and ankles. Then the foot is scanned in 10 sec. Above mentioned 5 landmarks are detected and labeled automatically. Four more landmarks are detected automatically based on the curvature of the foot surface. Seventeen foot dimensions are calculated from the scanned data and landmarks in 5 more sec. Millions data points and 9 landmark coordinates are saved (Fig.3 (b)). Consequently, the homologous foot model (Fig. 3(c)) can be calculated automatically.

Table 1 compares foot dimensions calculated by the scanner and measured by an expert using the traditional method. The difference was significant for all dimensions, but the MAD (mean absolute difference) was within 1.0 mm for most of them. Repeatability of measurements obtained by the scanner is as good as that for the manual measurements.

©CARS/Springer. All rights reserved.

This system is purchasable from I-Ware Laboratory Co, Ltd., and over 20 systems have been installed in shoe retailers and manufactures in Japan, Korea, US, and Germany.

Table 1: Difference between the traditional method and INFOOT (unit: mm)
*: p<0.05, **: p<0.01, ns: not significant.

		Mean by INFOOT	Mean by trad. method.	Difference	paired t-test	Correlation coefficient
2	Ball girth	242.0	240.3	-1.7	**	0.988
1	Foot length	241.9	243.1	1.1	**	0.997
10	Instep length	177.3	176.9	-0.4	ns	0.989
11	Fibular instep l.	158.3	155.5	2.8	**	0.991
3	Foot breadth	99.9	99.8	-0.1	ns	0.992
7	Heel breadth	64.0	63.6	0.5	**	0.996

4.2 A large foot database

An important feature of INFOOT system is automatic generation of a homologous foot model. Another feature is information services related to human body forms. These information services are based on our original technologies and put into practice by I-Ware Laboratory Co, Ltd (patent pending).

Usually, foot data measured by a scanner located in a shop belongs to the shop. Our proposal is that measured data should be accessible from the customer him/herself. Personal information including name and address must be managed by the shop, and copy of information which does not violate the privacy is sent to the common database server with the customer's agreement. Sent information is ID number, birth year, measured date, stature and foot data. If a customer has measured his/her foot by this system before, the customer can present his/her ID number to a clerk of a shop. The clerk can download the customer's foot data from the database server, and utilize it to select or recommend well-fitting shoes to the customer. In electronic commerce, consumers select the brand/design from a shoes catalogue and specify their ID number for the foot data. Consequently, the consumer would get well-fitting shoes. A free viewer of 3D foot data has been distributed from I-Ware Laboratory web site (http://www.i-ware.co.jp/). Consumers can download their foot data and the viewer, and enjoy browsing 3D foot data on a PC.

4.3 Advantages

This idea for creating foot database is different from the traditional anthropometric surveys. A large amount of data is gathered by ubiquitous foot scanners used in the business for selecting or manufacturing well-fitting shoes. These data must be handled with the agreement of every customer. With this strategy, a large foot database would be created with a small project budget. The information service business does not started yet, but data for over 700 feet are stored in the database during a trial service of 6 months.

It is a very important and useful feature of INFOOT system to store the foot data with homologous shape models. With homologous models, it is possible (1) to obtain the shape distribution map, (2) to calculate the average form, and (3) to generate standard deviation forms on the distribution map.

©CARS/Springer. All rights reserved.

4.4 Known problems

There are two problems for this database strategy. One is the quality control and the other is the biased sampling. Quality management of the measurement equipment is not so difficult, whereas the quality management of the measurement protocol is difficult. We should control the quality of measurers in landmarking and instruction to subjects. With a proper protocol, a measurer should instruct to a subject "Stand naturally and look straight ahead. Distribute your weight equally on your left and right feet." For controlling the subject's gaze, INFOOT system displays the measured shape on the screen on real time. The subject watches the screen naturally, thus their posture becomes stable. For controlling the subject's weight balance, we plan to install a weight sensor to the footstep of INFOOT system. It is very difficult to control the quality in landmarking. We are developing a new method to reduce the number of landmarks to be located by the measurer. In the present system, 5 anatomical landmarks must be identified by a measurer. Using the new method, only MT and MF are needed to be identified.
Handling the biased sampling is also difficult. Females, younger subjects, and subjects in higher social classes would be over represented, when we use the proposed system. We can get the location of the measurement equipment, gender and the age of subjects, but cannot get any information on the birthplace, ethnic group, social class, education level, or occupation. To complement under represented strata, a measurement project by public organization may be efficient, and it need not be a big project.

5. Conclusion

With homologous models, average form and the standard deviation forms can be easily calculated. Software libraries for homologous modeling were developed and application software to model the foot form was also developed using the libraries. This software was incorporated into a compact and low-cost foot scanner, and the scanning systems have been installed in some shoe retailers. With the scanning system, retailers can select well-fitting shoes for customers, and customers can enjoy browsing their foot shape data or shopping in electronic commerce. A large database can be constructed by using this system with special care for quality control and biased sampling.

References

1. M. Bayley, "The Use of 3D Body Normalisation to Enable Powerful Data Analysis Technique," *Scanning 3D - Human Modeling*, Paris, 2001.
2. M. Mochimaru, M. Kouchi, and M. Dohi, "Analysis of 3D human foot forms using the FFD method and its application in grading shoe last," *Ergonomics*, Vol. 43, pp. 1301-1313, 2000.
3. M. Kouchi and M. Mochimaru, "Development of a new dressmaking dummy based on a 3d human model," *Scanning 3D - Human Modeling*, Paris, 2001.
4. M. Kouchi and M. Mochimaru, "Analysis of 3D Human Face Forms and Spectacle Frames Based on Average Forms," *SAE Digital Human Modeling for Design and Engineering*, Munich, 2002.
5. T. W. Sederberg, "Free-From Deformation of Solid Geometric Models," *ACM SIGGRAPH'86 in Computers & Graphics*, Vol.20, pp. 151-160, 1986.
6. M. Mochimaru and M. Kouchi, "Development of a low cost foot scanner for custom shoes by the FFD," *Scanning 3D - Numerisation 3D*, Paris, 2001.

©CARS/Springer. All rights reserved.

A Web3D based CAESAR viewer

Sandy Ressler, Qiming Wang
National Institute of Standards and Technology, 100 Bureau Drive, STOP 8940
Gaithersburg MD 20899
sressler@nist.gov, qwang@nist.gov

Abstract

The CAESAR (Civilian American and European Surface Anthropometry Resource) project completed in 2002 has collected 3D scans of over 5000 subjects. We have created a 3D interface, the NIST CAESAR Viewer (NCV), utilizing the Virtual Reality Modeling Language (VRML) to provide 3D access via the Web. In addition to simply viewing the 3D scans we have augmented the display of the body with interactive anthropometric landmarks and contour line displays. The landmarks and viewpoints associated with the landmarks are automatically placed onto the body as a visual anthropometric glossary. Display of the contours boundaries are adjusted by the user moving sagittal, coronal and transverse cutting planes. This paper describes the functionality of the evolving NCV viewer.

Keywords: VRML, Web3D, anthropometry

1. Introduction

The NIST CAESAR Viewer (NCV) enables users to view and manipulate the display of CAESAR 3D body scans. NCV is a work in progress and several versions of the interface exist with varying functionality. The key advantage of NCV is that users, with appropriate access to the CAESAR database of bodies, can view the surface scans on inexpensive PCs or any computing platform with a VRML [1] browser. Anthropometric landmarks are easily visualized by showing the landmark locations on the body. It is a natural extension to create 3D illustrations of the landmarks by placing them on 3D computer generated bodies. Figure 1 illustrates the display of a single body with landmarks and contours. In addition to simple displays of the bodies, users can view multiple bodies and the data associated with the anthropometric landmarks. The user can toggle the display of landmarks, contour lines or the body surface as desired.

The NCV provides the anthropometry standards community a way of producing 3D illustrations for data visualization, and facilitates communication among members. In addition creation of a 3D anthropometric glossary allows non-professionals a simple way of introducing anthropometric concepts. As the NCV becomes more robust we intend on using it as a low-cost tool for anthropometric measurements and analysis of 3D scans.

DISCLAIMER: Mention of trade names does not imply endorsement by NIST.

©CARS/Springer. All rights reserved.

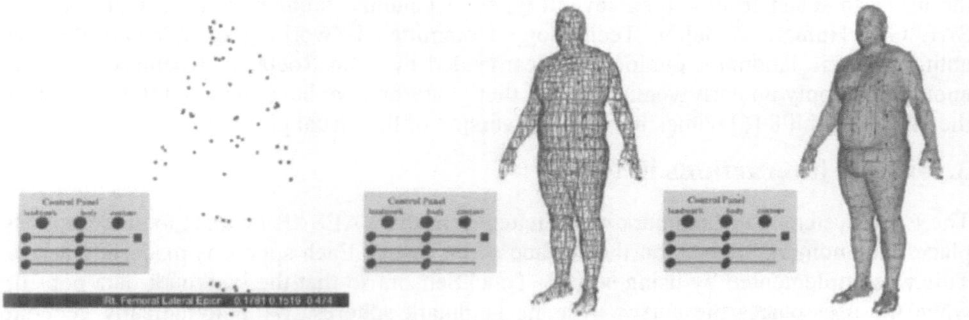

Fig 1. : Body with landmarks, contours and surfaces toggled on.

2. System evolution and background

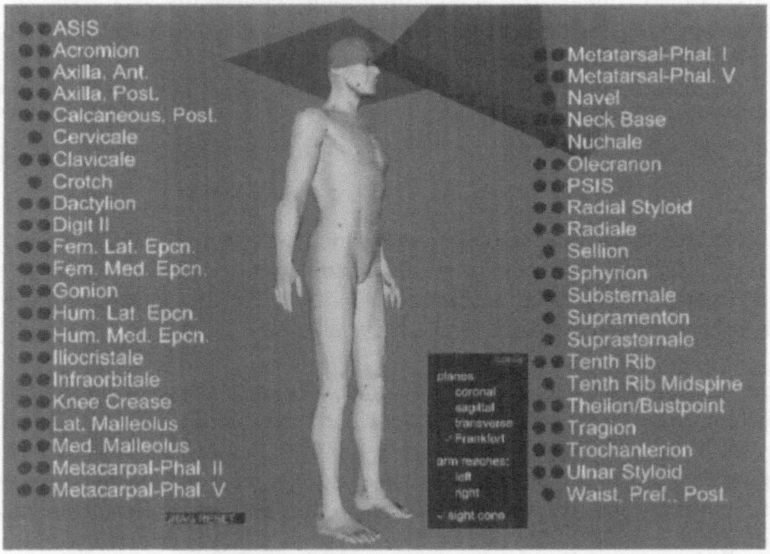

Fig 2. : AnthroGloss screen layout with Frankfort plane and sight cone indicators turned on.

Before our direct involvement in the use of CAESAR body scans we created a system called "AnthroGloss" [2] shown in Figure 2, which uses a synthetically created body. We placed anthropometric landmark spheres on the body by hand, a laborious process. In AnthroGloss users select a sphere causing a change in the viewpoint and the name of the selected landmark appears in a large size font in the middle of the display. The list of landmarks can be repositioned by dragging the entire column of names. Reference planes can be toggled on and off via the control panel. The glossary system also allows users to toggle on or off a variety of display indicators. These include the Frankfort plane, and a sagittal, coronal and transverse cutting planes. The planes were derived from illustrations in *Anthropometric Methods* [3]. Arm reach volumes, partial spherical areas, can also be displayed. The areas for the arm reaches were based on standard illustrations [4,5]. Also,

©CARS/Springer. All rights reserved.

the user can select from among several types of landmark nomenclatures. Currently the SAE G13 Human Modeling Technology Committee is working on a comprehensive anthropometric landmark dictionary, spearheaded by John Roebuck. Roebuck was kind enough to supply an early version of this dictionary and we have included this version of the SAE AIR 5408 [6] names in our latest version of the visual glossary.

3. Display interactions in NCV

The NCV system uses landmark coordinates from the CAESAR data set to automatically place the landmark spheres on the surface of the scans. Each sphere is made interactive. This was implemented by using VRML TouchSensors so that the landmark data pops up when the user places the cursor over the landmark spheres. We automatically generate points of view, using VRML Viewpoint Nodes, associated with each landmark to allow the user to get close-up views of the landmarks in context of the body. We generate the viewpoints by surrounding the body with an enclosing cylinder and drawing a vector from the landmark to the cylinder. The intersection point between the vector and the cylinder becomes the viewpoint for that landmark. The end result is a system that automatically generates views of the landmark spheres, places them on the body and automatically generates associated viewpoints for each landmark. These interactive bodies are the equivalent of our previous "AnthroGloss" body however they are now generated automatically for each CAESAR body rather than manually constructed for a particular synthetic body.

Figure 3 illustrates the most complex version of the system. This version includes the ability to toggle on or off body textures, landmarks, and contours. It also provides the ability to select a color for the entire body. Labels for the control slider change as appropriate to match the particular functionality selected.

The controls currently available to the user allow for the display of multiple (up to 10) bodies. The control panel operates on the "current" body indicated by a box surrounding the body. The "current" body is selected by simply clicking the body. Contour lines associated with sagittal, coronal and transverse cutting planes can be displayed. When the user selects a cutting plane an animated display of the contour cut plane is created and the user can drag the cutting plane through the body watching the effect on the contour. Finally the user can measure distances on the contour display by selecting start and end points on the contour lines. The distances are in the same units as the original CAESAR data.

©CARS/Springer. All rights reserved.

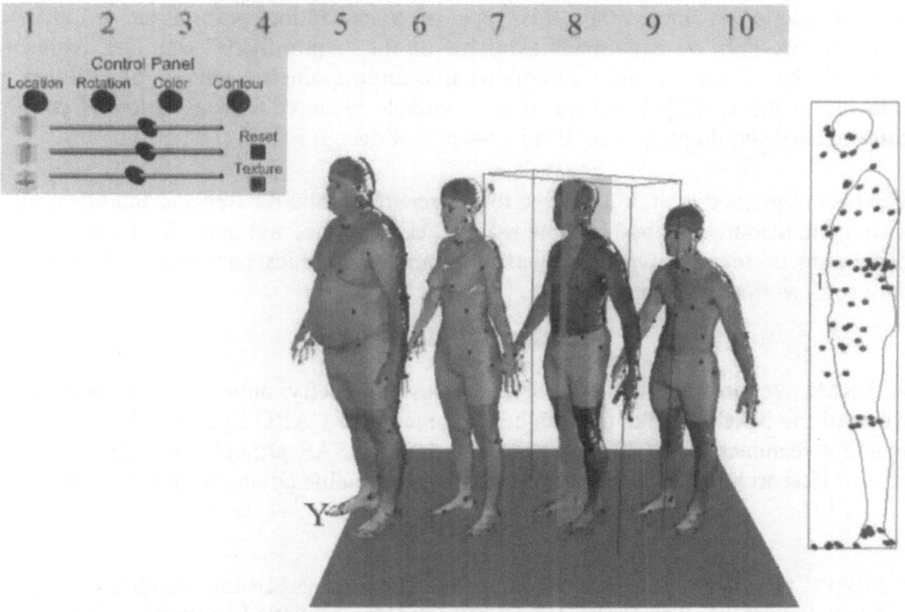

Fig. 3: Textured body display with multiple bodies and contours.

4. Issues, problems and future work

Currently there are only three widely used VRML browsers, CosmoPlayer (www.sgi.com/software/cosmo/player.html), Contact (www.blaxxun.com) and Cortona (www.parallelgraphics.com). CosmoPlayer is a discontinued product, for PCs, and is no longer maintained, however it is supported by SGI for their IRIX workstations. Contact and Cortona are both being actively developed and expanded. It is often a challenge to create VRML content that plays satisfactorily in multiple browsers. The NCV display generally does play back correctly but does on occasion exhibit idiosyncrasies due to the different behavior of the browsers. It may be more effective to use a proprietary Web3D technology such as Viewpoint (www.viewpoint.com) or Shockwave 3D (www.macromedia.com), as these are both available on a number of common platforms and may provide superior displays and download times via geometric compression.

We have also begun to examine the advantages of using a large format wall size 3D display. True 3D is achieved by the use of LCD shutter glasses and the image is projected life size. We use a pair of FakeSpace Rave [7] walls arranged in a corner configuration. The life-size nature of the display gives the user an intuitive perception the physical size of the human who was scanned. Standing in front of a 3D life-size gives one a powerful sense of presence and a clear sense of the size and distances of the data. Interaction with data in this 3D space remains problematic. However we expect to tackle that issue in the future through the use of new input devices.

©CARS/Springer. All rights reserved.

We also intend on integrating this type of visualization with a set of children's anthropometric data we have made available on the "AnthroKids" web site. AnthroKids [8] data is based on the only comprehensive anthropometric survey of children ever conducted in the USA [9] and remains a valuable resource. Visualization of children's anthropometry should prove useful for a variety of design issues.

We expect to make the NCV available to the general public for free and intend on making it a valuable resource for both people using CAESAR data and other 3D body scans. The proliferation of inexpensive high quality computer graphics hardware will make NCV more useful as time goes on.

Acknowledgements

The VRML versions of the CAESAR bodies (geometry only) were created by Eric Paquett of the NRC. Thanks to Kathleen Robinette (of CARD Lab and CAESAR project leader) for feedback on NCV and explaining the CAESAR project, and John Roebuck (of Roebuck Research & Consulting) for providing invaluable advice on anthropometry.

References

1. ISO/IEC, "The Virtual Reality Modeling Language," International Standard ISO/IEC 14772-1:1997.
2. Sandy Ressler, "A Web-based 3D Glossary for Anthropometric Landmarks," Proceedings of HCI International 2001, New Orleans, LA, August 5-10, 2001.
3. Roebuck Jr., J. A. "Anthropometric Methods: Designing to Fit the Human Body," Human Factors and Ergonomics Society, 1993.
4. Dreyfuss H. Associates. "The Measure of Man and Woman," Whitney Library of Design, 1993.
5. Woodson, W.E., Tillman, B., Tillman, P. "Human Factors Design Handbook second edition," McGraw Hill, 1992.
6. Roebuck Jr., J. A. "DRAFT 6 of Sample Visual Index Illustrations for AIR 5408 Dictionary of Anthropometric Landmarks, Lines and Planes for Computer Human Modeling," SAE G13, 2001.
7. Fakespace Systems Inc, http://www.fakespacesystems.com/workspace1.htm
8. NIST, AnthroKids - Anthropometric Data of Children, ovrt.nist.gov/projects/anthrokids
9. Snyder, R.G., Schneider, L. W., Owings, C. L., Reynolds, H. M., Golomb, D. H., Schork, M. A., "Anthropometry of Infants, Children, and Youths to Age 18 for Product Safety Design," University of Michigan Ann Arbor, UM-HSRI-77-17, 1977.

©CARS/Springer. All rights reserved.

Some tools for understanding anthropometry

Johan F.M. Molenbroek
Delft University of Technology
Landbergstraat 15, 2628 CE Delft, The Netherlands
j.f.m.molenbroek@io.tudelft.nl

Abstract

Two decades of experiences in education in engineering anthropometry to students in Industrial Design Engineering and to Industries resulted in useful guidelines for the developing of 3D-tools .

Keywords: 3D-anthropometry, education, tools

1. Introduction

During the 2 last decades we experienced several ways of learning students and companies about anthropometry.
First thoughts were that learning some knowledge about the normal distribution and percentiles would help especially if as an example a list with the values of mean, sd, p5 and p95 about Flying-Personnel 1954 was given.
But you can't go on with designing everything in Holland for American Pilots. We were happy with the publication of the German Din 33402. But after a while we compared the stature (with the body weight the only available anthropometry at that time in Holland at the beginning of the eighties) young adults of age 20 between German and the Netherlands. The conclusion was a higher value for the stature of 2% for all percentiles for females and 3,5 % for males of that age group. With that knowledge we created a educational standard for students called DINED, which meant to show we used the German DIN as well as Dutch data. In fact it was included in an a6-paper form in a small pocketbook called 'Kleine Ergonomische Datensamlung' [1], which was given for free to all students by the faculty. This student standard was meant to be used in the education of design engineering to learn about percentiles, correlation, adding and subtracting of measurements and to have a reasonable estimation of some variables for Dutch adults, children and elderly.

2. DINED

DINED was soon used as a standard in the Netherlands by the industry especially because it was attached to the Dutch Standard NEN1813 for office furniture and it was published in all kind of handbooks. Now after 17 years of using we can evaluate this simple tool.
We learned the following [2]:
-Percentiles were still just added despite of our efforts to include an algorithm about how to add or subtract two normal distributed measurements taking care of their correlation.

©CARS/Springer. All rights reserved.

-Because we published P5 and P95 after 5 years the users (designers and companies) didn't use any other percentiles; we called that the P5 syndrome.
-Because this DINED-table was more or less 1 dimensional, users were not triggered to think in 2 or 3 D.
-Because it was mainly presented as meant for adults of age 20-60, populations were not split or added in spite of our efforts to include an algorithm about this subject. For example if you are designing for a Dutch nursing home the population mostly consist of 75% female en 25 % male, which influences the anthropometry of the mixed group.
-The information about the secular trend was very popular and raised many comments and some improvements. This means a graph with a timeline is better then to mention just some figures.
-The information about variance, variation and correlation was to compact and should be illustrated
-Some variables were not popular: handwidth with thumb was included and people were asking for handwidth metacarpal; afterwards it was understandable.
-Some variables could easy be calculated like the vertical legroom from the sum of the popliteal height and the thigh clearance, but that was mostly not understood by students and mostly asked by industry.
-Calculations of percentiles can better be done graphically
-The user forgets the influence of the posture and the task
-The best lesson is that users always forget the influence of the correlation with the second and the third dimensions
-Also important for other teachers might be that we always saw ergonomics as one of the four discipline of the industrial design engineering. The other three are formgiving, innovation management and engineering. Anthropometry is seen as a very essential part of ergonomics. This means we include the knowledge of anthropometry in various stages of the process of product development.

3. AIS Anthropometric Information System

After our experiences with DINED we set up a digital system; first in DOS and later under Windows and currently a JAVA-applet is developed on http://dutoh60.io.tudelft.nl
In this design we want to overcome the lack of knowledge in anatomy by the users by showing pictures. We want to overcome the lack of knowledge of what we call the anthropometric design process by stimulate the user/designer to follow a stepwise process. For example they have to say something about the following points in a sequence:

- some demographic parameters of population where to design for
- a posture that will be used
- possible manual handling that will occur
- which are the relevant product or workplace dimensions
- which are in accordance the relevant human dimension
- what are the critical values
- what is the intercorrelation between the relevant dimensions
- what are the available anthropometrical sources
- what is needed to be estimated
- what are additional factors for clothing or posturing?

©CARS/Springer. All rights reserved.

This means in most cases that the needed data are not complete and must be estimated. That is why we found in handbooks of Roebuck and Anthropometric Source Book and developed ourselves calculation methods to make better estimations for designers. These formulas are includes in the AIS-software.

4. DINED digital

Because the development of AIS is slow we had in the meantime some experiences with a faster system and based on Flash-software. This can be seen at http://www.io.tudelft.nl/research/ergonomics/build/. In this site it was easier to enter several populations. In the near future we have to decide which development is the most adequate for the users as well for the software developers.

5. ELLIPSE

Another tool that came up to make the 2 dimensional anthropometrical world more understandable for designers was the experience with the first scatterplots or bivariate normal distribution we saw in literature [3]. These were very useful but time consuming. This was the reason why we made this phenomenon also interactive. An example of recent use of ELLIPSE can be seen on the last page of this paper. In that particular case the hip width was shown in relation to the chest width, because that were two relevant dimensions for that posture and the critical manual handling.

6. Recommendations

To develop new tools for anthropometry it would be recommended to involve future users during the development process on regular bases. Experiences from the past with 1D and 2D-data learn that 3D data not only should be available for education but also the tools to use these data in the design process.

References

1. Lange, W., *Kleine Ergonomische Datensammlung,* Verlag TUV Rheinland, Dortmund, 1981.
2. Molenbroek, J.F.M. and A.I.M. Voorbij, "Aanzet tot een nieuwe Nederlandse antropometrie tabel voor lichaamsmaten; de DINED revisited" *Tijdschrift voor Ergonomie*, 26,3,25-30,2001.
3. Sittig, J. en H. Freudenthal, De Juiste Maat, lichaamsafmetingen van Nederlandse vrouwen als basis van een nieuw maatsysteem voor damesconfectiekleding. Stafleu, Leiden, 1951.

©CARS/Springer. All rights reserved.

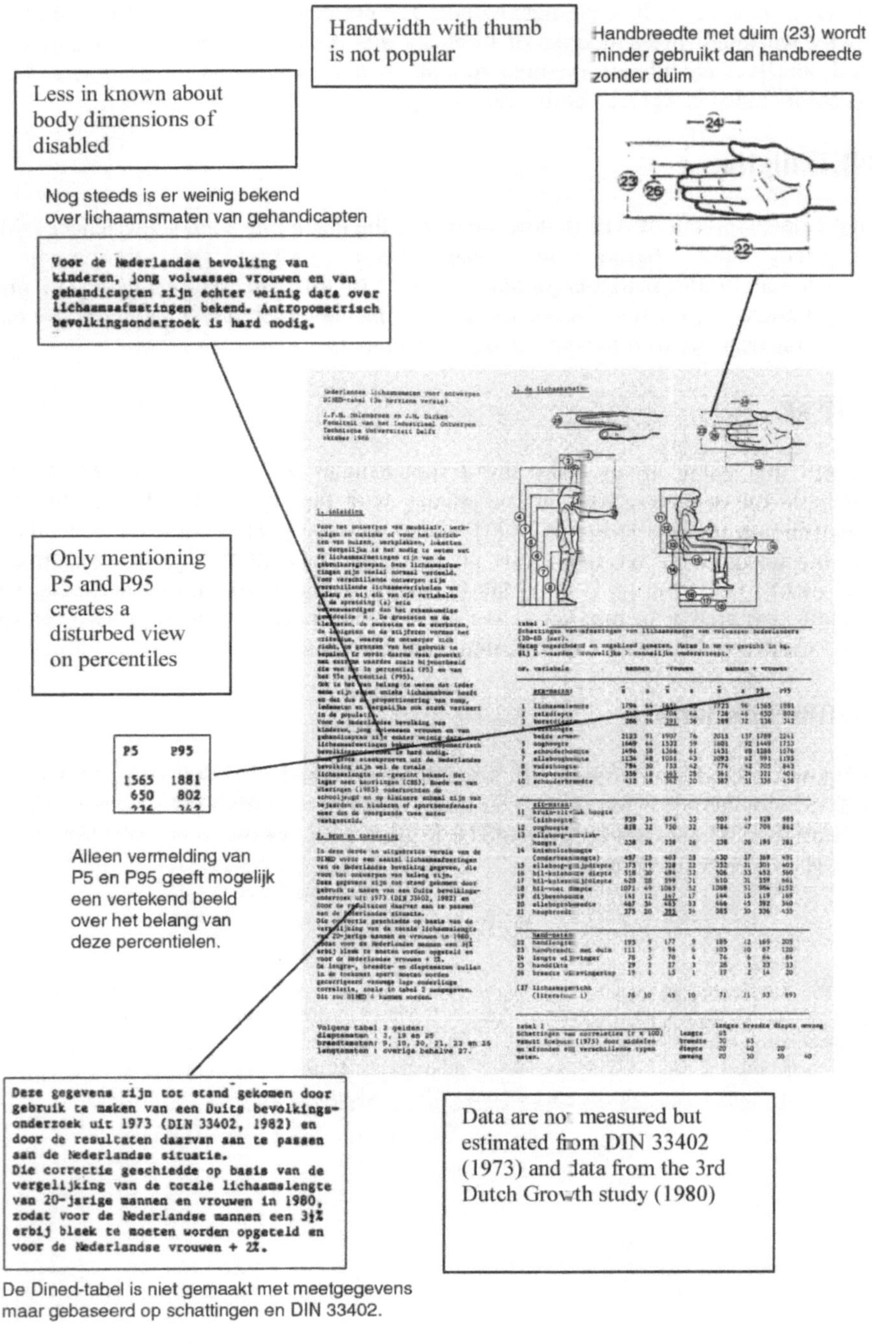
Handwidth with thumb is not popular
Handbreedte met duim (23) wordt minder gebruikt dan handbreedte zonder duim
Less in known about body dimensions of disabled
Nog steeds is er weinig bekend over lichaamsmaten van gehandicapten
Voor de Nederlandse bevolking van kinderen, jong volwassen vrouwen en van gehandicapten zijn echter weinig data over lichaamsafmetingen bekend. Antropometrisch bevolkingsonderzoek is hard nodig.
Only mentioning P5 and P95 creates a disturbed view on percentiles
P5 P95
1565 1881
650 802
Alleen vermelding van P5 en P95 geeft mogelijk een vertekend beeld over het belang van deze percentielen.
Deze gegevens zijn tot stand gekomen door gebruik te maken van een Duits bevolkingsonderzoek uit 1973 (DIN 33402, 1982) en door de resultaten daarvan aan te passen aan de Nederlandse situatie.
Die correctie geschiedde op basis van de vergelijking van de totale lichaamslengte van 20-jarige mannen en vrouwen in 1980, zodat voor de Nederlandse mannen een 3½% erbij bleek te moeten worden opgeteld en voor de Nederlandse vrouwen + 2%.
Data are not measured but estimated from DIN 33402 (1973) and data from the 3rd Dutch Growth study (1980)
De Dined-tabel is niet gemaakt met meetgegevens maar gebaseerd op schattingen en DIN 33402.

Figure 1: Dined 1984 -front page

©CARS/Springer. All rights reserved.

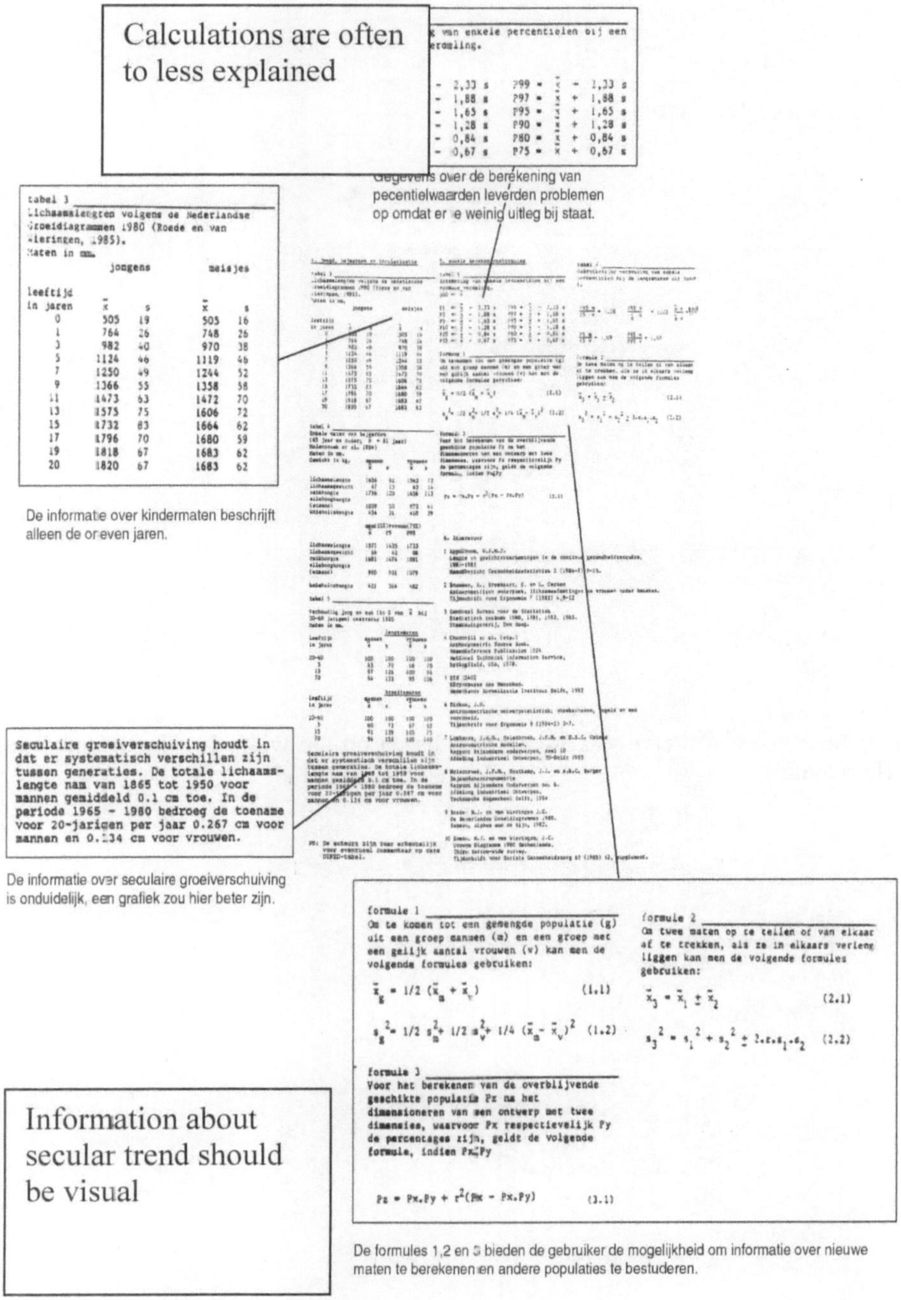

Figure 2: Dined 1984 back page

©CARS/Springer. All rights reserved.

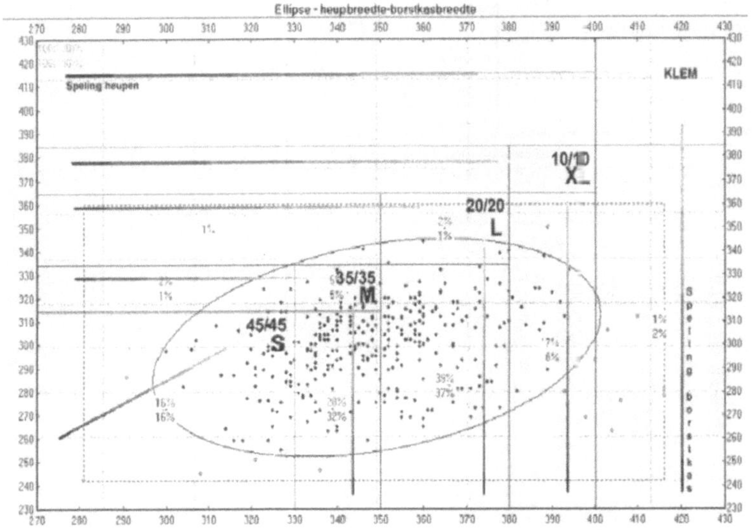

Figure 3: Four sizes of a cart seat are defined based cn hip width (vertical) and chest width (horizontal)

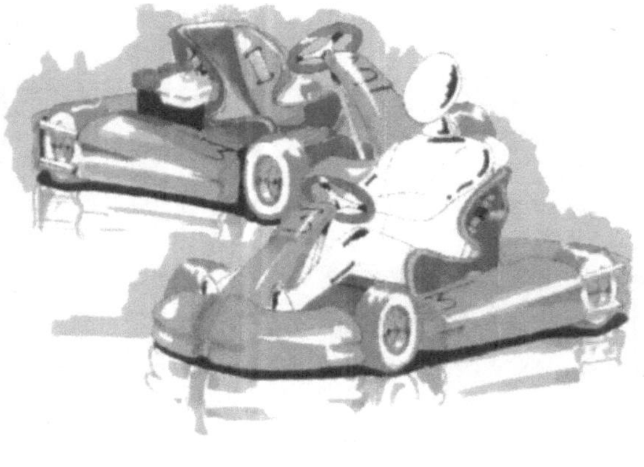

Figure 4: Concept of a the design of a cart in according to figure 3.

Telemedicine

CARS 2002 – H.U. Lemke, M.W. Vannier; K. Inamura, A.G. Farman, K. Doi & J.H.C. Reiber (Editors)
©CARS/Springer. All rights reserved.

A review: "In-Home Healthcare" projects in the USA

Gilbert B. Devey
Biomedical Engineering Program, National Science Foundation,
4201 Wilson Boulevard, Arlington VA 22230

Abstract

In 1995 the National Science Foundation opened the Internet (the World Wide Web) to public use and thereby released a technology that, arguably, in *less than a decade*, is impacting healthcare delivery much as Roentgen's discovery of the X-ray in 1895 advanced medical diagnosis and Fleming's discovery of penicillin in 1928 revolutionized the treatment of bacterial diseases. Contemporaneously with the opening of the Internet came the availability of broadband communications and computer networks, GHz desktop computers, high definition monitors, and massive computer memory — all at relatively low costs. Those technologies introduced the potential for the development of affordable devices and systems to enable consumers to access a wide range of healthcare services from the home, and to do so *interactively* with healthcare providers. Such devices and telemedicine systems have been described in a number of forums. The aging of the "baby boomers" and the increased longevity of the population have introduced the dimension of *prevention* in the design of In-Home Healthcare systems. No individual nor organization coordinates telemedicine/telehealth activities in the USA but several private sector and government programs support considerable research directed to the development of the necessary technologies for patient and provider acceptance of In-Home Healthcare systems.

Keywords: Home healthcare, telemedicine, aging

1. Introduction

Healthcare in the home is not a new concept. At the beginning of the 20th century it was quite common — the doctor even made house calls while toting his black bag. By the mid-1950s visits to the doctor's office, to a group practice, or to a hospital were rapidly becoming the norm. By the mid 1990s "high-tech home care" was being tested as a way to shorten hospital stays (presumably lowering the cost of care) and return the patient to the comfort and familiar environment of his/her home [1].

It is beyond the scope of this paper to cover past developments in Home Healthcare Systems. However, the report of the "Workshop on Home Care Technologies for the 21st Century" (April 7-9, 1999) provides an excellent description and analysis of the state-of-development of the field [2]. The White House Forum on "Technologies for Successful Aging", held October 4 and 5, 2000, focussed discussion on the "baby boomer" phenomena; namely, how are we to provide for the healthcare needs of a vastly larger

©CARS/Springer. All rights reserved.

retirement-age cohort in the face of the latest Census Bureau projections that place the 65+ population at 70.3 million in 2030, which is more than twice the number in 2000 [3]?

In-Home Healthcare development projects are funded by government research agencies and private foundations, academic research institutions, and industry. Not surprisingly, many projects involve the active participation of all of the foregoing stakeholders. Aggregate data is unavailable at the national level concerning financial support for, or the scope of the ongoing projects. However, government agencies do appear to sponsor a majority of the fundamental investigations for the development and validation of the new technologies required.. Several academic research universities have made investments in appropriate infrastructure developments (e.g. Adaptive House (U. Colorado); Aware Home (Georgia Tech); Age Labs (MIT); Smart Medical Home (U. Rochester)). As with all new health-related products, the ultimate success of the In-Home Healthcare concept will be influenced greatly by issues and events external to scientific and technical acumen: customer (patient and provider) satisfaction, regulatory body (FDA) approval, third-party (Medicare; private insurers) reimbursements, and legal matters (licensure; security/privacy).

Russell Coile contends, "The telemedicine revolution in medical care has taken off without a leader" [4]. Might the "leaderless" state of affairs perhaps resemble Adam Smith's *invisible hand* of capital, which, through the operation of our legislative system and its derivative regulatory bodies, has led a successful economic system lo these many years? The HIPAA legislation, with its standards setting requirements, is a recent example in the healthcare field that is expected to have enormous and positive impact on the development of In-Home Healthcare systems (and eHealth overall) [5][6].

2. Government "In-Home Healthcare" projects

A caveat. Government R&D programs in our field of interest typically have the words *disability* and/or *rehabilitation* in their titles, yet many of the potential beneficiaries of In-Home Healthcare may not be considered to be disabled nor require rehabilitation for a number of years after beginning to use "technologies for successful aging". Those persons are considered to be In-Home Healthcare participants, particularly as *prevention* is now a category receiving increased attention.

2.1 National Institute on Disability and Rehabilitation Research (NIDRR)

NIDRR, located in the Department of Education (DoED), supports a growing number of *Rehabilitation Engineering Research Centers* (RERCs) having the general objectives to study new or emerging technologies to solve rehabilitation problems, to demonstrate innovative models for the delivery of rehabilitation technology services, and to facilitate the delivery of such services. Note that *study of new or emerging technologies* is stressed in contrast to conducting *research for the development of new technologies*. A typical RERC is funded for a 5-year period up to $1million per year. During the first year of the project a plan is to be developed and implemented for ensuring that all new and improved technologies developed by the RERC are successfully transferred to the marketplace. In the third year of the project each RERC conducts a state-of-the-science conference on its area of research.

©CARS/Springer. All rights reserved.

Two RERC projects established in October 2001 are excellent examples of today's In-Home Healthcare concepts. They are:

- **Rehabilitation Engineering Research Center on Technology for Successful Aging**
  Project Director: William C. Mann, Ph.D.
  University of Florida, Gainesville

Projects being conducted by this RERC focus on the closely related areas of communications, home monitoring, and "smart" technologies. The driving technology is developing rapidly and requires an understanding of current and emerging technology areas, including wireless technology, computers, sensors, user interfaces, control devices, and networking. Successful integration of this technology into products and systems for older persons requires an understanding of their complex health, independence, and quality-of-life issues. The RERC-Tech-Aging tests currently available home monitoring products and demonstrates their effectiveness in relation to independence, quality of life, and health related costs. The RERC also identifies needs and barriers to home monitoring and communication technology, and addresses needs of special populations including rural-living, elders, and people aging with disability. The RERC-Tech-Aging brings together national expertise to meet this challenge, including major universities, (Univ. Wisconsin; Univ. Buffalo) industry leaders (Motorola) working in this area, major aging-related organizations, federal agencies that relate to funding or services in this area, other NIDRR-funded projects, and organizations that assist in identifying study participants.

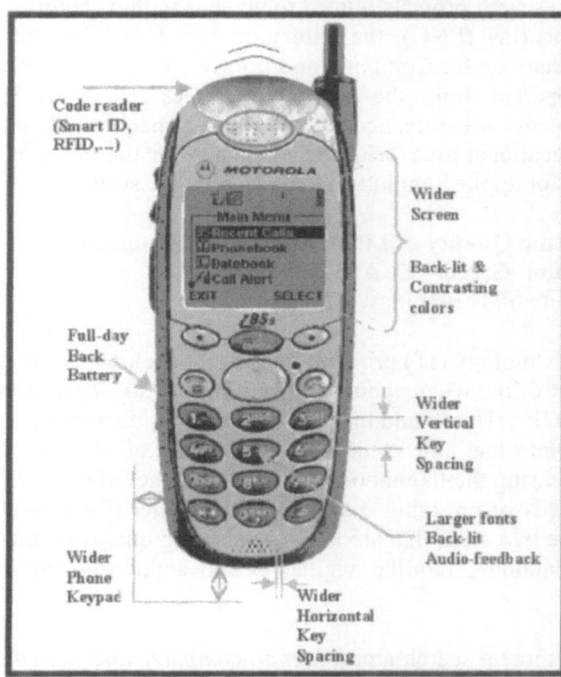

Figure 1. Cell Phone, University of Florida

As depicted in Figure 1, the Cell Phone was selected as the technology agent best suited for the client population as a) elders are accustomed to phones, b) the cell phone is the most portable and mobile device, c) sell phone technology has better chances for acceptability than other technologies, and d) computer and IP data network capability are on board.

©CARS/Springer. All rights reserved.

• RERC on Mobile Wireless Technologies for Persons with Disabilities
Project Director: Helena Mitchell
Georgia Institute of Technology, Atlanta

The overall goal of this investigation is to promote the independence and autonomy of people with disabilities, with two primary aims: 1) ensure equitable access to mobile wireless products and services by people with disabilities; and 2) investigate promising applications of mobile wireless technologies in support of employment, independent living, and community integration of people with disabilities [8].

2.2 National Science Foundation (NSF)

NSF provides support for a variety of research projects related to persons with disabilities primarily in the Directorate for Engineering (ENG), the Directorate for Education and Human Resources (EHR), and the Directorate for Computer and Information Science and Engineering (CISE). As will be apparent from the several examples below, NSF objectives are to seek solutions to problems or to advance knowledge in a specific field of science, engineering discipline, or educational area, with the outcomes for the example projects expected to have the potential for application in In-Home Healthcare systems.

• The Aware Home: Sustaining the Quality of Life for an Aging Population
Principal Investigator: Gregory D. Abowd, Ph.D.
Georgia Institute of Technology, Atlanta

This 5-year $1,599,997 Information Technology (IT) project focuses on development of a domestic environment that is cognizant of the whereabouts and activities of its occupants and can support them in their everyday life. The PI and his team will design, demonstrate, and evaluate a series of domestic services that aim to maintain the quality of life for an aging population, with the goal of increasing the likelihood of a "stay at home" alternative to assisted living that satisfies the needs of an aging individual and his/her distributed family. In particular, the PI will explore two areas that are key to sustaining quality of life for an independent senior adult: maintaining familial vigilance, and supporting daily routines.

This research will lead to advances in three research areas: *human-computer interaction; computational perception; and software engineering.* To achieve the desired goals, the PI will conduct the research and experimentation in an authentic domestic setting, a novel research facility called the Residential Laboratory recently completed next to the Georgia Tech campus. Together with experts in theoretical and practical aspects of aging, the PI will establish a pattern of research in which informed design of ubiquitous computing technology can be rapidly deployed, evaluated and evolved in an authentic setting. Special attention will be paid throughout to issues relating to privacy and trust implications. The products of this project are to be transitioned to researchers and practitioners interested in performing more large-scale observations of the social and economic impact of Aware Home technologies.

©CARS/Springer. All rights reserved.

• Using Context-Recognition for Preventative Medicine in the Home

Principal Investigator: Steven Intille. Ph.D.
Massachusetts Institute of Technology, Cambridge.

This 3-year, $319,916 Information Technology (IT) project, is investigating new technologies for "just-in-time" preventative health education in the home. Prior work on using computer telephony to deliver health education and counseling to people in their homes being extended to mobile computing devices. Algorithms are being investigated that passively and actively collect data from healthy users of mobile computing devices and process that data to identify patterns of everyday activity using probabilistic models. The activity of each person will be used to present preventative health information and counseling at "teachable moments" -- the times when that information is most likely to impact the user's health-related decision-making. A prototype system for elderly individuals interested in improving their exercise level and diet will be collaboratively developed by technologists and medical professionals. A participatory design process will be used to ensure the devices are easy to use, even for those who are not computer literate. The prototype system is to be evaluated in a small focus group study.

2.3 Centers for Medicare and Medicade Services (CMS)

Georgetown University Medical Center has been awarded a grant by the Health Care Financing Administration (HCFA) to participate in a demonstration project involving fee-for-service Medicare patients aged 65 or older. The award, effective February 1, 2001, enables a five-year study of innovative technologies to care for patients with congestive heart failure (CHF). The Principal Investigator of the project is James C. Welch, MD, MBA.

Through a combination of in-home visits, telephone monitoring, and discussions with the CHF' patient's physician, the care managers will be helping to assure that patients stay at the optimal level of health possible with this chronic disease.

High-tech innovations will assist the care managers in performing their duties. The first of these innovations will be a *home-monitoring device* by HomMed Corporation that is attached to a

- scale
- blood pressure cuff
- pulse oximeter.

The pulse oximeter counts the pulse and measures the oxygen saturation level in the blood by means of light passing through the finger. Each day at a prescribed time, the patient will be reminded by a prerecorded voice in the monitoring device that it is time to take their vital signs. The monitoring device will also ask the patient two or three yes-no questions about their perceived level or functioning for that day, such as: "Are you feeling better or worse than yesterday?"

Another high tech innovation to be employed by the care managers is a paperless operating environment. Currently, the efforts of home health nurses and others who work in the community are frequently delayed by lack of access to key information. The

©CARS/Springer. All rights reserved.

program will be using an Internet-based software application called Canopy that supplies a wealth of information to the care managers on laptop computers. For example, the daily results from the home monitoring devices will allow the care managers to see who has suddenly gained 3-5 pounds overnight, a sign of potential worsening of disease that need immediate intervention with diuretics and renewed dietary education.

It is hoped the 1,500 participants trial will demonstrate that high-tech (Internet-based) as well as "high-touch" (providing increased contact with health care providers) can both improve the quality of patients' lives and reduce the high cost to the Medicare program.

3. Conclusion

Although incomplete, this brief review of In-Home Healthcare projects in the USA provides a strong indication that, properly applied, currently available technologies and the newer capabilities "on the drawing hoard" hold high promise to meet the needs of the projected demographic revolution currently in progress.

Acknowledgements

My great appreciation is expressed to William C. Mann and Sumi Helal for providing information and graphic materials about the RERC on *Technology for Successful Aging,* to Betty Levine for materials about the *Medicare Demonstration Project*, and to Jeff Collmann for his briefing on the CPRI Toolkit. I am indebted to Kevin Cleary and Audrey Kinsella for their constructive suggestions and sound advice on matters of content and format of the presentation.

The views expressed herein are those of the author and do not represent the position of the National Science Foundation

References

1. Arras, J. D., and Dubler, N. N. "Ethical and Social Implications of High Tech Home Care", *Bringing the Hospital Home*, 99. 1-30, The Johns Hopkins University Press, 1995.
2. Winters, J. and Herman, B. "Report: Workshop on Home Care Technologies for the 21st Century". Catholic University of America and Center for Devices and Radiological Health, Food and Drug Administration, April 7-9, 1999.
3. Feussner, J. R., Aisen, M. L. "Proceedings: Technologies for Successful Aging", *Journal of Rehabilitation and Development,* VOL. 38, NO. 1, 2001 (Supplement).
4. Coile, R. C., Jr. *The Paperless Hospital: Healthcare in a Digital Age*, p. 205, Health Administration Press, Chicago, 2002.
5. Ibid., pp. 253-281.
6. CPRI Toolkit, "Managing Information Security in Health Care, Version 3". Computer-based Patient Record Institute. 2002 (http://www.cpri-host.org/toolkit/toc.html).
7. Interagency Committee on Disability Research. (http://www.ncddr.org/icdr/).
8. Rehabilitation Engineering Research Centers, H133E010106.
9. URL: http://www.naric.com/search/pd/indextype.html.
10. Ibid, H133E010804.

CARS 2002 – H.U. Lemke, M.W. Vannier; K. Inamura, A.G. Farman, K. Doi & J.H.C. Reiber (Editors)
©CARS/Springer. All rights reserved.

Home health monitoring and diabetes: a web-based approach to achieving better control

Betty A. Levine[a], Adil Alaoui[a], Ming-Jye Hu[a], Karen Smith[b], Stephen Clement[b], Alan Neustadtl[c], Seong K. Mun[a]
[a] ISIS Center, Georgetown University Medical Center, Washington DC, 20007
[b]Endocrinology, Georgetown University Medical Center, Washington DC, 20007
[c]Department of Sociology, University of Maryland, College Park, MD 20742

Abstract

MyCareTeam is a web-based application designed to facilitate self-monitoring and improve care provider monitoring of individuals with diabetes while improving communications between patients and their care providers. Authorized users of MyCareTeam access patient data via a secure socket layer (SSL) connection. A stand-alone application was developed to read the glucose readings directly from different manufacturer's glucose meters and create a data file of those values on the patient's local personal computer. Once securely connected to the MyCareTeam web site, the patient uploads the data file to the secure database. The data is automatically analyzed and presented in multiple formats to the patient and available to their care provider when he/she next visits MyCareTeam. A sixteen patient pilot study was undertaken at Georgetown University Medical Center using the MyCareTeam application to show technical feasibility. The patients that used the web site more frequently improved their diabetes control more than those that used it sporadically. Larger clinical trials are underway at the Boston VA in Massachusetts and Windber Medical Center in Pennsylvania.

Keywords: Home monitoring, e-health, diabetes

1. Introduction

Home monitoring of patients with a chronic disease is an area where telemedicine and tele-monitoring devices can make a tremendous impact on both the quality and cost of care. The daily regiments required of patients with a chronic disease are often burdensome and difficult for patients to maintain on their own. Studies have shown that close monitoring of patients with a chronic disease like diabetes by health care providers can improve clinical outcomes and quality of life, while reducing costs associated with complications of their disease. These studies also demonstrate, however, that patients require <u>intensive</u> support from health care providers in order to follow the rigorous treatment protocols necessary to achieve noticeably good results [1,2]. The cost and time required for intensive support from health care providers is prohibitively expensive using today's standards of care.

At Georgetown University, we have developed MyCareTeam, an interactive web-based disease management tool. MyCareTeam focuses on improving health outcomes of

©CARS/Springer. All rights reserved

patients with chronic diseases through better disease management, online monitoring by care providers, improved self-management, and education. The self-monitoring tools, educational resources, and on-line support communities available at MyCareTeam enable people with a chronic disease to take control of their health. MyCareTeam was designed to improve health outcomes by improving patient compliance through education, preventing complications through swift and effective intervention, and providing integrated data management.

While MyCareTeam can be applied to many diseases, our pilot application is for diabetes, a serious chronic disease affecting almost 16 million Americans and costing over 98 billion dollars annually [3,4]. MyCareTeam has also been piloted for kidney failure patients performing peritoneal dialysis at home and the development of MyCareTeam for the management of other chronic diseases is under investigation.

2. Methods

A patient with diabetes is often asked to check his/her blood sugar level as much as three to five times a day using a standard blood glucose meter. They do this by pricking their finger, or other part of their body, to get a small drop of blood that is placed on a reading strip into the glucose meter. The meter comes back with a reading of how much sugar is currently in the blood. The glucose meter, depending on manufacturer and model, can store from 10 – 1000 readings in its memory. In our study, patients were asked to connect their glucose meters to their personal computers weekly and run a small application to transfer the glucose readings from the glucose meter to their computer. Once the glucose readings are stored in a file on the computer, the patient goes to the MyCareTeam web site and uploads the glucose readings to the secure database accessible through the web site.

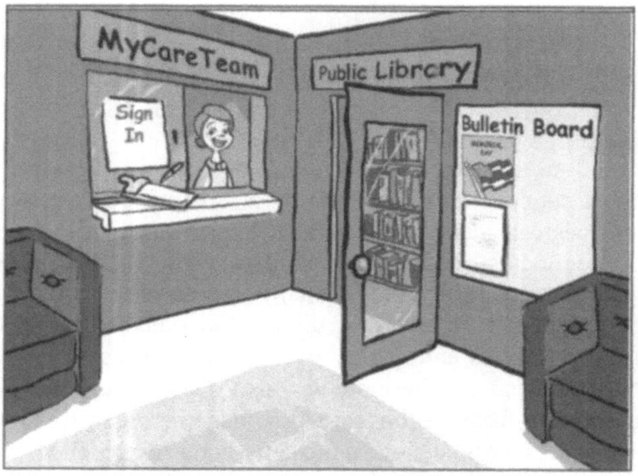

Figure 1.0 Lobby of MyCareTeam

MyCareTeam was designed to provide patients an easy, friendly, and familiar user interface that provides them access to their chronic disease data. Patients use a standard

©CARS/Springer. All rights reserved.

Internet browser to access MyCareTeam. The look and feel of MyCareTeam simulates a visit to a medical clinic. The patient enters the web site through the front door of the building and once inside can read the current notices on the bulletin board, get educational materials, or sign-in with the receptionist (see Figure 1.). Once they have entered the secure site using their username/password combination they are given a brief synopsis of their current health (see Figure 2.). Based on recent clinical data like blood glucose readings or lab values, MyCareTeam automatically analyzes the data and presents the results in a user-friendly format. Patients are made aware of alerts relating to their data as well as positive results like an average blood sugar level within the target range. There is also a section reminding patients of upcoming lab tests or office visits.

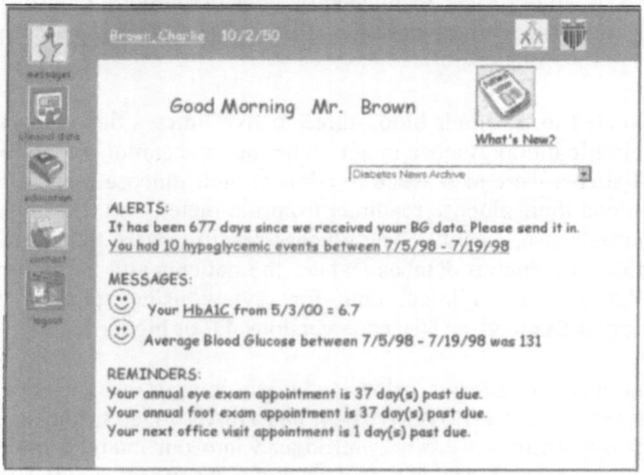

Figure 2.0 Synopsis of patient's current health

MyCareTeam also provides an easy, friendly, and automated interface for care providers. As the care provider enters the site with their username/password combination, they are presented with three lists of their current patients. The first list is patients requiring immediate attention due to an alert value in their latest data, also called the alert list. The second list is patients that have sent in new data but the care provider has not checked it yet, also called the new data list. Patients can appear in both the alert and new data lists, but reviewing the patients from either list clears them out of both lists. This maintains a current triage system for care providers so that they know which patients require attention when they first enter MyCareTeam. The third list is a complete listing of all patients associated with the current care provider.

MyCareTeam contains an on-line messaging system that provides secured messaging between the care provider and his/her patients. Care providers can review messages from all their patients when they first log in or review messages specific to a given patient while reviewing that patient's record. With the triage systems put in place to simplify the care provider's interaction with MyCareTeam, care providers can read through a patient's record in at most two to five minutes. Telephone contacts with patients are minimized; they now communicate via the messaging and comment sections of MyCareTeam.

©CARS/Springer. All rights reserved

3. Pilot Study

Sixteen patients with diabetes were enrolled in a six-month non-randomized pilot study of MyCareTeam at Georgetown University Medical Center. The study consisted of diabetic patients who failed to obtain glycemic control with conventional follow-up. Glycemic control is monitored through quarterly blood tests known as HbA1c or glycosylated hemoglobin. HbA1c measures the level of long-term glucose control, over two to three months. It is the best predictor of risk for future diabetes complications. Our goal was to show the effectiveness of the technology by reducing HbA1C by one point over six-months. An HbA1c value of less than seven is considered good control for people with diabetes. In our study the average baseline HbA1c for the entire patient population was 10.95.

Patients were directed to test their blood three to five times a day using an AccuChek© Complete™ electronic blood glucose meter. The meter accumulates up to 1000 readings in its memory. Patients were also asked to connect their glucose meters to their personal computers, download their glucose readings from the meter, and transmit the readings to the MyCareTeam database, weekly. The glucose readings were transferred over a point-to-point connection to a central database where the patients and their care providers had secure access (SSL) to the clinical data for review using standard Web browsing technologies (Internet Explorer or Netscape versions 4.0 or higher.)

In the statistical analysis of our pilot study, an attempt was made to establish a relationship between the use of MyCareTeam and HbA1c. Due to the small sample size, multivariate control measures were not introduced into our analytic models. Instead, a simple "before-after" research design was used and a dependent samples *t*-test to assess if there were statistically significant differences comparing the arithmetic averages of the measures at baseline and six months. All tests report the achieved *p-value* for a one-tailed matched pair *t-test* comparing averages at baseline and six-months later. A one-tailed *t*-test was selected because of the literature that shows that close monitoring of individuals with diabetes by health care providers improves clinical outcomes [1,2].

4. Results

Ten out of the sixteen patients regularly sent their data to the MyCareTeam database, three never sent in any data, and three sent it in sporadically. Eight patients checked their data online at least twice a month, while eight checked their data once a month or less. Therefore, we then split the users into groups identified as "Heavy" or "Light" users based on their usage patterns. At the end of the six-month trial we exceeded our initial goal of reducing HbA1c by one point.

Table 1.0 presents the average HbA1c results for 'All', 'Heavy', and 'Light' users. The average baseline HbAlc for all sixteen patients was 10.95 and their average six-months HbAlc was 8.73. HbAlc was reduced by 2.22 percentage points in the total group, *p-value* = 0.0005. Differences between Heavy (n=8) versus Light (n=8) users were evaluated for

©CARS/Springer. All rights reserved.

inter group differences based upon utilization of MyCareTeam. Heavy users had a baseline HbAlc of 10.83 compared to 11.08 in the Light users. Heavy users' six month HbAlc was reduced to 7.68 compared to 9.79 in Light users. Heavy users had a significant six month HbAlc reduction of 3.15 points, *p-value* = 0.01 compared to a 1.28 points reduction of HbAlc in light users, which was not significant.

Type of user	Average HbA1c at Baseline	Average HbA1c at 6 months	Difference	p-value
All users	10.95	8.73	2.22	0.0005
Heavy users	10.83	7.68	3.15	0.01
Light users	11.08	9.79	1.28	not significant

Table 1. Average HbA1c at baseline and six-months and the resultant drop

5. Conclusion

Our pilot study has shown that using MyCareTeam has enabled patients with diabetes to achieve better control of their diabetes. Even with a small sample size, the change in HbA1c was statistically significant. MyCareTeam automatically analyzes data and presents it to both patients and their care providers in a timely, easily understandable format. Increased interactions between patients and care providers, automated analysis of clinical data, and the presentations of the analyzed data provide the education and encouragement needed to help patients achieve good glycemic control. Two larger randomized control trials of MyCareTeam have begun at the Veterans Administration Healthcare System in Boston, Massachusetts and the Windber Medical Center in Windber, Pennsylvania.

Acknowledgements

This project was funded in part from The Advanced Medical Technology and Network Systems Research, U.S. Army, contract number DAMD17-94-V-4015

References

1. The Diabetes Control and Complications Trial Research Group: The effect of intensive treatment of diabetes on the development and progression of long-term complications in insulin-dependent diabetes mellitus. N Engl J Med 1993; 329:977-986
2. UK Prospective Diabetes Study Group (UKPDS 33 & 38) Lancet 352; 837-853 1998 & BMJ 317: 703-713, 1998.
3. National Diabetes Fact Sheet: National estimates and general information on diabetes in the United States. U.S. Department of Health and Human Services, Centers for Disease Control & Prevention. National Center for Chronic Disease Prevention and Health Promotion. Nov 1998.
4. Diabetes: A Serious Public Health Problem At-A-Glance 2000. U.S. Department of Health and Human Services, Centers for Disease Control and Prevention. 2000.

©CARS/Springer. All rights reserved.

The communication concept of a regional stroke unit network based on encrypted image transmission and the DICOM-Mail standard

Engelmann U[a], Schroeter A[a], Schweitzer T[b], Meinzer HP[a]

[a] German Cancer Research Center, Division Medical & Biological Informatics
Im Neuenheimer Feld 280, 69120 Heidelberg, Germany
U.Engelmann@DKFZ-Heidelberg.de
[b] Steinbeis-Transferzentrum Medizinische Informatik, Im Neuenheimer Feld 517, 69120 Heidelberg, Germany, URL: www.chili-radiology.com

Abstract

This paper describes the communication concept for a regional stroke network for the exchange of medical images and reports. The data transfer is realized with regular e-mail (SMTP). DICOM images are sent as DICOM compliant attachments. Private key encryption is used to ensure data security and privacy. All used protocols are standardized or de-facto standards and allow vendor-independent communication. Different problems and options of the concept realization are discussed.

Keywords: Teleradiology, DICOM, security

1. Introduction

Time is one of the most important factors in the diagnosis, therapy and prognosis of apoplexy or stroke (time is brain!). The German federal state Rhineland-Palatinate (Rheinland-Pfalz) took the political decision to support the establishment of a state-wide competence network. The main purpose is to enable fast and reliable distribution of medical images for the purpose of stroke diagnosis and therapy.

The first step is establishing (and funding) of a pilot network connecting the referring hospitals in Neustadt and Worms with the competence centers in Ludwigshafen and Mannheim. Basic requirements have been defined in the request for proposals (RFP) which was organized by a health care consultant company (Pergis, Ludwigshafen, Germany) and a group of subcontracted teleradiology experts. Key requirements of the RFP were the following:

Full DICOM compliance for the exchange of data with imaging modalities. Storage of data in databases, advanced functions for the display and analysis of medical images from different modalities. This means, that not a dedicated special purpose communication system, but an integrated system was required.

©CARS/Springer. All rights reserved.

The standard data transfer should be realized via E-Mail (SMTP) and the new DICOM supplement 54. The main reason for that was that e-mails can be sent through firewalls without any changes in their rule-sets. Another reason was the availability of standard encryption methods for e-mail.

The system should support autorouting and the automatic protocol conversion between DICOM and SMTP. All transmitted data must be encrypted. All communication channels must work with existing and future firewall solutions without security reductions.

Several teleradiology and PACS vendors submitted proposals. The selection process was based on the presentation of the solution and proof of concept with software demonstrations. The winner was the Steinbeis Transferzentrum Medizinische Informatik, a technology transfer company in Heidelberg, Germany, with a dedicated software architecture based on their CHILI (tele-) radiology product family.

2. Method

CHILI is a radiological workstation with powerful teleradiology functionality, supporting various protocols and de-facto standards for image distribution and interactive teleconferencing of medical images [1]. One important feature of the system is its security concept and the implemented data protection measures based on symmetric and public key encryption [2].

One of the supported transfer protocols is SMTP (simple mail transfer protocol). Thus, users can submit medical images and additional data as regular e-mails. They can also receive data in different formats (DICOM, JPEG, GIF, etc.) from communication partners who can submit images as attachments from a plain mail client only.

Most of the requested functionality of the RFP was already available in the CHILI software. Some additional features had to be implemented for the project, such as the automatic encryption/decryption of mails, and automatic protocol conversions between DICOM/SMTP. Data security measures, key management based on public key encryption and open standards have been implemented. The flexible protocol conversion to and from e-mail allows easy extension of the teleradiology network to other data types and can provide the basis for a general telemedicine network.

3. Main concepts

The principle components of the network are shown in figure 1. Referring hospitals (without expertise in neuroradiology, neurology and neurosurgery) are equipped with one or several CHILI workstations (PCs running Linux). One is acting as a CHILI server and the other are CHILI clients. The server receives the images from the imaging modalities (e.g. CT), PACS or a DICOM workstation via DICOM protocol [3]. The server stores the data in a relational database. The CHILI clients are connected to this database and can view and process the stored data. Teleconferences between all CHILI workstations are possible.

©CARS/Springer. All rights reserved.

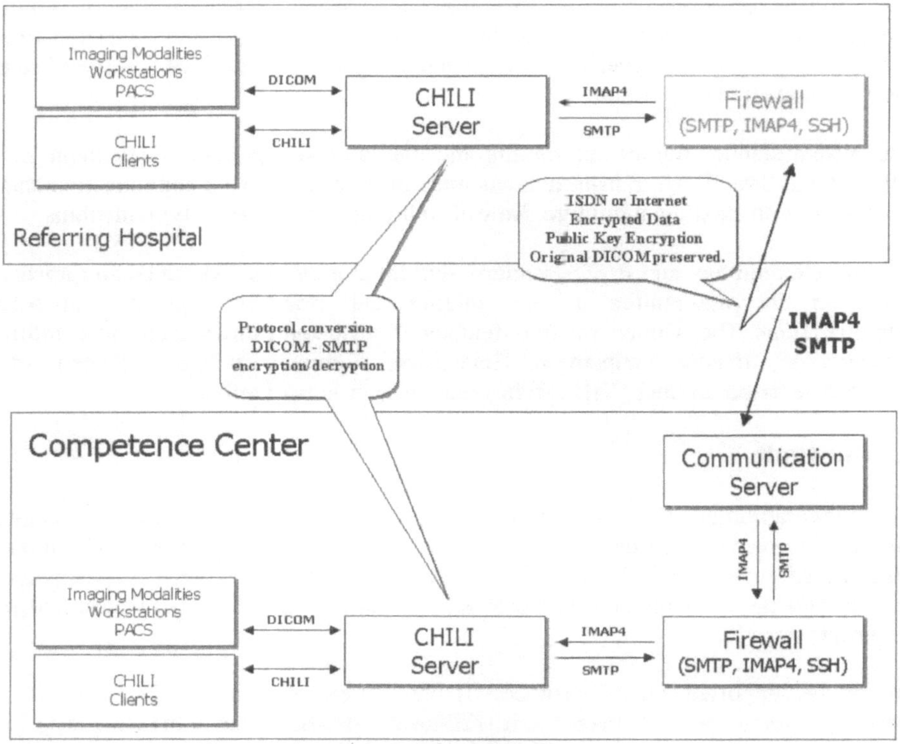

Figure 2. Protocols between the components

The data is submitted to the competence centers via e-mail, using the *Simple Mail Transfer Protocol* (SMTP) [4, 5]. The first versions of SMTP could only transfer 7-bit text messages. The *Multipurpose Internet Mail Extensions* (MIME) allows the transmission of multipart messages with many kinds of data [6]. The DICOM standard defines in supplement 54 the *DICOM MIME Type* [7]. This allows to transmit medical images via e-mail in a standardized way.

As DICOM images do contain patient data, it is not allowed (by different national and international laws) to transmit the data as clear text over unprotected communication lines. Thus, data protection measures have to be taken into account. One of the implemented methods of our communication concept is to encrypt and sign the mails, resp. parts of it. Galvin et al. define in RFC 1847: *Security Multiparts for MIME* how parts of e-mail can be signed and encrypted [8]. We used *MIME Security with OpenPGP* for the realization [9, 10]. The data is signed with the private key of the submitting person to protect authenticity and integrity of the data. The public key of the receiver is used to encrypt the data [2].

©CARS/Springer. All rights reserved.

We have to take into account that we are submitting large amounts of data. The mail gateways usually limit the size of mails which are processed. Thus, all data is splitted into several mails of acceptable size automatically.

The submission process can be activated either by a user or automatically by a so-called autorouter. Different rules can be defined how and to whom the data should be sent and when. A problem is that no user is sitting at the workstation when data is sent automatically. This means that the submitted data cannot be signed by a person. Thus, we use a private key of the workstation (or institution) to create the signature of the data which protects authenticity and integrity of the data.

The transmission starts when the DICOM data has been converted into a set of encrypted e-mails. The CHILI server of the referring hospital (see figure 1) sends the data out to the external network (ISDN or Internet) over an optional firewall. The SMTP port of the firewall is usually open for data exchange.

The communication server at the competence center receives and temporary stores the incoming data from the referring hospitals. Usually, this server is located outside the hospital LAN in front of a firewall. The teleradiology servers inside the competence centers (behind the firewall) fetch the data periodically via IMAP from the communication server [11].

The fetched data is removed from the communication server and decrypted and re-converted into standard DICOM files and stored in the database of the local CHILI server. Visible and audible alarms inform the personnel of new incoming data which can be reported directly with the viewer of the CHILI workstation (client or server). The autoroutes can be configured to forward the data to one or several other workstations in the competence center. DICOM workstation can also query and retrieve data from the CHILI server.

Results and other information can easily be replied to the sender of the data via the user interface of the CHILI program. The digital signature of the reporting physician is used to ensure the authenticity of the report. The replies are again sent as encrypted e-mails to the communication server in front of the firewall. The CHILI server of the referring hospital is then fetching the answer and integrates the report into the local database where it is stored and viewed with the related series of the image data.

It is very important is to control the completeness and correctness of the data transfers. All transfers are logged at both sites. Furthermore, sender and receiver can see the progress of the data transfer. A meta-protocol has been implemented on top of SMTP for reliable and secure transfer of confirmations (logging!) and possible failure repair measures, such as autorouting to another competence center. Automatic fail over between the communications servers at different locations has been implemented in this way.

The realized CHILI system is not only a dedicated emergency tool. But also a radiological workstation which can be used for reporting in daily routine. Additional clients can be connected to the server if necessary. All clients can perform interactive teleconferences in-

©CARS/Springer. All rights reserved.

house without the need of sending the data to the other workstation. Other options, such as long term archiving, distribution of images in the intranet, mobile clients, or 3D visualization modules [12,13] can be integrated into the "emergency system" easily.

4. Discussion

The system has been implemented as described. It is an open concept and based on standards. This ensures the data exchange with other systems. Nevertheless, there were from time to time several options possible. We used OpenPGP for the data encryption. An alternative to this was S/MIME [14]. We choose OpenPGP because it is at the current state easy to implement and as it was as popular as S/MIME. But the latter will be implemented later (see below).

Autorouting of data speeds up the transmission from the modality to the competence center. A limitation of this approach is, that the data is then signed by a machine with a machine signature instead of a person. We think that this is acceptable.

Another problem is when many people can be the receiver of the data. This means that the sender has to know the name of the person at the other side.

Currently, all public signatures are distributed by the CHILI system itself. The private keys are stored at the workstation and activated by a pass-phrase. The system is prepared to use digital signatures on cards, such as a health professional card. It is not yet clear which trust center will be chosen as provider for the certified signature cards. The price of the signatures is an important issue as a university hospital would need about 20-30 cards for the radiology department only. A budget has not been foreseen for this so far.

The *Sphinx project* launched by German authorities (BSI) aims to improve secure email exchange. The projects technological base is the protocol *TeleTrust e.V. MailTrusT Version 2*. This includes the standards S/MIME, X.509v3 and others [15]. Proprietary products are already on the way, but with the *project Ägypten* there is now also a Free Software solution going to be realized for popular mail user agents [16]. The integration of this software into our architecture is planned as well.

The aim of the *GNU Privacy Project* is to develop free encryption software for everybody [17]. This project is supported by two German ministries (Bundesministerium für Wirtschaft und Technologie and Bundesministerium des Inneren). It is planned to integrate the resulting free software tool *GNU Privacy Guard* as well into our realized infrastructure to achieve as much interoperability as possible.

5. Conclusion

The realized teleradiology network meets the requirements of the RFP for the stroke unit network. The network can easily be extended and scaled. Redundancy of all critical system components provides high availability.

©CARS/Springer. All rights reserved.

The data security concept and flexible protocol conversion allow an easy extension of the teleradiology network to other data types. They can provide the basis for a general telemedicine network.

Acknowledgements

The pilot project *Teleradiology (Stroke-Unit in Rheinland-Pfalz)* is funded by the *Ministerium für Arbeit, Soziales, Familie und Gesundheit* in Mainz, Rheinland-Pfalz, Germany.

References

1. Steinbeis-Transferzentrum Medizinische Informatik. CHILI: Second Generation Teleradiology and Telecardiology. http://www.chili-radiology.com/.
2. Baur HJ, Engelmann U. Saurbier F, Schröter A, Baur U, Meinzer HP. How to deal with Security and Privacy Issues in Teleradiology. Computer Methods and Programs in Biomedicine, 53, 1 (1997) 1-8.
3. NEMA Standards Publication PS 3.1-15. Digital Imaging and Communications in Medicine (DICOM). National Electrical Manufacturers Association, 2101 L Street, N.W., Washington, D.C. 20037, 2000.
4. Resnick P (ed). RFP 2822: Internet Message Format. April 2001. http://www.ietf.org/rfc.html.
5. Wood D. Programming Internet Email. O'Reilly: Sebastopol 1999.
6. Borenstein N, Freed N. RFC 1521: MIME (Multipurpose Internet Mail Extensions) part one: Mechanisms for specifying and describing the format of Internet message bodies, September 1993. http://www.ietf.org/rfc.html.
7. DICOM Standards Committee, Digital Imaging and Communications in Medicine (DICOM). Supplement 54: DICOM MIME Type. http://medical.nema.org/Dicom/supps/sup54_pc.pdf.
8. Galvin J, Murphy S, Crocker S, Freed N. RFC 1847: Security multiparts for MIME: Multipart/signed and multipart/encrypted, October 1995. http://www.ietf.org/.
9. Elkins M, Del Torto D, Levien R, Roessler T. RFC 3156: Mime security with openPGP, August 2001. http://www.ietf.org/rfc.html.
10. Callas J, Donnerhacke L, Finney H, Thayer R. RFC 2440: OpenPGP message format, November 1998. http://www.ietf.org/rfc.html.
11. Mullet D, Mullet K. Managing IMAP . O'Reilly: Sebastopol 2000.
12. Engelmann U, Schröter A, Schwab M, Eisenmann U, Meinzer HP. Openness and Flexibility: From Teleradiology to PACS. In: Lemke HU, Vannier MW, Inamura K, Farman AG (Eds). CARS'99. Amsterdam: Elsevier (1999) 534-538.
13. Engelmann U, Schröter A, Schwab M, Eisenmann U, Bahner ML, Delorme S, Hahne H, Meinzer HP. The Linux-based PACS project at the German Cancer Research Center. Lemke HU, Inamura K, Farman AG, Doi K (Eds). CARS 2000: Computer Assisted Radiology and Surgery. Proceedings of the 14th International Congress and Exhibition. Amsterdam: Elsevier (2000) 419-424.
14. Ramsdell, B. RFC 2633: S/MIME Version 3 Message Specification, June 1999. http://www.ietf.org/rfc.html.
15. Bundesamt für Sicherheit in der Informationstechnik. Sphinx Project. http://www.bsi.de/aufgaben/projekte/sphinx/index.htm.
16. The GNU Privacy Guard. Projekt Ägypten. http://www.gnupg.org/aegypten/tech.en.html.
17. Das GNU Privacy Projekt (GnuPP). http://www.gnupp.de/start.html.

©CARS/Springer. All rights reserved.

Framework for systematic assessment of the regional HUSpacs after the reengineering of hospital and external processes

Harno K[a], Roine R[b], Pohjonen H[c], Kinnunen J[c], Kauppinen T[c]
[a] Helsinki University Central Hospital, Department of Medicine, Administration,
[b] Helsinki University Central Hospital, Administration,
[c] Helsinki University Central Hospital, Department of Radiology, Finland

Abstract

Installing one of the largest regional PAC systems de novo in the Hospital District of Helsinki and Uusimaa (HUS) with 1, 4 million inhabitants has several potential benefits as the financially inefficient intermediate steps to digital radiography are eliminated. However, the capital costs to achieve this filmless digital environment within the existing three university hospitals, four regional hospitals and 32 communal health centres of HUS are enormous. It has been suggested that by re-engineering the x-ray service processes the number of stages in the overall process may be cut down by at least 25 %. This also speeds up the transfer time between processes. Since the number of imaging procedures in HUS reaches annually figures of 1.000.000, this points to the possibility that genuine cost savings may be achieved. The aim of the assessment is to study the effectiveness of the HUSpacs regarding its capacity to improve the quality of health care, to increase the equity of access to health care and to reduce the cost of delivering health care. This may be achieved by designing a framework for the systematic assessment of HUSpacs. A brief description of the regional integration of PACS with the planned security solution will be presented.

Keywords: Regional PACS, clinical processes, assessment

1. Introduction

Many telemedicine applications in radiology have been proven to result in savings through avoidance of unnecessary patient transfer or patient travel. Teleradiology is evolving from a point-to-point application to a universal network closely resembling the Internet. A picture archiving and communication system (PACS) that uses digital data held in a single or distributed database and is accessible through a network, offers new interfaces and gateways to healthcare facilities. This enables hospitals and clinics to reengineer new seamless clinical processes both within hospitals and between remote health care institutions. The high cost of PACS implies that they have to be shown to improve health and be cost-effective before wide-spread adoption. So far, this has not been the case, probably partly because previous studies have focused on organizational and not regional PACS installations utilizing the same common infrastructure.

©CARS/Springer. All rights reserved.

HUSpacs has been in operation in two clinics of the Helsinki University Central Hospital for over two years and seven hospitals have become filmless by the end of last year. The regional HUSpacs is planned to be completed by the year 2003. Installing one of the largest regional PAC systems de novo in the Hospital District of Helsinki and Uusimaa (HUS) with 1, 4 million inhabitants has several potential benefits as the financially inefficient intermediate steps to digital radiography are eliminated. By reducing the need for x-ray film, processing chemicals and archiving x-ray films should result in savings on material costs.

However, the capital costs to achieve this filmless digital environment within the existing three university hospitals, four regional hospitals and 31 communal health centres of HUS are enormous. It has been suggested that by re-engineering the x-ray service processes the number of stages in the overall process may be cut down by at least 25 %. This also speeds up the transfer time between processes. Since the number of imaging procedures in HUS reaches annually figures of 1.000.000, this points to the possibility that genuine cost savings may be achieved. After the implementation of the HUSpacs the improvement in effectiveness and cost-effectiveness of clinical care must be proven. The aim of the present study is to design a framework for the systematic assessment of HUSpacs.

2. Methods

The requirements for the infrastructure and design of the integrated PAC delivery system are based on local short-term archives and a centralized long-term or back-up archive. The regional wide architecture and integration plans include a regional reference data base system or patient information directory (PID), which facilitates access to patient information (including images, requests and reports).

There are agreed standards of using HL-7 (Health Level 7) and DICOM standards to integrate different modalities, RIS and HIS in sharing patient and study information across the regional network. Hospital Information Systems in all the regional hospitals comply with these standards, but pre IHE standards prevent information systems of health centres from communicating with HIS systems. The reference data base or PID is therefore needed for images to be delivered between secondary care and primary care, or a web-server may be used for self ordered images in health centres.

Data security is enforced by user ID's and passwords; authentication by smart cards is planned. The patient's consent is always needed for viewing images by means of the patient information directory.

When the idea of the regional digital imaging and archiving system in HUS was introduced its exact aims and applications were first defined. The more general requirements for HUSpacs were flexibility in respect to demand for services and resources, efficacy in production performance and ability to conform to the guidelines on security and confidentiality.

©CARS/Springer. All rights reserved.

Virtually most work processes by clinicians in today's hospital environment are impacted by imaging results. Efficient clinical practices demand that many elements of business processes in health care be successful and efficient. HUSpacs will only be as effective as the way it is used. Therefore, we designed a programme for the implementation defining the utilization of the HUSpacs system for clinicians, information technology staff and imaging. The broad outlines of this programme include the following:

(1) New model processes were first reengineered by applying a new software program (Process Guide, QPR Limited) for the design of these processes in the following departments - outpatient department, clinical wards, operating theatres and accident & emergency department of the Hospital District of Helsinki and Uusimaa. These model processes included three strategic options with estimated economic impacts: take the rule, make the rules and break the rules. Taking the rule was to conform to the existing way of working and the awaited financial advantage was greatest with the last choice.
Traditional hospital care processes impacted include admissions and ancillary support services. However, clinical care processes now include care planning, processing of physicians orders, medication administration and clinical documentation.
The process models were intended to steer the different departments after installing HUSpacs to re-design the way clinicians were presently working in the hospitals and promote both intranet as well as extranet consultation procedures. The strategic options were distributed to HUSpacs project groups and heads of the departments at least six months before implementing HUSpacs.

(2) **Positive outcomes** for HUSpacs were defined and thereafter converted to framework factors. The outcomes must provide either (a) reduced costs of care, (b) improved access of patients to care, (c) increased quality of care at the same or lower cost than alternatives, (d) improved quality of life for patients or (e) reduced clinical risk.

(3) For each new process the following **framework factors** will be applied in the final assessment of HUSpacs – quality factors, organizational factors and cost factors.

(4) The **assessment criteria** were based on demands and characteristics required from the framework factors. These assessment criteria were thereafter broken down into measurable quantities and accountable concepts.

(5) External steering of the assessment and evaluation of the results will be performed by independent observers.

3. Assessment procedure

Quality factors, which will be assessed in the processes during the HUSpacs study, will be

Positive outcome -> increased quality of care
Factor -> Quality factor
    Criteria -> Imaging diagnosis

©CARS/Springer. All rights reserved.

1. *Define the accuracy of imaging diagnosis inside and outside the radiological department.*

Firstly, radiological diagnosis after processing of digital data from digital archives can be compared with conventional x-ray reporting from images in radiological departments of two university hospital clinics.
Secondly, the accuracy of clinical diagnosis made by experienced orthopaedic surgeons and cardiologists from conventional x-ray films and HUSpacs system will be determined.

Positive outcomes -> increased quality of care and reduced costs
Factor -> Quality factor
Criteria -> Work flow

2. *Determine the speed of consultation and the decision making process effect on costs*

A signed report or similar transferred after imaging from the radiological departments of two hospitals with or without PACS (conventional reporting systems) to (a) clinicians in the same hospital or (b) general practitioners in health centres. The logistics of reporting between the two systems is tested.

Besides the decision making process, also the most efficient way of treating a health problem will be tackled by an open effectiveness analysis – either cost-effectiveness (CEA) or cost-benefit analysis (CBA).

Positive outcomes -> increased quality of care and improved quality of life for patients
Factor -> Quality factor
Criteria -> Access to care

3. *Specify the access of patients to required standard of care and the quality effect*

Patients treated and imaged in a district general hospital of HUS are randomly compared in respect to their access to specialized services of HUS (university hospital services). Half of the patients receive radiological consultations via HUSpacs and the other half are treated according to current local practice.

A standardized generic health state classification system will be chosen to measure the essential components of the quality of well-being. This choice should possess discriminatory power before the intervention and also detect changes in health status afterwards.

Organizational factors relate to the transformation of the mode of actions clinicians are using after the implementation of HUSpacs.

Positive outcomes -> increased quality of care at lower cost and improved quality of life for patients

©CARS/Springer. All rights reserved.

Factor -> Organizational factor
Criteria -> Process chain logistics

1. *Define the access time for clinicians to imaging results and its effects*

OD of hospitals and health centres in different organizations with and without (conventional use of x-ray films) access to HUSpacs system are compared in respect to speed of imaging result introduction and utilization of these results to clinical treatment. The maturity of the reengineered model processes to utilize the enhanced information flow will be tested and the total costs of this will be specified.

A standardized generic health state classification system will be chosen to measure the essential components of the quality of well-being. This choice should possess discriminatory power before the intervention and also detect changes in health status afterwards.

Positive outcomes -> reduced costs of care
Factor -> Organizational factor
Criteria -> Acceptability and utilization

2. *Clinical change management and productivity*

This refers to the willingness of clinicians to use computer terminals for viewing HUSpacs instead of x-ray films in outpatient departments and during ward rounds in clinics and district hospitals as well as in health centres. Estimating the costs from the new model processes allows assessment of productivity effects gained by the use of HUSpacs. The process with the least costly course of action producing equivalent benefits may be determined (cost-minimisation analysis).

Cost factors pertain to direct costs, which will be calculated according to a method specifically designed for assessing telemedicine. Direct costs can occur either within the health system (e.g. personnel costs, internal and external service charges, material expenses and rental) or to the patient (e.g. travel costs, other health-care costs and the cost of arranging home help).

(1) The service costs must lower clinical risk or lower diagnosis/treatment costs to cover the additional expense for the HUSpacs service
(2) The overhead costs of the repayment/depreciation of the HUSpacs equipment must be covered by the revenue generated or saved by the new radiology service
(3) The HUSnet charges of imaging services must be absorbed without making the price that has to be charged for services uncompetitive

4. Summary

The aim of the assessment is to study the effectiveness of the HUSpacs regarding its capacity to improve the quality of health care, to increase the equity of access to health care and to reduce the cost of delivering health care.

CARS 2002 – H.U. Lemke, M.W. Vannier; K. Inamura, A.G. Farman, K. Doi & J.H.C. Reiber (Editors)
©CARS/Springer. All rights reserved.

Evaluation of PACS and radiology services in 8 selected hospitals within the reference model program SaxTeleMed, using activity based costing and a generic business model (Marburg Model)

J. Böttcher[1], K. J. Klose[2]
[1] *pphc* Patient Process Healthcare Consulting GmbH, Ammersbek, Germany
[2]Philipps-University Marburg, Germany

Keywords: PACS evaluation, Activity Based Costing (ABC), Marburg hospital reference model

Abstract

The Free State of Saxony has set out a special reference model program SaxTeleMed for telematics in the public health system. A special focus was set to an evaluation in order to be able to transfer the knowledge and experience of the reference model program to other hospitals and medical centers but also to support a guideline for further result oriented funding. A new evaluation method, based on a generic hospital reference model, simulation technique and activity based costing had been developed and applied to 8 different institutions.

1. Introduction

The evaluation of PACS is facing a series of problems:
PACS is not a modality like e.g. CT or MR or in other words not a "product innovation"

- PACS like other IT-Sytems is a process-innovation, which means that conventional cost-benefit analysis from the product-innovation field can't be used.
- Business and medicine typically involve decisions about performing actions, whereas radiology involves decisions about obtaining information. Little has been done until now for the evaluation of information availability
- Until know, the knowledge about the real cost of secondary services in a hospital like radiology, pathology etc is very limited and in most cases, costs are mixed up with historical based reimbursement-figures.

However, the unknown cost structure of own services is a general problem not only in hospitals but also in industry. Traditional cost accounting systems and controlling have evolved primarily to serve the function of inventory valuation and external audiences.
With increased complexity of services, patient requirements, quality demands and external changes more than 50% of cost are handled as overhead and assumed cost and in general inappropriate cost information. In industry already for more than decade "process costs"

©CARS/Springer. All rights reserved.

or the more advanced "activity based costing ABC" and "activity based management ABM" has replaced the traditionally cost accounting or controlling at least for management decisions concerning make or buy, pricing and used process technology [1].

2. Method

In healthcare the success of activity based costing was limited as the process is opposed to industry not well structured and process data not available on easy ways. In order to make use of enormous amount but unstructured and fragmented patient and process information in a hospital, a generic business model "Marburg Model" was developed to integrate and to validate the available information according to figure 1.

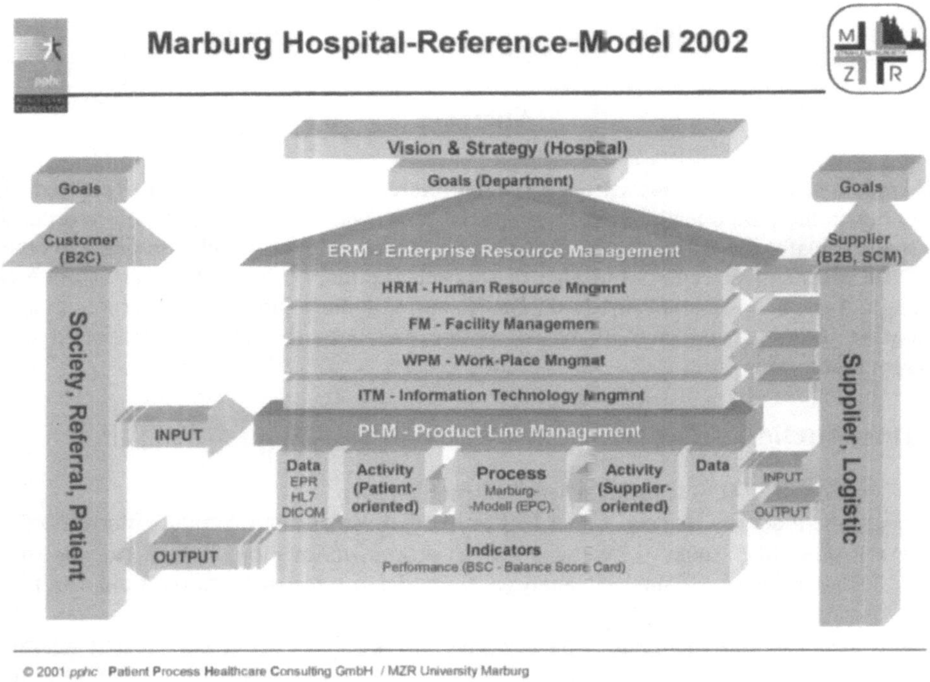

Figure 1: Marburg Hospital Reference Model

The main concept is build on a generic and fractal 3-step business process chain: Customer – Business Unit (Department) – Supplier. Complex Organization can be build up just by lining up several reference models on a line.

For the external representation two segments were integrated:

- Customers: Internal and external referrals e.g. requesting radiological services as the Input with a certain output and performance characteristic.
  The output is measured with the well known balance score card approach (BSC) covering the financial-, process-, customer- and learning-perspective)

©CARS/Springer. All rights reserved.

(this layer or view is also called "customer relation management" CRM in industry)

- Suppliers: Bought-in services from external departments for own radiological products or services, like e.g. external archiving or application service providing ASP for a complete outsourced IT-concept.
(this layer or view is also called "supply chain management" SCM in industry)

The Marburg Model [2] was designed as a business object module with the following internal modules
(see middle part in figure 1):

- Vision and Strategy of the entity, eg. hospital
- Goals and Measures of a center or department, e. g. radiology
- ERM = Entity Resource Management consisting of
- Organization and Management covering Human Resource Management (HRM), including shift- and allocation-management
- Facility Management (Plant- and Building- Management including operation and maintenance)
- WPM = Work-Place-Management: Equipment and Workspot-Design
- ITM = IT-Infrastructure: HW, SW, Workflow, Network, IT-Security
- PLM = Product Line Management, which designs and defines products and services of the department (like Standard-X-ray, Special-X-ray, Cross-Sectional, clinical conferences, Tele-Services, Education and Training, Research)

For the Process, Activity, Data and Output representation the well known ARIS-model (Architecture of Integrated Information Systems) [3] of Prof. Scheer (IDS AG) was used and adapted:

- Process: event driven process chain (epc) for all defined products and services, based on the IHE technical frame work
- Data: models of data structure for communication and elements like HL7, DICOM
- Activity: Catalogue of defined common subprocess like registration, scheduling, reporting, archiving, etc.
- Output: Time of Procedure, Intermediate Report, Conference, Final Report

The activity section had been divided in a patient- and supplier-oriented part.

3. Results

The evaluation was done in 8 selected hospitals of the reference model program SaxTeleMed in the Free State of Saxony:
The evaluation was done in a separate pre- and post-phase concerning the PACS-Implementation, starting end of 2000. For each phase and hospital a complete process documentation from request at referral side to final result presentation again referral side was done. For all phases and hospitals the data was collected in the same manner and matched with the Marburg Model for the described views.

©CARS/Springer. All rights reserved.

4. Conclusion

A fit to a generic and common business model (Marburg Model) was possible, even with the wide variety of organisation, size of hospitals and variation of way of working for the listed hospitals. Particular the use of specialised views to a common data core allowed to verify and recognize misinterpreted data. Manually measured data have as well known in hospitals, a limited accuracy. However, even online data are not always true and have to be checked carefully.

In most hospitals more data in the Hospital Information System HIM was available as known by staff. In addition, the documentation on the supplier side, supplied to the user but also in the development area, was limited. The fragmentation of data, even within closed systems is a standard. Staff reduction in hospital support areas like IT is already critical. The motivation is high but the capacity doesn't allow to serve all necessary tasks. This is a risk for future hospital operation.

Using a model with a business object structure allows to combine data from different sources and use it for multiple purposes. Finally, the costs for individual radiological services can be calculated and the dependencies from external factors can be determined by sensitivity analysis. Simulation also works in scenario-discussions as an enabler for process innovation [4].

5. Outlook

The data collected in this study will be used for further szenario-discussions in 2002.

Acknowledgement

This project is supported by the Ministry of Health, Free State of Saxony, Germany.

References

1. Baker, J., Activity-Based Costing and Activity-Based Management for Health Care
2. Aspen Publication Gaithersburg, Maryland 1998
3. Böttcher, J., Klose, K. J. Bewertung und Evaluierung von PACS auf Basis von Activity-based Costing (ABC) einschliesslich telemedizinischer Anwendungen, in Jäckel (Hrsg.) Telemedizinführer Deutschland 2002
4. Scheer, A.-W. Wirtschaftsinformatik. Referenzmodelle für industrielle Geschäftsprozesse Springer Verlag, Berlin-Heidelberg New York, 1998
5. Schrage, M., Serious Play – How the world best companies simulate to innovate
6. Harvard Business School Press 2000

CARS 2002 – H.U. Lemke, M.W. Vannier; K. Inamura, A.G. Farman, K. Doi & J.H.C. Reiber (Editors)
©CARS/Springer. All rights reserved.

Displaying and analysing DICOM waveforms on Java based cell phones and PDAs

M. Kroll [a], J. Riesmeier [b], K. Melzer [a], K. Annacker [a], H.-G. Lipinski [a], D. H. W. Grönemeyer [c]
[a] University of Applied Sciences Dortmund/Germany
[b] OFFIS e. V. Oldenburg/Germany
[c] Institute for Microtherapy, University of Witten-Herdecke/Germany

Abstract

Since mobile devices such as PDAs or mobile phones are no longer restricted to run native applications but are also capable of running Java applications, the demand for platform independent applications is growing. However, some devices running a Java implementation are not powerful enough to analyse DICOM waveforms directly but need to contact a server machine to delegate this complex tasks. In order to overcome the weakness of common GSM wireless networks we use high-speed wireless networks to accomplish the analysis of waveform objects on mobile devices.

Keywords: Java, DICOM, waveform

1. Introduction

Since Mobile Information Devices (MID) such as cell phones and Personal Digital Assistants (PDA) are capable of running Java applications the area for platform independent applications is now also covering mobile devices. Together with the high data transfer rates of third generation wireless networks such as GPRS (General Packet Radio Service) or HSCSD (High Speed Circuit Switched Data) mobile information devices are able to perform sophisticated tasks in medicine. We have investigated whether present mobile devices can be used to process DICOM waveforms [1] and, therefore, enable physicians and cardiologists to view and even analyse patient related data in a location independent manner.

The DICOM waveforms specification defines six different types of waveforms such as basic voice audio, 12-lead electrocardiogram (ECG), general electrocardiogram, ambulatory electrocardiogram, hemodynamic and basic cardiac electrophysiology objects. The implementation discussed in this paper is able to handle the 12-lead and basic ECG waveform objects only.

With the emerging Java 2 Micro Edition (J2ME) a wide range of devices can be used to view and analyse DICOM waveforms without the need to create device specific implementations of the application. With our software solution we want to demonstrate that the above described medical task can be performed using standard hardware and does not require cost-intensive hardware which can only be used for waveform analysis.

©CARS/Springer. All rights reserved.

2. Material and Methods

In order to create a platform independent solution for currently available devices we used the Mobile Information Device Profile (MIDP) [2] of J2ME. This is the first existing Application Programming Interface (API) available for mobile information devices supported by a wide range of device manufacturers. The J2ME technology was initially presented at the Java One Conference in 1999. This technology enabled us to run our application without any modification on mobile devices such as Motorola Accompli 008, Siemens SL45i, Nokia Communicator 9210 and on all devices running the Palm Operating System (PalmOS).

In some cases where the computing power of a cell phone is not strong enough to decode a DICOM waveform object directly on the device we still need to communicate to a server machine that is used for pre-processing the waveform object. Since the minimum requirements for a MIDP compliant runtime environment are specified according to the capabilities of regular mobile phones, the use of a MIDP implementation on smart phones or PDAs seems to be unchallenged. The PDA device class will be covered by the new, not yet specified / available PDA Profile (PDAP) [3] offering much more options to a developer than MIDP does. For those mobile information devices providing significantly more computing power compared to regular cell phones such as the Nokia Communicator or Palm powered PDAs, the server machine acts as a file server only since the devices can perform the decoding internally.

3. Results

First we had to distinguish more and less powerful MIDP platforms and, therefore we divided our implementation into two parts (a client and a server). Our first solution covers Java enabled cell phones where the DICOM waveform objects are transmitted in a pre-processed form. A second solution for smart phones and PDAs decodes the waveform objects directly on the mobile device. We call the first approach "Cell Phone solution" and the second one "PDA solution".

3.1 The "Cell Phone solution"

For the "Cell Phone solution" the server machine acts as both a file and a pre-processing server. The user of the mobile application is able to connect to the server and select a DICOM waveform object to be displayed on the mobile device. Storing the waveform objects that needs to be displayed and analysed on the cell phone is performed using an Internet portal that is set up at the University of Applied Sciences Dortmund/Germany.

In order to get access to the file storage archive the user has to authenticate himself by entering a valid username and password. After the user has successfully logged in waveform objects can be uploaded to and deleted or downloaded from the portals file storage archive using a standard web browser.
Moreover, the user can extend the signal analysis algorithms that are available on the server by adding so called plug-ins to the plug-in space on the server. Both the file and the analysis algorithm can be selected using the client software running on a mobile

©CARS/Springer. All rights reserved.

device. Upon selection of a 12-lead ECG signal, for instance, the DICOM waveform object is pre-processed on the server, converted to a proprietary file format and transferred to the mobile device via GPRS or HSCSD wireless networks at a rate of 40-50 kbit/s using a HTTP (Hypertext Transfer Protocol) connection. Compared to the standard GSM (Global System for Mobile Communications) network the data rate is about 4-5 times faster, i. e. the transfer time is quite satisfying. The received waveform object can then be viewed on the device and an appropriate analysis algorithm can be selected from the plug-in space on the server. In this case the selected signal is analysed on the server using the selected algorithm before it is sent to the mobile device. This solution is used for mobile phones such as SL45i and Accompli 008, but can also be used with smart phones and PDAs. Figure 1 shows the client/server communication scenario described above.

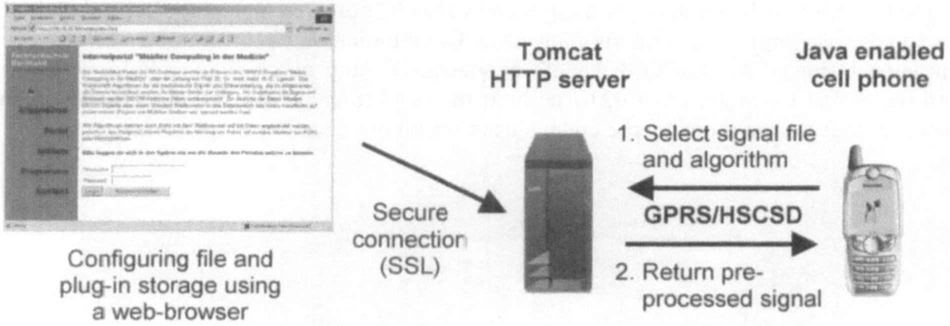

Fig. 1: Scenario showing how waveforms are displayed and analysed on mobile devices.

For the latter two device classes providing more processing power we have implemented the second, so called, "PDA Solution". In this case the server machine also acts as an algorithm and file server and both DICOM files and algorithms can be downloaded to the client device. The client connects to the portal in the same manner as described for the cell phones requiring the user to authenticate first. After selecting an algorithm or file, it is transmitted directly to the to the PDA or smart phone and stored in the persistent storage area of the device. Now the waveform objects stored in the Record Management System (RMS) or on a removable media card such as MulitMedia, SecureDigtal or CompactFlash of the mobile device can be displayed and analysed without a need to connect to a server since decoding is performed on the device itself. The algorithms are added to the algorithm database of the client device and are available for further analysis without connecting to the server again.

In order to decode the DICOM waveform objects we have implemented a toolkit that can be used with the Java 2 Standard Edition for the server implementation and with the Java 2 Micro Edition for the clients. Because of the shortcomings of the J2ME language specification we have divided platform specific implementations into two parts which are dynamically loaded depending on the platform. This toolkit enabled us to use the same source code for decoding waveform objects on the server and the client. Since the HTTP requests that are queried by a mobile device need to be responded by a server we have

©CARS/Springer. All rights reserved.

used Tomcat [4], a Java Servlet engine, that is not only capable of responding to requests sent from a mobile device but also to HTTP requests of a conventional web browser. This fact enabled us to view DICOM waveforms also using a standard web browser.

3.2 The "Cell PDA solution"

For the PDA solution we created an application that is based on the kAWT (Kilobyte Abstract Windowing Toolkit) [5] subset that is available for the Palm organiser running the Jbed virtual machine [6]. Using the kAWT subset, our application can be used with other AWT implementations without any modification. The DICOM waveform viewer application can also be run on the desktop computer, but desktop applications are not the main focus of this project. Mobile Java virtual machine implementations supporting AWT we have tested with our application are the Personal Java [7] based virtual machine implementation of Insignia [8] running on a PocketPC powered Compaq iPaq and Nokia's Personal Java implementation running on a Communicator 9210. Figure 2 shows our implementation of the DICOM waveform viewer running on an iPaq, a Palm organizer and the Nokia Communicator 9210 without the need to adapt the software for hardware specific issues. The same source code is used for all three supported platforms.

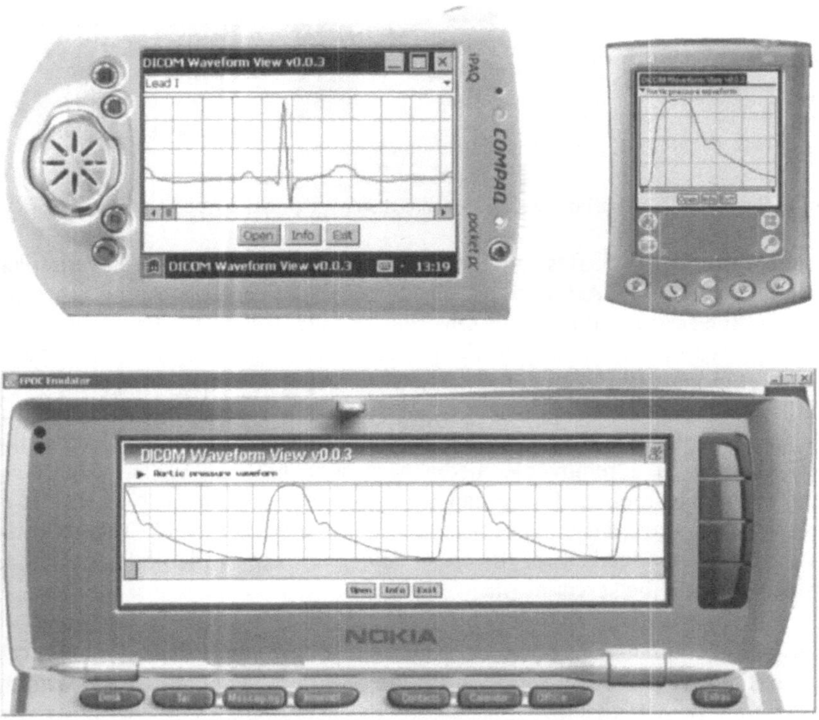

Fig. 2: DICOM waveform viewer on different mobile device platforms such as PocketPCs, Palm organisers and the Nokia Communicator 9210.

©CARS/Springer. All rights reserved.

4. Conclusion

Our approach presented in this paper enables physicians and cardiologists to view and even analyse waveforms such as ECGs in a location independent manner using standardised hardware. The client/server implementation illustrates the platform independence of Java based applications and demonstrates that currently available Mobile Information Devices running a J2ME virtual machine are capable of performing powerful medical tasks. Using the Tomcat Servlet Engine the server cannot only provide pre-processed waveform objects for MIDP devices but also for standard web browsers.

Although the language specification of J2ME is not as complex as the Java 2 Standard Edition used for desktop and server machines it is sufficient to implement a DICOM toolkit that can be used on J2ME devices in order to decode waveforms directly in a adequate time.

Acknowledgements

The project presented in this paper has been supported by the Ministry of Education, Science, and Research, Duesseldorf (North Rhine Westfalia) Germany, (TRAFO 514-80081801/Lipinski).

References

1. NEMA Standards Publication PS 3.x, "Digital Imaging and Communications in Medicine (DICOM)", National Electrical Manufacturers Association, 2101 L Street, N. W., Washington, D. C. 20037, 1992-2001.
2. Sun Microsystems Inc., "Mobile Information Device Profile (MIDP) for the J2ME Platform", http://www.jcp.org/aboutJava/communityprocess/final/jsr037/index.html, 2000.
3. Sun Microsystems Inc. "Personal Digital Assistant Profile (PDAP) for the J2ME Platform", http://www.jcp.org/jsr/detail/75.jsp, 2002.
4. Apache Software Foundation, "Jakarta Tomcat", http://jakarta.apache.org/tomcat/index.html, 1999-2002.
5. Haustein Stefan, Kroll Michael, "kAWT – The Kilobyte Abstract Windowing Toolkit", http://www.kawt.de/, 1999-2002.
6. Esmertec Inc., "Jbed Microedition CLDC", http://www.esmertec.com/, 2002.
7. Sun Microsystems Inc., "Personal Java (Pjava)", http://java.sun.com/products/personaljava/, 2002.
8. Insignia Solutions, Jeode PDA Edition, http://www.insignia.com/products/jeode_pda.asp, 2002.

Special Session on Electronic Health Record

CARS 2002 – H.U. Lemke, M.W. Vannier; K. Inamura, A.G. Farman, K. Doi & J.H.C. Reiber (Editors)
©CARS/Springer. All rights reserved.

Secure and future proof electronic health records over the Internet

Bernd Blobel
University Hospital Magdeburg
Leipziger Str. 44, 39120 Magdeburg, Germany

Abstract

Shared care concepts such as managed care or disease management require extended communication and co-operation between all parties directly or indirectly involved in the patient's care. The informational view on the shared patient is established by a comprehensive electronic health record (EHR) which has to be communicable, interoperable, and portable. Due to the lifetime of such an EHR, the underlying architecture must be open, flexible, and future proof. Because of the sensitivity of personal medical information, EHR and its communication have to be established and performed trustworthy. The solution consists of components reflecting constraint models according to the ISO Reference Model – Open Distributed Processing by inheritance and overriding mechanisms. The paper presents the latest technology introduced for meeting the challenges mentioned. Architectural principles and security solutions introduced are issues of ongoing standardisation efforts the author participates into.

Keywords: Electronic health record; security, components

1. Introduction

Shared care as the answer to the challenge for efficient and high quality care requests extended communication and co-operation between all partners directly or indirectly involved in the patient's care. The same patient is served by GPs and specialised practitioners, by hospitals with ATD departments, medical departments such as surgery, radiology, or clinical laboratories, with wards and financial departments, by aftercare and rehabilitation organisations, but also by pharmacies, insurance companies, etc. Nowadays, such health providers use different information systems more or less enabled to mutually communicate. Dealing with the same patient for different purposes, these parties realise special views on a comprehensive documentation about information and processes related to that patient. Therefore, an electronic health record (EHR) as kernel application is the gold standard for health information systems' interoperability.

2. A future proof EHR architecture

During the last five to ten years, different advanced EHR architectures have been developed which have been summarised, e.g., in [1]. Following, an advanced future proof architectural approach to health information systems including EHR systems will be presented which has harmonised and improved the currently available solutions.

©CARS/Springer. All rights reserved.

2.1. Component based architectures

Information systems intent to reflect organisational, functional, technological, and content constraints. Furthermore, they have to enable interoperability not only at data but also at functional or even knowledge level. The architecture meeting these challenges should consist of generic, encapsulated, persistent pieces which are accessible via interfaces and inherit or override their properties. These properties are met by objects. While objects are defined originally as

$$\text{Object} = \text{attributes} + \text{operations} \quad (1)$$

the constraints are represented by object-object interactions and cannot be invoked via interfaces. Components on the other hand are characterised by

$$\begin{aligned}\text{Component} = \; & \text{attributes} + \text{operations} + \text{structural constraints} + \\ & \text{operational constraints} + \text{events} + \text{multi-interfaces} * \\ & \text{scenarios} + \text{safety} + \text{reliability} + \text{security} + \ldots\end{aligned} \quad (2)$$

Therefore, the EHR architecture has to meet the component paradigm.

The different EHCR approaches established have been harmonised combining modern development paradigms and the huge domain knowledge expressed in other models, standards and R&D-project outcome. This has been done using the generic component approach developed by the Magdeburg Medical Informatics Department at mid-nineties [6]. Starting point of the approach is the ISO Reference Model – Open Distributed Processing (ISO RM-ODP) [2].

2.2. The ISO Reference Model – Open Distributed Processing

Depending on the requirements and needs of the user and his underlying models, concepts, etc., information systems have to offer different views on the real world within their development, implementation, and maintenance phase. For keeping the systems manageable in the phases mentioned, different level of granularity of considering the real world systems can be considered. In order to meet all of the possible requirements, an information system will enable all of the necessary views (different levels of abstraction) on the system that is supported, at all levels of granularity that are required. According to the ISO RM-ODP, the views concern the enterprise view, the information view, the computational view, the engineering view and the technology view. The granularity concerns concepts, relations network, aggregations and details. Regarding the corporate structure, the whole healthcare establishment, the relation between structural units, the departments, and procedural steps can be distinguished.

Components can perform state transitions regarding their level of granularity or their level of abstraction, respectively. The state transition has to follow strict rules for preserving consistency and integrity of the system and its views [3]. This state transition is realised through specialisation, generalisation, or association as well as by different constraints dedicated to the component. Composition or decomposition might be provided by separating at least some constraints from the basic component.

©CARS/Springer. All rights reserved.

2.3. Model driven architectures

Regarding concepts, other architectural approaches group systems and their components into domains with the same objective of keeping development and maintenance of comprehensive health information systems manageable. A domain is characterised by components of a system grouped by common organisational, logical, and technical properties. This could be done for common policies (policy domains) which are discussed in section 3, for common environments (environment domains), or common technology (technology domains) [1, 2]. To enable context-sensitive information system architectures as well as the presentation of domain-specific or view-specific knowledge, components and their corresponding object adapter must be managed in a flexible way according to the users' needs. The emerging CORBA 3 environment provides specifications and methods to fulfil those requirements [4]. Using these methods such as valuetypes, persistent state services, portable object adapter, or CORBA component model, the models describing the different levels of abstraction and granularity mentioned above can be developed and implemented. Starting from platform independent models and platform independent domain models dealing with the domain specific knowledge expressed as constraints and relations, platform specific models as well as platform specific domain models are derived from the unspecific ones. The unspecific models are called object models. Specific models have to meet constraints. Models representing constraints in content, datatypes, procedures, etc., are called archetypes. Therefore, specific models are called archetype models. Object model and archetype models can be derived from complex models or vice versa. Instantiation of archetype models and object model are bound together at runtime. The archetypes concern any concepts such as medical specialities, organisational restrictions or personal peculiarities. So different concepts within one view (abstraction level) or related to different view on a system can be specified. For binding the models in an unambiguous way, digital signature mechanisms might be deployed. This way for providing safety of the EHCR components will be extended towards reliability and security services. In that context, concepts for establishing both communication and application security services must be specified in archetypes. In actual EHR approaches, the Unified Modeling Language (UML) is used to model the components and the Extensible Markup Language (XML) schemata are deployed to express the different views explained before.

3. Security models for healthcare

Considering security threats, requirements, and solutions, security policies must be defined, negotiated, agreed on, stated, and controlled. A policy describes the legal framework including rules, regulations and ethical aspects, the organisational and administrative framework, functionalities, claims and objectives, the principals (human users, devices, applications, components, objects) involved, agreements, rights, duties, and penalties defined as well as the technological solution implemented for collecting, recording, processing and communicating data in information systems. For describing policies, methods such as policy templates or formal policy modelling might be applied.

3.1. The generic security model as specialisation of the generic component model

To manage security in distributed systems, two security concepts have to be supported: the concept of communication security between two or more principals (e.g., components) and the concept of application security within one component. Communication security

©CARS/Springer. All rights reserved.

services comprise strong mutual authentication and accountability (auditability) of principals involved, integrity, confidentiality and availability of communicated information as well as some notary's services. As result of the authentication procedure, authorisation for having access to the other principal has to be decided. Application security services concern accountability, authorisation and access control regarding data and functions, integrity, availability, confidentiality of information recorded, processed and stored as well as some notary's services and audit.

3.2. Concepts for roles and authorisation

Because it is impossible to assign authorisation and access rights within extended domains to any principal specifically, principals are grouped for assigning authorisation and access rights according to the role group members play. Grouping is performed according to defined attributes characterising the group. Such attributes could be qualifications and skills as prerequisites for assigned roles, commonly accepted groups (general professions, legally-defined or regulation-defined groups), etc.

For assigning authorisation and access control to specific principals as group members, attribute certificates must be bound to ID certificates. The Public Key Infrastructure (PKI) needed has been standardised internationally by ISO with the recently approved ISO TDS 17090 "Public Key Infrastructure" [5] and at European scale by CEN/ISSS (Comité Europeéan de Normalisation/Information Society Standardisation System) and ETSI (European Telecommunications Standards Institute) with the European Electronic Signature Standard Initiative (EESSI) [6]. Beside the technical harmonisation, the European Union performed also a legal harmonisation for establishing electronic signatures: the EU 99/93/EC "Directive on Electronic Signatures". Contrary to the harmonisation for ID-related certificates, attributes such as specialties, subspecialties and medical disciplines as well as related authorisations (rights and duties) are mostly different. If, e.g., prescriptions are a privilege for Germany's doctors, in Norway this activity is performed by nurses. Therefore, before an agreed terminology and ontology has been introduced, the services (acts) being provided are a better characteristic for defining harmonised roles. Such services are, e.g., observation, physical examination, prescription, nuclear treatment, surgical treatment, anaesthetic preparation, collection of specimen, order, billing. Part 2 of the ISO TDS 17090 defines structure and content of health-related attribute certificates [5].

Considering roles, two specialisations of roles might be distinguished: organisational or structural roles on the one hand and functional roles on the other hand. Organisational roles are established by relationships between entities such as organisations and/or persons. The structure-related role of an health professional (HP) defines his/her position in the organisational hierarchy of the institution reflecting responsibility and competence of the professional. Functional roles are created by acts. The function-related role of an HP immediately reflects the position in the healthcare process, i.e., the concrete HP-patient relationship. Both roles define the rights and duties of an HP in an Health Care Establishment (HCE). Because HPs fulfil obligations in both the organisational and the functional framework, the resulting access control model combines these two views. According to the codes of conduct, the data protection legislation and the European Data Protection Directive, in most of the democracies the function role dominates the access control model in health information systems. Details are given in [7].

CARS 2002 – H.U. Lemke, M.W. Vannier; K. Inamura, A.G. Farman, K. Doi & J.H.C. Reiber (Editors)
©CARS/Springer. All rights reserved.

4. The HARP Cross Security Platform

Real interoperability leads to a closer connection of both communication and application security services. Within the European HARP project funded by the European Commission within the Information Society Technologies (IST) Programme, partners from Greece, Germany, Norway, United Kingdom and The Netherlands specified, developed and implemented enhanced security solutions and Trusted Third Party (TTP) services for Internet-based communication and applications [8]. The HARP project's objective is building up entirely secure, component-based applications in client-server environments over the Web.

To provide platform independence of solutions in HARP as a real three tiers architecture, the design pattern approach of developing a middleware-like common cross platform called HARP Cross-Security Platform (HCSP) has been used. In HCSP, platform-specific security features have been isolated. Using XML as an abstraction layer, communication in different environments is enabled. According to the component paradigm, an interface definition of a component providing a platform-specific service specifies how a client accesses a service without regard of how that service is implemented. So, the HCSP design isolates and encapsulates the implementation of platform-specific services behind a platform-neutral interface as well as reduces the visible complexity. Deploying proper Enhanced TTP (ETTP) services, it helps to endorse policies by mapping them on processing components [8].

HARP's embedding security into any application to be instantiated over the web-based environment outlined above is based on object oriented programming principles. It is based on Internet technology and protocols solely. The trustworthiness needed has been provided by applying only certified components which are tailored according to the principal's role. In fine-grained steps, it establishes its complete environment required, avoiding any external services possibly compromised. After strong mutual authentication based on smartcards and TTP services, the security infrastructure components are downloaded and installed to be used for implementing the components needed to run the application as well as to transfer data input and output. The SSL protocol deployed to initiate secure sessions is provided by the Java Secure Socket Extension API. The applets and servlets for establishing the local client and the open remote database access facilities communicate using the XML standard set including XML Digital Signature. Because messages and not single items are signed, the messages are archived separately for accountability reasons meeting the legislation and regulations for health. Policies are dynamically interpreted and adhered to the components. All components applied at both server and client site are checked twice against the user's role and the appropriate policy: firstly in context of their selection and provision and second in context of their use and functionality. Applet security from the execution point of view is provided through the secure downloading of policy files, which determine all access rights in the client terminal. This has to be seen on top of the very desirable feature that the local, powerful, and versatile code is strictly transient and subject to predefined and securely controlled download procedures. All rights corresponding to predefined roles are subject to personal card identification with remote mapping of identity to roles and thereby to corresponding security policies with specific access rights.

©CARS/Springer. All rights reserved.

5. Future proof and component based EHR systems

Summarising all system-theoretical paradigms and architectural principles, a specification schema for secure EHR components has been established which consists of an object model and several archetype models. The latter reflect the different constraints related to concepts, conditions, and relations considered. By that way, technical constraints such as hardware, operating system, and protocol-related dependencies can be specified as well as managed and finally implemented at runtime. So, openness, interoperability, flexibility, and portability are provided. The expression of the models is performed using the XML standard set. The creation, implementation, and processing of such components has been realised by developing a set of generic specification and tools established as generic applets and servlets.

A generic applet consists, e.g., of the subcomponents GUI and interface controller, smartcard controller, XML signing and XML processing components, communication component applying the Java SSL (Secure Socket Layer) extension, and last but not least the data processing and activity controller. Beside equivalent subcomponents and an attribute certificate repository at the server side, policy repository, policy solver and authorisation manager have been specified and implemented as a “light weight Resource Access Decision Service”. More details as well as evaluation results are given in a book currently prepared to be published in May 2002 at IOS Press, Amsterdam.

Acknowledgement

The author is in debt to the European Commission for funding as well as to the international and national HARP project partners for their support and their kind co-operation.

References

1. B. Blobel: Evaluation and harmonisation of EHCR architecture approaches. World Markets Series BUSINESS BRIEFING: Global Healthcare 2002, pp. 18-22.
2. ISO/IEC 10746-2 “Information Technology – Open Distributed Processing – Reference Model: Part 2: Foundations”.
3. B. Blobel: Application of the Component Paradigm for Analysis and Design of Advanced Health System Architectures. *International Journal of Medical Informatics* **60** (3) (2000) 281-301.
4. J. Siegel: Quick CORBA3. Wiley Computer Publishing, John Wiley & Sons, Inc., New York, Chichester, Weinheim, Brisbane, Singapore, Toronto, 2001.
5. ISO DTS 17090 “Public Key Infrastructure, Part 1 – 3”, 2001.
6. European Electronic Signature Standard Initiative: www eessi.org
7. B. Blobel, F. Roger-France: A Systematic Approach for Analysis and Design of Secure Health Information Systems. *International Journal of Medical Informatics* **62** (3) (2001) pp. 51-78.
8. The HARP Consortium: http://www.ist-harp.org

CARS 2002 – H.U. Lemke, M.W. Vannier; K. Inamura, A.G. Farman, K. Doi & J.H.C. Reiber (Editors)
©CARS/Springer. All rights reserved.

Patient-oriented visualisation and interaction in a three dimensional environment

Kai Köchy, René Tschirley, Steffen Märkle
Dept. of Computer Graphics & Computer Assisted Medicine
Technical University Berlin, Germany
cg@cs.tu-berlin.de

Abstract

The PREPaRe system is a patient-oriented internet-based information system that is able to store, combine, process and visualize all types of medical data that are part of a "personal electronic medical record". This paper describes the visualization and interaction aspects of the PREPaRe system which is designed with respect to the user's needs. Special attention is given to the visualization of and interaction within a three-dimensional virtual hospital.

Keywords : Visualisation, interaction, electronic patient record

1. Introduction

As described in [1], computers are used in medicine to improve quality and efficiency in healthcare processes. Increasingly, medical institutions integrate computer generated image data into an "electronic patient record" (EPR).

Existing software systems are designed either for medical and administration personnel or for patients. The apparent reason is that understanding real world medical data needs a-priori knowledge which the medical and administration personnel have but the patient is not acquainted with. As a consequence, software for expert users offers detailed information about the patient's medical data which are stored in the patient's EPR.

If interested, patients should have the possibility of participating more actively in their personal health care process. Participation starts with the dialog between patient and physician and continues at home where the patient can review the dialog utilising his patient record. Available software for patients offers visual information not on their own data but on exemplary data.

Designed to bridge the gap between both types of applications the PREPaRe system provides the patient with access to his/her medical data. Therefore, the PREPaRe system needs an intuitive and convenient user interface.

©CARS/Springer. All rights reserved.

2. Concept

The PREPaRe system tries to realize a virtual hospital which is a three-dimensional virtual environment, as proposed in [2]. Besides the hospital's facilities (see Figure 1) which represent a macro world, anatomical structures of the patient, a micro world, are visualised. Combination of the macro world and the micro world creates a unique immersive environment. The following techniques for visualisation of three dimensional data are commonly utilized:

- surface rendering of polygonal data, e.g. the virtual hospital or segmented medical volume data with colorisation of volumes of interest
- volume rendering, e.g. ray casting
- visualisation of slices of 3D volume data
- blending semitransparent objects

The system designer has to choose a set of presentation algorithms which may be useful for the understanding of the medical data. Parameters have to be predefined or generated by the computer. The set of presentations is offered to the user by a menu where the user can choose from different types of visualization.

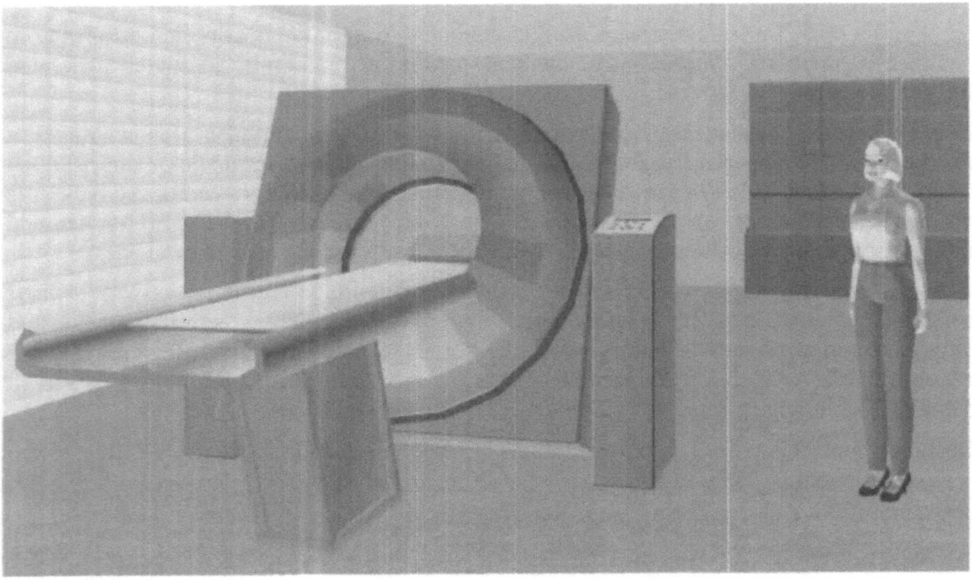

Figure 1: Three-dimensional virtual hospital

©CARS/Springer. All rights reserved.

Interaction is an integral component of the PREPaRe system. Derived from a classification of Mine [3] interaction in virtual worlds can be divided into movement (navigation), selection and manipulation (scaling):

- Navigation
  Inside the virtual hospital, the patient can navigate through the departments. There interaction with doctors, nurses, administration personnel and other patients can take place, as described in [4].
- Selection
  Looking at the visualization of an anatomic feature, the patient is able to select the different types of material, e.g. bones, cartilage, muscle tissue, blood vessels, nerves, fat and skin.
- Manipulation
  Tools for changing the representation of the visualized data are available. For example, a virtual magnifying glass allows an X-ray view through the given data set. Other tools are e.g. region/volume of interest.

In a three-dimensional world, there are six degrees of freedom (DOF) for navigation and at least six degrees of freedom for manipulation of an object. It is obviously necessary to focus on only a few degrees of freedom, because an input device should be no more difficult to use than a mouse. The number of DOFs left still requires a context switch between navigation, selection and manipulation.

Visualisation and user interaction differ for patients and medical personnel. Different representation of the same medical data have to be generated. For medical personnel the visualisation's accuracy is more important than usability and vividness. For the patient the accuracy can be neglected to some extent. Usability of the system and clearness of the visualisation have to be placed in the foreground. Considering the needs of patients, the user interface has to follow certain requirements :

- 3D interface for immersion

  A virtual environment is the natural way of recognizing and examining spatial representations of anatomic information and can be accomplished even on a home PC. A virtual world in which the anatomic information is presented creates an immersive multidimensional holistic view of the Personal Electronic Medical Record's (PEMR) medical image data. Furthermore, the data may be embedded in surgical simulations so that the patient can be shown possible therapies.

- Menus for interaction guidance

  When offering visualization methods to the patient which are commonly used by experts, knowledge about the algorithms and the parameters has to be provided by the computer system. As described above the predefined set of presentations is offered to the user by a menu.

©CARS/Springer. All rights reserved.

- Virtual hand for selection

  A natural way to select and interact with objects in any environment is to point and grasp with the hand. The PREPaRe system's user interface is intended to be intuitive and so the user is offered a virtual hand for interaction. Navigation in the virtual environment as well as selection and manipulation of the objects in the environment are available with this cursor.

- Visual feedback

  The user shall always be aware of what he/she is doing, e.g. when a user selects an object for manipulation, it is highlighted.

Summarizing the requirements, it can be reasoned that the complexity of the task can only be handled by reducing the available options to the user. Furthermore the information about the medical context of the data can be used to generate visualization scenarious for the patient .

3. Realisation

A description of usage shall illustrate the user interface A patient has been at a clinical institution for examination. The three-dimensional data acquired were stored in the electronic patient record where the physician in charge accessed them for diagnostic purposes. After a visit at the physician, the interested patient wants to review the data and the physician's diagnosis.

First he/she connects to the PREPaRe system from a home PC. Verification of identity can be accomplished either with a combination of username/password or an electronic authentification card, which employs mechanisms such as the health professional card (HPC) [5]. Then the patient enters the virtual hospital which is a three-dimensional clone of the real hospital. The patient navigates individually to the radiology department where the data were acquired. Navigation can be performed by simple two axis movement of the mouse. As the PREPaRe system is based on the patient's electronic healthcare record, it provides all information about the actual medical case. Therefore, if requested, the user may be guided by an agent. Help agents can be invoked at any information counter or by a context sensitive menu.

Arriving at the department, the patient enters the examination room, seeing a visualization of his medical data. A virtual menu offers standard visualization techniques, such as surface reconstruction of skin and bone tissue (Figure 2) or direct volume rendering of CT data (Figure 3).

©CARS/Springer. All rights reserved.

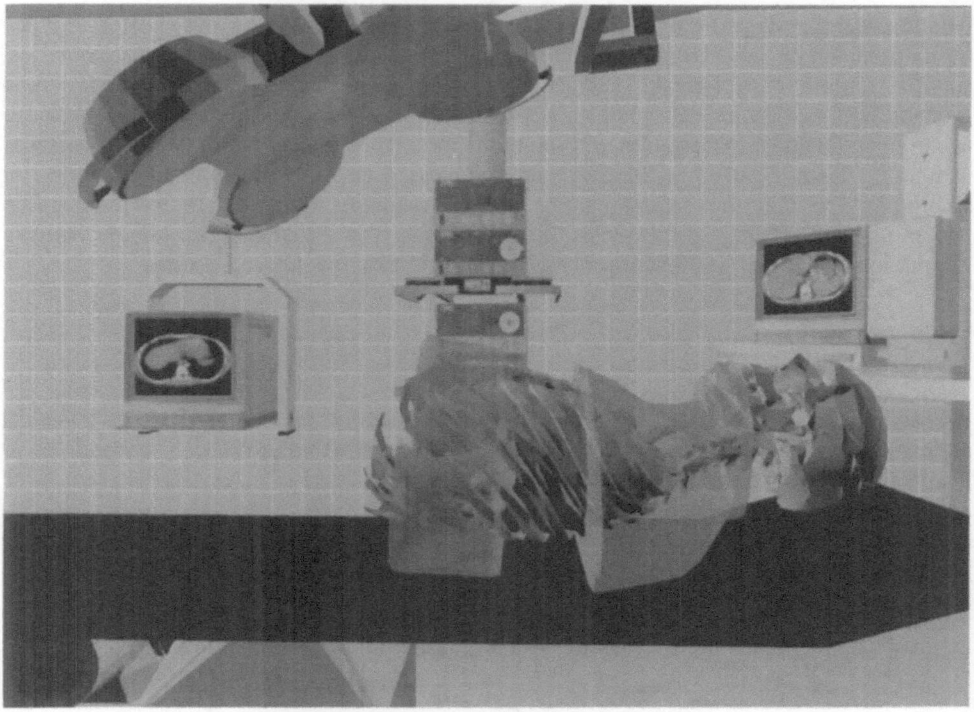

Figure 2: Surface reconstruction of bone and skin

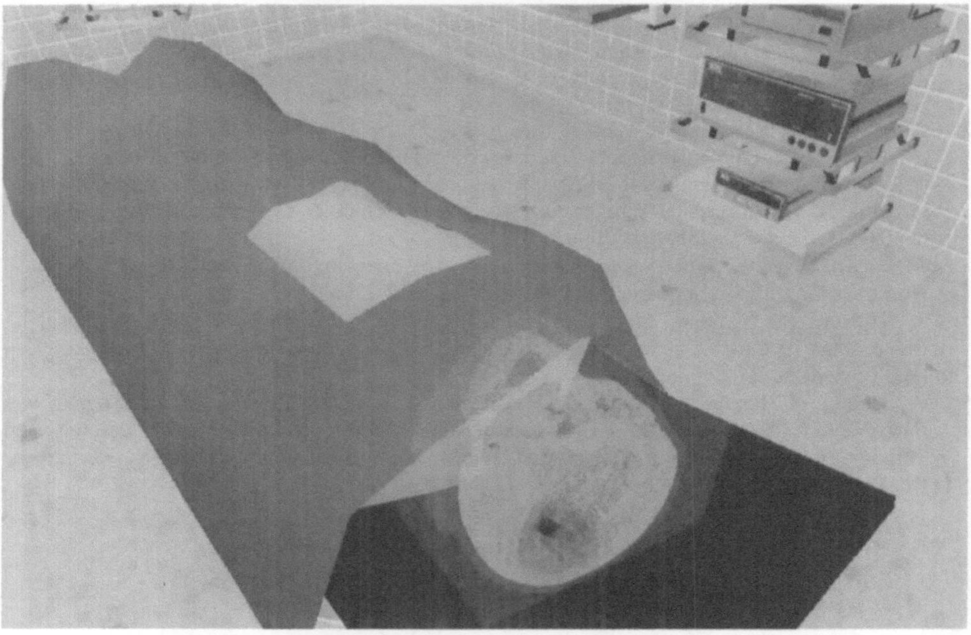

Figure 3: Volume rendering applying maximum intensity projection

©CARS/Springer. All rights reserved.

Due to preprocessing of the medical data, areas of interest can be shown. Different types of material can be selected and will be explained: links to external information databases, such as online encyclopedias, offer information about anatomical structures. As a precondition, all of the data's voxels have to be classified during preprocessing. In order to accomplish this task, registration and segmentation algorithms in combination with digital anatomic atlases are used. If desired, the preprocessed data may be embedded in surgical simulations so that the patient can be shown available therapies. In addition, when becoming part of the virtual world, the patient can also experience an almost realistic impression of the real healthcare processes as a visitor to the virtual hospital.

4. Conclusion

Interaction in the PREPaRe system provides an intuitive user interface that allows a patient to experience health care as an integrated process that is not only carried out in wards and hospitals but continues at home.

Provision of 3D models of hospitals, 2D, 3D and 4D visualization of medical data and interactive therapy simulation, enables the patients to virtually visit the health care center at will.

The presented interaction concept enables the patient to view and understand his/her medical data using a complex visualization tool until now only available to experts.

References

1. S. Märkle, K. Köchy, R. Tschirley, H. U. Lemke: *The PREPaRe system - Patient Oriented Access to the "Personal Electronic Medical Record"*, in: Proceedings of CARS 2001 Computer Assisted Radiology and Surgery, H. U. Lemke et al. (Eds), Excerpta Medica Int. Congress Series, Elsevier Science B.V., pp. 849-854, 2001.
2. J. Becker, R. Tschirley, S. Märkle: *Construction of a 3D information system for hospital environments*, in: From PACS to Internet / Intranet Information-Systems, Multimedia and Telemedicine Proceedings of the 18th international EuroPACS Conference, Graz, 2000. Hrsg. G. Gell, A. Holzinger, M. Wiltgen Österreichische Computer Gesellschaft, Wien, ISBN 3-85403-144-0, pp. 232-238, Sep. 2000.
3. M. R. Mine, *Virtual Environment Interaction Techniques*, in: ACM SIGGRAPH 97, Course Notes No. 29 : "Programming Virtual Worlds", pp. 212-227, 1997.
4. J. Wilhelmy, S. Märkle: *Virtual actors for a patient oriented virtual hospital,* to appear in: Proceedings of CARS 2002 Computer Assisted Radiology and Surgery, H. U. Lemke et al. (Eds), Springer, 2002.
5. A. Schurig, H. Heuser, R. Wedekind: *Introduction of the Health Professional Card (HPC) into the SAXTELEMED-Project,* in: Proceedings of CARS 2001 Computer Assisted Radiology and Surgery, H. U. Lemke et al. (Edts), Excerpta Medica Int. Congress Series, Elsevier Science B.V., pp. 849-854, 2001.

CARS 2002 – H U. Lemke, M.W. Vannier; K. Inamura, A.G. Farman, K. Doi & J.H.C. Reiber (Editors)
©CARS/Springer. All rights reserved.

Do EHR communication standards account for imaging communication needs?

François Mennerat[a], Joël Chabriais[b]
[a] PROREC-France, Paris
[b] Hôpital Necker, Paris

Keywords: Communication, EHRcom, DICOM.

1. Introduction

Over the past decade, a growing number of technical specifications regarding Electronic Health Records (EHRs) have appeared, as a consequence of various initiatives. GEHR (Good European Health Record) as a result of a European R&D project, somehow continued in the Synapse and Synex projects, and eventually the Australian "Good Electronic Health Record". CEN[1] prestandard ENV 12265 "Electronic Healthcare Record Architecture" (1996), followed in 2000 by ENV 13606 "Electronic Healthcare Record Communication" (EHRcom) being currently revised into a full standard; but other CEN documents also impact EHRs. DICOM Structured Reporting is another example of an EHR.

More recently, part of the Reference Information Model (RIM) of Health Level Seven (HL7) consists in a Clinical Document Architecture (CDA) that aims at forming the basis for messages consistent with the rest of their version 3. Other significant though less well-known sets of specifications may be proposed here and there.

The relationships between GEHR, CEN, and HL7 —that propose generic solutions to facilitate communication and data exchange between stakeholders— are relatively easy to identify. Various ways are used for collaboration between those teams and bodies.
With its Structured Reporting, DICOM offers a solution well that satisfies the sectorial needs of imaging specialists. How does it fits into generic solutions.

2. Preliminary issues

2.1 What is an Electronic Health Record

In several CEN documents, a health care record is defined as a "repository of information regarding the health of a subject of care", an electronic health care record, being a "health care record in computer readable form".

2.2 What are the roles of an EHR?

According to the above definition, the role of an EHR is firstly to store information, but rather, and more precisely, personal health data elements.

[1] Comité Européen de Normalisation (European Standardisation Committee)

©CARS/Springer. All rights reserved.

At the same time, an EHR plays a fundamental part in the communication between health care providers. It is the source and the destination of clinical messages exchanged between parties involved in health care provision. But achieving communication between remote EHR systems, does not imply that these systems are interoperable. The need is to send out messages that can be read by the receiver, understood, interpreted, classified, stored, re-used, etc.

In this perspective, in order to permit the repeated processing of the data, structuring the information provides an extraordinary added-value: when it comes to data interchange, the concern is not simply to send, and to receive envelopes, but to use their content in the most clinically meaningful way. This consideration also applies to the next issue.

2.3 What does "interoperability" of EHRs mean?

Somme sort of communication between dissimilar systems may well be achieved, but the communication process is not complete, making it somehow meaningless, if those systems are not interoperable. Interoperability is a feature common to two or more EHR systems, that allows data to be exchanged between them so that those data sent out by one system can be recognised and processed by another system without any particular human intervention being necessary. As a consequence, full interoperability between systems A and B means that system B can use in the same way the data received from system A as its own native data.

In practice, however, and given the current technological state of most EHR systems, it may occur that interoperability is only partial. For instance, a text document has a format that cannot be recognised by the receiver system without a specific operation being performed following a human command; or else, it has no structure at all (such as an ASCII file).

A message may well be properly received by a system, with its sender being acknowledged, the subject of care identified, and even the nature of its content outlined, without it being possible to process this actual content, simply because such an ability is not granted by the functions present in the receiver system. An image can be received by a system that cannot open it because it does not comply with the standards this system is based upon.

Even the use of XML for messages, though so often put forward as THE definitive remedy to any interoperability concerns, does not warrant that a remote system can process the content of a message, as long as the DTD used does not fit the internal structure of the target repository.

Full interoperability also implies that in order to preserve their entire clinical meaning, any personal health data must be conveyed together with their contextual references: any missing part jeopardise their meaning and relevance. Thus, any loss of meaning appears as a clue that interoperability is not complete.

©CARS/Springer. All rights reserved.

2.4 Is the nature of the message content univocal?

In other terms, is there a way to reconcile the different specific perspectives of the various medical specialities and health care professions take in defining the content, and moreover the basic structure, of the messaged exchanged? Radiologists, and other images specialists are acknowledged as pioneers in the domain. But clinical messages are not meant to carry only images and imaging reports. Terminology issues are also raised: could the thesaurus used in pathology sum up the needs of any health care profession? Obviously not.

Surgeons might also be tempted to view the whole medical knowledge through their sole expertise. Why not cardiologists? Indeed such provocative questions outline the need for a generic architecture for messages exchanged between EHRs structured according to the specific needs of any profession.

2.5 Structure of messages vs. structure of EHRs

In order to receive properly (XML)-structured messages, an EHR system needs at least that a browser acts at the interface, so that the content of the message can be read. It is so transformed for storage into the basic format (plain text, etc.) accepted locally by the local EHR system.

In this circumstance, no actual consistency is sought between the structured content of the successive messages received, and the internal organisation of the information within the EHR system itself: only the current content is deemed of any interest. Thus, theoretically, setting a message structure may have no impact on the record structure.

However, it is understandable that in order to get the most of the successive messages received, the structured content of which may be stored in the record, it makes it soon useful to structure the content of the record in a way that matches as much as possible the structure of the messages content. Thus, an unexpected effect of standardising the messages, is that it eventually almost inevitably impacts the structure of the EHRs.

3. A generic architecture

It results from the considerations above that there exists a need for a generic architecture. Such an architecture should allow for communication of health data items using messages exchanged between EHRs held in various facilities by a variety of professionals with their own knowledge, perspective, competence, expertise, and terminology. It makes it possible to exchange any kind of information between different authorised stakeholders. The introductory section above set a broad outline of the current situation with regard to existing standards.

It appears clearly that today, the only document world-wide having a nearly *de jure* standard status, is the European pre-standard ENV 13606 "EHRcom" [1]. A pre-standard keeps an experimental status over a three-year probationary period, after which it is likely to be revised into an actual standard, based on the experience gained by its implementers. This pre-standard has four parts:

1. Extended architecture and domain model
2. Domain term list

©CARS/Springer. All rights reserved.

3. Distribution rules
4. Message for the exchange of record information

Indeed, this generic architecture does not conflict with standards specific to domains such as imaging, but rather it permits for a wide variety of messages contents, including images, digitised signals, text —enriched or not—, etc.

4. EHRcom and DICOM Structured Reporting

When imaging specialists exchange digitised images, or structured text regarding the former documents, within their professional community, it proves relatively easy for them to adhere to the same basic conventions. It is possible, though usually not very likely, that the transfer of images is needed outside this imaging specialists professional community. Not the least because it would imply that the equipment —hardware and software— of the receiver makes him able to properly read such documents.

In most cases, only the reports —structured or not— are deemed of interest to the non-specialist. However, no particular data type are earmarked to be part of EHRcom Record Components. Thus nothing opposes DICOM objects (images or SRs) being considered Components (i.e. message "payloads") according to ENV 13606. The only potential issue could be that occasionally headers are found duplicated, and subsequently inconsistent.

5. Conclusion

DICOM and HL7 are already closely co-operating to make their standards used jointly. With its version 3 Clinical Document Architecture (CDA), to the design of which European experts have brought a significant contribution, HL7 aims at proposing solutions consistent with their other message formats to exchange clinical data. In Europe, CEN had published in 2000, with a status of pre-standard, a set of specification specific to EHR communication. As it had been meant from the start, it is now being revised into a standard, building upon experience gained in several instances of implementation, and also taking account of the developments fostered under the aegis of HL7, as well as other much valuable works that have taken place in Australia —with GEHR—, and elsewhere. It can now be contemplated that a consensus may appear at the world level for a standard to be used for communication between Electronic Health Records at large. This will encompass the any kind of data, including images, and any kinds of digitised signals.

References

1. CEN. *ENV 13606 Health Informatics - Electronic health care record communication (Parts 1 to 4)*. 2000. http://www.centc251.org
2. DICOM WG10. *DICOM Structured Reporting (SR) objects and XML - Extensible Markup Language, HL7 v3.0 RIM - Reference Information Model, HL7 Clinical Document Architecture*. 2001-04-03.
3. DICOM WG10. *DICOM Strategic Document*. 2001-07-10. http://medical.nema.org/dicom/geninfo/dicomstrategy\105/StrategyJuly0601.htm
4. DICOM WG10. *DICOM Strategic Direction for Image Distribution*. White paper, 2002-04-10.